HUMAN ANATOMY

LABORATORY TEXTBOOK

HUMAN ANATOMY

LABORATORY TEXTBOOK

FOURTH EDITION

Harold J. Benson

Pasadena City College

Kathleen P. Talaro

Pasadena City College

WCB **Wm. C. Brown Publishers**

Dubuque, Iowa • Melbourne, Australia • Oxford, England

Book Team

Editor *Colin H. Wheatley*
Developmental Editor *Jane DeShaw*
Production Editor *Kay J. Brimeyer*
Designer *Jeff Storm*
Art Editor *Joyce E. Watters*
Photo Editor *Carol Judge*

Wm. C. Brown Publishers

A Division of Wm. C. Brown Communications, Inc.

Vice President and General Manager *Beverly Kolz*
National Sales Manager *Vincent R. Di Blasi*
Assistant Vice President, Editor-in-Chief *Edward G. Jaffe*
Director of Marketing *John W. Calhoun*
Marketing Manager *Elizabeth Robbins*
Advertising Manager *Amy Schmitz*
Director of Production *Colleen A. Yonda*
Manager of Visuals and Design *Faye M. Schilling*

Design Manager *Jac Tilton*
Art Manager *Janice Roerig*
Publishing Services Manager *Karen J. Slaght*
Permissions/Records Manager *Connie Allendorf*

Wm. C. Brown Communications, Inc.

Chairman Emeritus *Wm. C. Brown*
Chairman and Chief Executive Officer *Mark C. Falb*
President and Chief Operating Officer *G. Franklin Lewis*
Corporate Vice President, President of WCB Manufacturing *Roger Meyer*

Anatomy and Physiology Laboratory Textbooks

Benson,
Gunstream,
Talaro,
Talaro
}
Complete Version—Cat, 5th edition
Intermediate Version—Cat, 3rd edition
Intermediate Version—Fetal Pig, 2nd edition
Short Version, 5th edition

Gunstream,
Benson,
Talaro,
Talaro
}
Essentials Version

Benson,
Talaro
}
Human Anatomy, 4th edition

Contents

Preface

This fourth edition of the *Human Anatomy Laboratory Textbook* has essentially the same format as the three previous editions. Human anatomical illustrations are provided for labeling, and cat anatomical illustrations are provided for reference in performing anatomical studies in dissections. Laboratory Report sheets are located in the back of the book that provide pertinent questions and space for recording labeling information. The Laboratory Reports can be removed from the book and submitted to the instructor for evaluation.

Although the basic format has not changed, we have made changes in the Table of Contents, the Histology Atlas, cat muscle dissection, and the use of eponyms. All these changes, and a few other minor ones, have been requested by our critical readers and other users of the book.

The principle change in the Table of Contents involves moving the material from the former Exercise 9 (Nerve and Muscle Tissues) to Parts 4 and 5. Most users of the manual felt that the study of muscle tissues fits best in Part 4 (Skeletal Muscles), and the study of nerve cells is more effective when studied in Part 5 (The Nervous System). This change added one more exercise to the total number in the manual.

Although the previous Histology Atlas was well received, we felt that it needed further expansion and textual information. New photomicrographs of tissues of the skin, receptors, eye, ear, tooth development, salivary glands, digestive tract, spleen, urinary bladder, gallbladder, lymphoid tissues, and reproductive organs have been added. To make the Atlas more meaningful we have included on each page a brief text to call the student's attention to significant structures. In the previous edition only photomicrographs with labels were provided on each page. To make this possible it was necessary to completely reorganize the Atlas and replace every illustration. The extended comprehensiveness of this section of the book should form a broader foundation for histological studies in the laboratory.

To improve the clarity of the cat muscle dissections in Part 4 we have added colored photographs of all the cat muscles and changed the dissection instructions. We are endebted to Dr. Ralph W. Stevens, III, of Old Dominion University for the excellent photographs. The dissection instructions for the cat muscles were provided by Dr. Thomas M. O'Connor of Washburn University of Topeka. The contributions of these two men are greatly appreciated.

Since most of the newly published anatomy textbooks have been deemphasizing eponyms in favor of more descriptive terminology, we, too, have decided to conform to this practice. Instead of terms such as Eustachian tube, Stensen's duct, and Volkmann's canal, we have adopted the more acceptable terms such as auditory tube, parotid duct, and perforating canal. For cross-referencing we have included the eponyms in parentheses after the newer terms that are set in bold type.

In addition to the above changes there are many minor textual changes that have been made to expand terminology and improve clarity. Some minor changes have also been made on the Laboratory Report sheets. The remainder of the book remains pretty much the same as the previous edition.

An Instructor's Handbook is available that provides setup information and time allotments for each experiment and answers to the questions on the Laboratory Reports. A set of eighty Kodachrome $2'' \times 2''$ histology slides is available, at no cost, to institutions that adopt the manual. A legend for using the slides accompanies the set. Also, in an effort to meet the needs of those professors who, for precautionary measures, do not use the experiments that involve handling blood, a video on blood cell counting, identification, and typing is offered at no cost to qualified adopters of the manual.

Although an attempt has been made to incorporate all suggestions made by users of this book, it was necessary to postpone some of the changes for the next edition. In addition to acknowledging the contributions of Dr. Stevens and Dr. O'Connor, we are also indebted to Frank Hollenberg of Clemson University and Dr. Beverly A. Marcum of California State University, Chico. We feel certain that users of this book will also appreciate their contributions.

List of Reviewers

Thomas M. O'Connor
Washburn University

Frank Hollenberg
Clemson University

Beverly A. Marcum
California State University, Chico

Introduction

The exercises in this laboratory guide consist, essentially, of three kinds of activities: (1) illustration labeling, (2) dissections, and (3) cytological and histological studies. Upon the completion of these assignments, questions on the Laboratory Reports will be answered to test your understanding of the work. The following suggestions should be helpful.

Labeling As you glance through the manual you will note that most of the illustrations are not labeled. To label each illustration it is necessary to read the text in the manual very carefully. You will discover that all significant anatomical structures are printed in **bold type** (occasionally, in *italics*) and are carefully described so that identifying the structures on the illustrations is not difficult. This method of labeling a diagram by reading the text is a learning experience that helps you to remember anatomical minutiae. Incorrectly labeled illustrations usually indicate a lack of comprehension.

Once the illustrations are labeled they can be useful to you in two other ways. First of all, the illustrations are often used for reference purposes in dissections or examinations of anatomical specimens. This is particularly true in the skeletal and nervous systems. Secondly, the illustrations can be used for review purposes. If the number legends of the labels are covered over as you mentally attempt to name the structures on illustrations, you can easily determine your level of understanding. Periodic reviews of this type during the semester will be very helpful.

In general, the labeling of illustrations will usually be performed prior to coming to the laboratory. In this way the laboratory time will be used primarily for dissections and microscopic examinations.

Dissections Once the illustrations of an exercise are labeled, the next step is to study the organs of a system on a cadaver or other animal. Although cadavers are obviously best, the cat has been selected for this course because of its availability and similarity to human anatomy. In many instances fresh organs, such as lungs, kidneys, and hearts, from other animals are also dissected. When doing a dissection you will be expected to find specific structures . . . often the same ones labeled on the illustrations.

Histological Studies Unless cytological and histological studies are made of the various organs of the body, complete anatomical understanding cannot occur. The realization that all organs function at the cellular level makes microscopic anatomy the basis of all subsequent physiological study.

For assistance, in performing histological studies, become familiar with the Histology Atlas that can be found on pages 165 through 200. If drawings are required, execute them with care, and label those structures that are significant.

Laboratory Reports These sheets, which are located at the back of the manual, are used to evaluate your understanding of each exercise. On these sheets you will record the labels for each illustration and answer questions pertaining to dissections or the text. Approximately one week after the dissections are completed in the laboratory, the Reports will be collected, graded, and returned to you.

Since these record sheets are located at the back of the manual, *it is recommended that they be removed from the binding as soon as you begin to record information.* Trying to shift from the front of the book to the back is very inconvenient and time-consuming. It is also recommended that the torn perforations along the binding edge of each sheet be trimmed with a pair of scissors prior to handing in. These ragged edges make handling of the sheets very difficult. Any drawings that are made on separate paper should be handed in at the same time.

Once these Laboratory Reports are corrected and returned to you, it will be possible for you to correct the illustrations and determine how well you understand the specific unit. You will also be able to use these sheets for review purposes when studying for tests.

Independent Study This laboratory manual is only a tool intended to help you to learn human anatomy. It can only be of value to you if you are willing to work with it. If, by yourself, you struggle through the problems it presents, you will learn this material. The easier route of letting someone else solve the problems may satisfy the requirement of getting the Laboratory Report completed on time, but it will do you little benefit at examination time. You are taking this course to learn anatomy, no one else can learn it for you.

Some of the laboratory experiments included in this text may be hazardous if materials are handled improperly or if procedures are conducted incorrectly. Safety precautions are necessary when you are working with chemicals, glass test tubes, hot water baths, sharp instruments, and the like, or for any procedures that generally require caution. Your school may have set regulations regarding safety procedures that your instructor will explain to you. Should you have any problems with materials or procedures, please ask your instructor for help.

Part 1 Some Fundamentals

This unit, which consists of only three exercises, attempts to accomplish two things: (1) to equip you with some of the basic anatomical terminology that you will need to get started, and (2) to present an overview of the systems and organs of the body that are going to be studied in greater detail as we progress through the book.

When you start Exercise 1 scan the entire exercise before attempting to label any of the illustrations. Note that the first two pages consist of descriptive terminology, followed by an *Assignment* on the third page which describes what you are to label. This, in turn, is followed by additional descriptive text, and another Assignment on page 5. After all the illustrations in the exercise have been labeled, you will transfer the label numbers from the legends of each illustration to the *Laboratory Report* sheet, which is located in the back of the manual on page 279. Once the Laboratory Report is completed, it can be turned in to your instructor for evaluation or self-graded if a key is made available.

1 Anatomical Terminology

Anatomical description would be extremely difficult without specific terminology. A consensus prevails among many students that anatomists synthesize multisyllabic words in a determined conspiracy to harass the beginner's already overburdened mind. Naturally, nothing could be further from the truth.

Scientific terminology is created out of necessity. It functions as a precise tool that allows people to say a great deal with a minimum of words. Conciseness in scientific discussion not only saves time, but it usually promotes clarity of understanding as well.

Most of the exercises in this laboratory manual employ the terms defined in this exercise. They are used liberally to help you to locate structures that are to be identified on the illustrations. If you do not know the exact meanings of these words, obviously you will be unable to complete the required assignments. First of all, read over all of the material carefully; then read the specific assignments for this exercise.

Relative Positions

Descriptive positioning of one structure with respect to another is accomplished with the following pairs of words. Their Latin derivations are provided to help you understand their meanings.

Superior and Inferior These two words are used to denote vertical levels of position. The Latin word *super* means *above;* thus, a structure that is located above another one is said to be superior. Example: The nose is *superior* to the mouth.

The Latin word *inferus* means *below* or *low;* thus, an inferior structure is one that is below or under some other structure. Example: The mouth is *inferior* to the nose.

Anterior and Posterior Fore and aft positioning of structures are described with these two terms. The word *anterior* is derived from the Latin *ante,* meaning *before*. A structure that is anterior to another one is in front of it. Example: Bicuspids are *anterior* to molars.

Anterior surfaces are the most forward surfaces of the body. The front portions of the face, chest, and abdomen are anterior surfaces.

Posterior is derived from the Latin *posterus,* which means *following*. The term is the opposite of anterior. Example: The molars are *posterior* to the bicuspids.

Cranial and Caudal When describing the location of structures on four-legged animals, these terms are often used in place of anterior and posterior. Since the word *cranial* pertains to the skull (Greek: *kranion,* skull), it may be used in place of anterior. The word *caudal* (Latin: *cauda,* tail) may be used in place of posterior.

Dorsal and Ventral These terms, as used in comparative anatomy of animals, assume all animals, including man, to be walking on all fours. The dorsal surfaces are thought of as *upper* surfaces, and the ventral surfaces as *underneath* surfaces.

The word *dorsal* (Latin: *dorsum,* back) not only applies to the back of the trunk of the body but may also be used in speaking of the back of the head and the back of the hand.

Standing in a normal posture, man's dorsal surfaces become posterior. A four-legged animal's back, on the other hand, occupies a superior position.

The word *ventral* (Latin: *venter,* belly) generally pertains to the abdominal and chest surfaces. However, the underneath surfaces of the head and feet of four-legged animals are also often referred to as ventral surfaces. Likewise, the palm of the hand may also be referred to as being ventral.

Proximal and Distal These terms are used to describe parts of a limb with respect to the point of reference such as the attachment of the appendage to the trunk of the body. *Proximal* (Latin: *proximus,* nearest) refers to that part of the limb nearest to the point of attachment. Example: The upper arm is the *proximal* portion of the arm.

Distal (Latin: *distare,* to stand apart) means just the opposite of proximal. Anatomically, the distal portion of a limb or other part of the body is that portion of the structure that is most remote from the point of reference (attachment). Example: The hand is *distal* to the arm.

Medial and Lateral These two terms are used to describe surface relationships with respect to the median line of the body. The *median line* is an imaginary line on a plane that divides the body into right and left halves.

The term *medial* (Latin: *medius,* middle) is applied to surfaces of structures that are closest to the median line. The medial surface of the arm, for example, is the surface next to the body because it is closest to the median line.

As applied to the appendages, the term *lateral* is the opposite of medial. The Latin derivation of this word is *lateralis,* which pertains to *side.* The lateral surface of the arm is the outer surface, or that surface furthest away from the median line. The sides of the head are said to be lateral surfaces.

Body Sections

To observe the structure and relative positions of internal organs it is necessary to view them in sections that have been cut through the body. Considering the body as a whole, there are only three planes to identify. Figure 1.1 shows these three sections.

Sagittal Sections A section parallel to the long axis of the body (longitudinal section) that divides the body into right and left sides is a *sagittal section.* If such a section divides the body into equal halves, as in figure 1.1, it is said to be a *midsagittal section.*

Frontal Sections A longitudinal section that divides the body into front and back portions is a *frontal* or *coronal section.* The other longitudinal section seen in figure 1.1 is of this type.

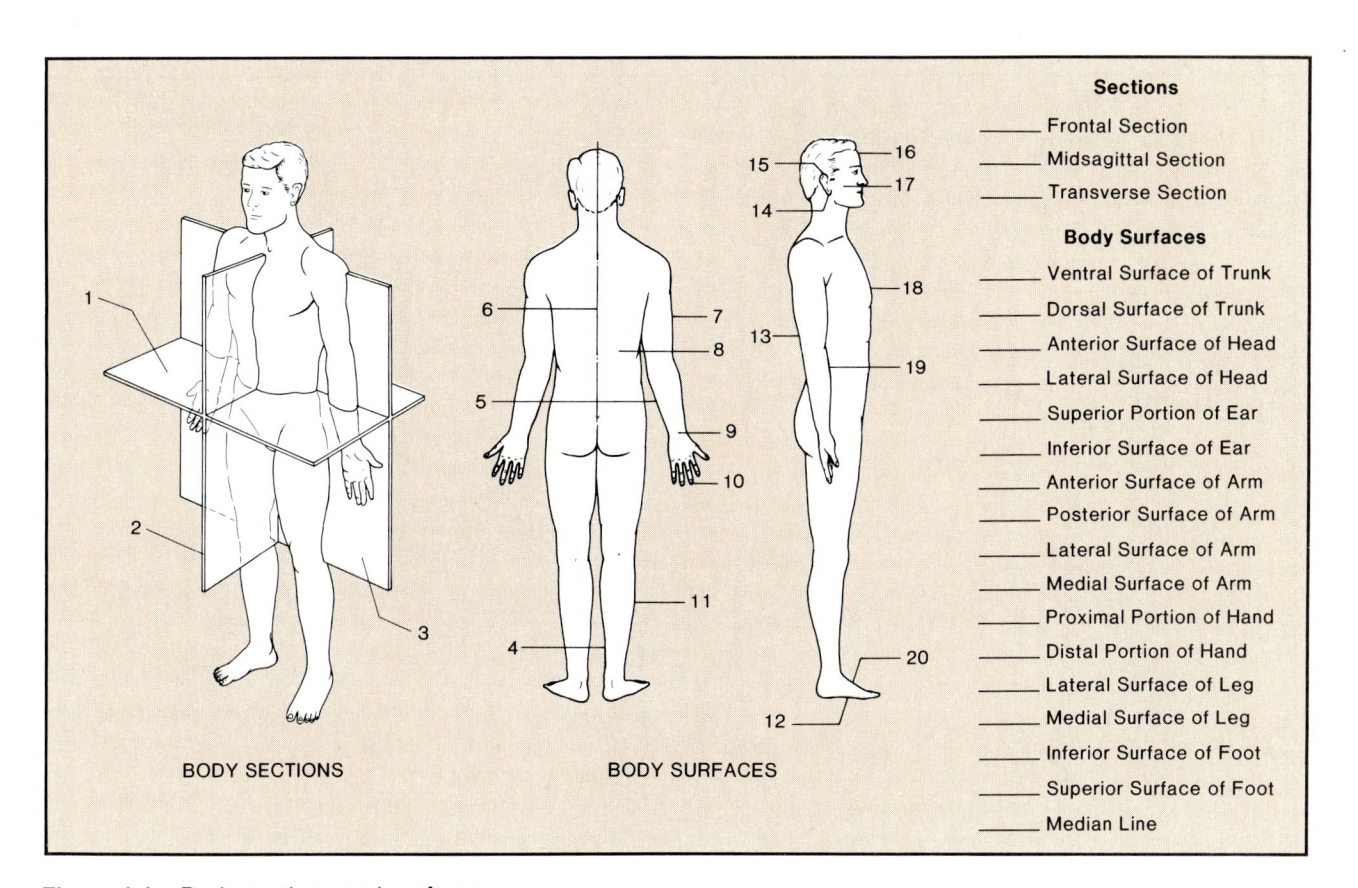

Figure 1.1 Body sections and surfaces.

Transverse Sections Any section that cuts through the body in a direction perpendicular to the long axis is a *transverse* or *cross section*. This is the third section shown in figure 1.1. It is parallel to the ground.

Although these sections have been described here only in relationship to the body as a whole, they can be used on individual organs such as the arm, finger, or tooth.

Assignment:

To test your understanding of the above descriptive terminology, identify the labels in figure 1.1 by placing the correct numbers in front of the terms to the right of the illustrations. Also, record these numbers on the Laboratory Report.

Regional Terminology

Various terms such as *flank, groin, brachium,* and *hypochondriac* have been applied to specific regions of the body to facilitate localization. Figures 1.2 and 1.3 pertain to some of the more predominantly used terminology.

Trunk

The anterior surface of the trunk may be subdivided into two pectoral, two groin, and the abdominal regions. The upper chest region may be designated as **pectoral** or **mammary** regions. The anterior trunk region not covered by the ribs is the **abdominal** region. The depressed area where the thigh of the leg meets the abdomen is the **groin.**

The posterior surface or dorsum of the trunk can be differentiated into the costal, lumbar, and buttocks regions. The **costal** (Latin: *costa,* rib) portion is the part of the dorsum that lies over the rib cage. The lower back region between the ribs and hips is the **lumbar** or **loin** region. The **buttocks** are the rounded eminences of the rump formed by the gluteal muscles; also called the **gluteal** region.

The side of the trunk that adjoins the lumbar region is called the **flank.** The armpit region that is between the trunk and arm is the **axilla.**

Upper Extremities

To differentiate the parts of the upper extremities, the term **brachium** is used for the upper arm and **antebrachium** for the forearm (between the elbow

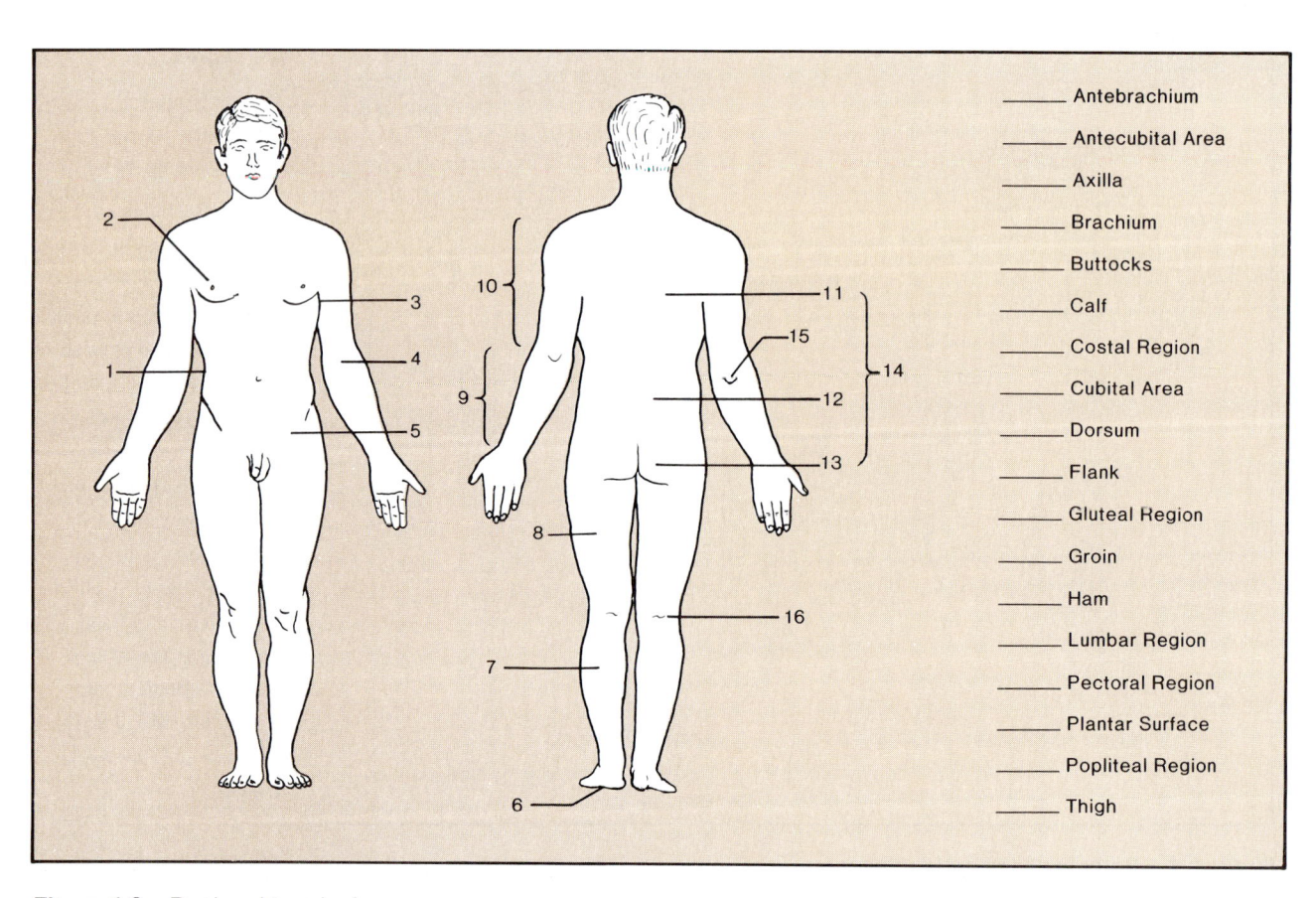

Figure 1.2 Regional terminology.

and wrist). The elbow area on the posterior surface of the arm is the **cubital** area. That area on the opposite side of the elbow is the **antecubital** area. It is also correct to refer to the entire anterior surface of the antebrachium as being antecubital.

Lower Extremities

The upper portion of the leg is designated as the **thigh,** and the lower fleshy posterior portion is called the **calf.** Between the thigh and calf on the posterior surface, opposite to the knee, is a depression called the **ham** or **popliteal** region. The sole of the foot is the **plantar** surface.

Abdominal Divisions

The abdominal surface may be divided into quadrants or into nine distinct areas. To divide the abdomen into nine regions one must establish four imaginary planes: two that are horizontal and two that are vertical. These planes and areas are shown in figure 1.3. The **transpyloric plane** is the upper horizontal plane which would pass through the lower portion of the stomach (pyloric portion). The **transtubercular plane** is the other horizontal plane that touches the top surfaces of the hipbones (iliac crests). The two vertical planes, or **right** and **left**

lateral planes, are approximately halfway between the midsagittal line and the crests of the hips.

The above planes describe the following nine areas. The **umbilical** region lies in the center, includes the navel, and is bordered by the two horizontal and two vertical planes. Immediately above the umbilical area is the **epigastric,** which covers much of the stomach. Below the umbilical zone is the **hypogastric** or *pubic area.* On each side of the epigastric is a right and left **hypochondriac areas.** Beneath the hypochondriac areas are the right and left **lumbar** areas. (Note that although we tend to think of only the lower back as being the lumbar region, we see here that it extends around to the anterior surface as well).

Assignment:

Label figures 1.2 and 1.3 and transfer these numbers to the Laboratory Report.

Laboratory Report

After transferring all the labels from figures 1.1 through 1.3 to the proper columns on Laboratory Report 1,2, answer the questions that pertain to this exercise.

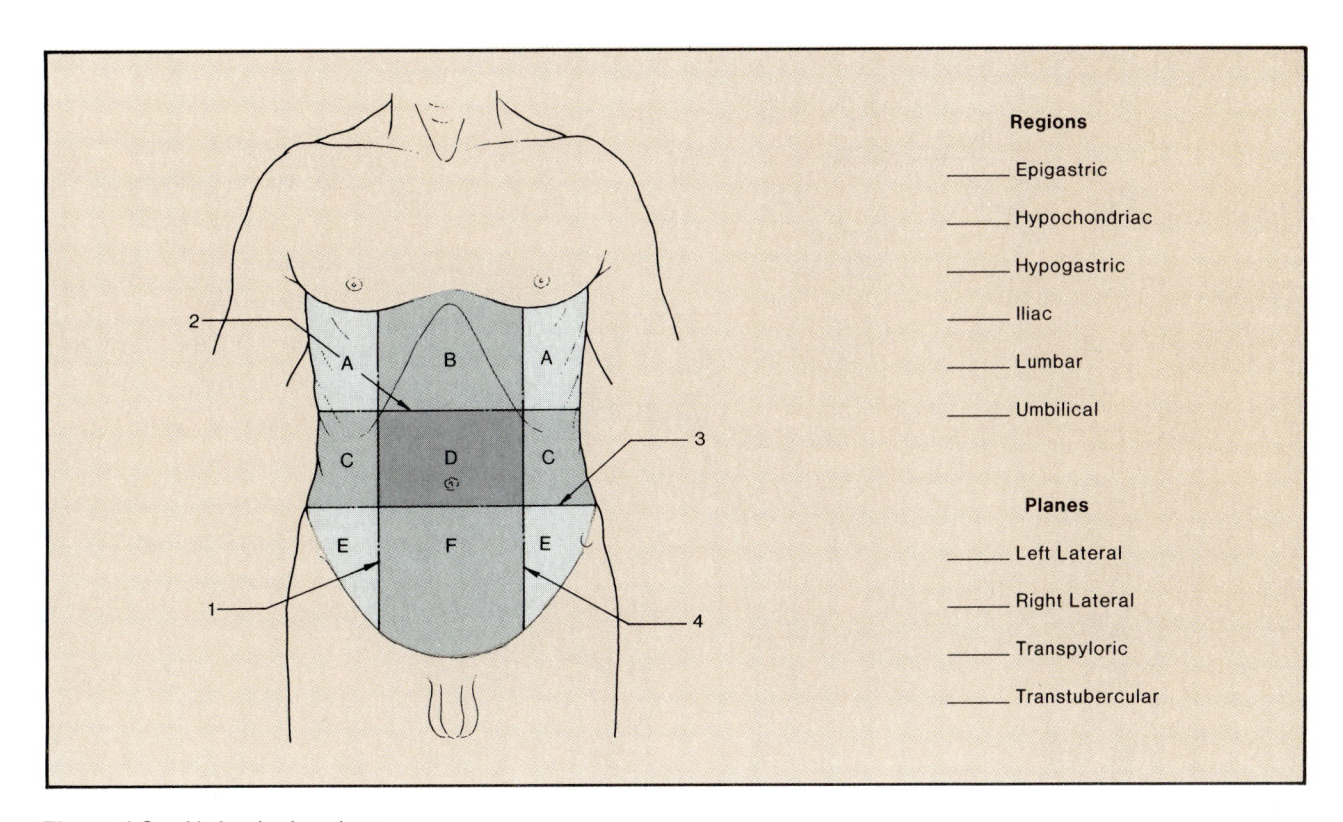

Figure 1.3 Abdominal regions.

Regions

_____ Epigastric

_____ Hypochondriac

_____ Hypogastric

_____ Iliac

_____ Lumbar

_____ Umbilical

Planes

_____ Left Lateral

_____ Right Lateral

_____ Transpyloric

_____ Transtubercular

2 Body Cavities and Membranes

All the internal organs, or *viscera,* are contained in body cavities that are completely or partially lined with smooth membranes. The relationships of these cavities to each other, the organs they contain, and the membranes that line them will be studied in this exercise.

Body Cavities

Figure 2.1 illustrates the seven principal cavities of the body. The two major cavities are the dorsal and ventral cavities. The **dorsal cavity,** which is nearest to the dorsal surface, includes the cranial and spinal cavities. The **cranial cavity** is the hollow portion of the skull that contains the brain. The **spinal cavity** is a long tubular canal within the vertebrae that contains the spinal cord. The **ventral cavity** is the large cavity that encompasses the chest and abdominal regions.

The superior and inferior portions of the ventral cavity are separated by a dome-shaped thin muscle, the **diaphragm.** The **thoracic cavity,** which is that part of the ventral cavity superior to the diaphragm, is separated into right and left compartments by a membranous partition or septum called the **mediastinum.** The lungs are contained in these right and left compartments. The heart, trachea, esophagus, and thymus gland are enclosed within the mediastinum. Figure 2.2 reveals the relationship of the lungs to the structures within the mediastinum. Note that within the thoracic cavity there exist right and left **pleural cavities** that contain the lungs, and a **pericardial cavity** that contains the heart.

The **abdominopelvic cavity** is the portion of the ventral cavity that is inferior to the diaphragm. It consists of two portions: the abdominal and pelvic

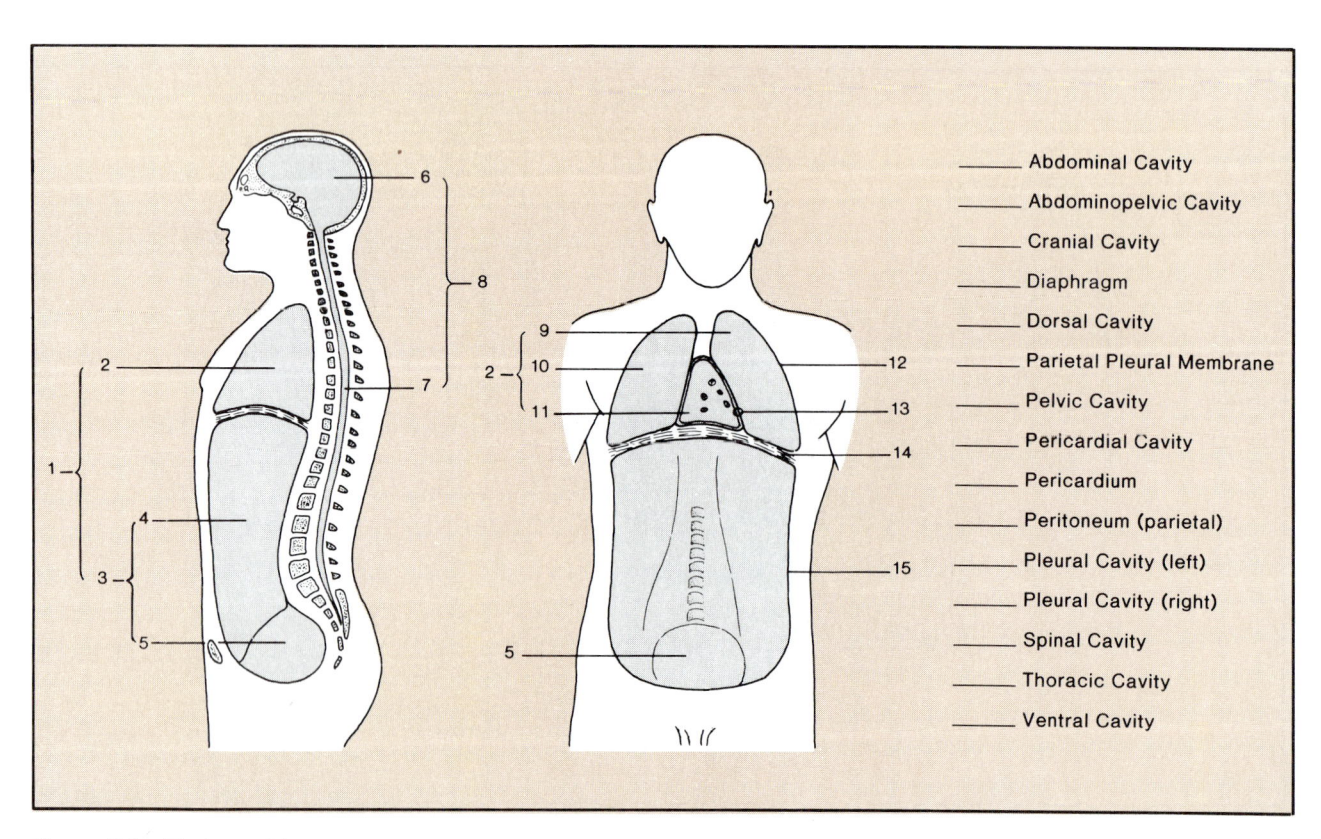

Abdominal Cavity

Abdominopelvic Cavity

Cranial Cavity

Diaphragm

Dorsal Cavity

Parietal Pleural Membrane

Pelvic Cavity

Pericardial Cavity

Pericardium

Peritoneum (parietal)

Pleural Cavity (left)

Pleural Cavity (right)

Spinal Cavity

Thoracic Cavity

Ventral Cavity

Figure 2.1 Body cavities.

cavities. The **abdominal cavity** contains the stomach, liver, gallbladder, pancreas, spleen, kidneys, and intestines. The **pelvic cavity** is the most inferior portion of the abdominopelvic cavity and contains the urinary bladder, sigmoid colon, rectum, uterus, and ovaries.

Body Cavity Membranes

The body cavities are lined with *serous membranes* that provide a smooth surface for the enclosed internal organs. Although these membranes are quite thin, they are strong and elastic. Their surfaces are moistened by a self-secreted *serous fluid* that facilitates ease of movement of the viscera against the cavity walls.

Thoracic Cavity Membranes

The membranes that line the walls of the right and left thoracic compartments are called **parietal pleurae** (*pleura,* singular). The lungs, in turn, are covered with **visceral (pulmonary) pleurae.** Note in figure 2.2 that these pleurae are continuous with each other. The potential cavity between the parietal and visceral pleurae is the pleural cavity. Inflammation of the pleural membranes results in a condition called *pleurisy.*

Within the broadest portion of the mediastinum lies the heart. It, like the lungs, is covered by a thin serous membrane, the **visceral pericardium,** or **epicardium.** Surrounding the heart is a double-layered fibroserous sac, the **parietal pericardium.** The inner layer of this sac is a serous membrane that is continuous with the epicardium of the heart. Its outer layer is fibrous, which lends considerable strength to the structure. A small amount of serous fluid produced by the two serous membranes lubricates the surface of the heart to minimize friction as it moves within the parietal pericardium. The potential space between the visceral and parietal pericardia is called the **pericardial cavity.**

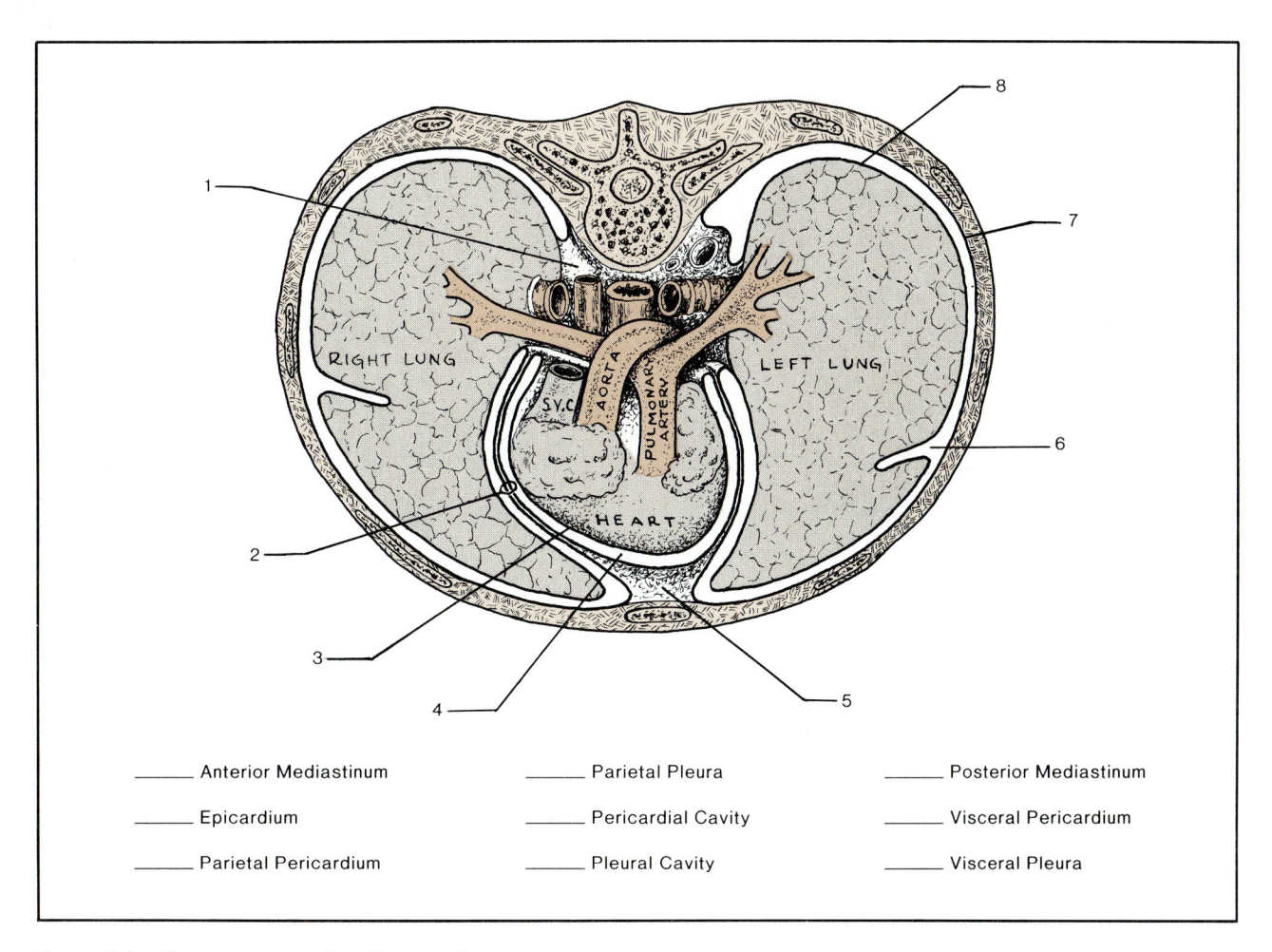

_____ Anterior Mediastinum	_____ Parietal Pleura	_____ Posterior Mediastinum
_____ Epicardium	_____ Pericardial Cavity	_____ Visceral Pericardium
_____ Parietal Pericardium	_____ Pleural Cavity	_____ Visceral Pleura

Figure 2.2 Transverse section through thorax.

Abdominal Cavity Membranes

The serous membrane of the abdominal cavity is the **peritoneum.** It does not extend deep down into the pelvic cavity, however; instead its most inferior boundary extends across the abdominal cavity at a level that is just superior to the pelvic cavity. The top portion of the urinary bladder is covered with peritoneum. In addition to lining the abdominal cavity, the peritoneum has double-layered folds called **mesenteries,** which extend from the dorsal body wall to the viscera, holding these organs in place. These mesenteries contain blood vessels and nerves that supply the viscera enclosed by the peritoneum. That part of the peritoneum attached to the body wall is the **parietal peritoneum.** The peritoneum that covers the visceral surfaces is **visceral peritoneum.** The potential cavity between the parietal and visceral peritoneums is called the **peritoneal cavity.**

Extending downward from the inferior surface of the stomach is a large mesenteric fold called the **greater omentum.** This double membrane structure passes downward from the stomach in front of the intestines, sometimes to the pelvis, and back up to the transverse colon where it is attached. Because it is folded upon itself it is essentially a double mesentery consisting of four layers. Protuberance of the abdomen in obese individuals is due to fat accumulation in the greater omentum. A smaller mesenteric fold, the **lesser omentum,** extends between the liver and the superior surface of the stomach and a short portion of the duodenum. Illustration B of figure 2.3 shows the relationship of these two omenta to the abdominal organs.

Assignment:

Label figures 2.1, 2.2, and 2.3.

Laboratory Report

Complete Laboratory Report 1,2 by answering the questions that pertain to this exercise.

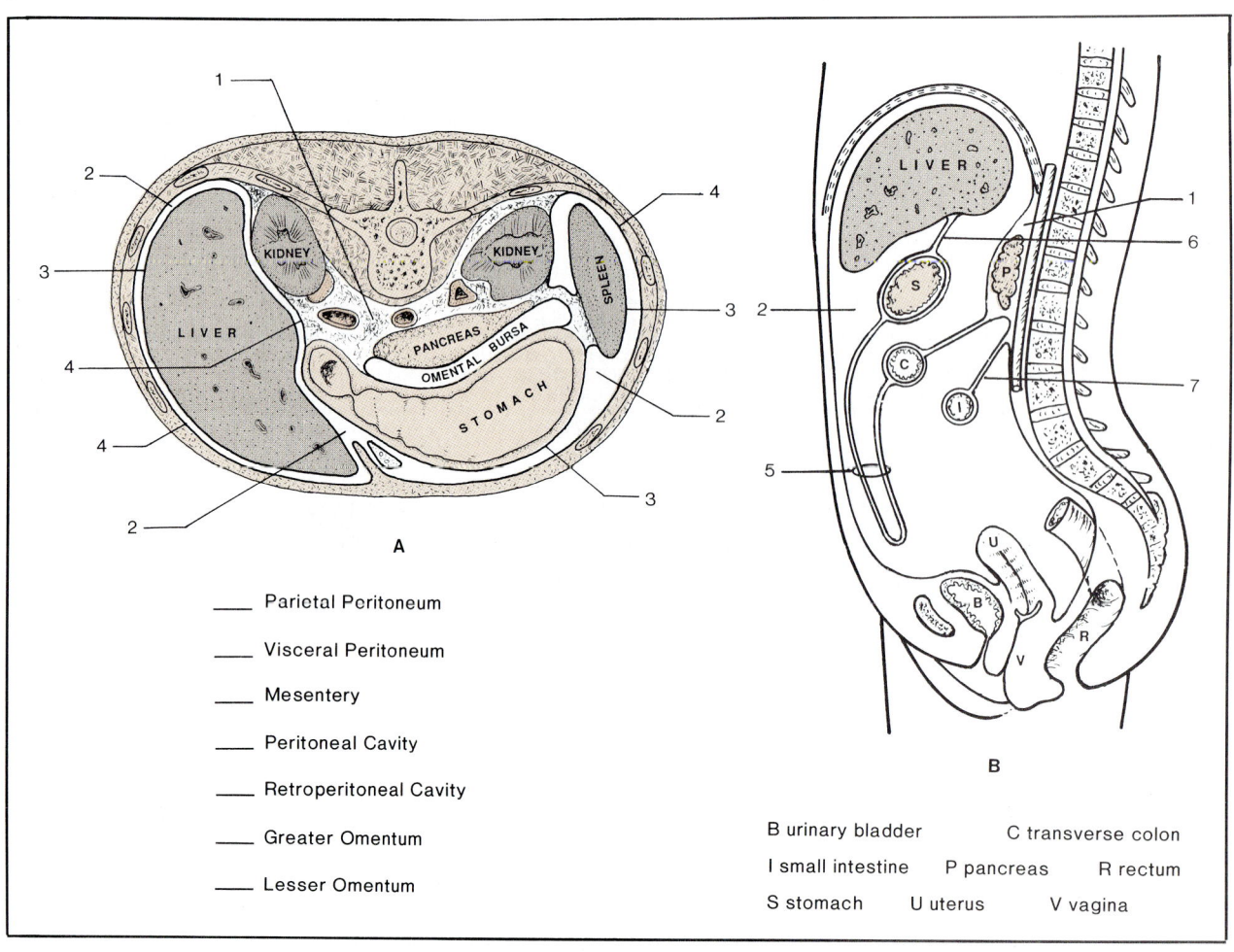

____ Parietal Peritoneum

____ Visceral Peritoneum

____ Mesentery

____ Peritoneal Cavity

____ Retroperitoneal Cavity

____ Greater Omentum

____ Lesser Omentum

B urinary bladder   C transverse colon

I small intestine   P pancreas   R rectum

S stomach   U uterus   V vagina

Figure 2.3   Transverse and longitudinal sections of the abdominal cavity.

Organ Systems: Rat Dissection 3

During this laboratory period we will dissect a freshly killed rat to perform a cursory study of the majority of the organ systems. Since rats and humans have considerable anatomical and physiological similarities, much will be learned here about human anatomy.

Before beginning the dissection, however, it will be necessary to review the eleven systems of the body. A brief description of each system follows. Keep in mind that an **organ** is defined as a structure composed of two or more tissues that performs one or more physiological functions. A **system,** on the other hand, is a group of organs that are directly related to each other functionally. Answer the questions on the Laboratory Report prior to doing the dissection.

The Integumentary System

The Latin word *integumentum* means covering. The surface of the body which consists of skin, hair, and nails comprises the integumentary system.

The skin's principal function is to prevent bodily invasion by harmful microorganisms. In addition to being a mechanical barrier, the skin produces sweat and sebum (oil) that contain antimicrobial substances for further protection.

The skin also aids in temperature regulation and excretion. The evaporation of perspiration cools the body. The fact that perspiration contains the same excretory products found in urine indicates that the kidneys are aided by the skin in the elimination of water, salts, and some nitrogenous wastes from the blood.

To some extent, the skin also plays a role in nutrition: Vitamin D forms in its deeper layers when a precursor in those cells is exposed to ultraviolet rays of sunlight.

As long as the skin is intact, the internal environment is protected, whereas serious damage to the skin (by burns, for example) may result in serous fluid and electrolyte imbalances.

The Skeletal System

The skeletal system forms a solid framework around which the body is constructed. It consists of bones, cartilage, and ligaments. This system provides support and protection for the softer parts of the body. Delicate organs such as the lungs, heart, brain, and spinal cord are protected by the bony enclosure of the skeletal system.

In addition to protection, the bones provide points of attachment for muscles, which act as levers when the muscles contract. This makes movement possible.

Two other important functions of the skeletal system are mineral storage and blood cell production. The mineral component of the bones provides a pool of calcium, phosphorous, and other ions that may be utilized to stabilize the mineral content of the blood. Both red and white blood cells originate in the red marrow of certain bones of the body.

The Muscular System

Attached to the skeletal framework of the body are muscles that make up nearly half the weight of the body. The skeletal muscles consist primarily of long multinucleated cells. The ability of these cells to shorten, when stimulated by nerve impulses, enables the muscles to move parts of the body in walking, eating, breathing, and other activities.

Two other kinds of muscle tissue exist in the body: smooth and cardiac. Smooth muscle tissue is the type found in the walls of the stomach, intestines, arteries, veins, urinary bladder, and other organs. Cardiac muscle tissue is found in the heart. Both types function like skeletal muscle fibers in that they perform work by shortening (contraction). However, while skeletal muscles are voluntarily controlled, smooth and cardiac muscle tissues are involuntarily regulated. Although skeletal muscles are primarily involved in limb movement, some skeletal muscles function in the reproductive, respiratory, and digestive systems.

The Nervous System

The nervous system consists of the brain, spinal cord, nerves, and receptors. While the nervous system has many functions, such as muscular control and regulation of circulation and breathing, its basic function is to facilitate adaptability: i.e., the ability to adjust to external and internal environmental changes.

To be able to adapt to environmental changes there are, first of all, a multitude of different kinds of **receptors** throughout the body that are activated by various kinds of stimuli. A receptor may be stimulated by changes in such things as pressure, chemicals, temperature, sound waves, or light. Once activated, nerve impulses pass along **conduction pathways** (nerves and spinal cord) to **interpretation centers** in the brain where recognition and evaluation of stimuli occur. Correct responses, which may be muscular, are then achieved by the nervous system via outgoing conduction pathways.

The Circulatory System

The circulatory system consists of the heart, arteries, veins, capillaries, blood, and spleen. The **heart** is a muscular pump that moves blood throughout the body. **Arteries** are thick-walled vessels that carry blood from the heart to the microscopic **capillaries** that permeate all the tissues. **Tissue fluid,** containing nutrients and oxygen, leaves the blood through the capillary walls and passes into the spaces between the cells. **Veins** are large blood vessels that convey blood from the capillaries back to the heart.

Thus, we see that this system provides transportation of various materials from one part of the body to another. In addition to the transportation of nutrients, oxygen, and carbon dioxide, the circulatory system transports hormones from glands, metabolic wastes from cells, and excess heat from muscles to the skin.

In addition to transporting all these substances, the blood is the body's primary defense against microbial invasion. The presence of phagocytic (cell-eating) white blood cells, antibodies, and special enzymes in blood prevents invading organisms from destroying the body.

The **spleen** is an oval structure on the left side of the abdominal cavity that acts to some extent as a blood reservoir. It also plays an important role in the removal of fragile red blood cells.

The Lymphatic System

The lymphatic system is a network of lymphatic vessels that returns tissue fluid from the intercellular spaces of tissues to the blood. This system is also responsible for the absorption of fats from the intestines. Although carbohydrates and proteins are absorbed directly into the blood through the intestinal wall, fats must pass first into the lymphatic system and then into the blood.

Once tissue fluid enters the lymphatic vessels it is called **lymph.** As this fluid moves through the lymphatic vessels it passes through nodules of lymphoid tissue called **lymph nodes.** Stationary phagocytic cells in these nodes remove bacteria and other foreign material, purifying the lymph before it is returned to the blood. Lymphocytes are also produced here.

Lymphoid tissue, as seen in the nodes, is also seen in the thymus gland, liver, spleen, tonsils, adenoids, appendix, Peyer's patches (in the digestive tract), and bone marrow. This diverse collection of lymphoidal tissue is collectively referred to as the **reticuloendothelial system,** an important component of the immune system.

The Respiratory System

The respiratory system consists of two portions: (1) the air passageways and (2) the respiratory portion. The actual exchange of gases between the blood and the air occurs in the respiratory portion. The lungs contain many tiny sacs called **alveoli,** which greatly increase the surface area for the transfer of oxygen and carbon dioxide in breathing. The passageways consist of the **nasal cavity, nasopharynx, larynx, trachea,** and **bronchi.**

The Digestive System

The digestive system includes the **mouth, salivary glands, esophagus, stomach, small intestine, large intestine, rectum, pancreas, liver,** and **gallbladder.** Its function is to convert ingested food to molecules that are small enough to pass through the intestinal lining into the capillaries and lymphatic vessels of the intestinal wall. This digestive process is achieved by hydrolysis of food molecules by **enzymes** produced in the digestive tract.

In addition to ingestion, digestion, and absorption of food, this system functions in the elimination of undigested materials. Since the contents of the digestive system contain many foreign, potentially harmful microorganisms, the digestive tract lining, like the integument, acts as a barrier to invasion of microorganisms.

The Urinary System

Cellular metabolism produces waste materials such as carbon dioxide, excess water, nitrogenous products, and excess metabolites. Although the skin, lungs, and large intestine assist in the removal of some of these wastes from the body, the majority of these products are removed from the blood by the **kidneys.** During this process of waste removal, the kidneys function to regulate the chemical composition of all body fluids to maintain homeostasis.

To assist the kidneys in excretion are the **ureters,** which drain the kidneys, the **urinary bladder,** which stores urine, and the **urethra,** which drains the bladder.

The Endocrine System

This system consists of a number of widely dispersed **endocrine glands** that dispense their secretions directly into the blood. These secretions, which are absorbed directly into capillaries within the glands, are called **hormones.**

Hormones perform such functions as integrating various physiological activities (metabolism and growth), directing the differentiation and maturation of the ovaries and testes, and regulating specific enzymatic reactions.

The endocrine system includes the following: the **pituitary, thyroid, parathyroid, thymus, adrenal, pancreas,** and **pineal glands.** The **ovaries,** **testes, stomach lining, placenta,** and **hypothalamus** also produce significant hormones.

The Reproductive System

Continuity of the species is the function of the reproductive system. Spermatozoa are produced in the testes of the male, and ova are produced by the ovaries of the female. Male reproductive organs include the **testes, penis, scrotum, accessory glands,** and various ducts. The female reproductive organs include the **ovaries, vagina, uterus, uterine** (Fallopian) **tubes,** and **accessory glands.**

Laboratory Report

Complete the Laboratory Report for this exercise. It is due at the beginning of the laboratory period in which the rat dissection is scheduled.

Rat Dissection

You will work in pairs to perform this part of the exercise. Your principal objective in the dissection is to *expose the organs for study, not to simply cut up the animal.* Most cutting will be performed with scissors. Whereas the scalpel blade will be used only occasionally, the flat blunt end of the handle will be used frequently for separating tissues.

Materials:

    freshly killed rat
    dissecting pan (with wax bottom)
    dissecting kit
    dissecting pins

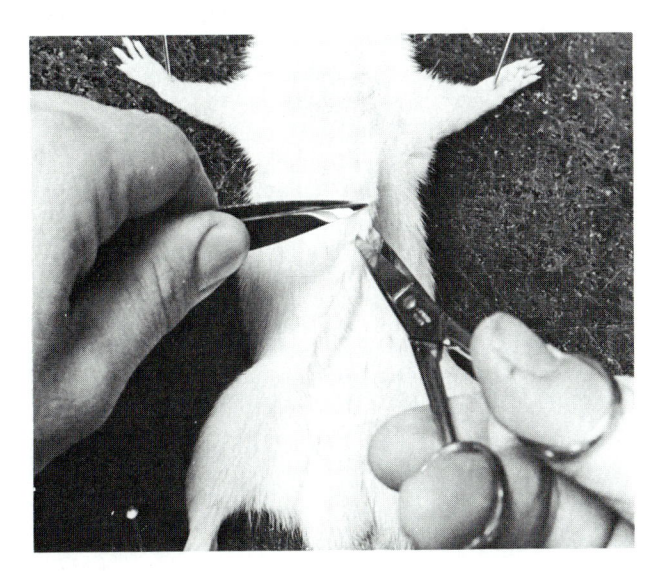

Figure 3.1 Incision is started on the median line with a pair of scissors.

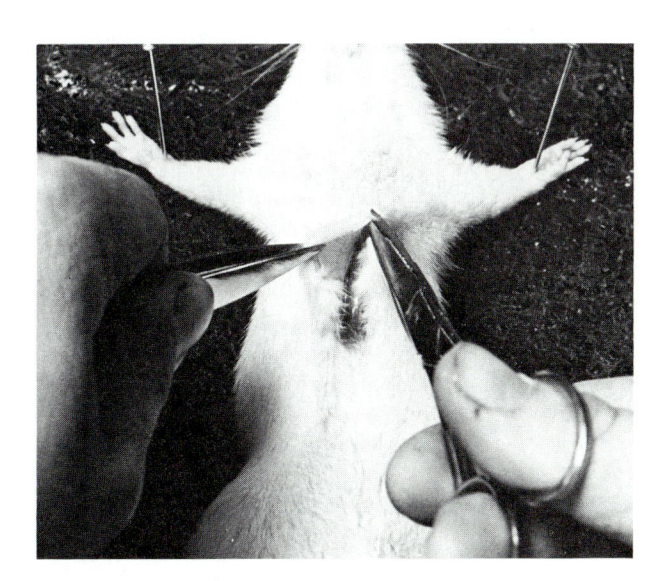

Figure 3.2 First cut is extended up to the lower jaw.

Skinning the Ventral Surface

1. Pin the four feet to the bottom of the dissecting pan as illustrated in figure 3.1. Before making any incision examine the oral cavity. Note the large **incisors** in the front of the mouth that are used for biting off food particles. Force the mouth open sufficiently to examine the flattened **molars** at the back of the mouth. These teeth are used for grinding food into small particles. Note that the **tongue** is attached at its posterior end. Lightly scrape the surface of the tongue with a scalpel to determine its texture. The roof of the mouth consists of an anterior **hard palate** and a posterior **soft palate.** The throat is the **pharynx,** which is a component of both the digestive and respiratory systems.

2. Lift the skin along the midventral line with your forceps and make a small incision with scissors as shown in figure 3.2. Cut the skin upward to the lower jaw, turn the pan around, and complete this incision to the anus, cutting around both sides of the genital openings. The completed incision should appear as in figure 3.3.

3. With the handle of the scalpel, separate the skin from the musculature as shown in figure 3.4. The fibrous connective tissue that lies between the skin and musculature is the **superficial fascia** (Latin: *fascia,* band).

4. Skin the legs down to the "knees" or "elbows" and pin the stretched-out skin to the wax. Examine the surfaces of the **muscles** and note that **tendons,** which consist of tough fibrous connective tissue, attach the muscles to the skeleton. Covering the surface of each muscle is another thin gray feltlike layer, the **deep fascia.** Fibers of the deep fascia are continuous with fibers of the superficial fascia, so that considerable force with the scalpel handle is necessary to separate the two membranes.

5. At this stage your specimen should appear as in figure 3.5. If your specimen is a female, the mammary glands will probably remain attached to the skin.

Opening the Abdominal Wall

1. As shown in figure 3.5, make an incision through the abdominal wall with a pair of scissors. To make the cut it is necessary to hold

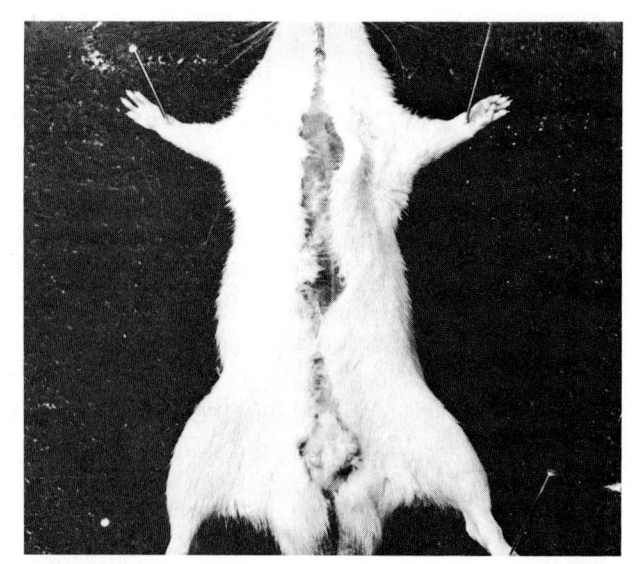

Figure 3.3 Completed incision from the lower jaw to the anus.

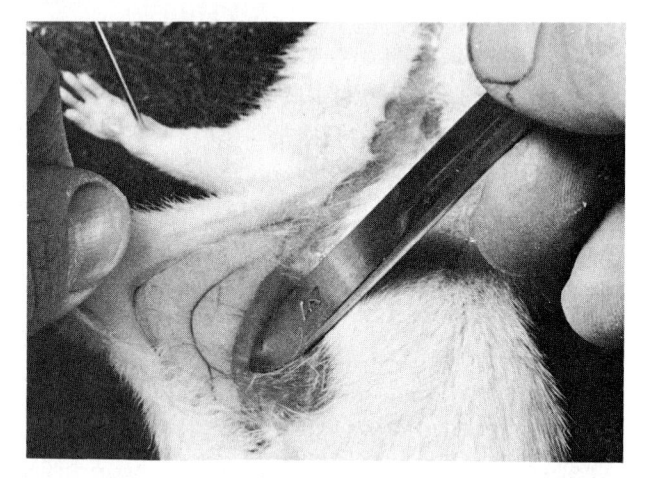

Figure 3.4 Skin is separated from musculature with scalpel handle.

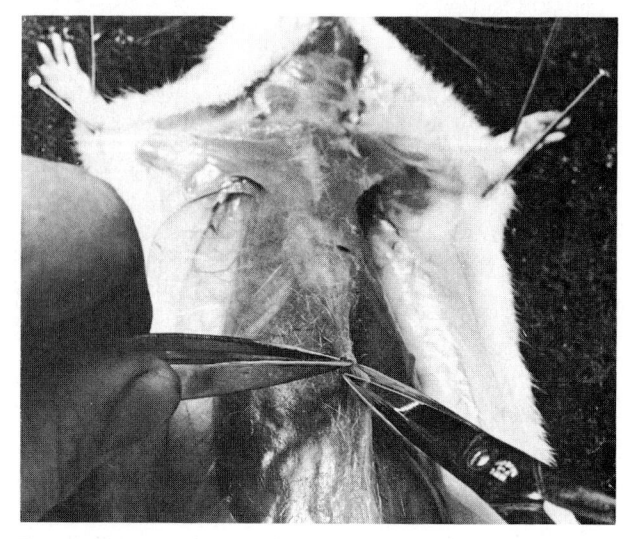

Figure 3.5 Incision of musculature is begun on the median line.

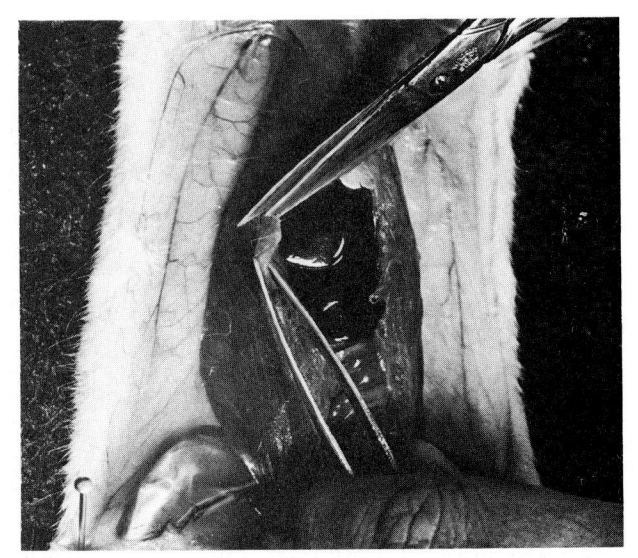

Figure 3.6 Lateral cuts at base of rib cage are made in both directions.

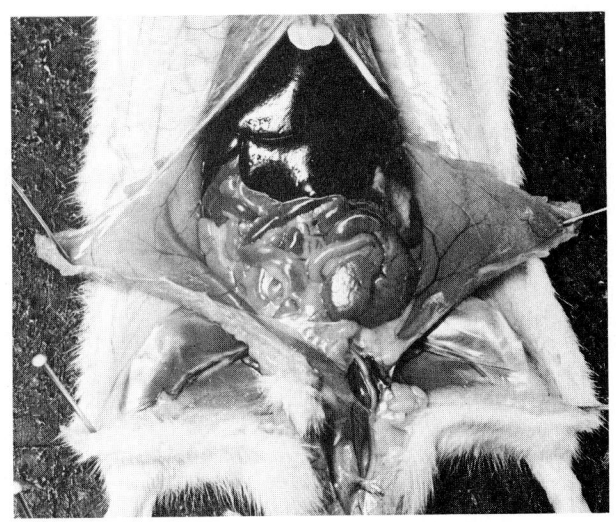

Figure 3.7 Flaps of abdominal wall are pinned back to expose viscera.

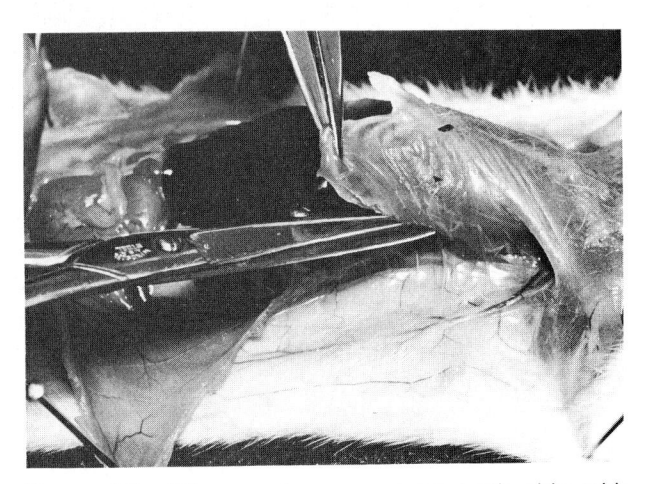

Figure 3.8 Rib cage is severed on each side with scissors.

the muscle tissue with a pair of forceps. **Caution:** Avoid damaging the underlying viscera as you cut.

2. Cut upward along the midline to the rib cage and downward along the midline to the genitalia.

3. To completely expose the abdominal organs make two lateral cuts near the base of the rib cage—one to the left and the other to the right. See figure 3.6. The cuts should extend all the way to the pinned-back skin.

4. Fold out the flaps of the body wall and pin them to the wax as shown in figure 3.7. The abdominal organs are now well exposed.

5. Using figure 3.9 as a reference, identify all the labeled viscera without moving the organs out of place. Note in particular the position and structure of the **diaphragm.**

Examination of Thoracic Cavity

1. Using your scissors, cut along the left side of the rib cage as shown in figure 3.8. Cut through all of the ribs and connective tissue. Then, cut along the right side of the rib cage in a similar manner.

2. Grasp the xiphoid cartilage of the sternum with forceps as shown in figure 3.10 and cut the diaphragm away from the rib cage with your scissors. Now you can lift up the rib cage and look into the thoracic cavity.

3. With your scissors, complete the removal of the rib cage by cutting off any remaining attachment tissue.

4. Now examine the structures that are exposed in the thoracic cavity. Refer to figure 3.9 and identify all the structures that are labeled.

5. Note the pale-colored **thymus gland,** which is located just above the heart. Remove this gland.

6. Carefully remove the thin **pericardial membrane** that encloses the **heart.**

7. Remove the heart by cutting through the major blood vessels attached to it. Gently sponge away pools of blood with Kimwipes or other soft tissues.

8. Locate the **trachea** in the throat region. Can you see the **larynx** (voice box) which is located at the anterior end of the trachea? Trace the trachea posteriorly to where it divides into two **bronchi** that enter the **lungs.** Squeeze the lungs

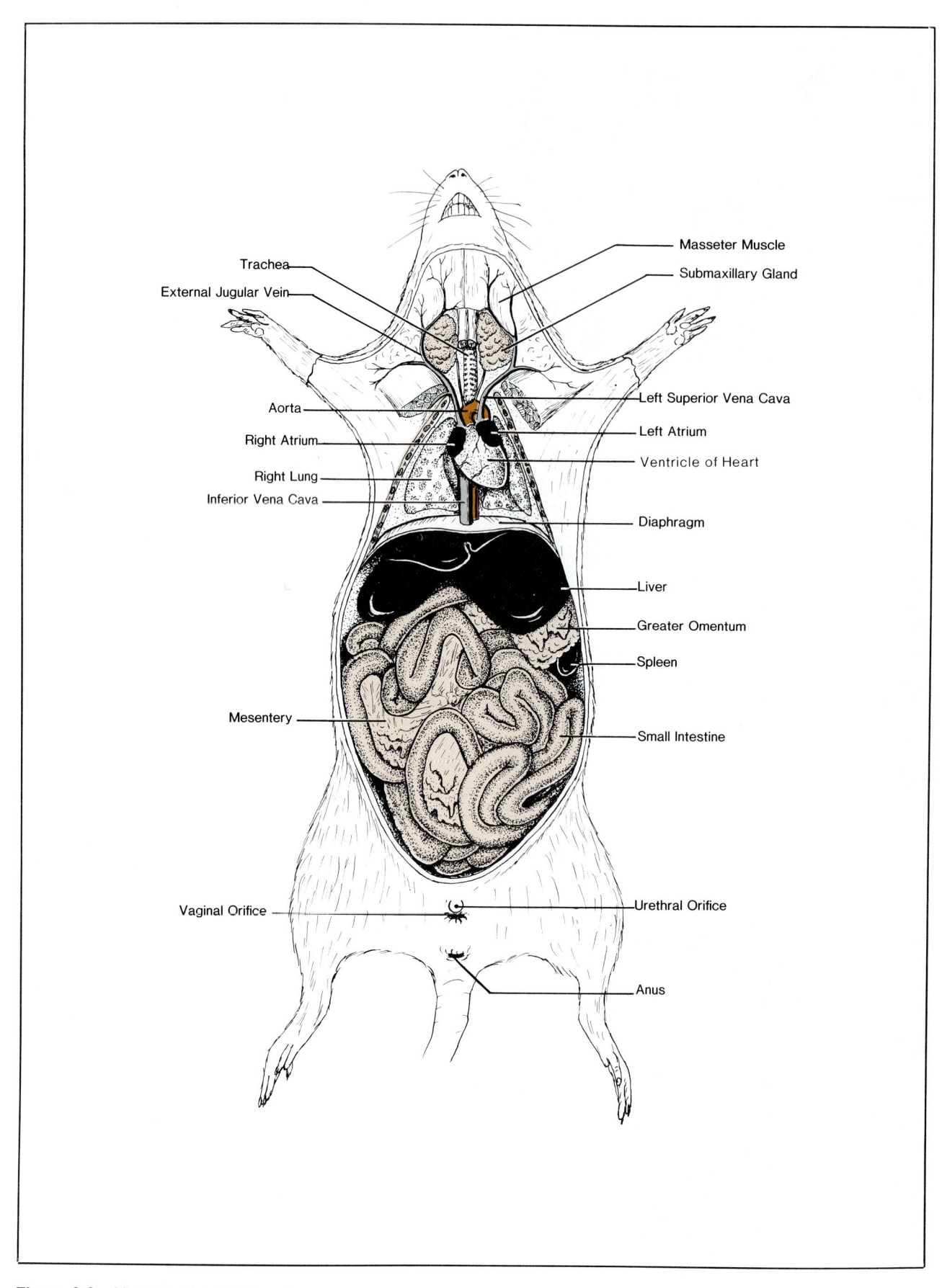

Figure 3.9 Viscera of a female rat.

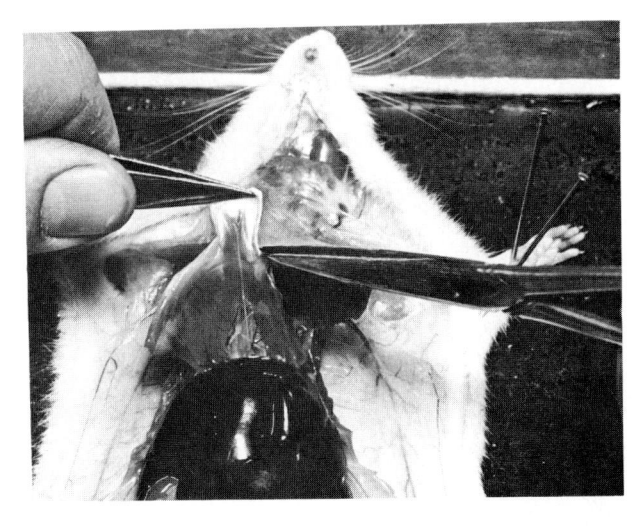

Figure 3.10   Diaphragm is cut free from edge of rib cage.

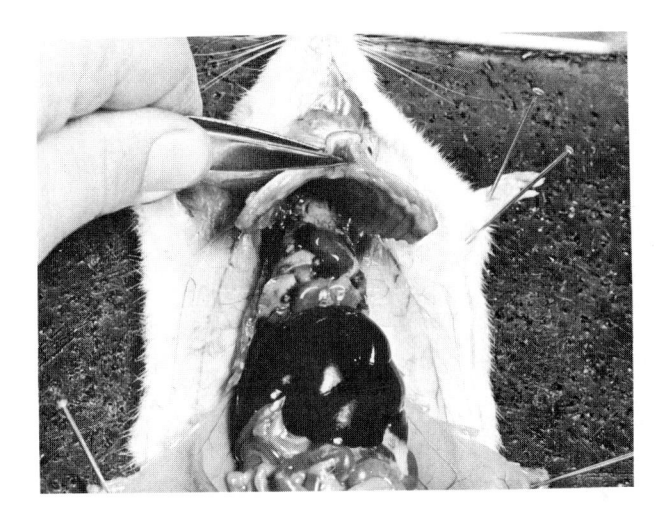

Figure 3.11   Thoracic organs are exposed as rib cage is lifted off.

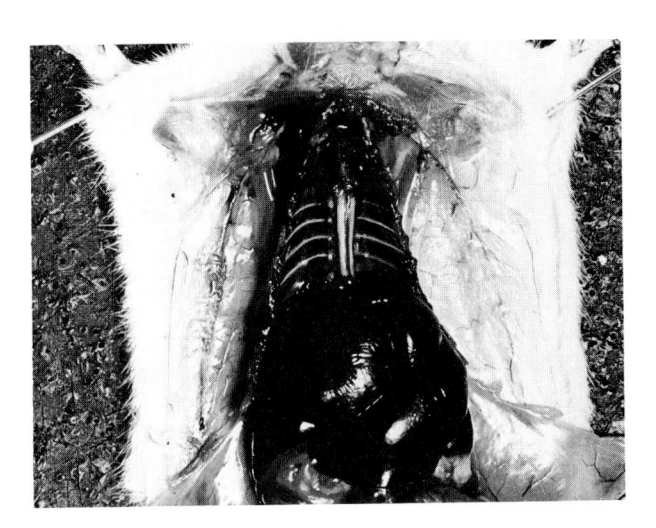

Figure 3.12   Specimen with heart, lungs, and thymus gland removed.

with your fingers, noting how elastic they are. Remove the lungs.

9. Probe under the trachea to locate the soft tubular **esophagus** that runs from the oral cavity to the stomach. Excise a section of the trachea to reveal the esophagus as illustrated in figure 3.13.

Deeper Examination of Abdominal Organs

1. Lift up the lobes of the reddish brown liver and examine them. Note that rats lack a **gallbladder.** *Carefully excise the liver* and wash out the abdominal cavity. The stomach and intestines are now clearly visible.

2. Lift out a portion of the intestines and identify the membranous **mesentery,** which holds the intestines in place. It contains blood vessels and nerves that supply the digestive tract. If your specimen is a mature healthy animal, the mesenteries will contain considerable fat.

3. Now lift the intestines out of the abdominal cavity, cutting the mesenteries, as necessary, for a better view of the organs. Note the great length of the small intestine. Its name refers to its diameter, not its length. The first portion of the small intestine, which is connected to the stomach, is called the **duodenum.** At its distal end the small intestine is connected to a large saclike structure, the **cecum.** The *appendix* in man is a *vestigial* portion of the cecum. The cecum communicates with the **large intestine.** This latter structure consists of the **ascending, transverse, descending,** and **sigmoid** divisions. The last of these portions empties into the **rectum.**

4. Try to locate the **pancreas,** which is embedded in the mesentery alongside the duodenum. It is often difficult to see. Pancreatic enzymes enter the duodenum via the **pancreatic duct.** See if you can locate this minute tube.

5. Locate the **spleen,** which is situated on the left side of the abdomen near the stomach. It is reddish brown and held in place with mesentery. Do you recall the functions of this organ?

6. Remove the digestive tract by cutting through the esophagus next to the stomach and through the sigmoid colon. You can now see the descending **aorta** and the **inferior vena cava.** The aorta carries blood posteriorly to the body tis-

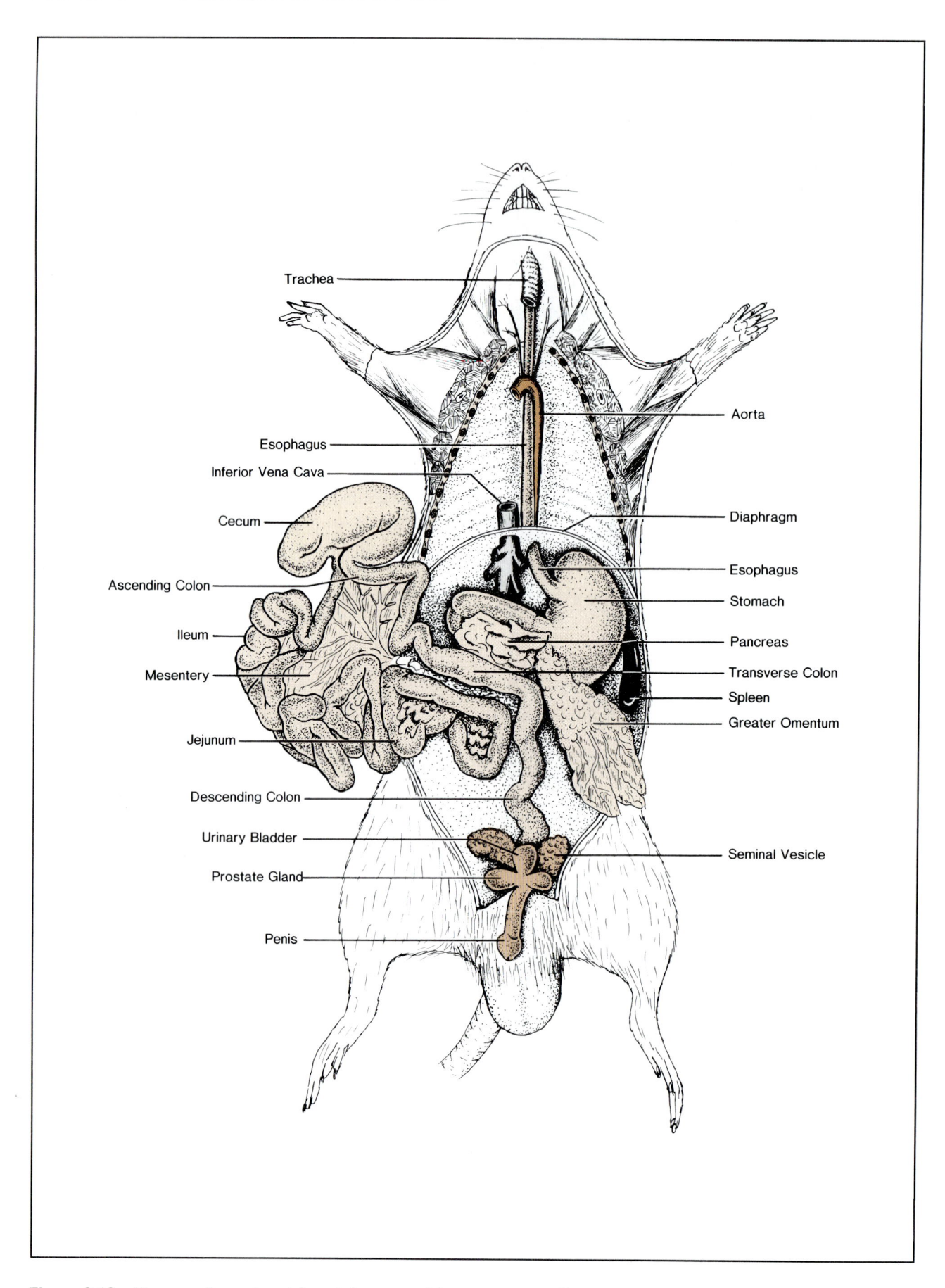

Figure 3.13 Viscera of a male rat (heart, lungs, and thymus removed).

sues. The **inferior vena cava** is a vein that returns blood from the posterior regions to the heart.

7. Peel away the peritoneum and fat from the posterior wall of the abdominal cavity. *Removal of the fat will require special care to avoid damaging important structures.* This will make the kidneys, blood vessels, and reproductive structures more visible. Locate the two **kidneys** and **urinary bladder.** Trace the two **ureters** which extend from the kidneys to the bladder. Examine the anterior surfaces of the kidneys and locate the **adrenal glands,** which are important components of the endocrine gland system.

8. **Female.** If your specimen is a female, compare it with figure 3.14. Locate the two **ovaries,** which lie lateral to the kidneys. From each ovary a **uterine tube** leads posteriorly to join the **uterus.** Note that the uterus is a Y-shaped structure joined to the **vagina.** If your specimen appears to be pregnant, open up the uterus and examine the developing embryos. Note how they are attached to the uterine wall.

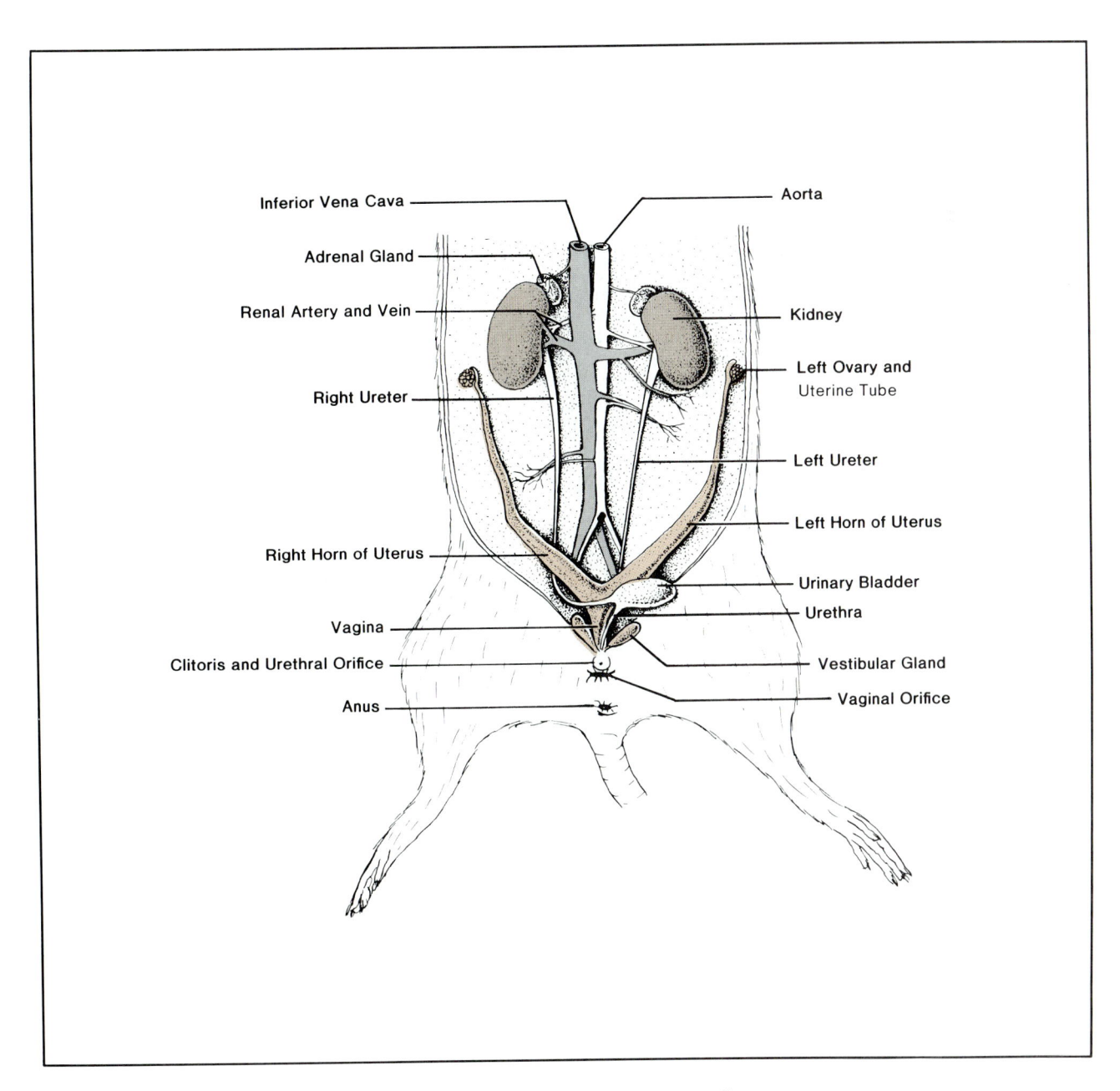

Figure 3.14 Abdominal cavity of a female rat (intestines and liver removed).

9. **Male.** If your specimen is a male, compare it with figure 3.15. The **urethra** is located in the **penis.**

Apply pressure to one of the **testes** through the wall of the **scrotum** to see if it can be forced up into the **inguinal canal.**

Carefully dissect out the testis, **epididymis,** and **vas deferens** from one side of the scrotum and, if possible, trace the vas deferens over the urinary bladder to where it penetrates the **prostate gland** to join the urethra.

In this cursory dissection you have become acquainted with the respiratory, circulatory, digestive, urinary, and reproductive systems. Portions of the endocrine system have also been observed. Five systems (integumentary, skeletal, muscular, lymphatic, and nervous) have been omitted at this time. These will be studied later. If you have done a careful and thoughtful rat dissection, you should have a good general understanding of the basic structural organization of the human body. Much that we see in rat anatomy has its human counterpart.

Clean-up Dispose of the specimen as directed by your instructor. Scrub your instruments with soap and water, rinse, and dry them.

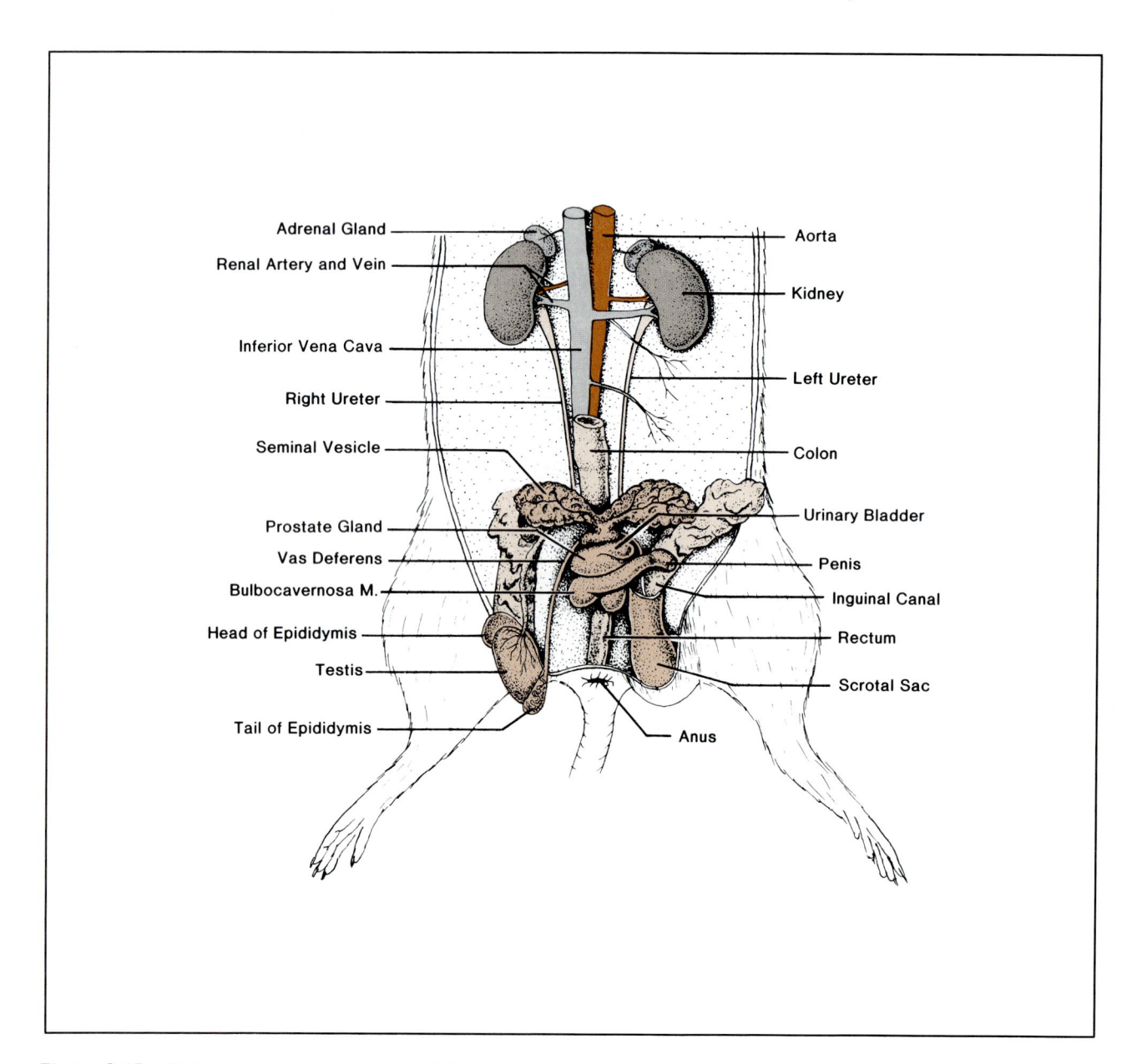

Figure 3.15 Abdominal cavity of a male rat (intestines and liver removed).

Part 2 Cells and Tissues

This unit consists of six exercises that pertain to the study of cells and tissues. Since considerable emphasis will be placed on histological studies throughout the course, this unit, which is very basic to anatomy and physiology, is extremely important.

The first exercise, which pertains to microscopy, should be studied prior to going to the laboratory. It is of a general nature, and attempts to provide some of the physical and mathematical reasons why certain techniques in microscopy work and others do not.

Exercise 5 and 6 relate to basic cellular structure and cell reproduction (mitosis). In Exercises 7 and 8, the epithelial and connective tissues will be studied. Exercise 9, which pertains to the skin, is included here because it contains many of the tissues studied in Exercises 7 and 8. In all of these laboratory studies, extensive references will be made to the Histology Atlas.

4 Microscopy

Many types of microscopes are available today to one who wishes to study cells and tissues: electron, phase-contrast, interference, and fluorescence microscopes are just a few examples. In this laboratory we will use the conventional brightfield microscope for our studies. This instrument, in spite of its limitations, is still the most widely used type of microscope in hospitals and clinical laboratories. In this exercise our concern will be with accepted procedures for using this instrument.

Microscopy can be fascinating or frustrating. Success in this endeavor depends to a considerable extent on how well you understand the mechanics and limitations of your microscope. It is the purpose of this exercise to outline procedures that should minimize difficulties and enable you to get the most out of your subsequent attempts at cytological microscopy.

Before entering the laboratory to do any of the studies on cells and tissues, it would be desirable if you answered all the questions on the Laboratory Report after reading over the entire exercise. Your instructor may require the Laboratory Report to be handed in prior to doing any laboratory work.

Care of the Instrument

Microscopes represent considerable expense and can be damaged rather easily if certain precautions are not observed. The following suggestions cover most hazards.

Transport When carrying your microscope from one part of the room to another, use both hands when holding the instrument, as illustrated in figure 4.1. If it is carried with only one hand and allowed to dangle at your side, there is always the danger of collision with furniture or some other object. And, incidentally, under no circumstances should one attempt to carry two microscopes at one time.

Clutter Keep your work station uncluttered while doing microscopic work. Keep unnecessary books, lunches, and other unneeded objects away from your work area. A clear work area promotes efficiency and results in fewer accidents.

Electric Cord Microscopes have been known to tumble off of tabletops when students have entangled a foot in a dangling electric cord. Don't let the light cord on your microscope dangle in such a way as to hazard entanglement.

Lens Care At the beginning of each laboratory period check the lenses to make sure they are clean. At the end of each lab session be sure to wipe any immersion oil off the oil immersion lens if it has been used. More specifics about lens care are itemized on pages 22 and 23.

Dust Protection In most laboratories dustcovers are used to protect the instruments during storage. If one is available, place it over the microscope at the end of the period.

Components

Before we discuss the procedures for using a microscope, let's identify the principal parts of the microscope as illustrated in figure 4.2.

Framework All microscopes have a basic frame structure that includes the **arm** and **base.** To this framework all other parts are attached. On many of the older microscopes the base is not rigidly at-

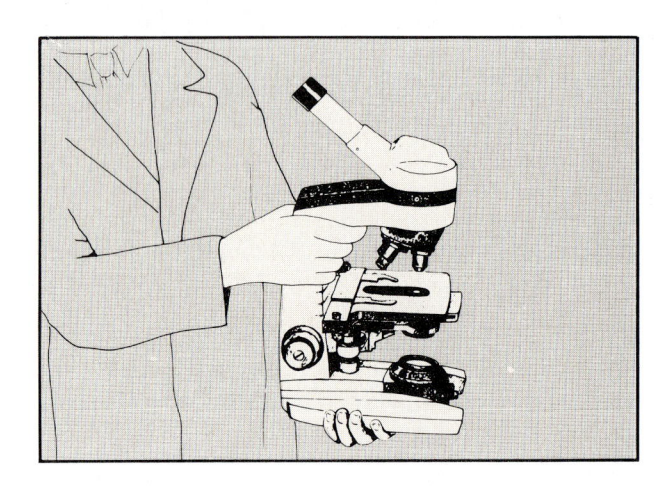

Figure 4.1 The microscope should be held firmly with both hands while carrying it.

tached to the arm as is the case in figure 4.2; instead, a pivot point is present which enables one to tilt the arm backward to adjust the eyepoint level.

Stage The horizontal platform that supports the microscope slide is called the **stage.** Note that it has a clamping device, the **mechanical stage,** which is used for holding and moving the slide around on the stage. Note, also, the location of the **mechanical stage control** in figure 4.2.

Light Source In the base of most microscopes is positioned some kind of light source. Ideally, the lamp should have a voltage control to vary the intensity of light. The microscope in figure 4.2 has the type of lamp that is controlled by a detached transformer unit (not shown). The light source on the microscope base in figure 4.4 has an electronic voltage control that is built into the lamp housing.

Many microscopes utilize a **neutral density filter,** in addition to a voltage control, to further reduce light intensity.

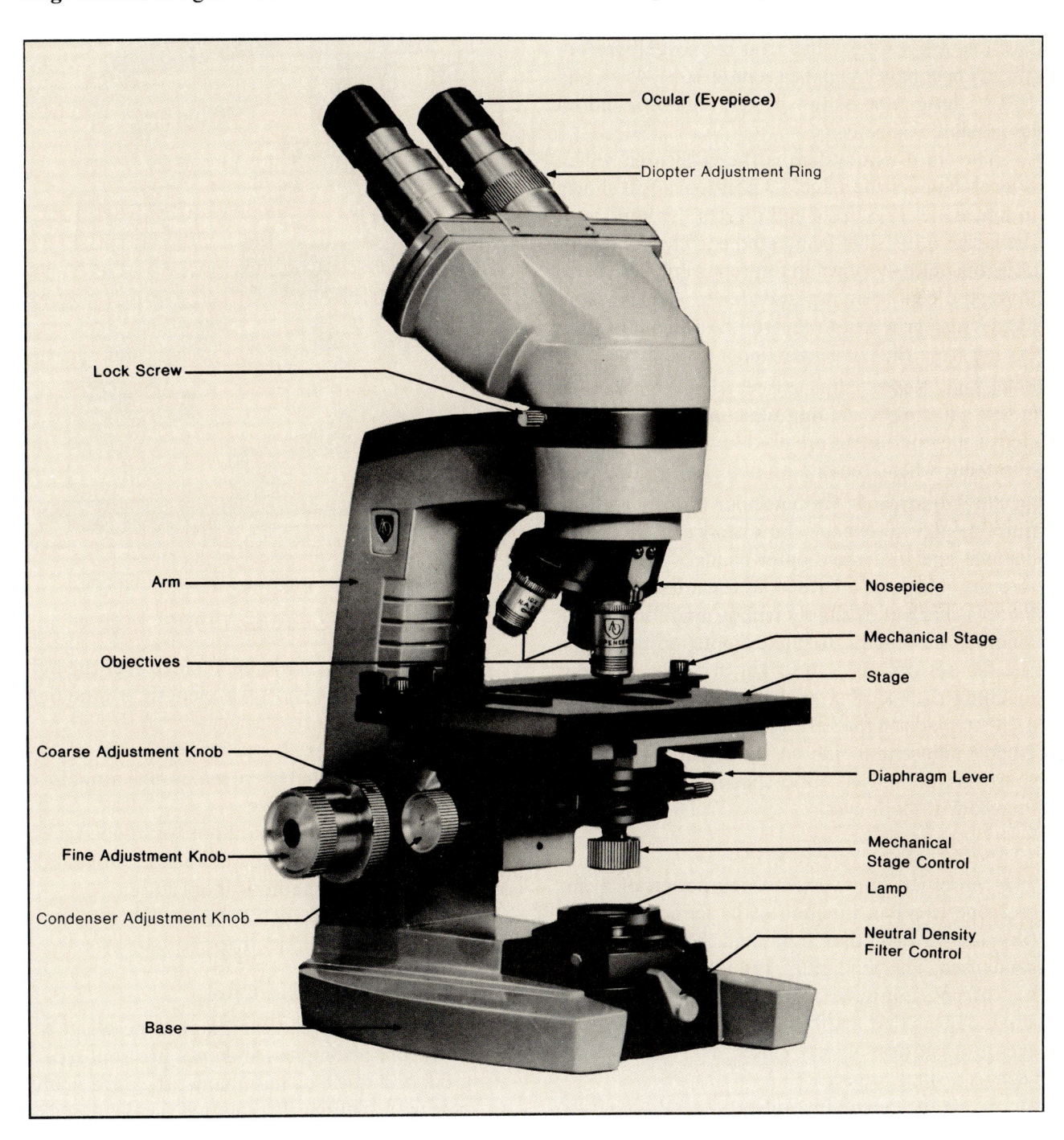

Figure 4.2 The compound microscope.

Lens Systems All microscopes have three lens systems: the oculars, objectives, and the condenser. Figure 4.3 illustrates the light path through these three systems.

The **ocular,** or eyepiece, which is at the top of the instrument, consists of two or more internal lenses and usually has a magnification of $10\times$. Although the microscope in figure 4.2 has two oculars (binocular), a microscope often has only one.

Three or more **objectives** are usually present. Note that they are attached to a rotatable **nosepiece,** which makes it possible to move them into position over a slide. Objectives on most laboratory microscopes have magnifications of $10\times$, $45\times$, and $100\times$, designated as **low power, high-dry,** and **oil immersion,** respectively.

The third lens system is the **condenser,** which is located under the stage. Its position is best shown in figure 4.3. It collects and directs the light from the lamp to the slide being studied. The **condenser adjustment knob** shown in figure 4.2 enables one to move the condenser up and down. A **diaphragm lever** is also provided to control the amount of light exiting from the condenser under the stage.

Focusing Knobs The concentrically arranged **coarse adjustment** and **fine adjustment knobs** on the side of the microscope are used for bringing objects into focus when studying an object on a slide.

Ocular Adjustments On binocular microscopes one must be able to change the distance between the oculars, and to make diopter changes for eye differences. On most microscopes the interocular distance is changed by simply pulling apart or pushing together the oculars. To make diopter adjustments, one focuses first with the right eye only. Without touching the focusing knobs, diopter adjustments are then made on the left eye by turning the knurled **diopter adjustment ring** on the left ocular until a sharp image is seen. One should now see sharp images with both eyes.

Resolution

The resolution limit, or **resolving power,** of a microscope lens is a function of its numerical aperture, the wavelength of light, and the design of the condenser. The maximum resolution of the best microscopes is around 0.2 μm. This means that two small objects that are 0.2 μm apart will be seen as separate entities; objects closer than that will be seen as a single object.

To get the maximum amount of resolution from a lens system, the following factors must be taken into consideration:

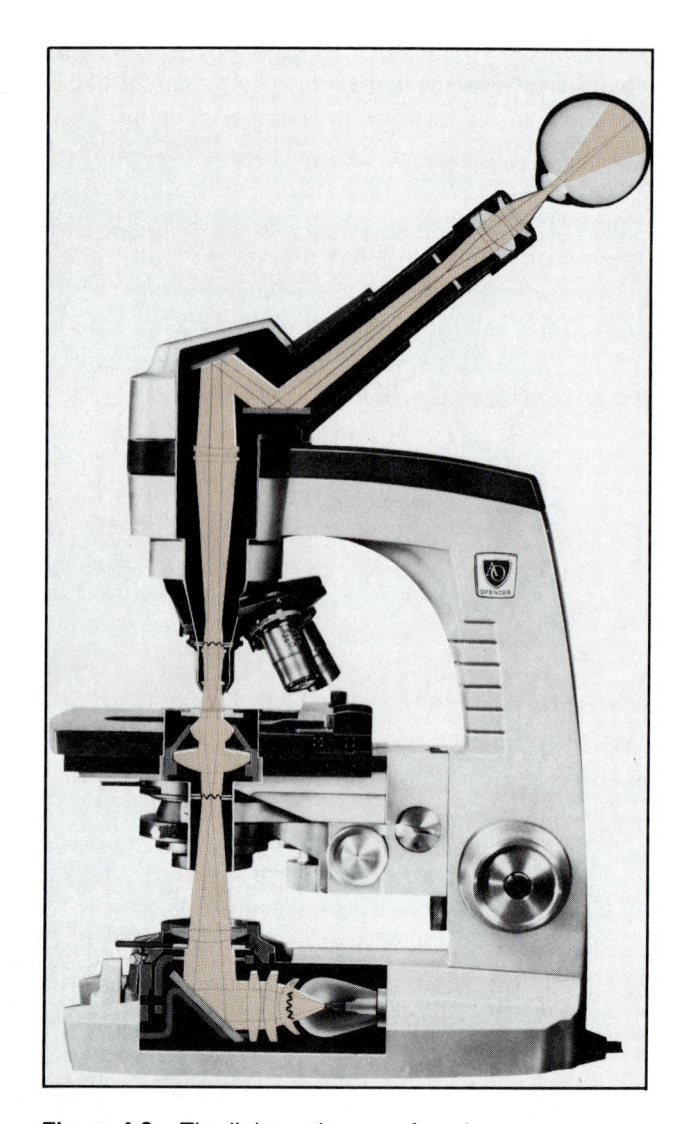

Figure 4.3 The light pathways of a microscope.

• A **blue filter** should be in place over the light source, because the short wavelength of blue light provides maximum resolution.

• The **condenser** should be kept at its highest position where it enables a maximum amount of light to enter the objective.

• The **diaphragm** should not be stopped down too much. Although stopping down improves contrast it reduces the numerical aperture.

• **Immersion oil** should be used between the slide and the $100\times$ objective.

Lens Care

Keeping the lenses of your microscope clean is a constant concern. Unless all lenses are kept free of dust, oil, and other contaminants, they are unable to achieve the degree of resolution that is intended. Consider the following suggestions for cleaning the various lens components.

Cleaning Tissues Only lint-free, optically safe tissues should be used to clean lenses. Tissues free of abrasive grit fall in this category. Booklets of lens tissue are most widely used for this purpose. Although several types of boxed tissues are also safe, *use only the type of tissue that is recommended by your instructor.*

Solvents Various liquids can be used for cleaning microscope lenses. Green soap with warm water works very well. Xylene is universally acceptable. Alcohol and acetone are also recommended, often with some reservations. Acetone is a powerful solvent that could possibly dissolve the lens mounting cement in some objective lenses if it were used too liberally. When it is used, it should be used sparingly. Your instructor will inform you as to what solvents can be used on the lenses of your microscope.

Oculars The best way to determine if your eyepiece is clean is to rotate it between the thumb and forefinger as you look through the microscope. A rotating pattern will be evidence of dirt.

If cleaning the top lens of the ocular with lens tissue fails to remove the debris, one should try cleaning the lower lens with lens tissue and blowing off any excess lint with an air syringe. *Whenever the ocular is removed from the microscope, it is imperative that a piece of lens tissue be placed over the open end of the microscope as illustrated in figure 4.5.*

Objectives Objective lenses often become soiled by materials from slides or fingers. A piece of lens tissue moistened with green soap and water or one of the other solvents mentioned will usually remove whatever is on the lens. Sometimes a cotton swab with a solvent will work better than lens tissue. At any time that the image on a slide is blurred or cloudy, assume at once that the objective you are using is soiled.

Condenser Dust often accumulates on the top surface of the condenser; thus, wiping it off occasionally with lens tissue is desirable.

Procedures

If your microscope has three objectives you have three magnification options: (1) low-power or 100× magnification, (2) high-dry magnification which is 450× with a 45× objective, and (3) 1000× magnification with the oil immersion objective. Note that the total magnification seen through an objective is calculated by multiplying the power of the ocular by the power of the objective.

Whether you use the low-power objective or the oil immersion objective will depend on how much magnification is necessary. Generally speaking, however, it is best to start with the low-power objective and progress to the higher magnifications as your study progresses. Consider the following suggestions for setting up your microscope and making microscopic observations.

Viewing Setup If your microscope has a rotatable head, such as the one being used by the two students in figure 4.6, there are two ways that you can use the instrument. Note that the student on the left has the arm of the microscope near him, and the other student has the arm away from her. With

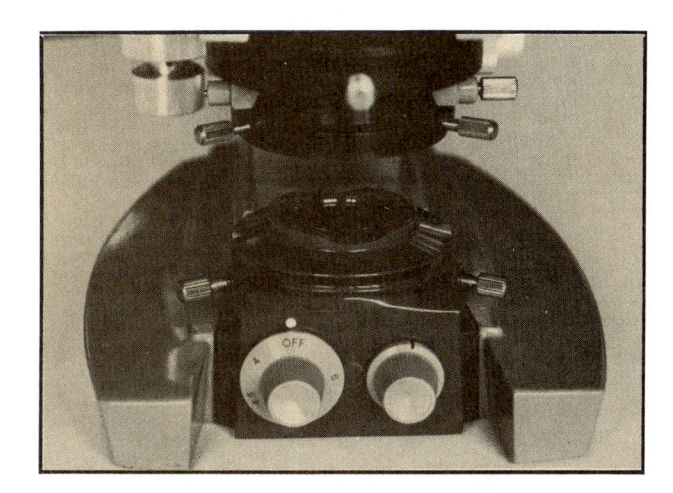

Figure 4.4 The left knob controls voltage; the other knob controls the neutral density filter.

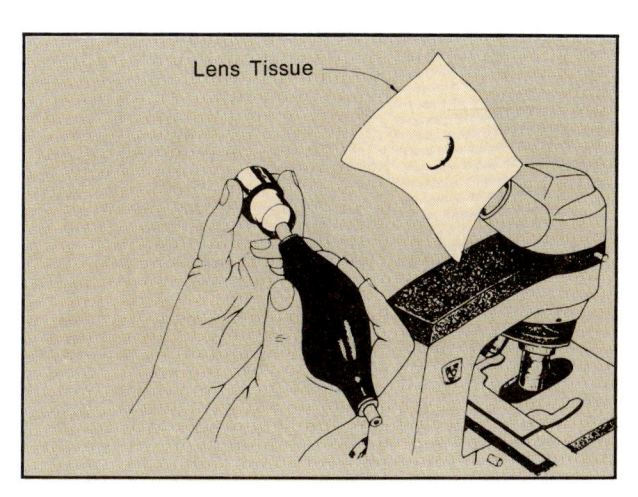

Figure 4.5 After cleaning the lenses, a blast of air from an air syringe removes residual lint.

this type of microscope, the student on the right has the advantage in that the stage is easier to observe. Note, also, that when focusing the instrument she is able to rest her arm on the table. The manufacturers of this type of microscope intended that the instrument be used in the way demonstrated by the young lady. If the head is not rotatable, it will be necessary to use the other position.

Low-Power Examination The main reason for starting with the low-power objective is to enable you to explore the slide to look for the object you are planning to study. Once you have found what you are looking for, you can proceed to higher magnifications. Use the following steps when exploring a slide with the low-power objective:

1. Position the slide on the stage with the material to be studied on the *upper* surface of the slide. Figure 4.7 illustrates how the slide must be held in place by the mechanical stage retainer lever.
2. Turn on the light source, using a *minimum* amount of voltage. If necessary, reposition the slide so that the stained material on the slide is in the *exact center* of the light source.
3. Check the condenser to see that it has been raised to its highest point.
4. If the low-power objective is not directly over the center of the stage, rotate it into position. Be sure that as you rotate the objective into position it clicks into its locked position.
5. Turn the coarse adjustment knob to lower the objective *until it stops*. A built-in stop will prevent the objective from touching the slide.

6. While looking down through the ocular or oculars, bring the object into focus by turning the fine adjustment focusing knob. Don't readjust the coarse adjustment knob. If you are using a binocular microscope, it will also be necessary to adjust the interocular distance and diopter adjustment to match your eyes.
7. Manipulate the diaphragm lever to reduce or increase the light intensity to produce the clearest, sharpest image. Note that as you close down the diaphragm to reduce the light intensity, the contrast improves and the depth of field increases.
8. Once an image is visible, move the slide about to search out what you are looking for. The slide is moved by turning the knobs that move the mechanical stage.
9. Check the cleanliness of the ocular, using the procedure outlined above.
10. Once you have identified the structures to be studied and wish to increase the magnification, you may proceed to either high-dry or oil immersion magnification. However, before changing objectives, *be sure to center the object you wish to observe.*

High-Dry Examination To proceed from low-power to high-dry magnification, all that is necessary is to rotate the high-dry objective into position and open up the diaphragm somewhat. It may be necessary to make a minor adjustment with the fine adjustment knob to sharpen up the image, but *the coarse adjustment knob should not be touched.*

If a microscope is of good quality, only minor focusing adjustments are needed when changing

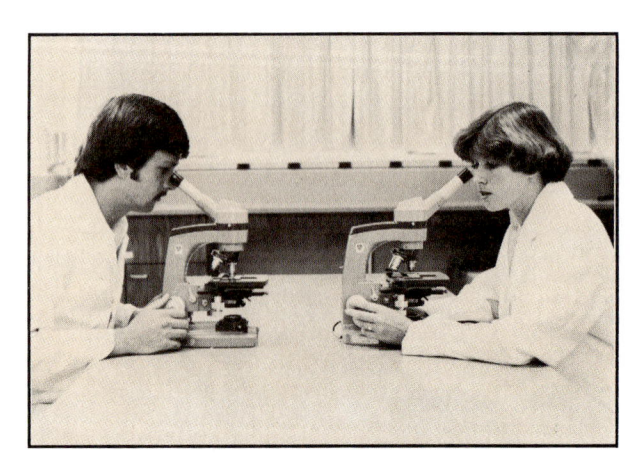

Figure 4.6 The microscope position on the right has the advantage of stage accessibility.

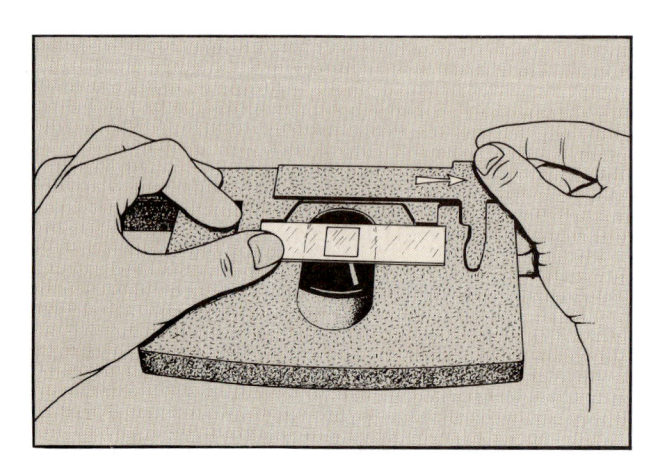

Figure 4.7 The slide must be properly positioned as the retainer lever is moved to the right.

from low power to high-dry, because all the objectives will be **parfocalized.** Nonparfocalized microscopes do require considerable focusing adjustments when changing objectives.

High-dry objectives should only be used on slides that have cover glasses; without them, images are often unclear. When increasing the lighting, be sure to open up the diaphragm first instead of increasing the voltage on your lamp; reason: lamp life is greatly extended when used at low voltage. If the field is not bright enough after opening the diaphragm, feel free to increase the voltage. A final point: keep the condenser at its highest point.

Oil Immersion Techniques The oil immersion lens derives its name from the fact that a special mineral oil is interposed between the lens and the microscope slide. The oil is used because it has the same refractive index as glass, which prevents the loss of light due to the bending of light rays as they pass through air. The use of oil in this way enhances the resolving power of the microscope. Figure 4.8 reveals this phenomenon.

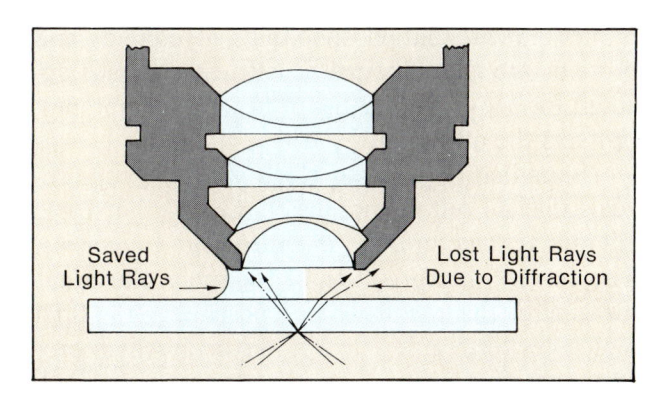

Figure 4.8 Immersion oil, having the same refractive index as glass, prevents light loss due to diffraction.

With parfocalized objectives one can go to oil immersion from either low power or high-dry. Once the microscope has been brought into focus at one magnification, the oil immersion lens can be rotated into position without fear of striking the slide.

Before rotating the oil immersion lens into position, however, a drop of immersion oil is placed on the slide. If the oil appears cloudy, it should be discarded.

When using the oil immersion lens it is best to open the diaphragm as much as possible. Stopping down the diaphragm tends to limit the resolving

power of the optics. In addition, the condenser must be at its highest point. If different colored filters are available for the lamp housing, it is best to use blue or greenish filters to enhance the resolving power.

Using this lens takes a little practice. The manipulation of lighting is critical. Before returning the microscope to the cabinet, all oil must be removed from the objective and stage. Slides with oil should be wiped clean with lens tissue, also.

Returning Microscope to Cabinet

When you take a microscope from the cabinet at the beginning of the period, you expect it to be clean and in proper working condition. The next person to use the instrument after you have used it will expect the same consideration. A few moments of care at the end of the period will ensure these conditions. Check over this list of items at the end of the period before you return the microscope to the cabinet:

1. Remove the slide from the stage.
2. If immersion oil has been used, wipe it off the lens and stage with lens tissue.
3. Rotate the low-power objective into position.
4. If the microscope has been inclined, return it to an erect position.
5. If the microscope has a built-in movable lamp, raise the lamp to its highest position.
6. If the microscope has a long attached electric cord, wrap it around the base.
7. Adjust the mechanical stage so that it does not project too far on either side.
8. Replace the dustcover.
9. If the microscope has a separate transformer, return it to its designated place.
10. Return the microscope to its correct place in the cabinet.

Laboratory Report

Before the microscope is to be used in the laboratory, answer all the questions on the Laboratory Report. Preparation on your part prior to going to the laboratory will greatly facilitate your understanding. Your instructor may wish to collect this report at the *beginning of the period* on the first day that the microscope is to be used in class.

Cell Study

Proceed to the cellular studies of Exercise 5.

5 Basic Cell Structure

As a prelude to the study of cellular physiology, it is essential to review cellular anatomy. An understanding of the nature of the plasma membrane and the roles of organelles such as mitochondria, ribosomes, and endoplasmic reticulum is of fundamental importance.

In the first portion of this exercise, a summary of the present knowledge of cellular structure and function is presented. This is followed by laboratory studies of epithelial cells.

Since much of the discussion in this exercise pertains to cellular structure as seen with an electron microscope, and since our laboratory observations will be made with a light microscope, there will be some cellular structures that cannot be seen in great detail in the laboratory.

To get the most out of this exercise *it is recommended that the questions on the Laboratory Report be answered prior to entering the laboratory.*

The Basic Design

Cytology, the study of cellular structure, has advanced at a rapid rate over the past decades with the use of electron microscopy and special techniques in the study of cellular physiology. The old notion of the cell as a "sac of protoplasm" has been supplanted by a much more dynamic model. A cell is now viewed as a highly complex miniature computer with an integrated, compartmentalized ultrastructure capable of communicating with its environment, altering its shape, processing information, and synthesizing a great variety of substances. It is largely through our advancing knowledge of the cellular organelles that this new viewpoint has emerged.

Figure 5.1 is a view of a pancreatic cell as it might appear if magnified by an electron microscope. This cell has been chosen for our study because it lacks the degree of specialization that is seen in many other cells, and so it can be considered illustrative of generalized cell structure. It contains the majority of organelles present in body cells and is also representative of an active secretory cell.

Although it is not possible to see the fine structure of many organelles with our ordinary light microscope, we are including descriptions of their appearance and current theories of function.

As the various cell structures are discussed in the following text, identify them in figure 5.1.

Plasma Membrane

The outer surface of every cell consists of an extremely thin, delicate *plasma membrane* or *cell membrane.* Chemical analyses of plasma membranes indicate that phospholipids, glycolipids, and proteins are the principal constituents. Lipids account for one-half the mass of plasma membranes, proteins the other half.

Examination with an electron microscope reveals that all cell membranes have a similar basic trilaminar structure, the so-called *unit membrane.* The current interpretation of the molecular organization of this membrane proposes that the lipid molecules form a double fluid layer in which protein and glycoprotein molecules are embedded. Figure 5.1 depicts an enlarged view of this fluid mosaic model (Singer-Nicholson 1972). Note that some of the proteins protrude externally, others protrude internally, and some extend through both sides of the membrane. This asymmetrical architecture appears to account for the external and internal differences in receptor sites that affect the permeability characteristics of the membrane.

Cell membranes are *selectively permeable* in allowing certain molecules to pass through easily and preventing other molecules from gaining entrance to the cell. Although cell membranes play both active and passive roles in molecular movements, experimental evidence seems to indicate that the movement of all molecules, including water, is assisted by the membrane.

Nucleus

Near the basal portion of the cell is a large spherical body, the *nucleus*. It is shown in figure 5.1 with a portion of its outer surface cut away. The substance of this body (*nucleoplasm*) is surrounded by a double-layered **nuclear envelope** that unlike other membranes, is perforated by pores of significant size. These openings provide a viable passageway between the cytoplasm and nucleoplasm.

A cell that has been stained with certain dyes will exhibit darkly stained regions in the nucleus called *chromatin granules*. These granules are visible even with a light microscope. They represent highly condensed DNA molecules that comprise part of the chromosomes. Current theories suggest that increased condensed chromosomal material indicates a metabolically less active cell.

The most conspicuous substructure of the nucleus is the **nucleolus.** Although nucleoli of different cells vary considerably in number and structure, they all consist primarily of RNA and function chiefly in the production of ribonucleoprotein for the ribosomes.

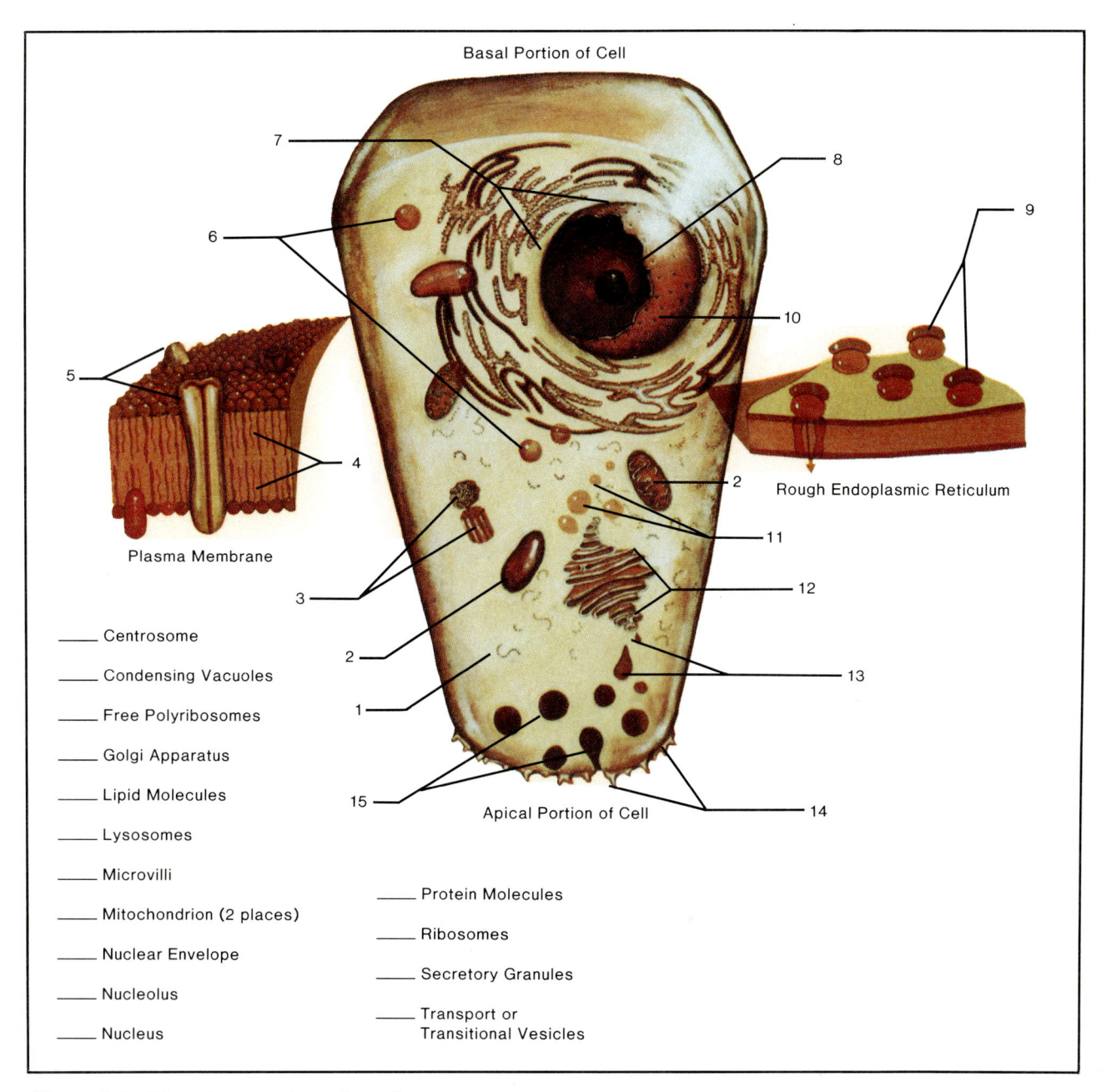

_____ Centrosome

_____ Condensing Vacuoles

_____ Free Polyribosomes

_____ Golgi Apparatus

_____ Lipid Molecules

_____ Lysosomes

_____ Microvilli

_____ Mitochondrion (2 places)

_____ Nuclear Envelope

_____ Nucleolus

_____ Nucleus

_____ Protein Molecules

_____ Ribosomes

_____ Secretory Granules

_____ Transport or Transitional Vesicles

Figure 5.1 The microstructure of a cell.

Cytoplasmic Matrix

Between the plasma membrane and nucleus is an area called the *cytoplasmic matrix,* or *cytoplasm.* This region is a heterogenous aggregation of many components involved in cellular metabolism. The cytoplasm is structurally and functionally compartmentalized by the numerous organelles, many of which are hollow and enclosed by unit membranes. A description of each of these cytoplasmic organelles follows.

Endoplasmic Reticulum The most extensive structure within the cytoplasm is a complex system of tubules, vesicles, and sacs called the *endoplasmic reticulum (ER).* It is a double-layered unit membrane that is somewhat similar to the nuclear and plasma membranes; in some instances it is continuous with these membranes. It appears to function, in part, as a microcirculatory system for the cell, providing a passageway for intracellular transport of molecules.

Detailed studies of cells have shown that ER may have surfaces that are smooth or rough. ER that is designated as **rough endoplasmic reticulum (RER)** is a fluid-filled canalicular system studded with ribosomes. It is the type illustrated in the magnified view on the right side of figure 5.1. RER is believed to be an important site of protein synthesis and storage. It is more developed in cells that are primarily secretory in function. **Smooth endoplasmic reticulum (SER)** also consists of multilayered unit membrane compartments but lacks ribosomes. It is thought that SER is active in various types of biosynthesis.

Ribosomes As stated above, ribosomes are small bodies attached to the surface of the RER. They are also scattered throughout the cytoplasm in rosettes and chains called **free polyribosomes.** Since they are only 170 Angstrom units (17 nanometers) in diameter they can be resolved only by electron microscopy.

The components for each ribosome originate in the nucleolus of the nucleus. They pass from the nucleolus through the pores of the nuclear membrane into the cytoplasm where they unite to form the completed ribosomal particle. Each ribosome consists of about 60% RNA and 40% protein. Their proposed structure is shown in figure 5.1.

Ribosomes are sites of protein synthesis and are particularly numerous in actively synthetic cells.

There is evidence to indicate that free polyribosomes are involved in synthesis of proteins for endogenous use; attached (RER) ribosomes are implicated in the synthesis of protein to be transported extracellularly (i.e., secretion).

Mitochondria The bean-shaped bodies with double-layered walls in figure 5.1 are *mitochondria.* These unit membrane structures are approximately 1×2–3 micrometers in size. Note that the inner membranes of these bodies have infoldings, called *cristae,* that serve to increase the inner surface area.

Mitochondria contain DNA and are able to replicate themselves. They also contain their own ribosomes. They are sometimes referred to as the "power plants" of the cell, since it is here that the energy-yielding reactions of oxidative respiration occur. Simply stated, these reactions oxidize glucose ($C_6H_{12}O_6$) to yield energy in the form of ATP:

$$C_6H_{12}O_6 + 6O_2 \rightarrow 6CO_2 + 6H_2O + ATP + Heat$$

Golgi Apparatus This unit membrane organelle is quite similar in basic structure to SER. In figure 5.1 it appears as a layered diamond-shaped stack of vesicles; in other cells it may appear differently. Although not shown in figure 5.1, it is connected to a portion of the RER.

Its primary role relates to the packaging, movement, and completed synthesis of products to be released by secretory cells. Proteins synthesized by the RER are pinched off into ovoid sacs, or **transitional vesicles** (label 11), which then coalesce with the cisternae of the Golgi apparatus proper. Here, further synthesis and completed processing of the secretory product take place. Completely processed materials accumulate at the apical end of the organelle and form **condensing vacuoles.** These membrane-bound bodies move to the apex of the cell where, as **secretory granules,** they are ultimately exocytosed. Figure 5.1 illustrates this process and how the granules fuse with the plasma membrane. The fate of the exocytosed product depends upon the cell type.

Lysosomes Oval sacs, such as the one in the upper left part of the cell in figure 5.1, contain digestive enzymes and are called *lysosomes.* These sacs consist of a single unit membrane and are believed to form by the pinching off of sacs from the Golgi apparatus. The contents of these organelles vary from cell to cell, but typically they include enzymes that hydrolyze proteins and nucleic acids.

The function of these organelles is not known for certain. It appears, however, that they act as disposal units of the cytoplasm, for they often contain fragments of mitochondria, ingested food particles, dead microorganisms, worn-out red blood cells, and any other debris that may have been taken into the cytoplasm. When the lysosome has performed its function, it is expelled from the cell through the plasma membrane.

In dying cells, the membrane of the lysosome disintegrates to release the enzymes into the cytoplasm. The hydrolytic action of the enzymes on the cell hastens the death of the cell. It is for this reason that these organelles have been called "suicide bags."

Centrosome At the far left of figure 5.1 are a pair of microtubule bundles that are arranged at right angles to each other. Each bundle, called a *centriole,* consists of nine triplets of microtubules arranged in a circle. The two centrioles are collectively referred to as the *centrosome.* Because of their small size, centrosomes appear as very small dots when observed with a light microscope. During mitosis and meiosis in animal cells centrioles play a role in the formation of spindle fibers that aid in the separation of chromatids. They also function in the formation of cilia and flagella in certain types of cells.

Cytoskeletal Elements

It now appears that a living cell has an extensive permeating network of fine fibers that contribute to cellular properties such as contractility, support, shape, and translocation of materials. Microtubules and microfilaments fall into this category.

Microtubules Molecules of protein (*tubulin*), arranged in submicroscopic cylindrical hollow bundles, the *microtubules,* are found dispersed through the cytoplasm of most cells. They converge especially around the centrioles to form aster fibers and the spindles that are seen during cell division (Exercise 6). They also play a significant role in the transport of vesicles from the Golgi apparatus to other parts of the cell.

Nerve cells that have long processes, called axons, utilize microtubules to transport vesicles and mitochondria. Movement of these organelles is from

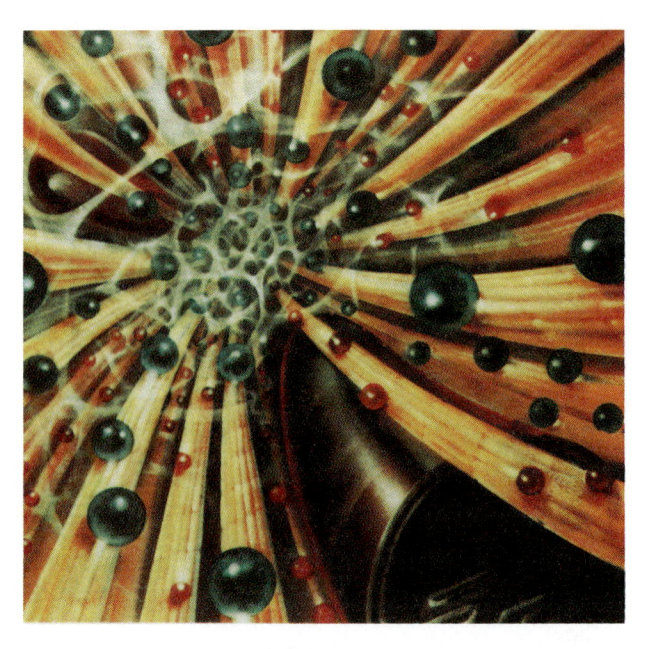

Figure 5.2 A computer-generated visualization of microtubules, vesicles, and mitochondria in a nerve cell. Vesicles and mitochondria are being propelled by the microtubules.

the cell body to the axon terminal, as well as from the terminal back to the cell body.

Figure 5.2 is a computer-generated image of how these microtubules might look where they enter an axon of a nerve cell. Note that various sized vesicles are propelled along the microtubules and that these vesicles move along the microtubules in both directions, *simultaneously.* The energy for vesicle transport is supplied by mitochondria. A portion of one is seen in the lower right quadrant; another is shown in the upper left quadrant.

Microfilaments All cells show some degree of contractility. Cytoskeletal elements responsible for this phenomenon are the *microfilaments.* These filaments are composed of protein molecules arranged in solid parallel bundles. They are most highly developed in muscle cells that are adapted for contraction. In other types of cells, they are present as interwoven networks of the cytoplasm and are relatively inconspicuous even in electron photomicrographs. Besides aiding in contractility, they also appear to be involved in cell motility and support.

Cilia and Flagella

Hairlike appendages of cells that function in providing some type of movement are either *cilia* or *flagella.* While cilia are usually less than 20 micrometers long, flagella may be thousands of micrometers in length. Cells that line the respiratory tract and uterine tubes have cilia (See illustration D in figures HA-2 and HA-31 of the Histology Atlas). The only human cells with flagella are the spermatozoa. Both cilia and flagella originate from centrioles, which explains why they both have microtubular internal structure similar to the centrioles.

Microvilli

Certain cells, such as the one in figure 5.1, have tiny protruberances known as *microvilli* on the apical or free surfaces. They may appear as a fine **brush border** (illustration C, figure HA-2) or as **stereocilia** (illustration B, figure HA-34) Both of these may be mistaken for cilia with a light microscope.

Each microvillus is an extension of cytoplasm enclosed by the plasma membrane. Microvilli are very common on cells lining the intestine and kidney tubules where they function to increase surface area of the cells for absorption of water and nutrients. Microvilli are not motile.

Laboratory Assignment

After labeling figure 5.1 and answering the questions on the Laboratory Report pertaining to cell structure and function, prepare a wet mount slide from some cells removed from the inside surface of your cheek. Use the following procedure:

Materials:

> microscope slides
> cover glasses
> toothpicks
> IKI solution

1. Wash a microscope slide and cover glass with soap and water.
2. Gently scrape some cells loose from the inside surface of your cheek with a clean toothpick. Try not to draw blood.
3. Mix the cells into a drop of IKI solution on the slide.
4. Cover with a cover glass.
5. After locating a cell under low power of your microscope, make a careful examination of the cell under high-dry magnification. Identify the *nucleus, cytoplasm,* and *cell membrane.*
6. Draw a few cells on the Laboratory Report, labeling the three structures.

Laboratory Report

Complete the first portion of Laboratory Report 5,6 that pertains to this exercise.

6 Mitosis

Growth of body structures and the repair of specific tissues occur by cell division. While many cells in the body are able to divide, many do not beyond a certain age. Cell division is characterized by the equal division of all cellular components to form two daughter cells that are identical in genetic composition to the original cell. Cleavage of the cytoplasm is referred to as *cytokinesis;* nuclear division is *karyokinesis,* or *mitosis.* Cells that are not undergoing mitosis are said to be in a "resting stage," or *interphase.*

During this laboratory period we will study the various phases of mitosis on a microscope slide of hematoxylin-stained embryonic cells of *Ascaris,* a roundworm. The advantage of using *Ascaris* over other organisms is that it has so few chromosomes.

To facilitate clarity in understanding this process it has been necessary to combine photomicrographs and diagrams in figures 6.1 and 6.2. However, before we get into the mitotic stages, let's see what takes place in the interphase.

The Interphase

Although a cell in the interphase stage doesn't appear to be active, it is carrying on the physiological activities that are characteristic of its particular specialization. The cell may be in one of two different phases: the G_1 phase or the S phase (G_1 for growth, S for synthesis). After a previous division, cells in the *S phase* begin to synthesize DNA, with each double-stranded DNA molecule replicating itself to produce another identical molecule. Most cells in the S phase will accomplish this replication within twenty hours and then divide. If division does not occur within this time frame, the cell is said to be in the *G phase* and will not divide again. Note in illustration 1, figure 6.1, that cells in the interphase stage exhibit a more or less translucent nucleus with an intact nuclear membrane.

Stages of Mitosis

The process of mitotic cell division is a continuous one once the cell has started to divide. However, for discussion purposes, the process has been divided

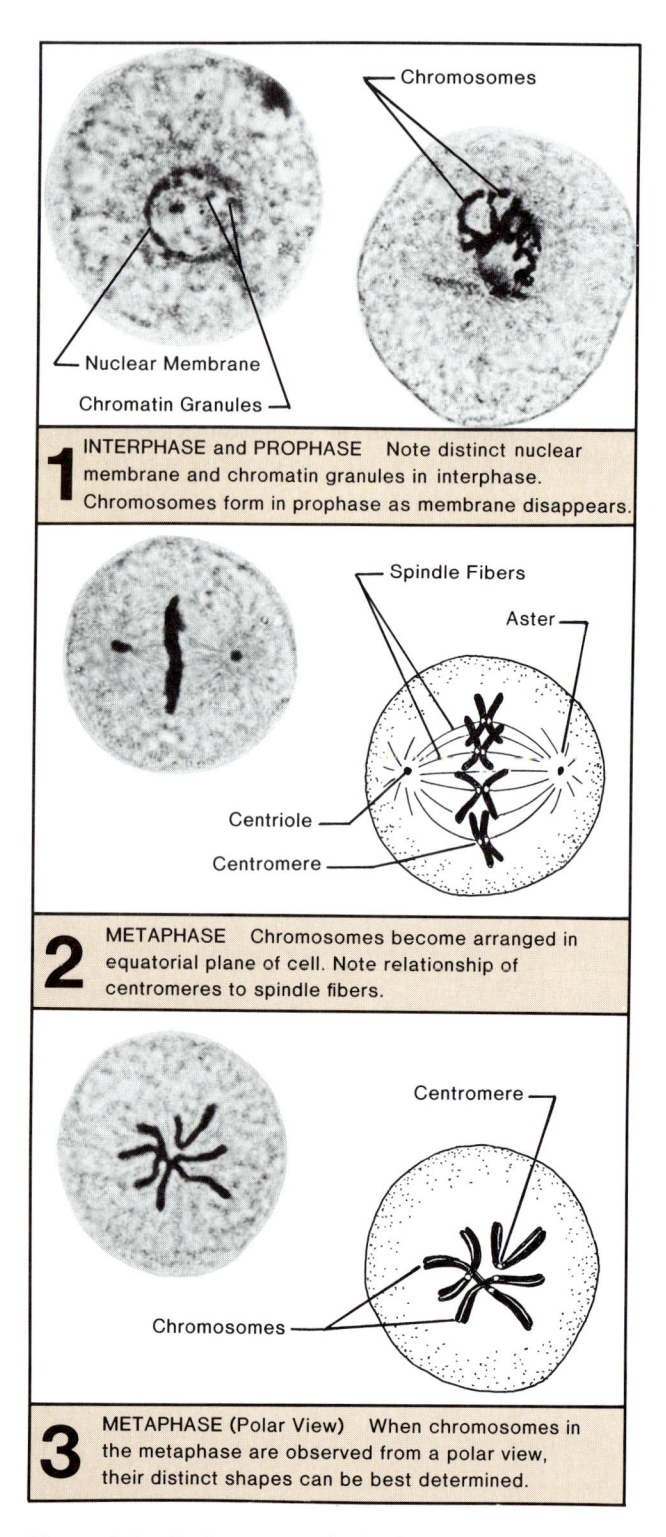

1 INTERPHASE and PROPHASE   Note distinct nuclear membrane and chromatin granules in interphase. Chromosomes form in prophase as membrane disappears.

2 METAPHASE   Chromosomes become arranged in equatorial plane of cell. Note relationship of centromeres to spindle fibers.

3 METAPHASE (Polar View)   When chromosomes in the metaphase are observed from a polar view, their distinct shapes can be best determined.

Figure 6.1   Early stages of mitosis.

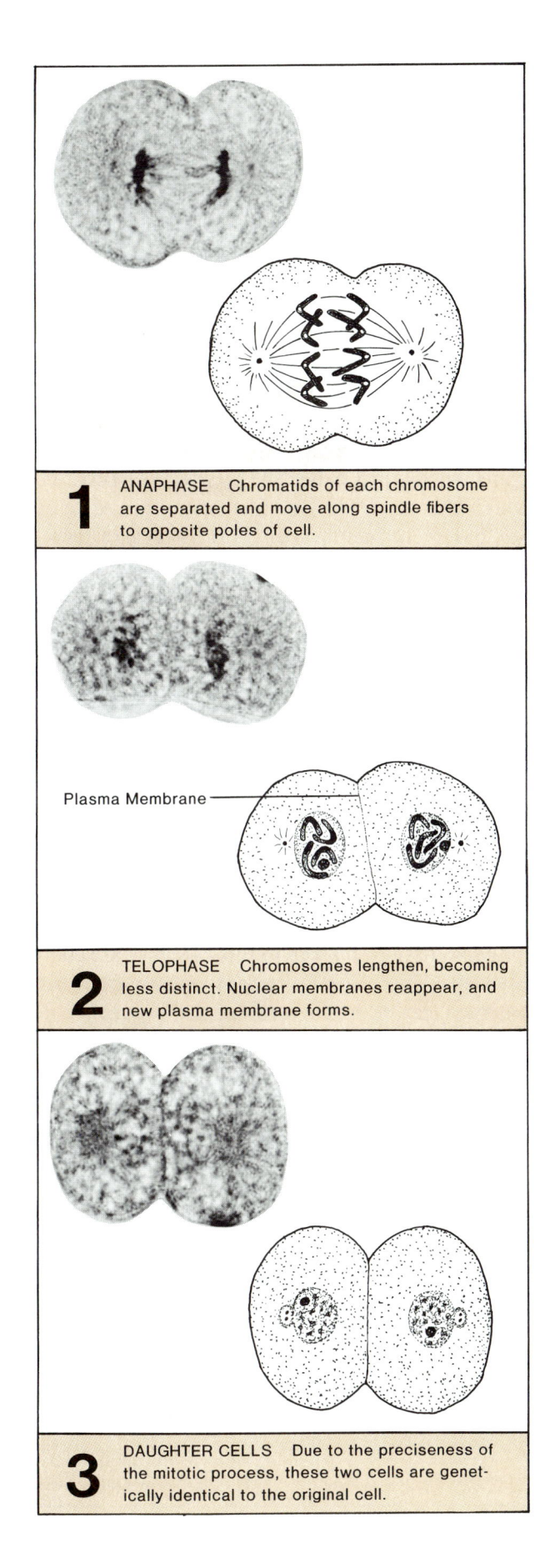

1 ANAPHASE Chromatids of each chromosome are separated and move along spindle fibers to opposite poles of cell.

Plasma Membrane

2 TELOPHASE Chromosomes lengthen, becoming less distinct. Nuclear membranes reappear, and new plasma membrane forms.

3 DAUGHTER CELLS Due to the preciseness of the mitotic process, these two cells are genetically identical to the original cell.

Figure 6.2 Later stages of mitosis.

into a series of four recognizable stages: prophase, metaphase, anaphase, and telophase. A description of each phase follows.

Prophase In this first stage of mitosis the nuclear membrane disappears, **chromosomes** become visible, and each **centriole** of the centrosome moves to opposite poles of the cell to become an **aster.** The dark-staining chromosomes are made up of DNA and protein. Each aster consists of a centriole and astral rays (microtubules). By the end of the prophase some of the astral rays from each aster extend across the entire cell to become the **spindle fibers.**

From the early prophase to the late prophase the chromosomes undergo thickening and shortening. During this time each chromosome has a double nature, consisting of a pair of **chromatids.** This dual structure is due to the replication of the DNA molecules during the interphase.

Metaphase During this stage the chromosomes migrate to the equatorial plane of the cell. Note in illustration 2, figure 6.1, that each chromosome has a **centromere,** which is the point of contact between each pair of chromatids and a spindle fiber.

Anaphase As indicated in illustration 1 of figure 6.2, the individual chromatids of each chromosome are separated from each other and move apart along a spindle fiber to opposite poles of the cell.

Telophase This stage begins with the appearance of a **cleavage furrow.** It is much like the prophase in reverse in that the chromosomes become less distinct and a new nuclear membrane begins to form around each set of chromosomes. In the late telophase the spindle fibers disappear and the centrioles duplicate themselves. When the nuclear membranes and newly formed cell membrane are complete the two new structures are referred to as **daughter cells.**

Laboratory Assignment

Examine a prepared slide of *Ascaris* mitosis (Turtox slide E6.24). It will be necessary to use both the high-dry and oil immersion objectives. Identify all of the stages and make drawings, if required. Identifiable structures should be labeled. Answer the questions on Laboratory Report 5,6 that pertain to mitosis.

7 Epithelial Tissues

Although all cells of the body share common structures such as nuclei, centrosomes, and Golgi apparatus, they differ considerably in size, shape, and structure according to their specialized functions. An aggregate of cells that are similar in structure and function is called a *tissue*. The science which relates to the study of tissues is called *histology*.

In this exercise we will study the different types of epithelial tissues. Prepared microscope slides from portions of different organs will be available for study. Learning how to identify specific epithelial tissues on slides that have several types of tissue will be part of the challenge of this exercise.

Epithelial tissues are aggregations of cells that perform specific protective, absorptive, secretory, transport, and excretory functions. They often serve as coverings for internal and external surfaces and they rest upon a bed of connective tissue. Characteristics common to all epithelial tissues are as follows:

• The individual cells are closely attached to each other at their margins to form tight sheets of cells lacking in extracellular matrix and vascularization.

• The cell groupings are oriented in such a way that they have an apical (free) surface and a basal (bound) region. The basal portion is closely anchored to underlying connective tissue. This thin adhesive margin between the epithelial cells and connective tissue is called the **basement lamina.** Although this structure was formerly referred to as the "basement membrane," it is not a true membrane. Unlike true membranes the basement lamina is acellular. In reality, it is a colloidal complex of protein, polysaccharide, and reticular fibers.

Differentiation of the various epithelia is illustrated in the separation outline, figure 7.1. The basic criteria for assigning categories are cell shape, surface specializations, and layer complexity. The three divisions (*simple, pseudostratified,* and *stratified*) are based on layer complexity. A discussion of each follows.

Simple Epithelia

Epithelial tissues that fall in this category are composed of a single cell layer that extends from the basement lamina to the free surface. Figure 7.2 illustrates three basic kinds of simple epithelia.

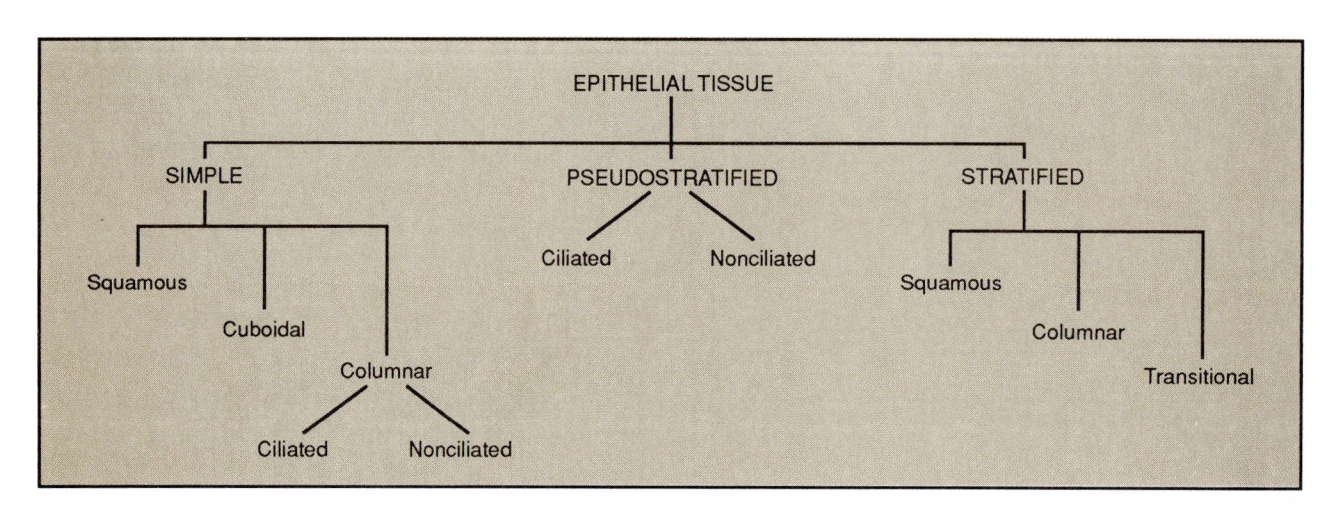

Figure 7.1 A morphologic classification of epithelial types.

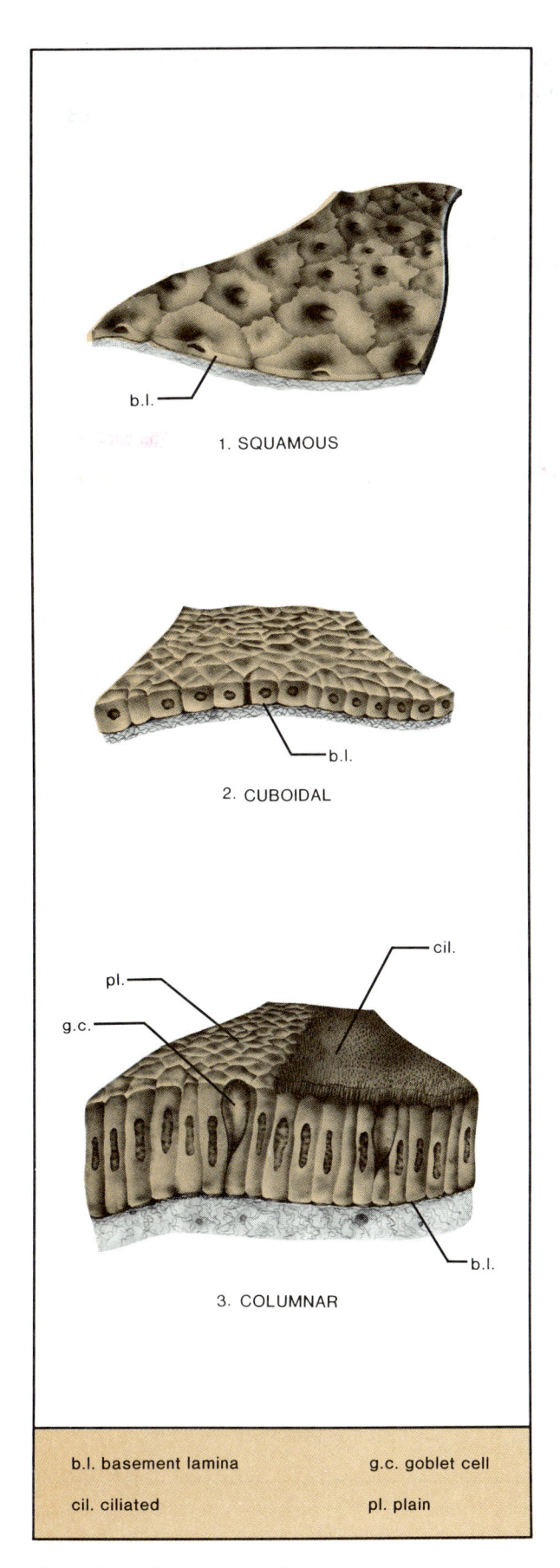

Figure 7.2 Simple epithelia.

1. SQUAMOUS

2. CUBOIDAL

pl.

g.c.

cil.

b.l.

3. COLUMNAR

| b.l. basement lamina | g.c. goblet cell |
| cil. ciliated | pl. plain |

Simple Squamous Epithelia These cells are very thin, flat, and irregular in outline. An example of this type is seen in illustration 1, figure 7.2. They form a pavementlike sheet in various organs that perform filtering or exchange functions. Capillary walls, alveolar walls in the lungs, the peritoneum, the pleurae, and blood vessel linings consist of simple squamous epithelia.

Cuboidal Epithelia Cells of this type are stout and blocklike in cross section, and hexagonal from a surface view (illustration 2, figure 7.2). Several glands (thyroid, salivary, pancreas), the ovary, and the lens of the eye (its capsule) contain cuboidal tissue.

Simple Columnar Epithelia Illustration 3, figure 7.2, reveals that cells of this type are elongated between their apical and basal surfaces; on their free surfaces they are polygonal. They may be functionally specialized for protection, secretion, or absorption. Specialized secretory cells in columnar epithelia, called **goblet cells,** produce the protective glycoprotein, *mucus.*

The linings of the stomach, intestines, and kidney collecting tubules consist of *plain* (nonciliated) columnar epithelial tissue. *Ciliated* columnar cells are seen lining the respiratory tract, uterine tubes, and portions of the uterus. Goblet cells may be present in both plain and ciliated columnar epithelia.

Another modification of the free surfaces of columnar cells is the presence of *microvilli.* These structures are seen as a *brush border* when observed with a light microscope under oil immersion. Columnar cells that line the small intestine and make up the walls of the collecting tubules in the kidney exhibit microvilli.

Stratified Epithelia

Squamous, columnar, and cuboidal epithelia that exist in layers are referred to as being *stratified.* Figure 7.3 illustrates four layered epithelia that have distinct differences.

Stratified Squamous Illustration 1, figure 7.3, is of this type. Note that while the superficial cells are distinctly squamous, the deepest layer is columnar; in some cases this layer is cuboidal. In between the basal cell layer and the squamous cells are successive layers of irregular and polyhedral cells.

Protection is the chief function of this type of tissue. Exposed inner and outer surfaces of the body, such as the skin, oral cavity, esophagus, vagina, and cornea, consist of stratified squamous epithelia.

Stratified Columnar This type of epithelium is shown in illustration 2, figure 7.3. Note that although the superficial cells are distinctly columnar, the deeper cells are irregular or polyhedral. Note also that the superficial columnar cells are variable in height.

Protection and secretion are the chief functions of this type of tissue. Distribution of stratified columnar is limited to some glands, the conjunctiva, the pharynx, a portion of the urethra, and the anus.

Transitional A unique characteristic of this type of stratified epithelium is that the surface layer consists of large, round, dome-shaped cells that may be binucleate. The deeper strata are cuboidal, columnar, and polyhedral.

Note in illustration 3, figure 7.3, that the deeper cells are not as closely packed as other stratified epithelia. Distinct spaces can be seen between the cells. This looseness of cells imparts a certain degree of elasticity to the tissue. Organs such as the urinary bladder, ureters, and kidneys (the calyces) contain transitional epithelium that enables distension due to urine accumulation.

Stratified Cuboidal Although no stratified cuboidal tissue is shown in figure 7.1, tissue of this configuration is seen in the ducts of sweat glands of the skin. The ducts in Illustration C, figure HA-9, show what stratified cuboidal looks like.

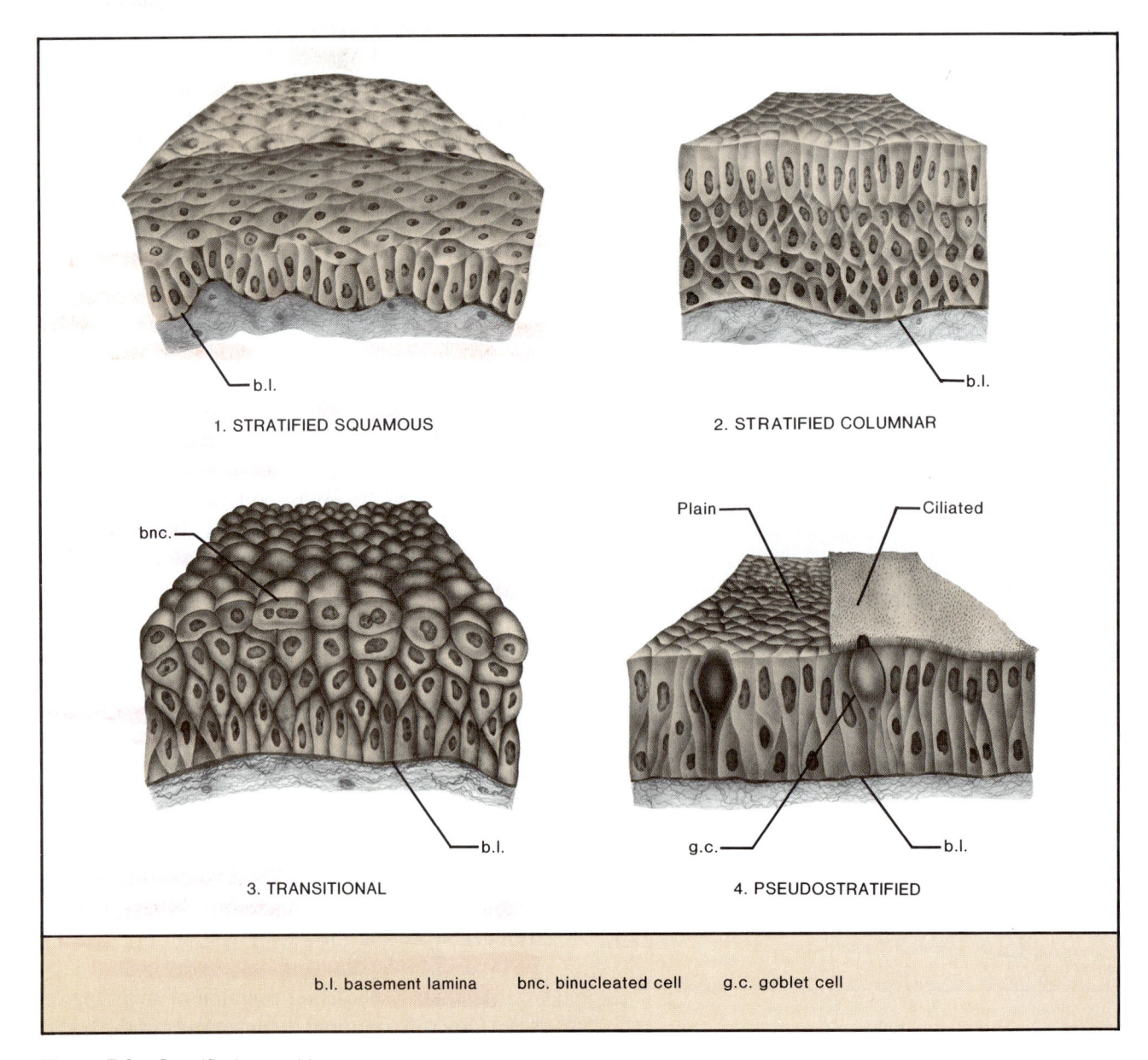

1. STRATIFIED SQUAMOUS

2. STRATIFIED COLUMNAR

3. TRANSITIONAL

4. PSEUDOSTRATIFIED

b.l. basement lamina   bnc. binucleated cell   g.c. goblet cell

Figure 7.3 Stratified, transitional, and pseudostratified epithelia.

Pseudostratified Epithelia

This epithelium presents a superficial stratified appearance because of the staggered nuclei as well as two different cell orientations. It is only one layer thick, however. Close examination will reveal that every cell is in contact with the basal lamina, but only the columnar types extend to the free surface. The smaller cells wedged between them have no free surface.

Two types are shown in illustration 4 of figure 7.3: plain and ciliated. The *plain,* or nonciliated, is found in the male urethra and parotid gland. The *ciliated* type lines the trachea, bronchi, auditory tube, and part of the middle ear. Since both types frequently produce mucus, they possess goblet cells.

Laboratory Assignment

Do a systematic study of each kind of epithelial tissue by examining prepared slides that should show the kinds of tissue you are looking for. Remembering that epithelial cells have a free surface and a basement lamina, always look for the tissue near the edge of a structure.

Note in the materials list below that *preferred* and *optional* lists of slides are given. The preferred list is of slides that are limited to the type of tissue being studied. If these are available, use them. If they are not available, use the optional slides, which are somewhat more difficult to use. The numbers listed in parentheses after each tissue are Turtox code numbers of slides that should reveal structures illustrated in the Histology Atlas.

Materials:

preferred slides: squamous (H1.1), stratified squamous (H1.14), cuboidal (H1.21), simple columnar (H1.31), pseudostratified ciliated (H1.32), and transitional (H1.41)

optional slides: skin (H11.12 or H11.14), trachea (H6.41), stomach (H5.415 or H5.425), ileum (H5.531), kidney (H9.11 or H9.15), and thyroid gland (H14.11, H14.12, or H14.13)

Squamous Epithelium Look for the flattened cells that are representative of this kind of tissue. Use figure HA-1 in the Histology Atlas for reference. The exfoliated cells are the same ones you studied in Exercise 5. Explore each slide first with the low-power objective before using the high-dry or oil immersion objectives. Make drawings if required.

Columnar Epithelium Consult figure HA-2 in the Histology Atlas for representatives of this group of epithelial cells. To see the **brush border** or **cilia** on these cells it will be necessary to study the cells with the high-dry or oil immersion objectives. Can you identify the **basement lamina** on each tissue?

Cuboidal Epithelium Illustrations A and B, figure HA-3, reveal the appearance of cuboidal tissue. If Turtox slide H1.21 is unavailable, use a slide of the thyroid gland for this type of tissue. Turtox slide H1.21 is usually made from the uterine lining of a pregnant guinea pig.

Transitional Tissue Illustrations C and D of figure HA-3 and illustration C, figure HA-30, provide good examples of this type of tissue. Note that the cells seem to be loosely arranged. Look for **binucleate cells.**

Ciliated Pseudostratified Columnar Epithelium The best place to look for this type of tissue is in a cross section of the trachea. Illustration D, figure HA-2, is the epithelium of the trachea.

Laboratory Report

Answer the questions on Laboratory Report 7,8 that pertain to the epithelial tissues.

8 Connective Tissues

Connective tissues include those tissues which perform binding, support, transport, and nutritive functions for organs and organ systems. Characteristically, all connective tissues have considerable amounts of nonliving extracellular substance that holds and surrounds various specialized cells.

The extracellular material, or *matrix,* is composed of fibers, fluid, organic ground substance, and/or inorganic components intimately associated with the cells. This matrix is a product of the cells in the tissue. The relative proportion of cells to matrix will vary from one tissue to another.

Several systems of classification of connective tissues have been proposed. Figure 8.1 reveals the system that we will use here. It is based on the nature of the extracellular material; in some cases there is a certain amount of overlapping of categories.

Connective Tissue Proper

Histologically, **connective tissue proper** is composed primarily of protein fibers, special cells, and a ground substance that varies among the several types. The fibers may differ in protein composition and density. From the standpoint of composition, fibers consist of either collagenous or elastin protein. There are three basic types of fibers: collagenous, reticular, and elastic. **Collagenous,** or *white fibers,* are relatively long, thick bundles seen in most ordinary connective tissues in varying amounts. **Reticular fibers** constitute minute networks of very fine threads. Although both collagenous and reticular fibers are composed of collagen, the reticular fibers stain more readily with silver dyes (*argyrophilic*). **Elastic fibers,** also called *yellow fibers,* are often found in the connective tissue stroma of organs that must yield to shape changes. These are the only fibers to contain elastin protein. All three types of fibers are seen in loose fibrous tissue (figure 8.2).

The **ground substance** usually consists of complex peptidoglycans that form an amorphous solution or gel around the cells and fibers. Chondroitin sulfate and hyaluronic acid are frequent components.

Cells or formed elements of connective tissue proper are of many types; examples are fibroblasts, adipose cells, mast cells, macrophages, and other blood cells, both fixed and wandering.

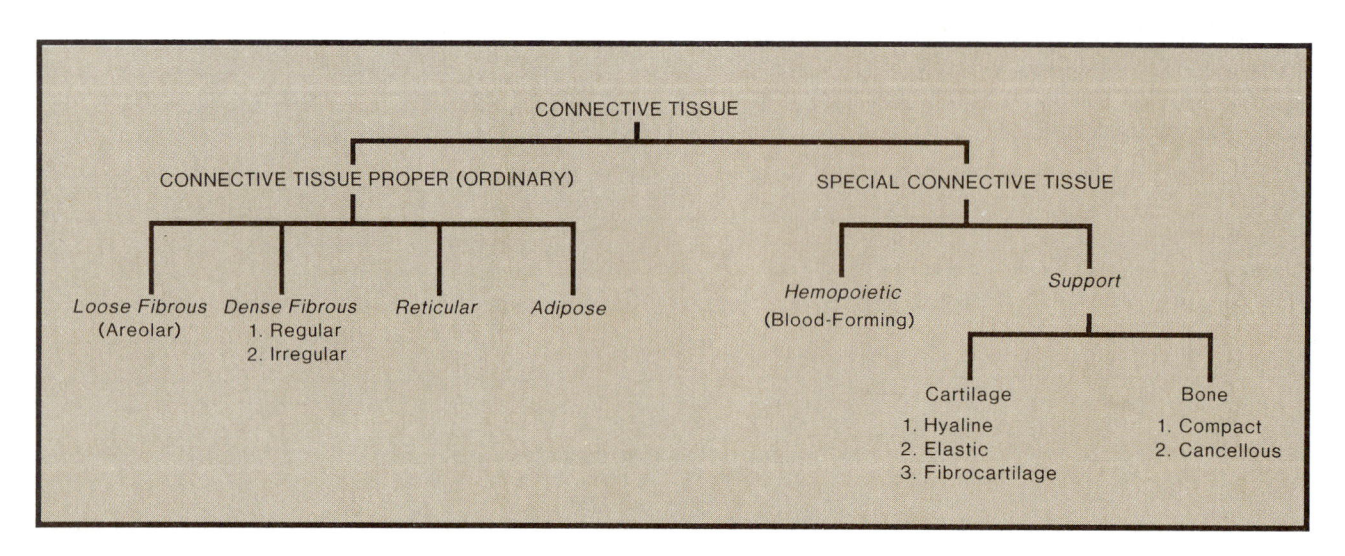

Figure 8.1 Types of connective tissue.

Loose Fibrous (*Areolar*) Connective Tissue

This is a widespread tissue that is interwoven into the stroma of many organs. The cells and extracellular substances of this tissue are very loosely organized. Because of the preponderance of spaces in this tissue, it is designated as *areolar* (a small space). It is highly flexible and capable of distension when excess extracellular fluid is present. The left-hand illustration in figure 8.2 depicts its generalized structure. Note the presence of **mast cells, macrophages,** and **fibroblasts.**

Three important functions are served by loose connective tissue: (1) it provides flexible support and a continuous network within organs, (2) it furnishes nutrition to cells in adjacent areas due to its capillary network, and (3) it provides an arena for activities of the immune system. It may be found beneath epithelia, around and within muscles and nerves, and as part of the serous membranes. The deep and superficial fasciae encountered in the rat dissection are of this type.

Adipose Tissue

Fat or adipose cells can be found in small groupings throughout the body; however, as they constitute a storage depot for fat, they frequently accumulate in large areas to make up the bulk of body fat. These latter areas are made up, essentially, of *adipose tissue.* There are various types of adipose tissue, but ordinary adipose is that most commonly found in humans. See figure 8.2.

Fat cells are very large and characterized by a spherical or polygonal shape; as much as 95% of their mass may be stored fat. As the process of fat deposition ensues, the cell cytoplasm becomes reduced and thin, and the vacuole, filled with lipids, appears as a large open space with a thin periphery of cytoplasm. The nucleus is displaced to one side, producing a signet ring appearance. A fine network of reticular fibers exists between the cells.

Fat tissue serves as a protective cushion and insulation for the body, in addition to being a potential source of energy and heat generator. Its rich vascular supply points to its relatively high rate of metabolism and turnover.

Reticular Tissue

This tissue (figure 8.3) is generally regarded as a network of reticular fiber elements within certain organs. As the fibers show a unique pattern and staining reaction, they can be identified as the supporting framework of many vascular organs such

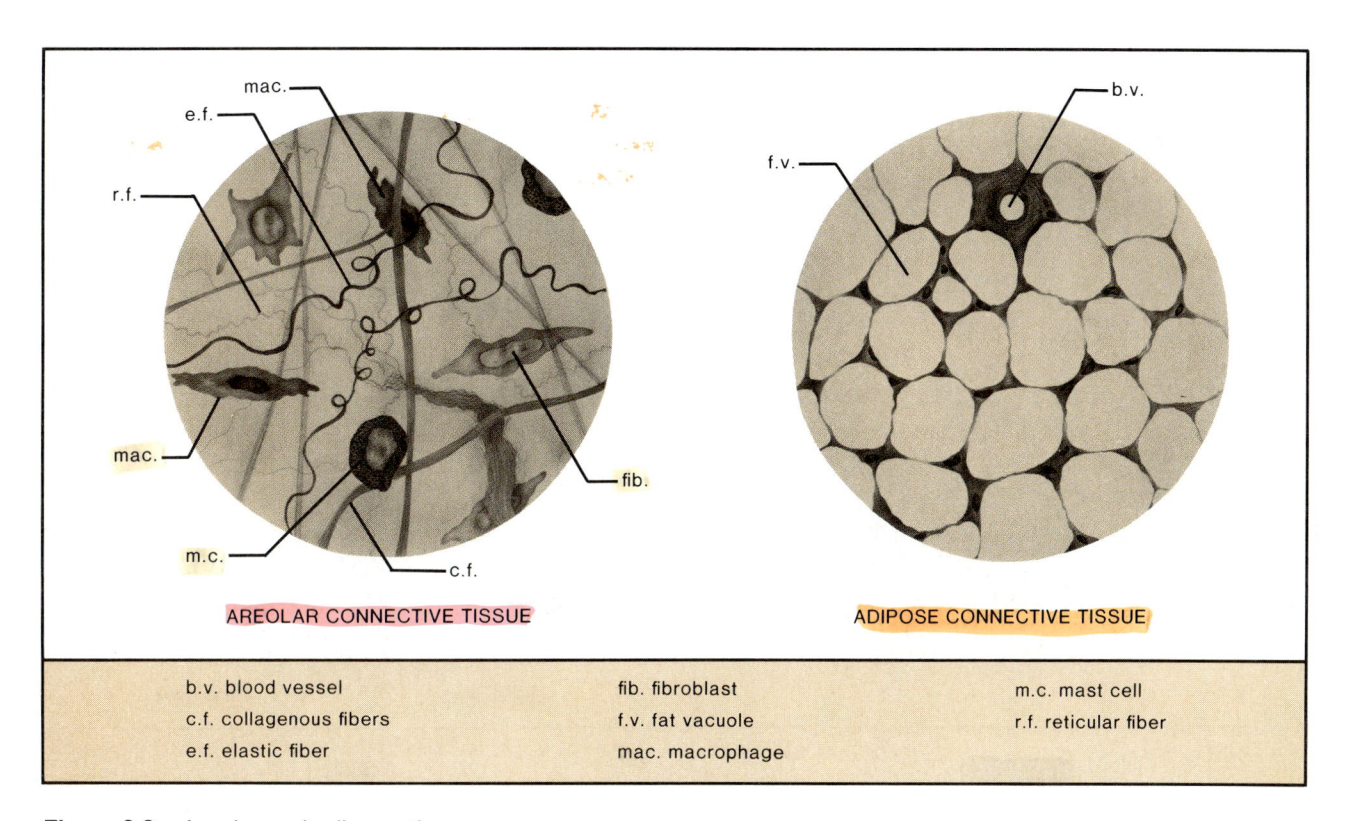

AREOLAR CONNECTIVE TISSUE

ADIPOSE CONNECTIVE TISSUE

b.v. blood vessel	fib. fibroblast	m.c. mast cell
c.f. collagenous fibers	f.v. fat vacuole	r.f. reticular fiber
e.f. elastic fiber	mac. macrophage	

Figure 8.2 Areolar and adipose tissues.

as the liver, lymphatic structures, hemopoietic tissue, and basement laminas. The left-hand illustration in figure 8.3 reveals the appearance of the reticulum of a lymph node.

Dense Fibrous (*White*) Connective Tissue

Tissue in this category differs from the loose variety in having a predominance of fibrous elements and a sparseness of cells, ground substance, and capillaries. According to the arrangement of fibers, this tissue can be separated into two groups: regular dense tissue and irregular dense tissue. The right-hand illustration in figure 8.3 reveals both types.

Dense regular connective tissue is the type found in tendons, ligaments, fasciae, and aponeuroses. It consists of thick groupings of longitudinally organized collagenous fibers and some elastic fibers. These tough strands have enormous tensile strength and are capable of withstanding strong pulling forces without stretching. Fibroblasts are the principal cells, although they are quite scarce.

Dense irregular connective tissue has the same kind of fibers that are woven into flat sheets to form capsules around certain organs. The sheaths that encircle nerves and tendons are of this type. A large portion of the dermis of the skin also consists of the dense irregular type.

Supporting Connective Tissues

As indicated in figure 8.1, the supporting connective tissues fall in the category of special connective tissues that include hemopoietic, cartilage, and bone tissues. Since our only concern with hemopoietic tissue will be with the formed elements in blood (Exercise 30), we will devote the remainder of this exercise to cartilage and bone tissues.

Cartilage and bone are adapted for the bearing of weight. Structural characteristics shared by these tissues include (1) a solid, flexible, yet strong extracellular matrix, (2) cells borne in matrix cavities called **lacunae,** and (3) an external covering capable of generating new tissue.

Cartilage

In general, cartilage consists of a stiff, plastic matrix that has lubricating as well as weight-bearing capability. As a result, it is found in areas requiring support and movement (skeleton and joints).

Basically, all three types of cartilage in man consist of cartilage cells, or **chondrocytes,** embedded within a matrix that contains ground substance and fibers. The proportion devoted to matrix

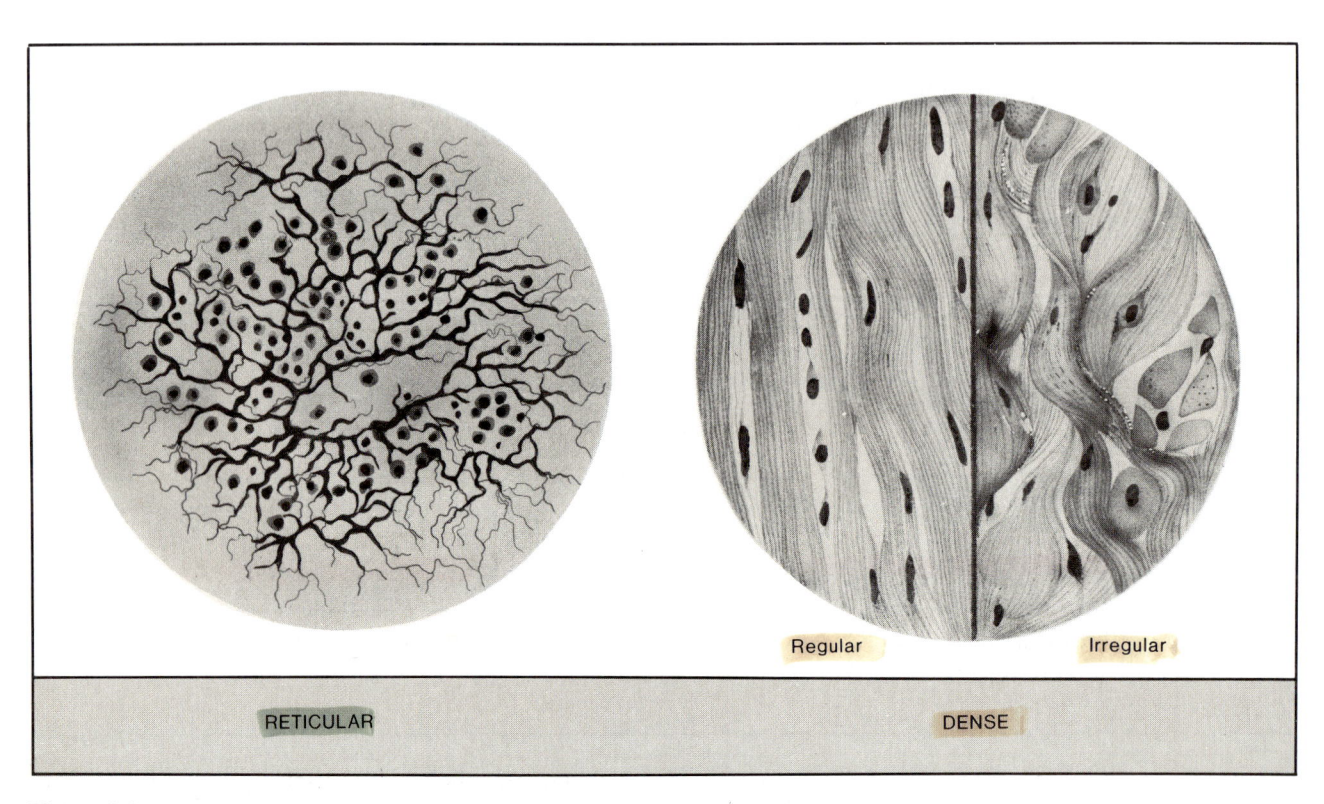

Regular   Irregular

RETICULAR   DENSE

Figure 8.3   Reticular and dense connective tissues.

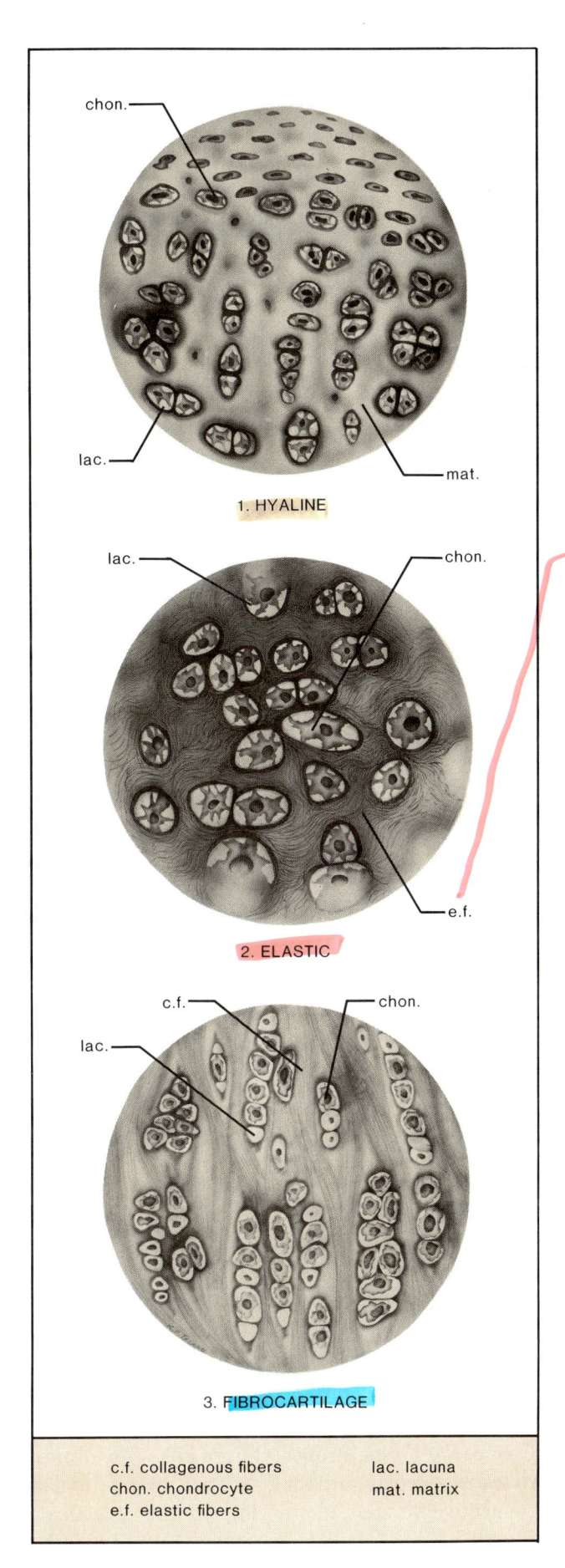

Figure 8.4 Types of cartilage.

1. HYALINE

2. ELASTIC

3. FIBROCARTILAGE

c.f. collagenous fibers
chon. chondrocyte
e.f. elastic fibers

lac. lacuna
mat. matrix

is much greater than that for chondrocytes. Unlike other connective tissues, cartilage is devoid of a vascular supply and receives all nutrients through diffusion. The three classes of cartilage are shown in figure 8.4.

Hyaline cartilage (illustration 1) is a pearly white, glasslike tissue that makes up a very large part of the fetal skeleton which is gradually replaced by bone, except for areas in the joints, ear, larynx, trachea, and ribs. The matrix is a firm, homogenous gel made up of chondroitin sulfate and collagen. Cells occur singly or in "nests" of several cells, the sides of which may be flattened. Often the areas directly around lacunae appear denser in sections.

Elastic cartilage (illustration 2) is similar in basic structure to hyaline cartilage, but differs in that it contains significant amounts of elastic fibers in its matrix. The result is a tissue that has highly developed flexibility and elasticity. The external ear (pinna), epiglottis, and the auditory tube are reinforced with this type of cartilage.

Fibrocartilage (illustration 3) differs from the other two types in that its chondrocytes are arranged in groupings between bundles of collagenous fibers. It serves a useful cushioning function in strategic joint ligaments and tendons. It is the major component, for instance, of the intervertebral disks of the vertebral column and of the symphysis pubis.

Bone Tissue

The tissue that makes up the bones of the skeleton meets all the criteria of connective tissue, yet it has many striking and unique features. It is hard, unyielding, very strong, and light. It is found in those parts of the anatomy that require weight-bearing, protection, and storage capacity.

In a sense, bone can be visualized as a living organic cement. It consists of specialized cells, blood vessels, and nerves that are reinforced within a hard ground substance made up of organic secretions impregnated with mineral salts. It arises during embryonic and fetal development from cartilage and/or fibrous connective tissue precursors. The initial organic matrix consists of collagen fibers that serve as a framework for the gradual deposition of calcium and phosphate salts by special bone cells, the *osteoblasts*. Far from being an inactive tissue, it is continuously being modified and reconstructed by both metabolic and external influences.

In macroscopic sections of bones, two frameworks are apparent: the solid, dense **compact bone,** which makes up the outermost layer, and the more porous **spongy,** or *cancellous,* **bone,** which is located internally. Each of these variations has a distinctive histological character.

Compact Bone

Upon close inspection of a cut section of the sternum viewed from a three-dimensional perspective (figure 8.5 in illustration A), it is apparent that compact bone (label 2) is permeated by a microscopic framework of tunnels, channels, and interconnecting networks that are surrounded by a hard matrix. Within this hollow network exist the living substances of bone that facilitate its nourishment and maintenance.

The functional and structural unit of compact bone is a cylindrical component called the **osteon** or Haversian system (label 9, illustration B). In the center of each osteon is a hollow space, the **central** (Haversian) **canal,** which contains one or two blood capillaries. Surrounding each central canal are several concentric rings of matrix called the **lamellae. Osteocytes,** which are responsible for secreting the lamellae, can be seen within small hollow cavities, the **lacunae.** Note that these cavities, which are oriented between the lamellae, have many minute hollow tunnels, called **canaliculi,** that radiate outward, imparting a spiderlike appearance. The canaliculi contain protoplasmic processes of the osteocytes.

If one follows the various levels of structure shown in figure 8.5, it should become evident that the network comprises a continuous communication system from the central canal to the lacunae and between adjacent lacunae via the canaliculi. Thus, the entrapped ostcocytes can receive nourishment and exchange materials within the hard space of the matrix. Intimate contact between the protoplasmic processes of adjacent osteocytes through the canaliculi makes all of this possible.

Groups of osteons lie in vertical array with adjacent lamellae separated at lines of demarcation called **cement lines.** Continuity between the central canals of adjacent osteons is achieved by **perforating** (Volkmann's) **canals** that penetrate the bone obliquely or at right angles.

Spongy Bone

This type of bone lies adjacent to compact bone and is continuous with it: there is no distinct line of de-

marcation between the two regions. Histologically, it presents a lesser degree of organization than compact bone. Illustration A reveals that its outstanding feature is a series of branching, overlapping plates of matrix called **trabeculae.** These are oriented so as to produce large, interconnecting cavelike spaces. These spaces function well in storage and as pockets to hold the blood-forming cells of the bone marrow; they also function in weight reduction. Note that the trabeculae are also randomly punctuated by the osteocyte-holding spaces, or lacunae, and that blood vessels meander through the large spaces between the trabeculae, bringing nourishment to nearby osteocytes.

The Periosteum

Contiguous with the outer layer of compact bone, and tightly adherent to it, is a thick, tough membrane called the **periosteum.** It is composed of an outer layer of fibrous connective tissue and an inner *osteogenic layer* that serves as a source of new bone-forming cells and provides an access for blood vessels. The periosteum is anchored tightly to compact bone by bundles of collagenous fibers that perforate and become firmly embedded within the outer lamellae. These minute attachments are called **Sharpey's fibers.**

Assignment:

Label figure 8.5.

Laboratory Assignment

Do a systematic study of each type of connective tissue by examining prepared slides that are available. Note that Histology Atlas references are indicated for each type of tissue.

Materials:

prepared slides: areolar (H2.13), adipose (H2.51), white fibrous (H2.115), yellow (elastic) fibrous (H2.125), reticular (H2.31), hyaline cartilage (H2.61), fibrocartilage (H2.63), elastic cartilage (H2.62), bone, x.s. (H2.735), and developing bone (H2.79)

Connective Tissue Proper (figure HA-4) Examine slides of areolar, adipose, fibrous, and reticular connective tissues, identifying all the structures shown in figure HA-4. Mast cells, which are seen in areolar tissue, secrete heparin and histamine. Macrophages are amoeboid cells that ingest bacteria, dead cells, and other materials.

Cartilage (figure HA-5) Study the three different types of cartilage, noting their distinct differentiating characteristics.

Bone (figure HA-6) When studying a slide of developing membrane bone, try to differentiate the osteoblasts from osteoclasts. Note that an osteoclast is a large multinucleate cell with a clear area between it and the bony matrix.

Laboratory Report

Complete Laboratory Report 7,8 by answering the questions that pertain to this exercise.

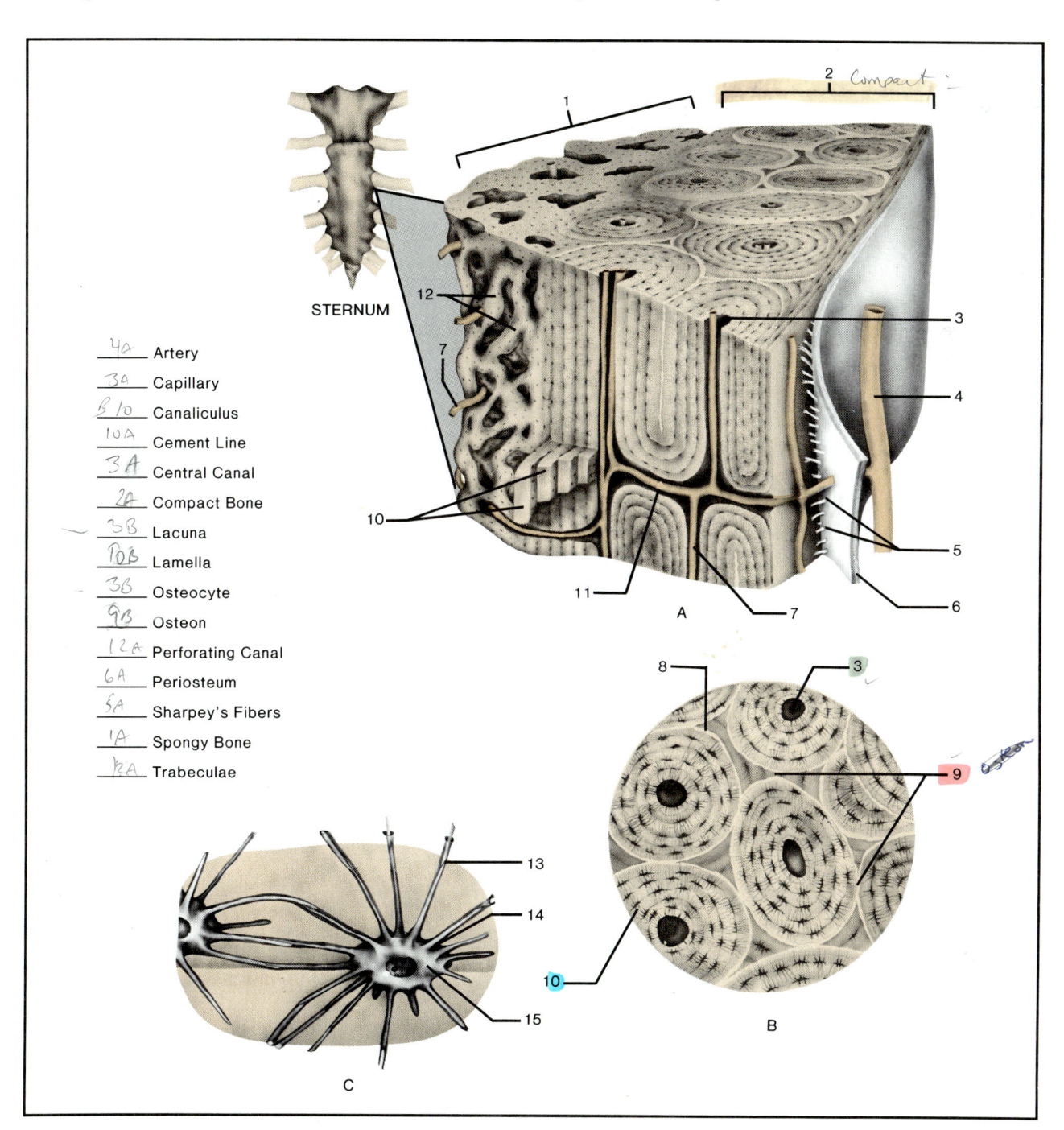

4A	Artery
3A	Capillary
B10	Canaliculus
10A	Cement Line
3A	Central Canal
2A	Compact Bone
3B	Lacuna
10B	Lamella
3B	Osteocyte
9B	Osteon
12A	Perforating Canal
6A	Periosteum
5A	Sharpey's Fibers
1A	Spongy Bone
12A	Trabeculae

Figure 8.5 Bone tissue.

9 The Integument

Since it is constructed of epithelial and connective tissues, a study of the skin at this time provides one with an opportunity to review experiences of the last two laboratory periods. During this laboratory period prepared slides of the skin will be available for study. Prior to examining the slides, however, figure 9.1 should be labeled from the descriptive text that follows. Note that the skin consists of an outer multilayered **epidermis** and a deeper **dermis.**

The Epidermis

The enlarged section of skin on the right side of figure 9.1 is the *epidermis.* Note that it consists of four distinct layers: an outer **stratum corneum,** a thin translucent **stratum lucidum,** a darkly stained **stratum granulosum,** and a multilayered **stratum spinosum** (mucosum).

All four layers of the epidermis originate from the deepest layer of cells of the stratum spinosum. This deep layer, which lies adjacent to the dermis, is called the **stratum germinativum** or *stratum basale.* The columnar cells of this deep layer are constantly dividing to produce new cells that move outward to undergo metamorphosis at different levels. The brown skin pigment, *melanin,* which is produced by stellate *melanocytes* of the stratum germinativum, is responsible for skin color. Skin color differences are due to the amount of melanin present.

The stratum corneum of the epidermis consists of many layers of the scaly remains of dead epithelial cells. This protein residue of dead cells is primarily *keratin,* a water-repellent material. As the cells of the stratum spinosum are pushed outward, they move away from the nourishment of the capillaries, die, and undergo *keratinization.* The *eleidin* granules of the stratum granulosum are believed to be an intermediate product of keratinization. The translucent stratum lucidum consists of closely packed cells with traces of flattened nuclei.

The Dermis

This layer is often referred to as the "true skin." It varies in thickness of less than a millimeter to over six millimeters. It is highly vascular and provides most of the nourishment for the epidermis. It consists of two strata, the papillary and reticular layers.

The outer portion of the dermis, which lies next to the epidermis, is the **papillary layer.** It derives its name from numerous projections, or **papillae,** which extend into the upper layers of the epidermis. In most regions of the body these papillae form no pattern; however, on the fingertips, palms, and soles of the feet they form regularly arranged patterns of parallel ridges that improve frictional characteristics in these areas.

The deeper portion, or **reticular layer,** contains more collagenous fibers than the papillary layer. These fibers greatly enhance the strength of the skin. The surface texture of suede leather is, essentially, the reticular layer of animal hides.

Subcutaneous Tissue

Beneath the dermis lies the subcutaneous tissue, or **hypodermis;** it is also referred to as the *superficial fascia.* It consists of loose connective tissue, nerves, and blood vessels. One of its prime functions is to provide attachment for the skin to underlying structures.

Hair Structure

Hair (*pili*) consists of keratinized cells that are compactly cemented together. Each shaft of hair (label 1) is surrounded by a tube of epithelial cells, the **hair follicle.** The terminal end of the hair shaft, or **root,** is enlarged to form an onion-shaped region called the **bulb.** Within the bulb is an involution of loose connective tissue called the **hair papilla.** It is through the latter structure that nourishment enters

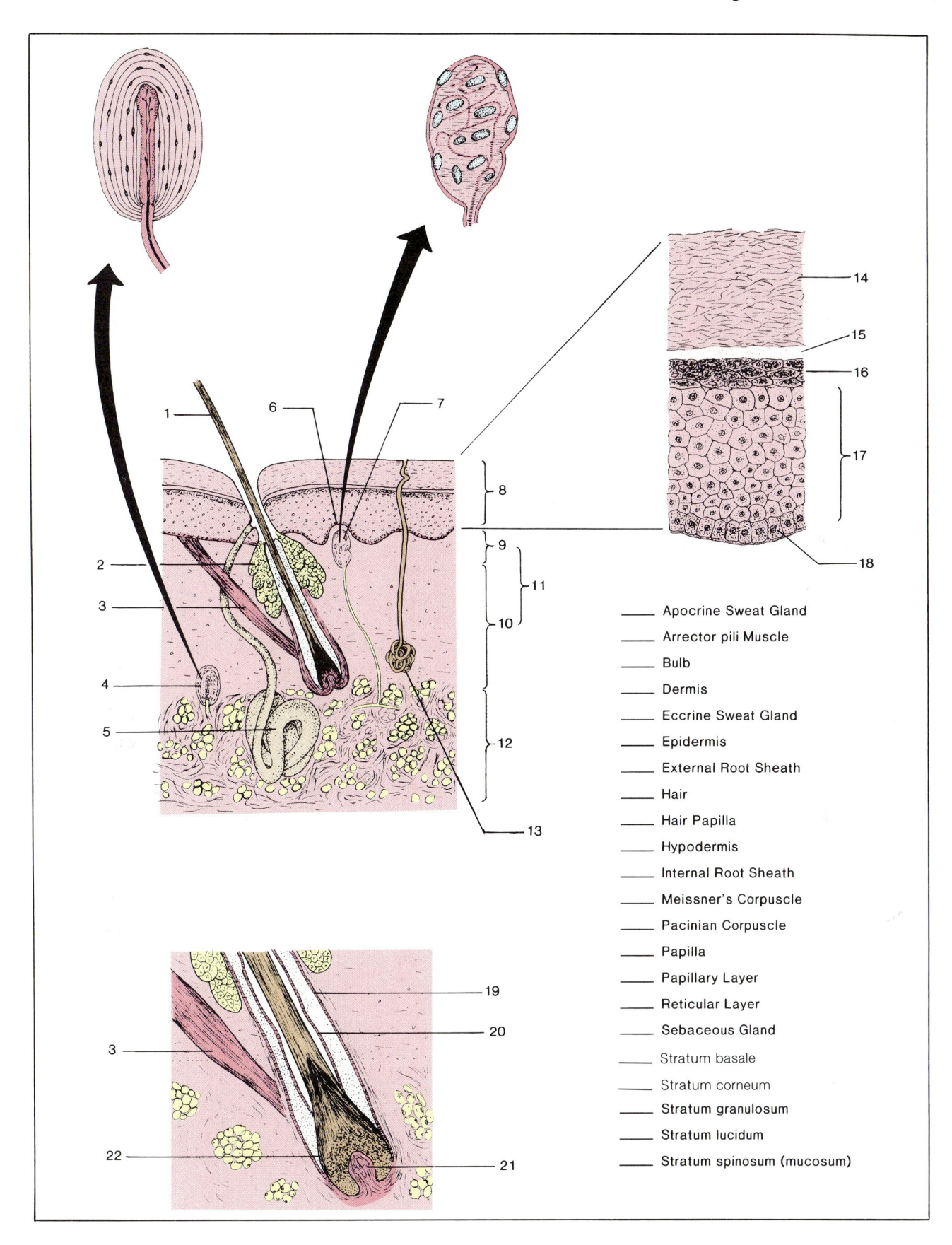

Figure 9.1 Skin structure.

_____ Apocrine Sweat Gland
_____ Arrector pili Muscle
_____ Bulb
_____ Dermis
_____ Eccrine Sweat Gland
_____ Epidermis
_____ External Root Sheath
_____ Hair
_____ Hair Papilla
_____ Hypodermis
_____ Internal Root Sheath
_____ Meissner's Corpuscle
_____ Pacinian Corpuscle
_____ Papilla
_____ Papillary Layer
_____ Reticular Layer
_____ Sebaceous Gland
_____ Stratum basale
_____ Stratum corneum
_____ Stratum granulosum
_____ Stratum lucidum
_____ Stratum spinosum (mucosum)

the shaft. The root of the hair is encased in an **internal root sheath** and an **external root sheath.**

Extending diagonally from the wall of the hair follicle to the epidermis is a band of smooth muscle fibers, the **arrector pili muscle.** Contraction of these muscle fibers causes the hair to move to a more perpendicular position, causing elevations on the skin surface commonly referred to as "goose pimples."

Glands

Two kinds of glands are present in the skin: sebaceous and sweat.

Sebaceous Glands

These glands are located within the epithelial tissue that surrounds each hair follicle. An oily secretion, called *sebum,* is secreted by these glands into the hair follicles and out onto the skin surface. Secretion is facilitated to some extent by the force of the arrector pili muscles during contraction. Sebum keeps hair pliable and helps to waterproof the skin.

Sweat Glands

Sweat glands are of two types: eccrine and apocrine. The small sweat glands that empty directly out through the surface of the skin are **eccrine sweat glands.** These glands are simple tubular structures that have their coiled basal portions located deep in the dermis. Except for the lips, glans penis, and clitoris, they are widely distributed throughout the body.

Although the composition of all eccrine secretions is similar, there are two different controlling stimuli. Almost everyone is aware that the sweat glands of some parts of the body, such as the palms and axillae, are affected by emotional factors. Glands in other regions, however, such as the forehead, neck, and back, are regulated primarily by thermal stimuli.

Apocrine sweat glands are much larger than the eccrine type and have their secretory coiled portions located in the hypodermis. Instead of emptying out onto the surface of the epidermis, all apocrine glands empty directly into a hair follicle canal. These glands are found in the axillae, scrotum of the male, female perigenital region, external ear canal, and nasal passages. While eccrine sweat is watery, the secretion of apocrine glands is a thick white, gray, or yellowish secretion. Malodorous substances in apocrine sweat are the principal contributors to body odors. Psychic factors rather than temperature changes primarily affect apocrine secretions.

Receptors

The receptors shown in figure 9.1 are Meissner's and Pacinian corpuscles. **Meissner's corpuscles** are located in the papillary layer of the dermis, projecting up into papillae of the epidermis. They function as receptors of touch. **Pacinian corpuscles** are spherical receptors with onionlike laminations and lie deep in the reticular layer of the dermis. Pacinian corpuscles are sensitive to variations in sustained pressure.

Laboratory Assignment

After labeling figure 9.1 and answering the questions on the Laboratory Report, proceed as follows:

Materials:

> prepared slide of the skin (H11.11, H11.12, or H11.14)

Examine prepared slides of sections through the skin and identify the structures seen in figures 9.1, HA-9, HA-10, and HA-11. Make drawings, if required.

Part 3 The Skeletal System

Many phases of medical science demand a thorough understanding of the skeletal system. Since most of the muscles of the body are anchored to specific loci on bones, it is imperative that the student of muscular anatomy know the names of many processes, ridges, and grooves on individual bones.

The study of the nervous and circulatory systems also depends to some extent on one's comprehension of the structure of the skeletal system. This is particularly true when studying the passage of nerves and blood vessels through openings in bones of the skull. Each passageway (foramen or meatus) has a name. A complete comprehension of the skeletal system includes a knowledge of the names of all these openings.

X ray technology is an important branch of medical practice that relies heavily on osteology. In dentistry, the structure of the mandible and surrounding facial bones is of particular importance in taking X rays of the teeth. In medicine, all parts of the skeleton must be thoroughly understood.

10 The Skeletal Plan

In this exercise we will study the structure of the skeleton as a whole and the anatomy of a typical long bone. Detailed examination of individual parts will follow in subsequent exercises.

Materials:

fresh beef bones, sawed longitudinally
articulated human skeleton

The adult skeleton is made up of 206 named bones and many smaller unnamed ones. They are classified as being long, short, flat, irregular, or sesamoid. The *long* bones include the bones of the arm, leg, metacarpals, metatarsals, and phalanges. The *short* bones are seen in the wrist and ankle. In addition to being shorter, the short bones differ from the long ones in another respect: they are filled with cancellous bone instead of having a medullary cavity. The *flat* bones are the protective bones of the skull. Those bones that are neither long, short, nor flat are classified as being *irregular*. The vertebrae and bones of the middle ear fall into this category. Round bones embedded in tendons are called *sesamoid* bones (the shape resembles sesame seeds). The kneecap is the most prominent one of this type.

Bone Structure

Bones contain cavities, holes, processes, depressions, and other variations that serve different purposes. Terms that pertain to the several kinds of **depressions** or **cavities** follow:

Foramen: An opening in a bone that provides a passageway for nerves and blood vessels.

Fossa: A shallow depression in a bone. In some instances the fossa is a socket into which another bone fits.

Sulcus: A groove or furrow.

Meatus: A canal or long tubelike passageway.

Fissure: A narrow slit.

Sinus (antrum): A cavity in a bone.

Any prominence on a bone may be referred to as a **process.** They exist in various shapes and sizes. The following are different types of processes:

Condyle: A rounded knucklelike eminence on a bone that articulates with another bone.

Tuberosity: A large roughened process on a bone that serves as a point of anchorage for a muscle.

Tubercle: A small rounded process.

Trochanter: A very large process on a bone.

Head: A portion supported by a constricted part, or *neck.*

Crest: A narrow ridge of bone.

Spine: A sharp slender process.

Figure 10.1 shows a long bone, the *femur,* that has been sectioned to reveal its internal structure. Linearly, it consists of an elongated shaft, the **diaphysis,** and two enlarged ends, the **epiphyses.** Where the epiphyses meet the diaphysis are growth zones called **metaphyses.** During the growing years a plate of hyaline cartilage, the **epiphyseal disk,** exists in this area. As new cartilage forms on the epiphyseal side it is destroyed and then replaced by bone on the diaphyseal side. The metaphysis, thus, consists of the epiphyseal disk, calcified cartilage, and bone during the growing years. At maturity the area becomes completely ossified and linear growth ceases.

Note that the central portion of the diaphysis is a hollow chamber, the **medullary cavity.** The compact bone tissue of the shaft provides ample strength, obviating the need for central bone tissue. This cavity is lined with a membrane called the **endosteum** that is continuous with the canals of the osteons. The entire medullary cavity and much of the cancellous bone of the extremities contain a fatty material, the **yellow marrow.** The cancellous bone of the epiphyses of the humerus and femur contains **red marrow** in the adult. The epiphyses of

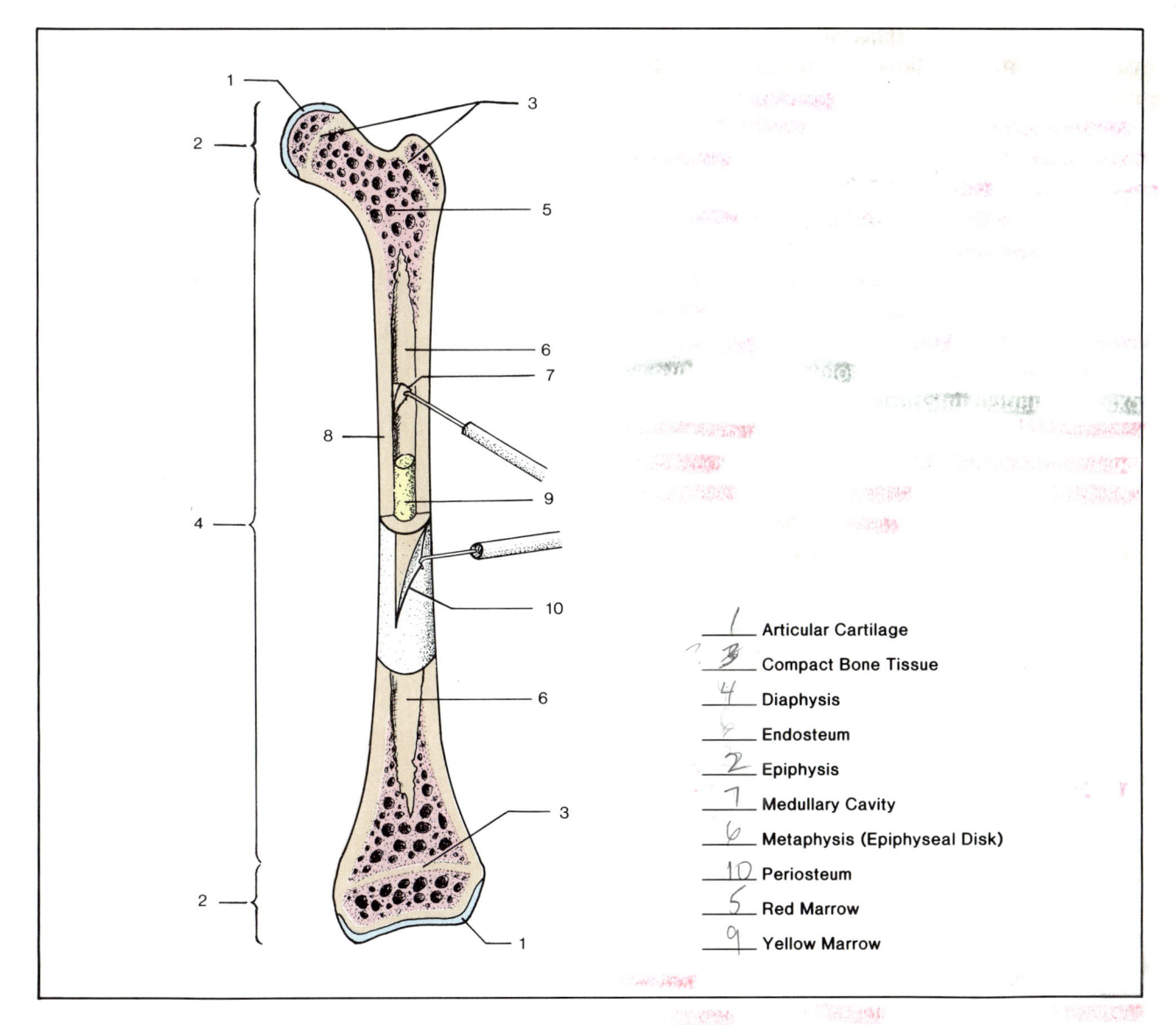

Figure 10.1 Long bone structure.

_1_	Articular Cartilage
_3_	Compact Bone Tissue
_4_	Diaphysis
_8_	Endosteum
_2_	Epiphysis
_7_	Medullary Cavity
_6_	Metaphysis (Epiphyseal Disk)
_10_	Periosteum
_5_	Red Marrow
_9_	Yellow Marrow

other long bones in the adult contain yellow marrow. Most red marrow in adults is found in the ribs, sternum, and vertebrae.

A tough covering, the **periosteum,** envelops the surfaces of the entire bone except for the areas of articulation. This covering consists of fibrous connective tissue that is quite vascular. The surfaces of each epiphysis which contact adjacent bones are covered with smooth **articular cartilage** that is of the hyaline type.

Assignment:

Figure 10.1: Identify the labels in this illustration.

Beef Bone Study: Examine a freshly cut section of bone. Identify all structures shown in figure 10.1. Probe into the periosteum near a torn ligament or tendon; note the continuity of fibers between the periosteum and these structures. Probe into the marrow and note its texture.

Bone Names

The bones of the skeleton fall into two main groups: those that make up the axial skeleton and those forming the appendicular skeleton.

Axial Skeleton The parts of the axial skeleton are the **skull, hyoid bone, vertebral column** (spine), and **rib cage.** The hyoid bone is a horseshoe-shaped bone that is situated under the lower jaw. The rib cage consists of twelve pairs of **ribs** and a **sternum** (breastbone).

Appendicular Skeleton This portion of the skeleton includes the upper and lower extremities and their girdles. Each **shoulder girdle** consists of a **scapula** (shoulder blade) and **clavicle** (collarbone). Each upper extremity consists of a **humerus** in the arm, two forearm bones, (the **radius** and **ulna**), and the **hand.** The radius is lateral to the ulna when the body is in anatomical position.

The **pelvic girdle** is formed by two bones, the **os coxae,** which are attached to the vertebral column (sacrum) posteriorly, and to each other on their anterior surfaces. The joint where the two os coxae are united anteriorly is the **symphysis pubis.** Each lower extremity consists of a femur, tibia, fibula, patella, and foot. The **femur** is the long bone of the thigh. The **tibia** (shinbone) is the largest bone of the leg. The **fibula** (calfbone) parallels the tibia, lateral to it. The **patella** is the kneecap.

Assignment:

Label the parts of the skeleton in figure 10.2 and identify them on an articulated skeleton.

Bone Fractures

When bones of the body are subjected to excessive stress, various kinds of fractures occur. The type of fracture that results will depend on the nature and direction of forces that are applied. Some of the more common types are illustrated in figure 10.3.

If the fracture is contained in the soft tissues and does not communicate in any way with the skin or mucous membranes, it is considered to be a **closed,** or **simple,** fracture. A majority of the fractures in figure 10.3 would probably fall in this category. If the fracture does communicate with the external surfaces, however, it is called an **open,** or **compound,** fracture. Fractures of this type may become considerably more difficult to treat because bone marrow infections (osteomyelitis) may result.

Fractures may also be complete or incomplete. **Incomplete fractures** are the type in which the bone is split, splintered, or only partially broken. Illustrations A, B, and C in figure 10.3 are of this type. When a bone breaks through on only one side as a result of bending, it is often referred to as a **green-**
stick
fracture.

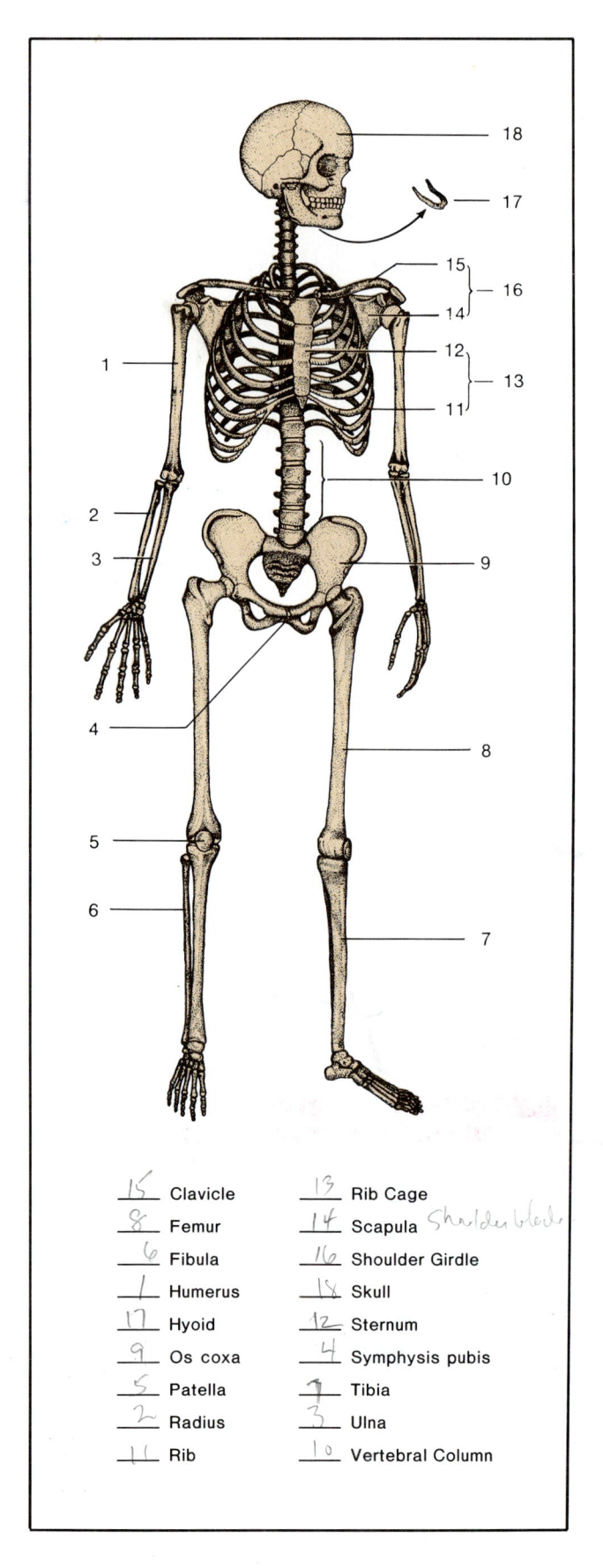

15	Clavicle	13	Rib Cage
8	Femur	14	Scapula Shoulder blade
6	Fibula	16	Shoulder Girdle
1	Humerus	18	Skull
17	Hyoid	12	Sternum
9	Os coxa	4	Symphysis pubis
5	Patella	7	Tibia
2	Radius	3	Ulna
11	Rib	10	Vertebral Column

Figure 10.2 The human skeleton.

stick fracture. These fractures are most common among the young. Linear splitting of a long bone may be referred to as a **fissured** fracture.

Complete fractures are those in which the bone is broken clear through. If the break is at right angles to the long axis, it is considered to be a **transverse** fracture. Breaks that are at an angle to the long axis are termed **oblique** fractures. If a fracture results from torsional forces, it may be referred to as a **spiral** fracture.

If a piece of bone is broken out of the shaft it is a **segmental** fracture. More extensive fractures, in which two or more fragments are seen, are designated as **comminuted** fractures. When bone fragments have been moved out of alignment, as in illustration G, the fracture may also be referred to as being **displaced.**

Severe vertical forces can result in compacted or compression bone fractures. If a broken portion of a bone is driven into another portion of the same bone it is referred to as a **compacted** fracture. This is often seen in femur fractures, such as in illustration J. **Compression** fractures (not shown) often occur in the vertebral column when vertebrae are crushed due to falls from excessive heights.

Assignment:

Identify the types of fractures illustrated in figure 10.3.

Complete the Laboratory Report for this exercise.

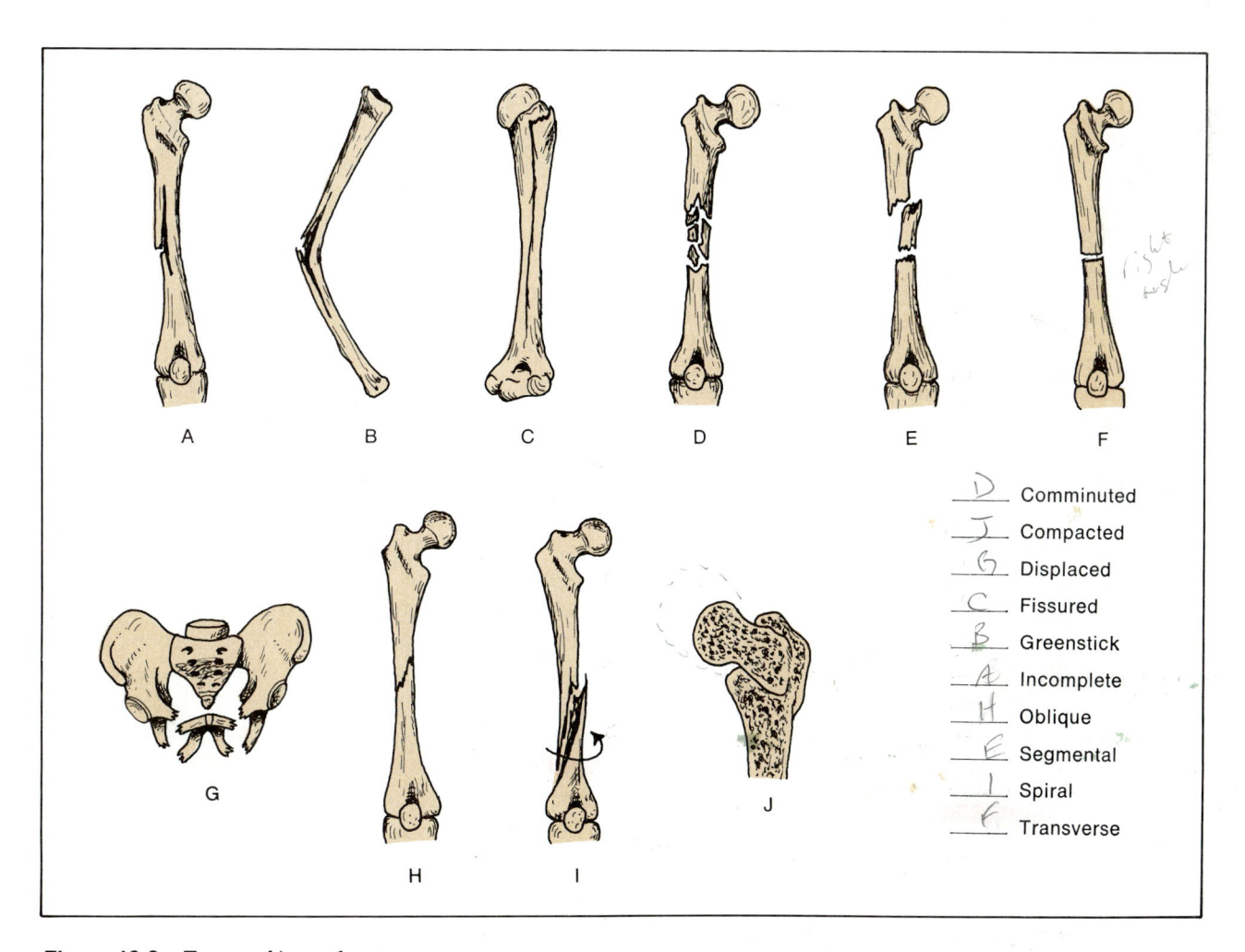

Comminuted   D

Compacted   J

Displaced   G

Fissured   C

Greenstick   B

Incomplete   A

Oblique   H

Segmental   E

Spiral   I

Transverse   F

Figure 10.3   Types of bone fractures.

11 The Skull

For this study of the skull, specimens will be available in the laboratory. As you read through the discussion of the various bones, identify them first in the illustrations and then on the specimens. Compare the specimens with the illustrations to note the degree of variance.

Care of Skulls

When you handle laboratory skulls be very careful to avoid damaging them. **Never use a pencil as a pointer.** Pencil marks must not be made on the bones. A metal probe or a pipe cleaner should be used instead. If a metal probe is used, **touch the bones very gently to avoid bone perforation** where bone is thin.

Materials:

> whole and disarticulated skulls
> fetal skulls
> metal probe or pipe cleaner

The Cranium

The portion of the skull that encases the brain is called the *cranium*. It consists of the following eight bones: a single frontal, two parietals, one occipital, two temporals, one sphenoid, and an ethmoid. All these bones are joined together at their margins by irregular interlocking joints called *sutures*. The lateral and inferior aspects of the cranium are illustrated in figures 11.1 and 11.2. A sagittal section of the cranium is seen in figure 11.6.

Frontal The anterior superior portion of the skull consists of the frontal bone. It forms the eyebrow ridges and the ridge above the nose. The most inferior edge of this bone extends well into the orbit of the eye to form the **orbital plates** of the frontal bone. On the superior ridges of the eye orbits are a pair of foramina, the **supraorbital foramina.** See figure 11.3.

Parietals Directly posterior to the frontal bone on the sides of the skull are the parietal bones. The lateral view of the skull actually shows only the left parietal bone. The right parietal is on the other side of the skull. The right and left parietals meet on the midline of the skull to form the **sagittal suture.** Between the frontal and each parietal bone is another suture, the **coronal suture.** Two semicircular bony ridges that extend from the forehead (frontal bone) and over the parietal bone are the **superior temporal line** and **inferior temporal line.** These ridges form the points of attachment for the longest muscle fibers of the *temporalis* muscle. Reference to figure 19.1 shows the position of this muscle (label 2). It is the upper extremity of this muscle that falls on the superior temporal line.

Temporals On each side of the skull, inferior to the parietal bones, are the temporals. These bones are colored yellow in figure 11.1. Each temporal is joined to its adjacent parietal by the **squamosal suture.** A depression, the **mandibular** (*glenoid*) **fossa,** on this bone provides a recess into which the lower jaw articulates. Pull the jaw away from the skull to note the shape of this fossa. The rounded eminence of the mandible that fits into this fossa is the **mandibular condyle.** Just posterior to the mandibular fossa is the ear canal, or **external acoustic meatus** (*acoustic:* hearing; *meatus:* canal or passage).

The temporal bone has three significant processes: the zygomatic, styloid, and mastoid. The **zygomatic process** is a long slender process that extends forward, anterior to the external acoustic meatus, to form a bridge to the cheekbone of the face. The **styloid process** is a slender spinelike process that extends downward from the bottom of the temporal bone to form a point of attachment for some muscles of the tongue and pharynx. This process is often broken off on laboratory specimens. The **mastoid process** is a rounded eminence on the inferior surface of the temporal just posterior to the styloid process. It provides anchorage for the *sternocleidomastoideus* muscle of the neck. Middle ear infections that spread into the cancellous bone of this process are referred to as *mastoiditis.*

Sphenoid The pink-colored bone seen in the lateral view of the skull, figure 11.1, is the sphenoid bone. Note in the inferior view, figure 11.2, that this bone extends from one side of the skull to the other. Identify the two greater wings, the orbital surfaces and the pterygoid processes of the sphenoid. Those parts that are on the sides of the skull in the "temple" region are the **greater wings of the sphenoid.** On the ventral surface (figure 11.2) are the **pterygoid processes of the sphenoid** to which the pterygoid muscles are attached. The **orbital surfaces of the sphenoid** (figure 11.3) make up the posterior walls of each eye orbit.

Ethmoid On the medial surface of each orbit of the eye is seen the ethmoid bone (label 6, figure 11.1). This bone forms a part of the roof of the nasal cavity and closes the anterior portion of the cranium.

Examine the upper portion of the nasal cavity of your skull. Note that the inferior portion of the ethmoid has a downward extending **perpendicular plate** on the median line. Refer to figure 11.6 (label 4). This portion articulates anteriorly with the nasal and frontal bones. Posteriorly, it articulates with the sphenoid and vomer. On each side of the perpendicular plate are irregular curved plates, the **superior** and **middle nasal conchae.** They provide bony reinforcement for the fleshy upper nasal conchae of the nasal cavity.

Occipital The posterior inferior portion of the skull consists primarily of the occipital bone. It is joined to the parietal bones by the **lambdoidal suture.** Examine the inferior surface of your laboratory skull and compare it with figure 11.2. Note the large **foramen magnum** that surrounds the brain stem in real life. On each side of this opening is seen a pair of **occipital condyles** (label 25). These two condyles rest on fossae of the *atlas,* the first vertebra of the spinal column.

Near the base of each occipital condyle are two passageways, the condyloid and hypoglossal canals. The opening to the **condyloid canal** is posterior to the occipital condyle. The **hypoglossal canal** is seen with a piece of wire passing through it. The hypoglossal canal provides a passageway for the hypoglossal (twelfth) cranial nerve.

Three prominent ridges form a distinctive pattern posterior to the foramen magnum on the oc-

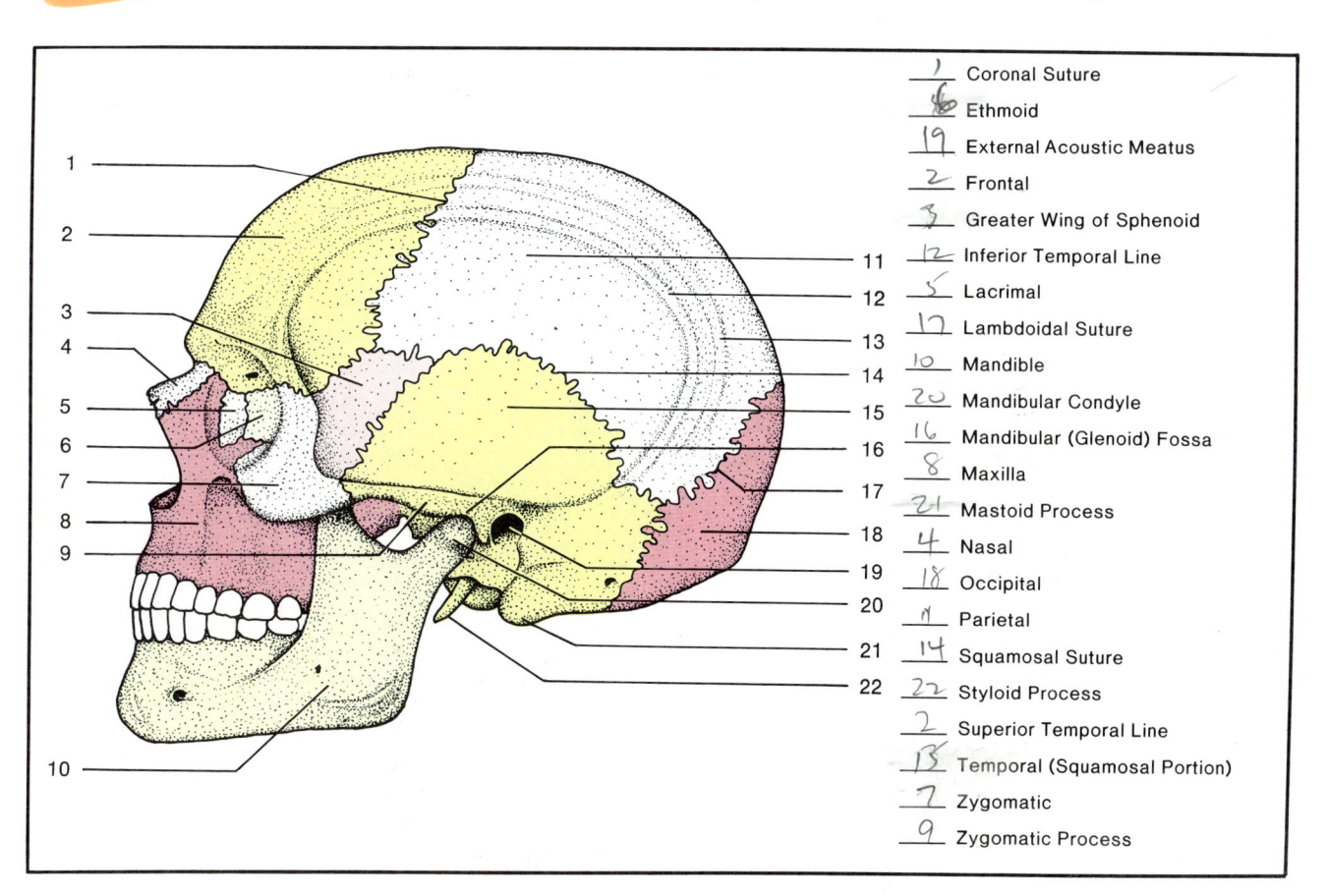

1	Coronal Suture
6	Ethmoid
19	External Acoustic Meatus
2	Frontal
3	Greater Wing of Sphenoid
12	Inferior Temporal Line
5	Lacrimal
17	Lambdoidal Suture
10	Mandible
20	Mandibular Condyle
16	Mandibular (Glenoid) Fossa
8	Maxilla
21	Mastoid Process
4	Nasal
18	Occipital
11	Parietal
14	Squamosal Suture
22	Styloid Process
2	Superior Temporal Line
13	Temporal (Squamosal Portion)
7	Zygomatic
9	Zygomatic Process

Figure 11.1 Lateral view of skull.

53

cipital bone. The **median nuchal line** is a ridge that extends posteriorly from the foramen magnum. It provides a point of attachment for the *ligamentum nuchae*. The **inferior** and **superior nuchal lines** lie parallel to each other. The inferior one lies between the foramen magnum and the superior nuchal line. These ridges form points of attachment for various neck muscles. Note that where the superior nuchal and median nuchal lines meet is a distinct prominence, the **external occipital protruberance.**

Foramina on Inferior Surface

Examine the inferior surface of your laboratory skull and compare it to figure 11.2 to identify the following foramina. The significance of these openings will become more apparent when the circulatory and nervous systems are studied.

Two foramina, the foramen ovale and foramen spinosum, are seen on each half of the sphenoid bone. The **foramen ovale** (label 6) is a large elliptical foramen that provides a passageway for the mandibular branch of the trigeminal nerve. Slightly posterior and lateral to it is a smaller **foramen spinosum,** which allows a small branch of the mandibular nerve and middle meningeal blood vessels to pass through the skull.

The temporal bone has five openings on its inferior surface. The **foramen lacerum** (label 21) is characterized by having a jagged margin. If a piece of wire (bent paper clip) is carefully inserted into the foramen lacerum as shown in figure 11.2, a passageway, the **carotid canal,** can be observed. It is through this canal that the internal carotid artery supplies the brain with blood. Just posterior to the carotid canal opening is an irregular slitlike opening, the **jugular foramen,** which allows drainage of blood from the cranial cavity, via the inferior petrosal sinus. A depression, the **jugular fossa** (label 10), is adjacent to it. The **stylomastoid foramen** is a small opening at the base of the styloid process. The **mastoid foramen** is the most posterior foramen on the temporal bone. This foramen is sometimes absent.

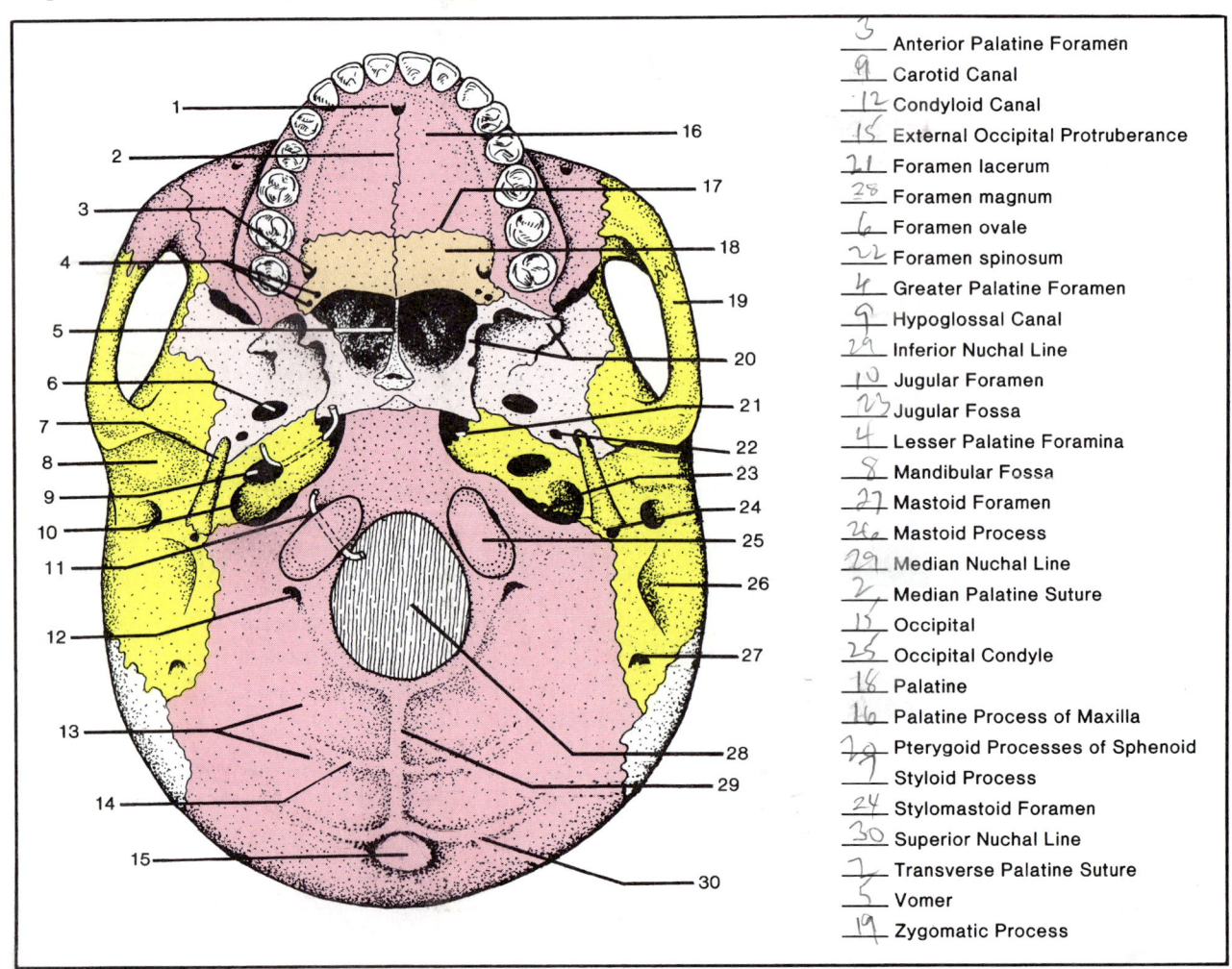

3	Anterior Palatine Foramen
9	Carotid Canal
12	Condyloid Canal
15	External Occipital Protruberance
21	Foramen lacerum
28	Foramen magnum
6	Foramen ovale
22	Foramen spinosum
4	Greater Palatine Foramen
9	Hypoglossal Canal
29	Inferior Nuchal Line
10	Jugular Foramen
23	Jugular Fossa
4	Lesser Palatine Foramina
8	Mandibular Fossa
27	Mastoid Foramen
26	Mastoid Process
29	Median Nuchal Line
2	Median Palatine Suture
13	Occipital
25	Occipital Condyle
16	Palatine
16	Palatine Process of Maxilla
19	Pterygoid Processes of Sphenoid
7	Styloid Process
24	Stylomastoid Foramen
30	Superior Nuchal Line
7	Transverse Palatine Suture
5	Vomer
19	Zygomatic Process

Figure 11.2 Inferior surface of skull.

Assignment:

Label all bones of the cranium in figure 11.1. Facial bones will be labeled later.

Except for the hard palate and vomer, label all structures in figure 11.2. Labeling of other structures will be completed later.

The Face

The face of the skull consists of thirteen bones fused together, plus a movable mandible. Of the thirteen fused bones, only one is not paired: the vomer. Figure 11.3 reveals a majority of the facial bones.

Maxillae The upper jaw consists of two maxillary bones (*maxillae*) that are joined by a suture on the median line. Remove the mandible from your laboratory skull and examine the hard palate. Compare it with figure 11.2. Note that the anterior portion of the hard palate consists of two **palatine processes of the maxillae. A median palatine suture** joins the two bones on the median line.

The maxillae of an adult support sixteen permanent teeth. Each tooth is contained in a socket, or *alveolus*. That portion of the maxillae that contains the teeth is called the *alveolar process*.

Three significant foramina are seen on the maxillae: two infraorbital and one anterior palatine. The **infraorbital foramina** are situated on the front of the face under each eye orbit. Nerves and blood vessels emerge from each of these foramina to supply the nose. The **anterior palatine** (incisive) **foramen** is seen in the anterior region of the hard palate just posterior to the central incisors.

Palatines In addition to the horizontal palatine processes of the maxillae, the hard palate also consists of two palatine bones. These bones form the posterior third of the palate. Locate them on your laboratory specimen. Note that each palatine bone has a large **greater palatine foramen** and two smaller **lesser palatine foramina.**

Assignment:

Label the parts of the hard palate in figure 11.2.

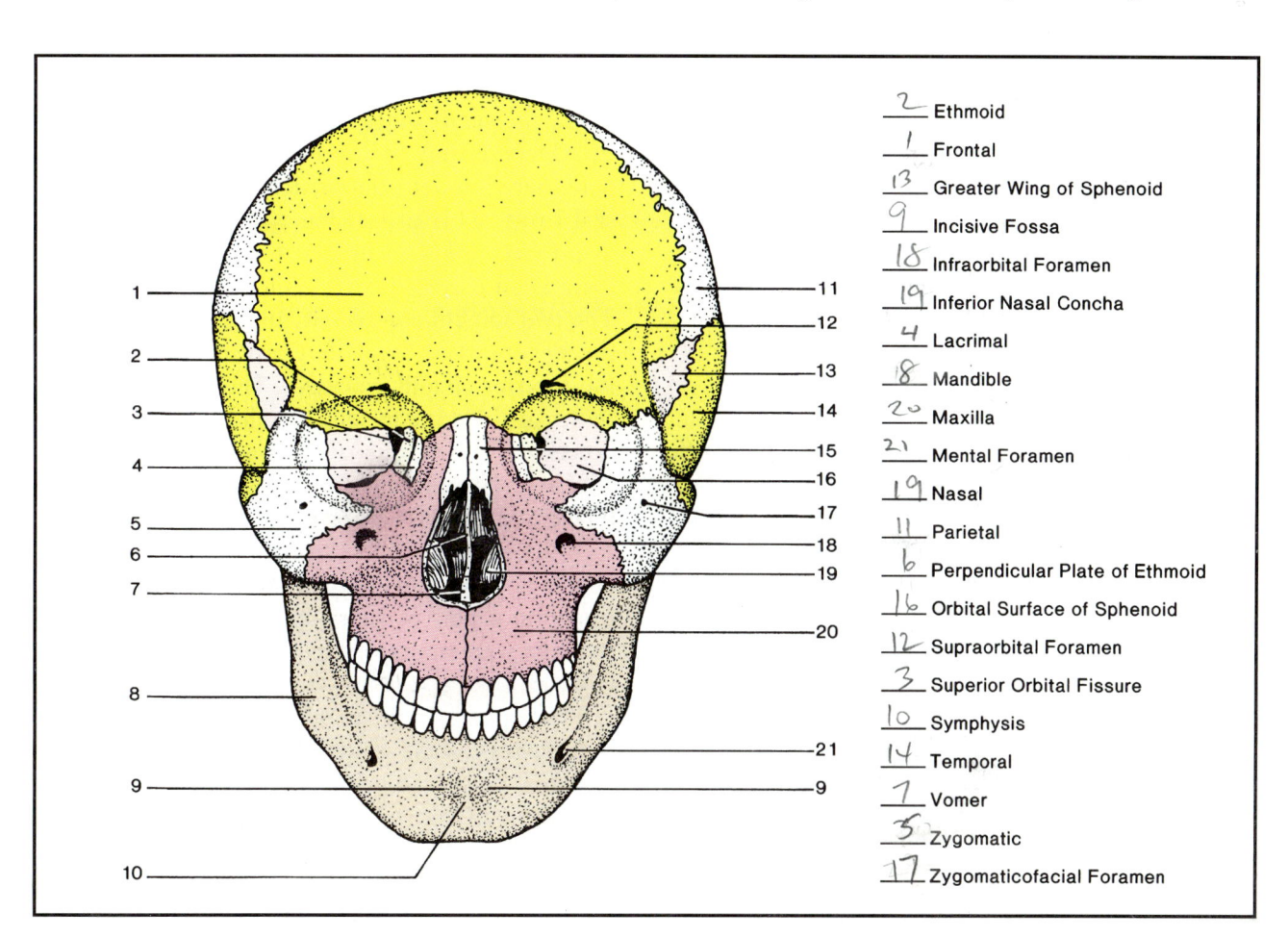

2	Ethmoid
1	Frontal
13	Greater Wing of Sphenoid
9	Incisive Fossa
18	Infraorbital Foramen
19	Inferior Nasal Concha
4	Lacrimal
8	Mandible
20	Maxilla
21	Mental Foramen
19	Nasal
11	Parietal
6	Perpendicular Plate of Ethmoid
16	Orbital Surface of Sphenoid
12	Supraorbital Foramen
3	Superior Orbital Fissure
10	Symphysis
14	Temporal
7	Vomer
5	Zygomatic
17	Zygomaticofacial Foramen

Figure 11.3   Anterior aspect of skull.

Zygomatics On each side of the face are two zygomatic (*malar*) bones. They form the prominence of each cheek and the inferior, lateral surface of each eye orbit. Each zygomatic has a small foramen, the **zygomaticofacial foramen.**

Lacrimals Between the ethmoid and upper portion of the maxillary bones are a pair of lacrimal (*lacrima:* tear) bones—one in each orbit. Locate a groove on the surface of each lacrimal bone that is continuous with a groove on the maxilla. This groove provides a recess for the *lacrimal duct* through which tears flow from the eye into the nasal cavity.

Nasals The bridge of the nose is formed by a pair of thin, rectangular nasal bones.

Vomer This thin bone is located in the nasal cavity on the median line. Its posterior upper edge articulates with the back portion of the perpendicular plate of the ethmoid and the rostrum of the sphenoid. The lower border of the vomer is joined to the maxillae and palatines. The *septal cartilage* of the nose extends between the anterior margin of the vomer and the perpendicular plate of the ethmoid. Locate this bone on figures 11.2, 11.3, and 11.6 as well as on your laboratory specimen.

Inferior Nasal Conchae The inferior nasal conchae are curved bones attached to the walls of the nasal fossa. They are situated beneath the superior and middle nasal conchae which are part of the ethmoid bone.

Assignment:

Label the vomer in figure 11.2.

Except for the parts of the mandible label all structures in figure 11.3 and the remaining facial bones in figure 11.1.

Floor of the Cranium

Now that all bones of the skull have been identified let's examine the inside of the cranium to note the significant structural details. Remove the top of your laboratory skull and compare the floor of the cranium with figure 11.4 to identify the following structures.

Cranial Fossae As you look down on the entire floor of the cranium note that it is divided into three large depressions called *cranial fossae*. The one formed

by the orbital plates of the frontal is called the **anterior cranial fossa.** The large depression made up mostly of the occipital bone is the **posterior cranial fossa.** It is the deepest fossa. In between these two fossae is the middle cranial fossa which is at an intermediate level. The middle cranial fossa, which is not labeled in figure 14.4, involves the sphenoid and temporal bones.

Ethmoid The ethmoid bone in the anterior cranial fossa is seen as a pale yellow structure between the orbital plates of the frontal bone. Note that it consists of a perforated horizontal portion, the **cribriform plate,** and an upward projecting process, the **crista galli** (cock's comb). The holes in the cribriform plate allow branches of the olfactory nerve to pass from the brain into the nasal cavity. The crista galli serves as an attachment for the *falx cerebri* (label 1, figure 26.1).

Locate the small **foramen cecum** that perforates the frontal bone just anterior to the ethmoid bone. This foramen provides a passageway for a small vein.

Sphenoid Note the batlike configuration of this bone, with the greater wings extending out on each side. The anterior leading edges of the wings are called the **small wings of the sphenoid.**

Observe that on the median line of the sphenoid there is a deep depression called the **hypophyseal fossa.** This depression contains the pituitary gland (*hypophysis*) in real life. Posterior to this fossa is an elevated ridge called the **dorsum sella.** The two spinelike processes anterior and lateral to the hypophyseal fossa that project backward are the **anterior clinoid processes.** The outer spiny processes of the dorsum sella are the **posterior clinoid processes.** The hypophyseal fossa, dorsum sella, and clinoid processes, collectively, make up the **sella turcica,** or *Turkish saddle*.

Just anterior to the sella turcica are a pair of openings called the **optic foramina.** These openings lead into a pair of short **optic canals.** Locate the latter on your laboratory specimen. The optic nerves pass through these canals from the eyes to the brain.

Extending from one optic foramen to the other is a narrow shelf called the **chiasmatic groove.** Locate it on your specimen. It is on this bony ledge that fibers of the right and left optic nerves cross over in the optic chiasma (label 3, figure 26.7).

Lying under each anterior clinoid process of the sphenoid is a **superior orbital fissure** (label 3, figure 11.4). Very little of it is shown in figure 11.4. Locate it on your laboratory specimen. Note that it is also seen in figure 11.3 (label 3). It enables the third, fourth, fifth (ophthalmic division), and sixth cranial nerves to enter the eye orbit from the cranial cavity. Certain blood vessels also pass through it.

Just posterior to the superior orbital fissure is the **foramen rotundum.** It provides a passageway for the maxillary branch of the fifth cranial (trigeminal) nerve. Just posterior and slightly lateral to the foramen rotundum is the large **foramen ovale.** The small foramen posterior and lateral to the foramen ovale is the **foramen spinosum.** The **foramen lacerum** (label 4) is formed between the margins of the sphenoid and temporal bones. Observe the proximity of the **carotid canal** (label 7) to the foramen lacerum.

Temporals The significant parts of the temporal bone to identify in figure 11.4 are the petrous, squamous, and mastoid portions. The **squamous**

portion of the temporal is that thin portion that forms a part of the side of the skull. The **petrous portion** (label 8) is probably the hardest portion of the skull. The medial sloping surface of the petrous portion has an opening to the **internal acoustic meatus.** This canal contains the facial and vestibulocochlear cranial nerves. The latter pass from the inner ear region to the brain. The **mastoid portion,** which contains the **mastoid foramen** and **mastoid process,** is the most posterior portion of the temporal bone.

Occipital Observe that this large bone has a semicircular groove called the **depression of the transverse sinus** (label 28). Blood of the brain collects in a large vessel in this groove. Locate the **jugular foramen** where the internal jugular vein takes its origin. It appears as an irregular slit between the anterolateral margin of the occipital bone and the

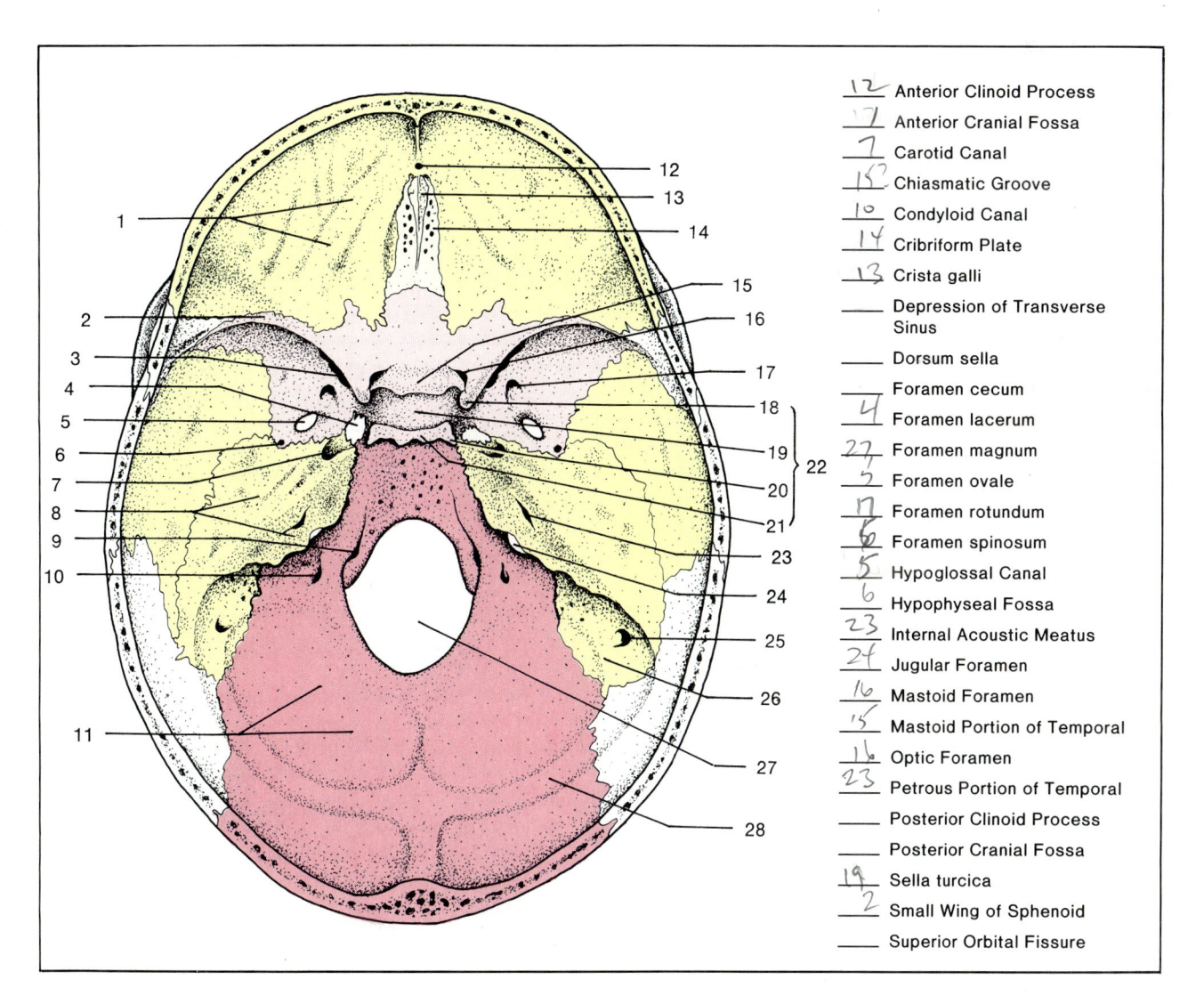

12	Anterior Clinoid Process
1	Anterior Cranial Fossa
7	Carotid Canal
15	Chiasmatic Groove
10	Condyloid Canal
14	Cribriform Plate
13	Crista galli
	Depression of Transverse Sinus
	Dorsum sella
	Foramen cecum
4	Foramen lacerum
27	Foramen magnum
5	Foramen ovale
17	Foramen rotundum
6	Foramen spinosum
5	Hypoglossal Canal
6	Hypophyseal Fossa
23	Internal Acoustic Meatus
24	Jugular Foramen
16	Mastoid Foramen
15	Mastoid Portion of Temporal
16	Optic Foramen
23	Petrous Portion of Temporal
	Posterior Clinoid Process
	Posterior Cranial Fossa
19	Sella turcica
2	Small Wing of Sphenoid
	Superior Orbital Fissure

Figure 11.4 Floor of cranium.

petrous portion of the temporal bone. Cranial nerves nine, ten, and eleven also pass through this foramen.

Identify the openings to the **condyloid** and **hypoglossal canals.** Reference to figure 11.2 establishes that the hypoglossal canal is the one that passes through the base of the occipital condyle. Explore these foramina with a slender probe or pipe cleaner to differentiate them.

Assignment:

Label figure 11.4.

Summary of Foramina of the Skull

Table 11.1 summarizes the more important foramina of the skull discussed in this exercise. Use this table for quick referencing.

The Paranasal Sinuses

Some of the bones of the skull contain cavities, the *paranasal sinuses,* which reduce the weight of the skull without appreciably weakening it. All of the sinuses have passageways leading into the nasal cavity and are lined with a mucous membrane similar to the type that lines the nasal cavities. The paranasal sinuses are named after the bones in which they are situated. Figure 11.5 shows the lo-

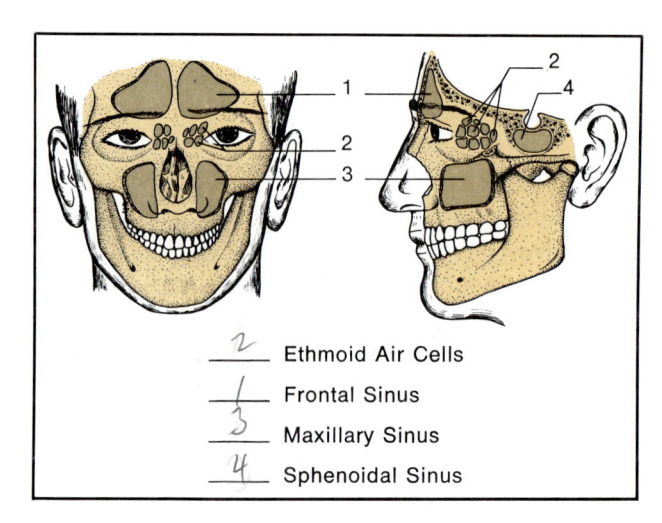

2	Ethmoid Air Cells
1	Frontal Sinus
3	Maxillary Sinus
4	Sphenoidal Sinus

Figure 11.5 The paranasal sinuses.

cation of these cavities. Above the eyes in the forehead are the **frontal sinuses.** The largest sinuses are the **maxillary sinuses,** which are situated in the maxillary bones. These sinuses are also called the *antrums of Highmore.* The **sphenoidal sinus** is the most posterior sinus seen in figure 11.5. Between the frontal and sphenoidal sinuses are a group of small spaces called the **ethmoid air cells.**

Assignment:

Label figure 11.5.

Answer the questions on the Laboratory Report that pertain to the bones of the face.

Table 11.1 Location and contents of skull foramina

Foramen	Location	Passageway for:
Anterior Palatine	maxillae	nasopalatine nerves descending palatine vessels
Carotid Canal	temporal bone	internal carotid artery
Foramen Lacerum	between sphenoid and temporal bones	internal carotid artery and plexus of sympathetic nerves
Foramen Magnum	occipital bone	brain stem
Foramen Ovale	sphenoid bone	mandibular nerve and accessory meningeal artery
Foramen Spinosum	sphenoid bone	branch of mandibular nerve
Greater Palatine	palatine bone	anterior palatine nerve and descending palatine vessels
Hypoglossal Canal	occipital bone	12th cranial nerve (hypoglossal)
Jugular	between temporal and occipital bones	inferior petrosal sinus, vagus n., glossopharyngeal n., accessory n., etc.
Mandibular	mandible	inferior alveolar nerve (branch of 5th cranial n.) and blood vessels
Mental	mandible	mental nerve and blood vessels

Sagittal Section

Visualization of the sinuses and many other structures in the center of the skull is greatly facilitated if a sagittal section of the skull is available for study. Figure 11.6 is of such a section. Note, first of all, how the frontal bone is hollowed out in the forehead region to form the **frontal sinus.** The **sphenoidal sinus** (pink bone) is revealed as a space of considerable size. Immediately above it is a distinct saddlelike structure, the **sella turcica.**

This section also shows best the relationship of the ethmoid to the vomer. The **ethmoid** is the pale yellow bone in the nasal region. The **vomer** is the uncolored bone that is shaped somewhat like a plowshare. Extending upward from the superior margin of the vomer is the **perpendicular plate of the ethmoid.** These two bones, combined, form a bony septum in the nasal cavity. The uppermost projecting structure of the ethmoid is the **crista galli.** The air cells of the ethmoid are not revealed in this section because they are not on the median line.

Note also the relationship of the bones of the palate to the vomer. The anterior portion of the hard palate is the **palatine process of the maxilla.** Posterior to it is the **palatine bone** (orange color). The vomer is fused to these two bones of the hard palate.

Assignment:

Label figure 11.6.

The Mandible

The only bone of the skull that is not fused as an integral part of the skull is the lower jaw, or *mandible.* Figure 11.7 reveals the anatomical details of this bone.

The mandible consists of a horizontal portion, the **body,** and two vertical portions, the **rami.** Embryologically, it forms from two centers of ossification, one on each side of the face. As the bone develops toward the median line, the two halves finally meet and fuse to form a solid ridge. This point of fusion on the midline is called the **symphysis**

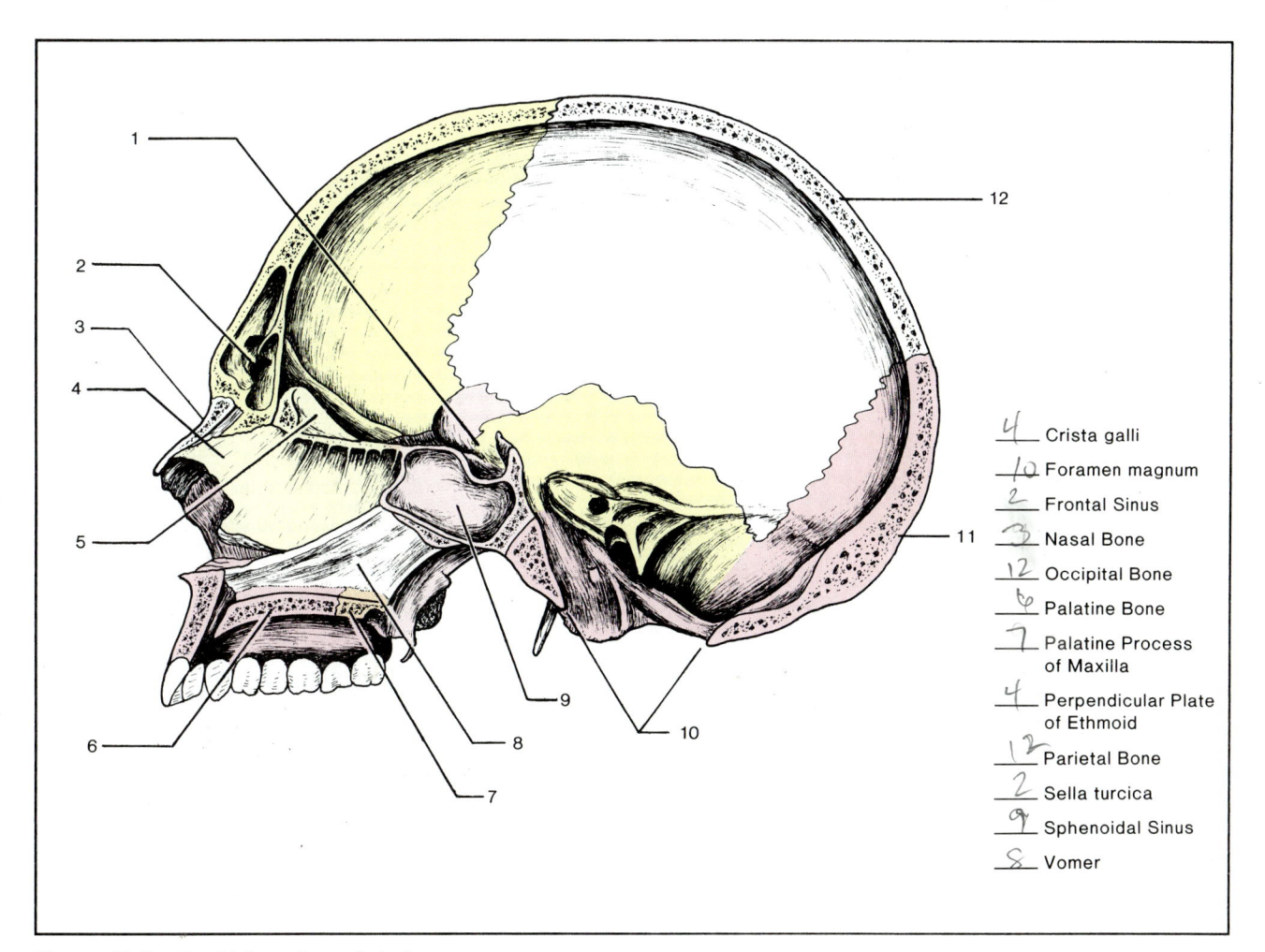

4	Crista galli
10	Foramen magnum
2	Frontal Sinus
3	Nasal Bone
12	Occipital Bone
6	Palatine Bone
7	Palatine Process of Maxilla
4	Perpendicular Plate of Ethmoid
12	Parietal Bone
2	Sella turcica
9	Sphenoidal Sinus
8	Vomer

Figure 11.6   Sagittal section of skull.

(label 10, figure 11.3). On each side of the symphysis are two depressions, the **incisive fossae.**

The superior portion of each ramus has a condyle, a coronoid process, and a notch. The **mandibular condyle** occupies the posterior superior terminus of the ramus. The process on the superior anterior portion of the ramus is the **coronoid process.** This tuberosity provides attachment for the *temporalis* muscle (see illustration A, figure 19.1). Between the mandibular condyle and the coronoid process is the **mandibular notch.** At the posterior inferior corners of the mandible, where the body and rami meet, are two protuberances, the **angles.** The angles provide attachment for the *masseter* and *internal pterygoid* muscles.

A ridge of bone, the **oblique line,** extends at an angle from the ramus down the lateral surface of the body to a point near the mental foramen. This bony elevation is strong and prominent in its upper part, but gradually flattens out and disappears, as a rule, just below the first molar. On the internal (medial) surface of the mandible is another diagonal line, the **mylohyoid line.** It extends from the

ramus down to the body. To this crest is attached a muscle, the *mylohyoid,* which forms the floor of the oral cavity. The bony portion of the body that exists above this line makes up a portion of the sides of the oral cavity proper.

Each tooth lies in a socket of bone called an *alveolus.* As in the case of the maxilla, the portion of this bone that contains the teeth is called the **alveolar process.** The alveolar process consists of two compact tissue bony plates, the *external* and *internal alveolar plates.* These two plates of bone are joined by partitions, or *septae,* which lie between the teeth and make up the transverse walls of the alveoli.

On the medial surfaces of the rami are two foramina, the **mandibular foramina.** On the external surface of the body are two prominent openings, the **mental foramina** (*mental:* chin).

Assignment:

Label figure 11.7 and all the parts of the mandible in figure 11.3.

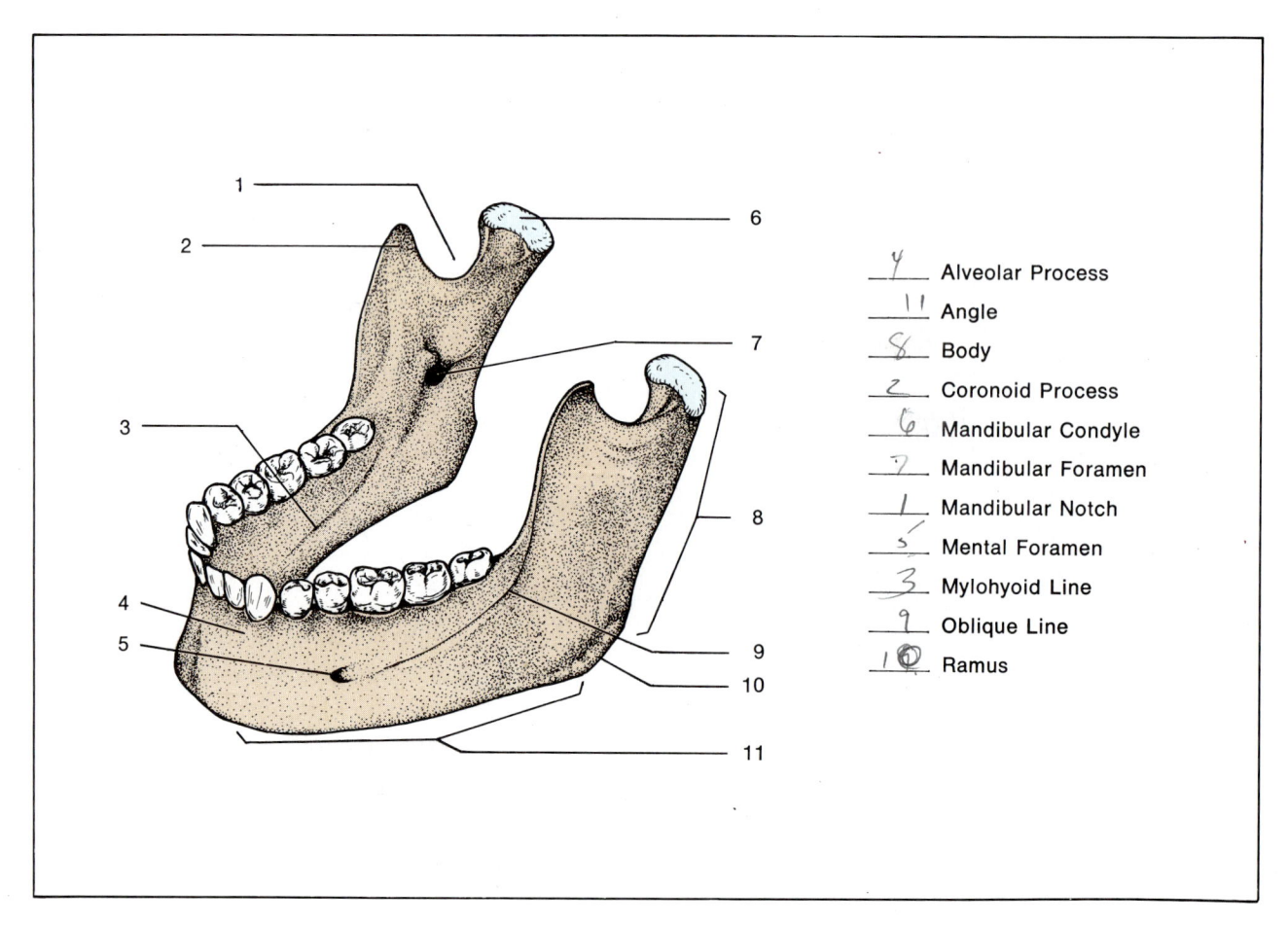

_4_	Alveolar Process
_11_	Angle
_8_	Body
_2_	Coronoid Process
_6_	Mandibular Condyle
_7_	Mandibular Foramen
_1_	Mandibular Notch
_5_	Mental Foramen
_3_	Mylohyoid Line
_9_	Oblique Line
_10_	Ramus

Figure 11.7 The mandible.

The Fetal Skull

The human skull at birth is incompletely ossified. Figure 11.8 reveals its structure. These unossified membranous areas, called *fontanels,* facilitate compression of the skull at childbirth. During labor the bones of the skull are able to lap over each other as the infant passes down the birth canal without causing injury to the brain.

There are six fontanels joined by five areas where future sutures of the skull form. The largest fontanel is the **anterior fontanel,** a somewhat diamond-shaped membrane that lies on the median line at the junction of the frontal and parietal bones. The **posterior fontanel** is somewhat smaller and lies on the median line at the junction of the parietal and occipital bones. Between these two fontanels on the median line is a membranous area where the **future sagittal suture** of the skull will form.

On each side of the skull, where the frontal, parietal, sphenoid, and temporal bones come together behind the eye orbit, is an **anterolateral fontanel.** Between the anterior and anterolateral fontanels can be seen a membranous line that is the area where the **future coronal suture** will develop. The most posterior fontanel on the side of the skull is the **posterolateral fontanel** that lies at the junction of the parietal, temporal and occipital bones. Between the anterolateral and posterolateral fontanels is a membranous line that will develop into the **future squamosal suture.** Ossification of these fontanels and membranous future sutures is usually completed in the two-year-old child.

Assignment:

Label figure 11.8.

Examine a fetal skull, identifying all of the structures in figure 11.8.

Complete the Laboratory Report for this exercise.

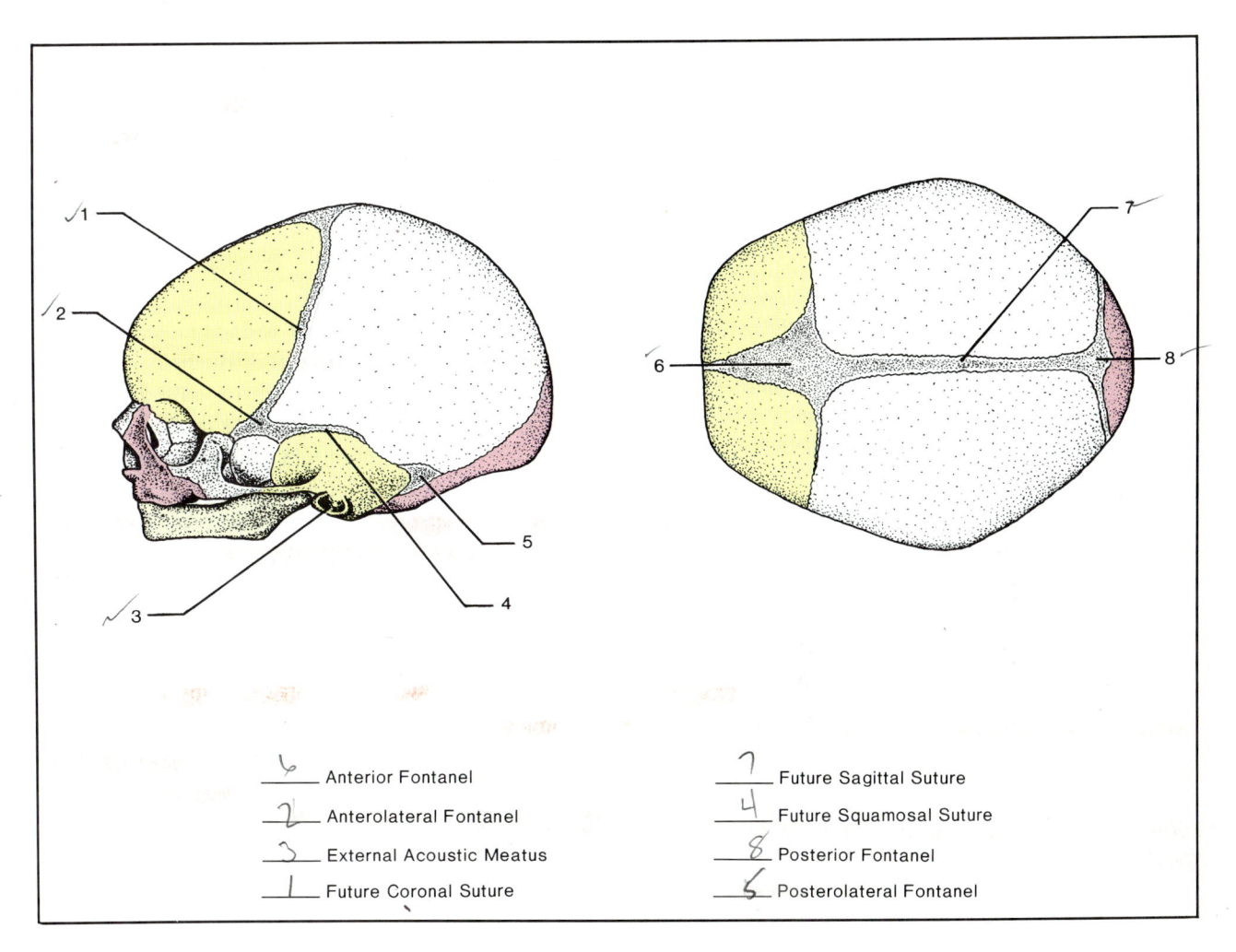

____6____ Anterior Fontanel

____2____ Anterolateral Fontanel

____3____ External Acoustic Meatus

____1____ Future Coronal Suture

____7____ Future Sagittal Suture

____4____ Future Squamosal Suture

____8____ Posterior Fontanel

____5____ Posterolateral Fontanel

Figure 11.8   The fetal skull.

12 The Vertebral Column and Thorax

The skeletal structure of the trunk of the body will be studied in this exercise. The vertebral column, ribs, sternum, and hyoid bone make up this part of the body.

Materials:

skeleton, articulated
skeleton, disarticulated
vertebral column, mounted

The Vertebral Column

The vertebral column consists of thirty-three bones, twenty-four of which are individual movable vertebrae. Figure 12.1 illustrates its structure. Note that the individual vertebrae are numbered from the top.

The Vertebrae

Although the vertebrae in different regions of the vertebral column vary considerably in size and configuration, they do have certain features in common. Each one has a structural mass, the **body,** which is the principal load-bearing contact area between adjacent vertebrae. The space between the surfaces of adjacent vertebral bodies is filled with a fibrocartilaginous **intervertebral disk.** The collective action of these twenty-four disks imparts a vital cushion effect to the spinal column.

In the center of each vertebra is an opening, the **vertebral** or **spinal foramen,** which contains the spinal cord. Projecting out from the posterior surface of each vertebra is a **spinous process.** On each side is a **transverse process.** These processes of the spinal column are joined to each other by ligaments to form a unified flexible structure. Various muscles of the body are anchored to them.

Extending backward from the body of each vertebra are two processes, the **pedicles,** which form a portion of the bony arch around the vertebral foramen. These structures are labeled in illustration C. The opening formed between the pedicles of adjacent vertebrae allows spinal nerves to emerge

from the spinal cord. These openings are the **intervertebral foramina** (label 26) of the vertebral column.

The posterolateral portions of each vertebra consists of two broad plates, the **laminae** (label 7). The two pedicles and two laminae constitute the **neural arch.**

Cervical Vertebrae The upper seven bones are the cervical vertebrae of the neck. The first of these seven is the **atlas.** Illustration A, figure 12.1, reveals the superior surface of this bone. Note that the spinal foramen is much larger here than on the lumbar vertebrae. Its larger size is necessary to accommodate a short portion of the brain stem that extends down into this space. Note that on each side of the spinal foramen is a depression, the **superior articular surface** (facet), which articulates with the skull. Which processes of the skull fit into these depressions?

Within each transverse process is a small **transverse foramen.** These foramina are seen only in the cervical vertebrae. Collectively, they form a passageway on each side of the spinal column for the vertebral artery and vertebral vein.

The second cervical vertebra is called the **axis.** It differs from all other vertebrae in having a vertical protrusion, the **odontoid process** (dens), which provides a pivot for the rotation of the atlas. When the head is turned from side to side, movement occurs between the axis and atlas around this process.

Thoracic Vertebrae Below the seven cervical vertebrae are twelve thoracic vertebrae. Observe that these bones are larger and thicker than the ones in the neck. The superior surface of a typical thoracic vertebra is seen in illustration C. A distinguishing feature of these vertebrae is that all twelve of them have facets on their transverse processes for articulation with ribs.

Lumbar Vertebrae Inferior to the thoracic vertebrae lie five lumbar vertebrae. The bodies of these

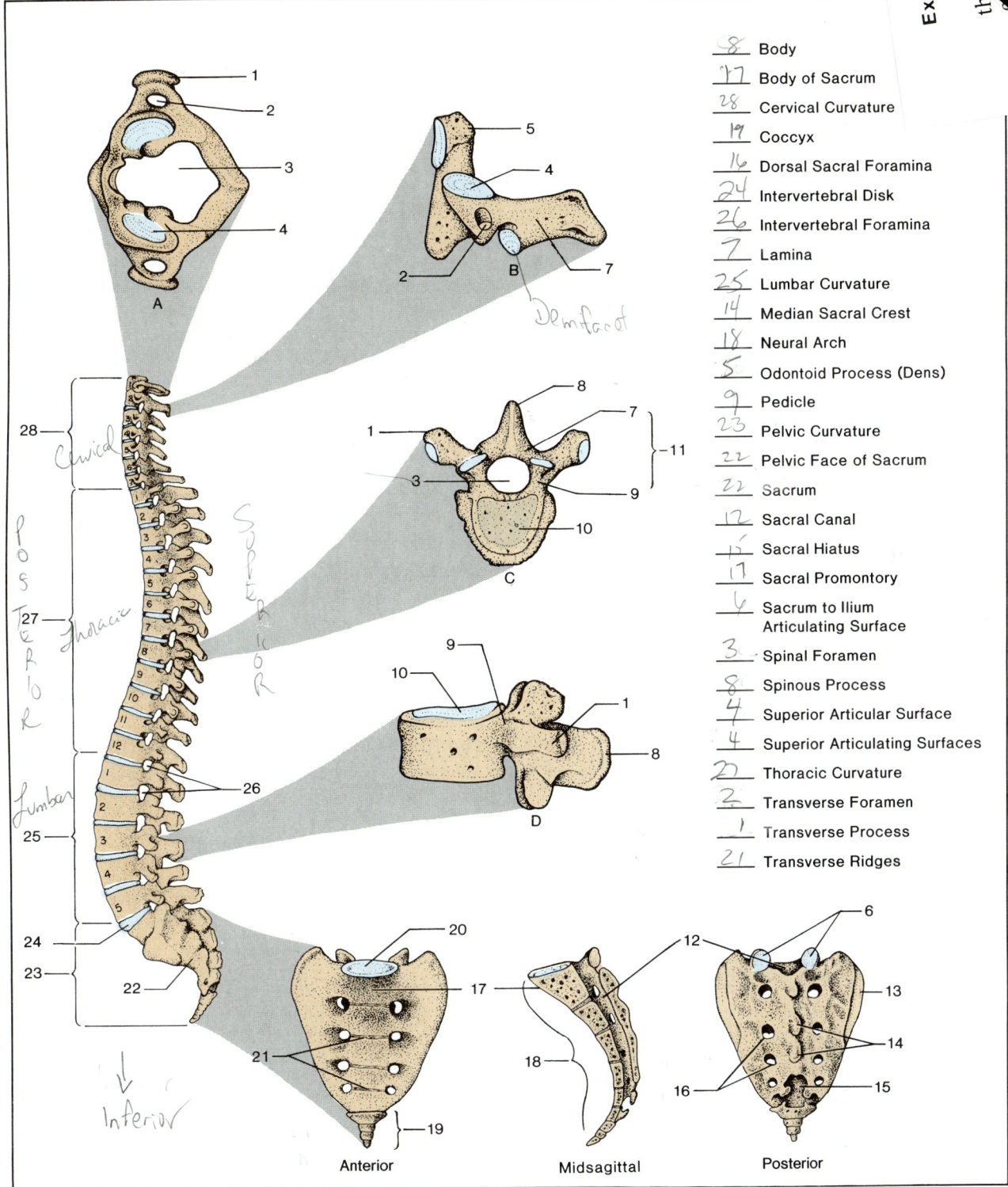

8	Body
17	Body of Sacrum
28	Cervical Curvature
19	Coccyx
16	Dorsal Sacral Foramina
24	Intervertebral Disk
26	Intervertebral Foramina
7	Lamina
25	Lumbar Curvature
14	Median Sacral Crest
18	Neural Arch
5	Odontoid Process (Dens)
9	Pedicle
23	Pelvic Curvature
22	Pelvic Face of Sacrum
22	Sacrum
12	Sacral Canal
15	Sacral Hiatus
17	Sacral Promontory
6	Sacrum to Ilium Articulating Surface
3	Spinal Foramen
8	Spinous Process
4	Superior Articular Surface
4	Superior Articulating Surfaces
20	Thoracic Curvature
2	Transverse Foramen
1	Transverse Process
21	Transverse Ridges

Demifacet

Cervical

POSTERIOR

Thoracic

SUPERIOR

Lumbar

Inferior

Anterior   Midsagittal   Posterior

Figure 12.1   The vertebral column.

bones are much thicker than those of the other vertebrae due to the greater stress that occurs in this region of the vertebral column. **Illustration D** is of a typical lumbar vertebra.

The Sacrum

Inferior to the fifth lumbar vertebra lies the sacrum. It consists of five fused vertebrae. Note that there are two oval **superior articulating surfaces** (facets) provide contact with articulating facets on the fifth lumbar vertebra. On its lateral surfaces are a pair of **sacrum to ilium articulating surfaces.** The intervertebral disk between the fifth lumbar vertebra and the sacrum contacts the flat surface of the **body of the sacrum.**

Note how the anterior aspect, or **pelvic face,** of the sacrum curves backward and that the body of the first sacral vertebra forms a protrusion called the **sacral promontory.** Observe, also, that four **transverse ridges** can be seen on the pelvic face that reveal where the five vertebrae are fused together.

Identify the **median sacral crest** (label 14) and the **dorsal sacral foramina** on the posterior surface. The neural arches of the fused sacral vertebrae form the **sacral canal,** which exits at the lower end as the **sacral hiatus.**

The Coccyx

The "tailbone" of the vertebral column is the coccyx. It consists of four or five rudimentary vertebrae. It is triangular in shape and is attached to the sacrum by ligaments.

Spinal Curvatures

Four curvatures of the vertebral column, together with the intervertebral disks, impart considerable springiness along its vertical axis. Three of them

are identified by the type of vertebrae in each region: the **cervical, thoracic,** and **lumbar curves.** The fourth curvature, which is formed by the sacrum and coccyx, is the **pelvic curve.**

Assignment:

Label figure 12.2.

The Thorax

The sternum, ribs, costal cartilages, and thoracic vertebrae form a cone-shaped enclosure, the *thorax.* Its components are illustrated in figures 12.2 and 12.3.

The Sternum The sternum, or breastbone, consists of three separate bones: the upper **manubrium,** the middle **gladiolus** (body), and the lower **xiphoid** (*ensiform*) **process.** The superior border of the manubrium has a depression called the **jugular** (presternal) **notch.** On its inferior border where the manubrium meets the body, a ridge called the **sternal angle** is formed.

On both sides of the sternum are notches (facets) where the sternal ends of the **costal cartilages** are attached. Note that the second rib fits into a pair of *demifacets* (*demi,* half) at the sternal angle.

The Ribs There are twelve pairs of ribs. The first seven pairs attach directly to the sternum by costal

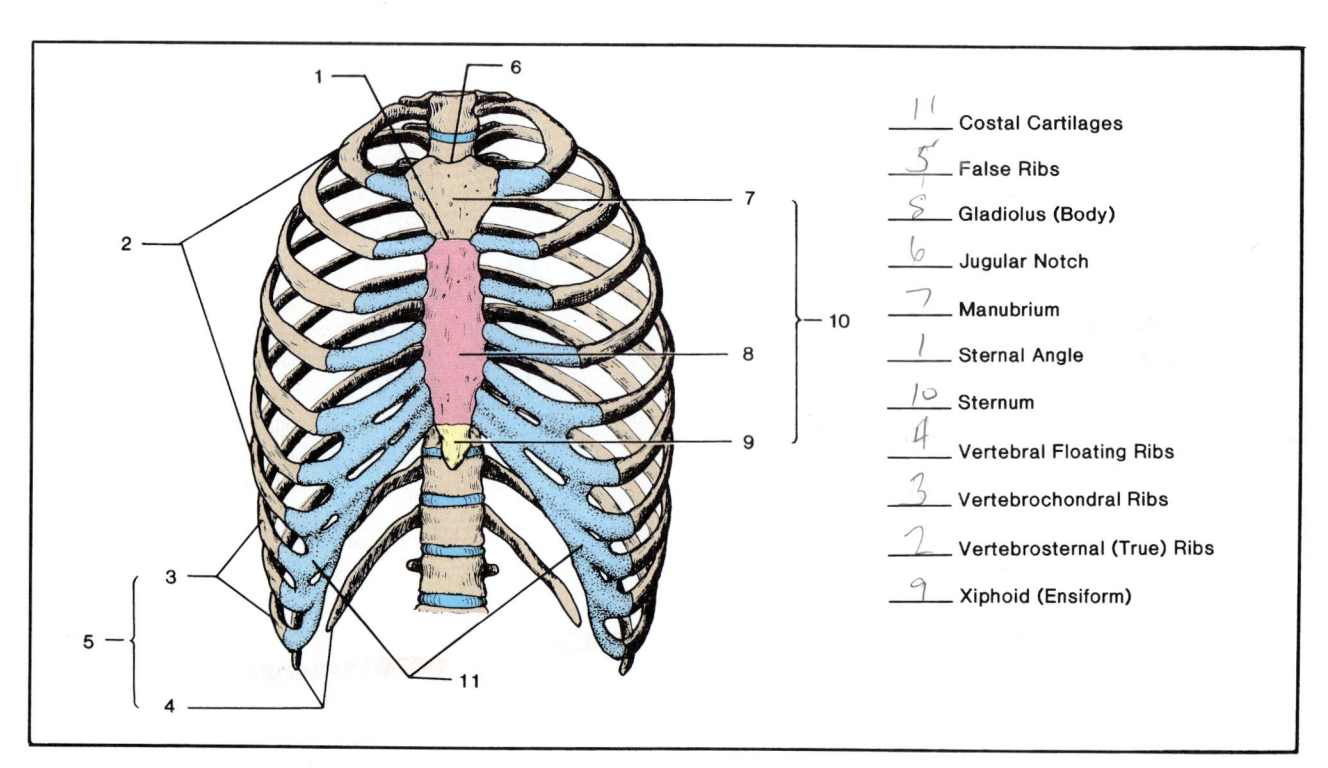

Answer	Label
11	Costal Cartilages
5	False Ribs
8	Gladiolus (Body)
6	Jugular Notch
7	Manubrium
1	Sternal Angle
10	Sternum
4	Vertebral Floating Ribs
3	Vertebrochondral Ribs
2	Vertebrosternal (True) Ribs
9	Xiphoid (Ensiform)

Figure 12.2 The thorax.

cartilages and are called **vertebrosternal** or *true ribs.* The remaining five pairs are called **false ribs.** The upper three pairs of false ribs, the **vertebrochondral ribs,** have cartilaginous attachments on their anterior ends but do not attach directly to the sternum. The lowest false ribs, the **vertebral** or *floating ribs,* are unattached anteriorly.

Figure 12.3 illustrates the structure of a central rib, a lateral view of a thoracic vertebra, and articulation details. Although considerable variability exists in size and configuration of the various ribs, the central rib reveals structures common to most ribs.

The principal parts of each rib are a head, neck, tubercle, and body. The **head** (label 15) is the enlarged end of the rib that articulates with the vertebral column. The **tubercle** (label 17) consists of two portions: an **articular portion** and a **nonarticular portion.** The **neck** is a flattened portion, about 2.5 cm long, between the head and tubercle. The **body** is the flattened curved remainder of the rib.

Note that the head of this rib has two **articular facets** on its medial surface that enable contact with two adjacent vertebrae. Between these two facets is a roughened **interarticular crest** to which ligamentous tissue is anchored. The 1st, 2nd, 10th,

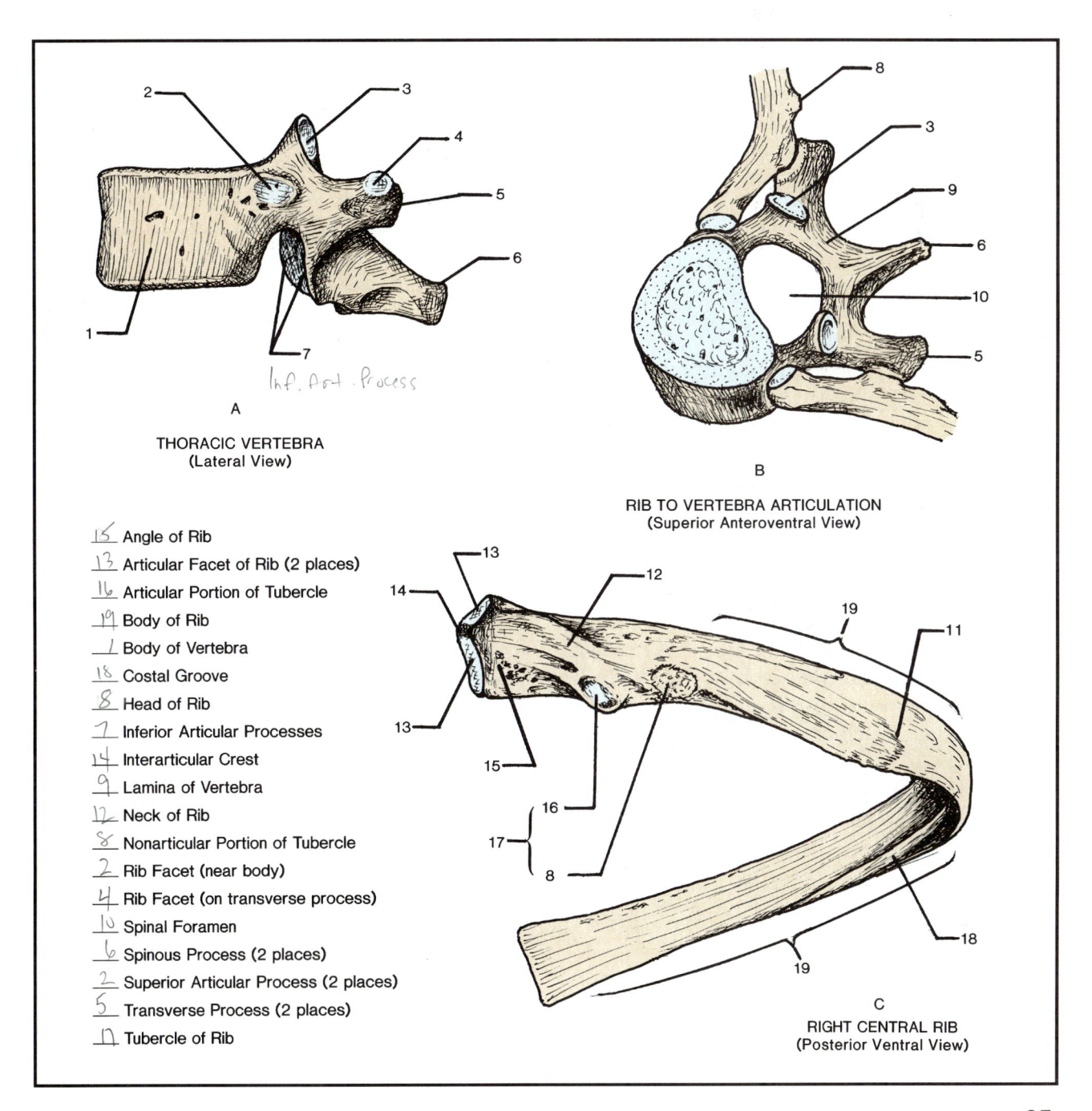

A

THORACIC VERTEBRA
(Lateral View)

Inf. Art. Process

B

RIB TO VERTEBRA ARTICULATION
(Superior Anteroventral View)

C

RIGHT CENTRAL RIB
(Posterior Ventral View)

15 Angle of Rib
13 Articular Facet of Rib (2 places)
16 Articular Portion of Tubercle
19 Body of Rib
1 Body of Vertebra
18 Costal Groove
8 Head of Rib
7 Inferior Articular Processes
14 Interarticular Crest
9 Lamina of Vertebra
12 Neck of Rib
8 Nonarticular Portion of Tubercle
2 Rib Facet (near body)
4 Rib Facet (on transverse process)
10 Spinal Foramen
6 Spinous Process (2 places)
2 Superior Articular Process (2 places)
5 Transverse Process (2 places)
11 Tubercle of Rib

Figure 12.3 Rib anatomy and its articulation.

11th, and 12th ribs have only a single articular facet on their heads.

Articulation of each rib occurs at two points on each vertebra, as shown in illustration B. Note that the articular portion of the tubercle contacts a facet on the transverse process.

The body of this rib has two landmarks: an angle and a costal groove. The **angle** is a ridge on the external surface that provides anchorage for the *iliocostalis* muscle of the back. Note that the portion between the angle and tubercle is rough and irregular; it is on this surface that another back muscle, the *longissimus dorsi,* is attached. Both of these muscles are shown in figure 20.2 (labels 8 and 9). The **costal groove** is a depression on the ventral side of the rib which provides a recess for the intercostal nerve and blood vessels.

In addition to revealing the location of the two rib facets, the lateral view of the thoracic vertebra (illustration A) also reveals the **superior articular process** which contacts the inferior articular process of the vertebra above it. On its underside are seen the two **inferior articular processes.**

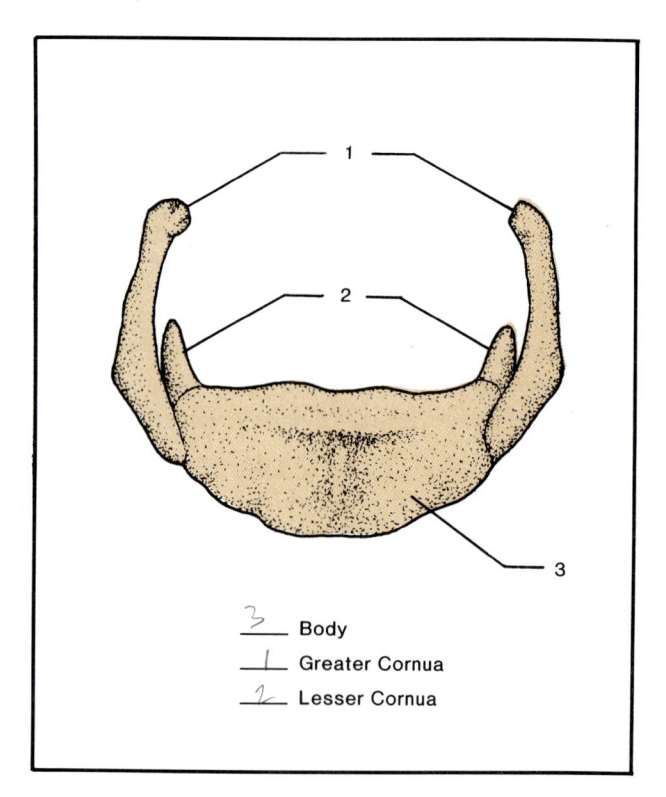

_____ Body
_____ Greater Cornua
_____ Lesser Cornua

Figure 12.4 The hyoid bone.

Assignment:

Label figures 12.2 and 12.3.

The Hyoid Bone

The hyoid bone is a horseshoe-shaped bone located in the neck region between the mandible and larynx. Although it does not articulate directly with any other bone, it is held in place by various ligaments and muscles. Figure 12.4 illustrates its structure.

The bone consists of five segments: a body, two greater cornua, and two lesser cornua. The massive central portion of the bone is the **body.** The two long arms that extend out from each side of the body are the **greater cornua** (*cornu,* singular). Note that the distal end of each greater cornu terminates in a tubercle.

The **lesser cornua** are the conical eminences that are located on the sides of the body superior to the bases of the greater cornua. These structures are separate bone entities that are connected to the body, and occasionally to the greater cornua, by fibrous connective tissue. These joints are usually diarthrotic (freely movable), but occasionally become fused (ankylosed) in later life.

The following muscles have points of attachment on the hyoid bone: *mylohyoideus, sternohyoideus, omohyoideus, thyrohyoideus, digastricus, hyoglossus, genioglossus,* and *constrictor pharyngis medius.*

Assignment:

Label figure 12.4.

Laboratory Report

Complete the Laboratory Report for this exercise.

The Appendicular Skeleton 13

In this exercise a study will be made of the individual parts of the upper and lower extremities.

Materials:

skeleton, articulated
skeleton, disarticulated
male pelvis and female pelvis

The Upper Extremities

Shoulder Girdle Figure 13.2 illustrates the upper arm and its attachment to the trunk. The **clavicle** is a slender S-shaped bone that articulates with the manubrium of the sternum on its medial end. The lateral end of the clavicle articulates with the scapula to form a portion of the shoulder joint. Important muscles of the shoulder attach to this bone.

The **scapula** of the shoulder girdle is a triangular bone that has a socket, the **glenoid cavity,** into which the head of the humerus fits. The scapula is not attached directly to the axial skeleton; rather, it is loosely held in place by muscles providing more mobility to the shoulder. Figure 13.1 illustrates the anatomical details of this bone. Note that on its

posterior surface there is an elongated diagonal ridge called the **scapular spine** (label 4), above which is a depression, the **supraspinatus fossa;** inferior to the spine is another depression, the **infraspinatus fossa.** On the anterior surface of the bone is a large depression called the **subscapular fossa** (label 13). These fossae provide anchorage for many shoulder muscles.

Two prominent processes, the acromion and coracoid, are best seen on the lateral aspect. The **acromion process** (label 10) provides a point of attachment for the clavicle; it lies posterior and superior to the glenoid cavity. The **coracoid process** lies superior and anterior to the same cavity.

The scapula is bounded by three margins. The **vertebral** (medial) **margin** is the convex margin on the left side of the posterior aspect. This border extends from the **superior angle** (label 2) down to the **inferior angle** at the bottom. The **axillary** (lateral) **margin** makes up the border opposite to the vertebral border; it extends from the glenoid cavity down to the inferior angle. The third border is the **superior margin** that extends from the superior angle to a deep depression called the **scapular notch.**

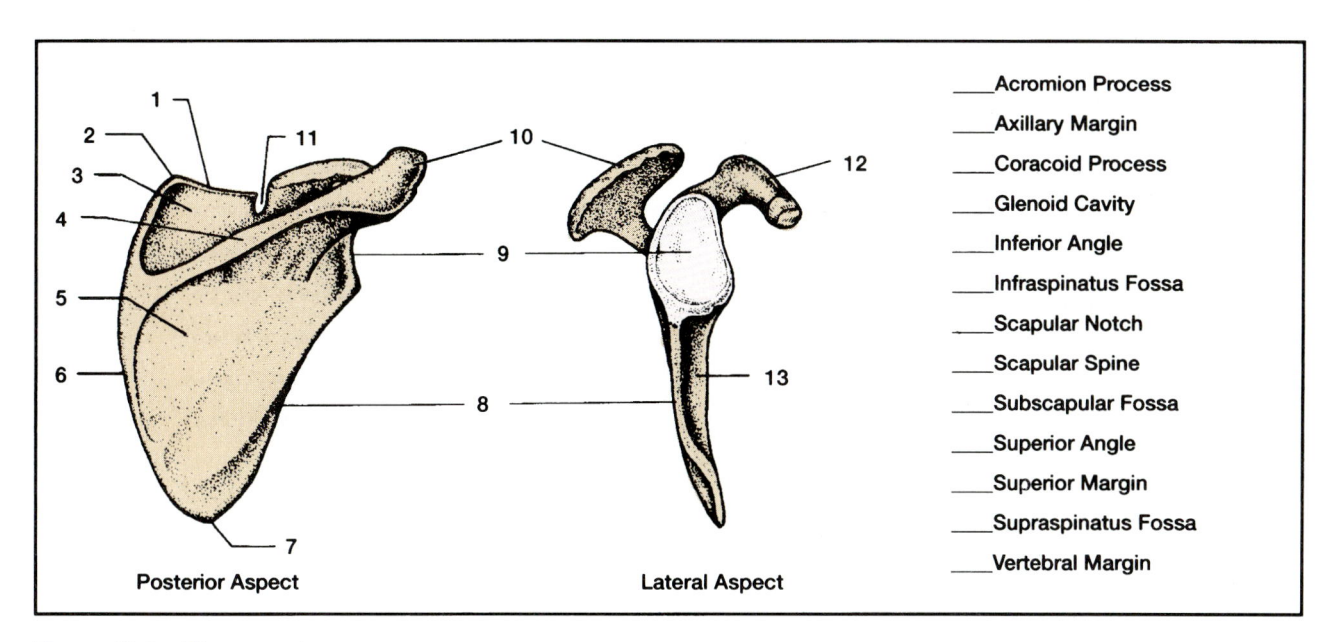

_____Acromion Process
_____Axillary Margin
_____Coracoid Process
_____Glenoid Cavity
_____Inferior Angle
_____Infraspinatus Fossa
_____Scapular Notch
_____Scapular Spine
_____Subscapular Fossa
_____Superior Angle
_____Superior Margin
_____Supraspinatus Fossa
_____Vertebral Margin

Posterior Aspect   Lateral Aspect

Figure 13.1 The scapula.

Assignment:

Label figure 13.1.

Upper Arm The skeletal structure of the upper arm consists of a single bone, the **humerus.** Its smooth rounded upper end, the **head,** fits into the glenoid cavity of the scapula. Just below the head is a narrowing section called the **anatomic neck.**

Inferior to the head and anatomic neck are two eminences, the greater and lesser tubercles. The **greater tubercle** is the larger process that is lateral to the **lesser tubercle.** Between the two tubercles is a depression, the **intertubercular groove.** The narrowing section below the two tubercles is the **surgical neck,** so named because of the frequency of bone fractures in this area.

The surface of the shaft of the humerus has a roughened raised area near its midregion that is the **deltoid tuberosity.** In this same general area is also an opening, the **nutrient foramen.**

The distal terminus of the humerus has two condyles, the capitulum and trochlea, which contact the bones of the forearm. The **capitulum** is the lateral condyle that articulates with the radius. The **trochlea** is the medial condyle that articulates with the ulna. Superior and lateral to the capitulum is

an eminence, the **lateral epicondyle.** On the opposite side (the medial surface) is a larger tuberosity, the **medial epicondyle.** Above the trochlea on the anterior surface is a depression, the **coronoid fossa.** The posterior surface of this end of the humerus has a depression, the **olecranon fossa.**

Assignment:

Label figure 13.2.

Forearm The radius and ulna constitute the skeletal structure of the forearm. Figure 13.3 shows the relationship of these two bones to each other and the hand.

The **radius** is the lateral bone of the forearm. The proximal end of this bone has a disk-shaped **head** which articulates with the capitulum of the humerus. The disklike nature of the head makes it possible for the radius to rotate at the upper end when the palm of the hand is changed from one position to another (pronation-supination, see illustrations H and I, figure 17.1). A few centimeters below the head on the medial surface is an eminence, the **radial tuberosity.** This process is the point of attachment for the *biceps brachii,* a muscle of

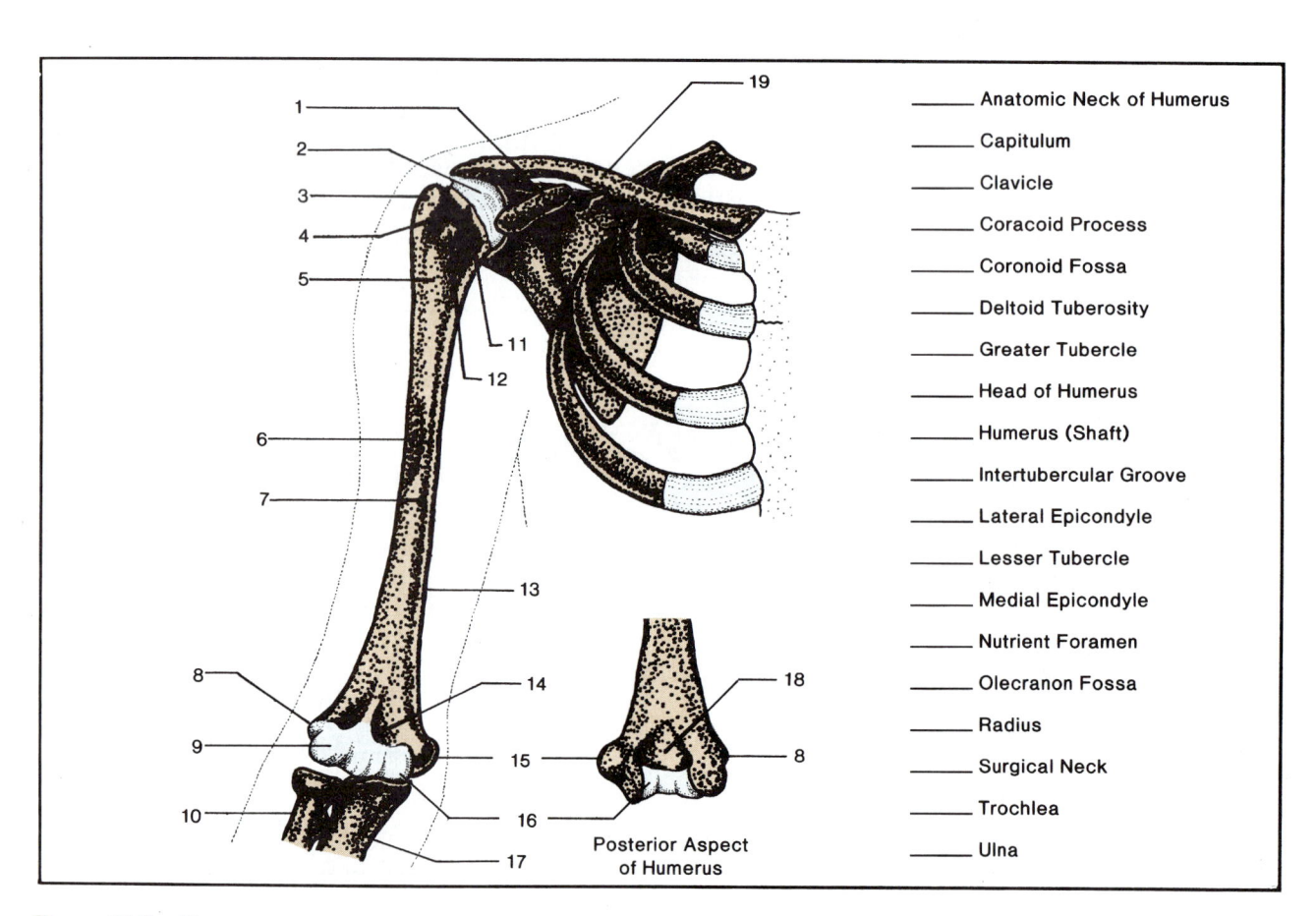

_____ Anatomic Neck of Humerus

_____ Capitulum

_____ Clavicle

_____ Coracoid Process

_____ Coronoid Fossa

_____ Deltoid Tuberosity

_____ Greater Tubercle

_____ Head of Humerus

_____ Humerus (Shaft)

_____ Intertubercular Groove

_____ Lateral Epicondyle

_____ Lesser Tubercle

_____ Medial Epicondyle

_____ Nutrient Foramen

_____ Olecranon Fossa

_____ Radius

_____ Surgical Neck

_____ Trochlea

_____ Ulna

Posterior Aspect of Humerus

Figure 13.2 The upper arm.

the arm. The region between the head and the radial tuberosity is the **neck** of the radius. The distal lateral prominence of the radius which articulates with the wrist is the **styloid process.** Locate this process on your own wrist.

The **ulna,** or elbow bone, is the largest bone in the forearm. A portion of the humerus in figure 13.3 has been cut away to reveal the prominence of the elbow which is called the **olecranon process.** Within this process is a depression, the **semilunar notch,** which articulates with the trochlea of the humerus. The eminence just below the semilunar notch on the anterior surface is the **coronoid process** (label 1). Where the head of the radius contacts the ulna is a depression, the **radial notch.** The lower end of the ulna is small and terminates in two eminences: a large portion, the **head,** and a small **styloid process.** The head articulates with a fibrocartilage disk which separates it from the wrist. The styloid pro-

cess is a point of attachment for a ligament of the wrist joint.

Hand Each hand consists of a carpus (wrist), a metacarpus (palm), and phalanges (fingers).

The **carpus** consists of eight small bones arranged in two rows of four bones each. Named from the lateral to medial aspects, the proximal (upper) carpal bones are the **navicular, lunate, triquetral,** and **pisiform.** The navicular and lunate articulate with the distal end of the radius. The names of the distal carpal bones from lateral to medial aspects are the **trapezium** (*greater multangular*), **trapezoid** (*lesser multangular*), **capitate,** and **hamate.**

The **metacarpus** consists of five metacarpal bones. They are numbered from one to five, the thumb side being one.

The **phalanges** are the skeletal elements of the fingers distal to the metacarpal bones. There are

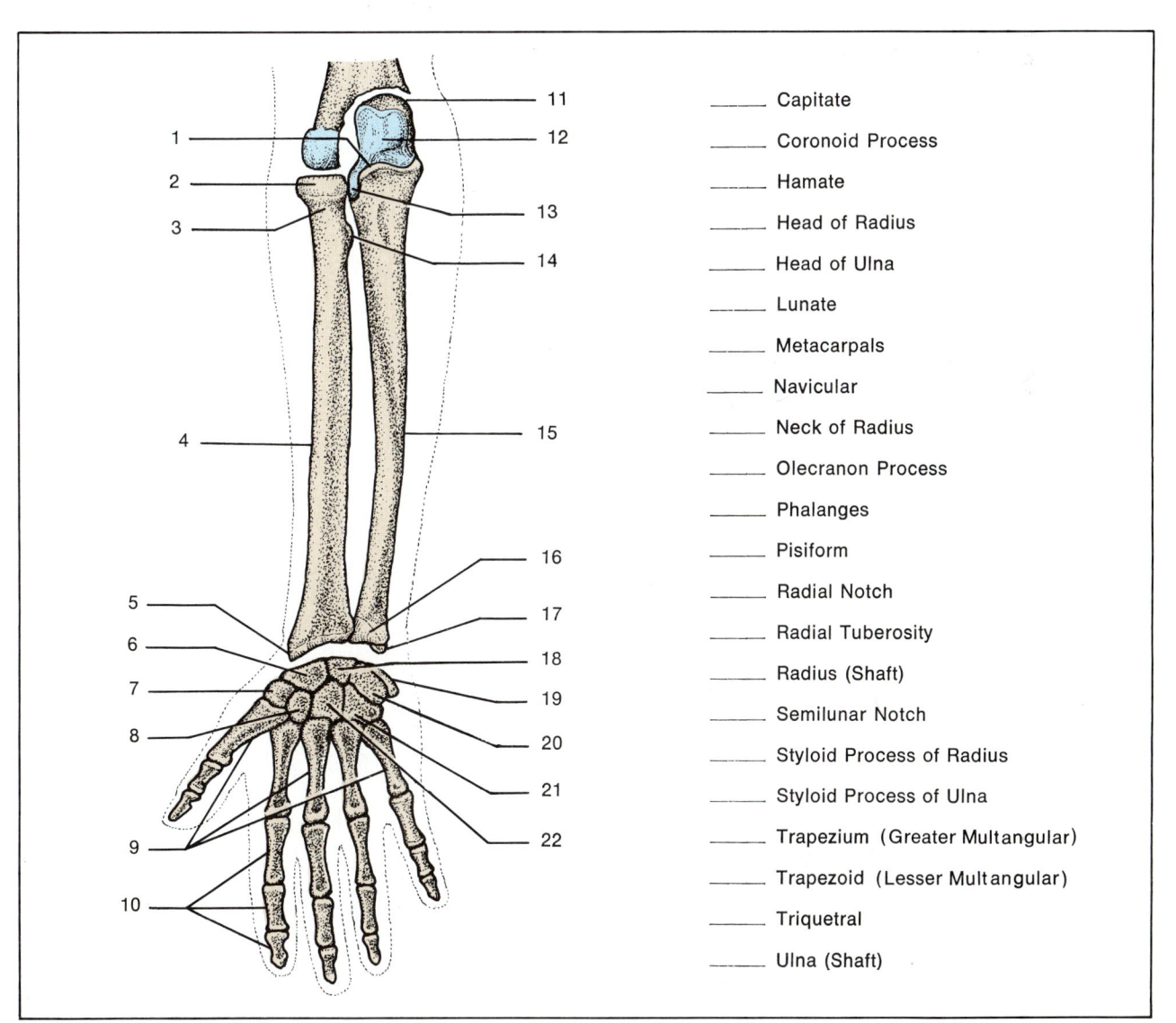

_____	Capitate
_____	Coronoid Process
_____	Hamate
_____	Head of Radius
_____	Head of Ulna
_____	Lunate
_____	Metacarpals
_____	Navicular
_____	Neck of Radius
_____	Olecranon Process
_____	Phalanges
_____	Pisiform
_____	Radial Notch
_____	Radial Tuberosity
_____	Radius (Shaft)
_____	Semilunar Notch
_____	Styloid Process of Radius
_____	Styloid Process of Ulna
_____	Trapezium (Greater Multangular)
_____	Trapezoid (Lesser Multangular)
_____	Triquetral
_____	Ulna (Shaft)

Figure 13.3 The forearm and hand.

three phalanges in each finger and two in the thumb.

Assignment:

Label figure 13.3.

Answer the questions on the Laboratory Report that pertain to the upper extremities.

The Lower Extremities

Pelvic Girdle The two hipbones (*ossa coxae*), articulate in front to form a bony arch called the *pelvic girdle*. The back of this arch is formed by the union of the hipbones with the sacrum and coccyx. The enclosure formed within this bony ring is the **pelvis** (Latin: *pelvis,* basin) Figure 13.5 illustrates one half of the pelvis and the right femur.

Figure 13.4 illustrates the lateral and medial views of the right os coxa. The large circular depression into which the head of the femur fits is the **acetabulum.** Note that each os coxa consists of three fused bones (ilium, ischium, and pubis) that are joined together in the center of the acetabulum. Although these ossification lines are readily discernible in young children, they are generally obliterated in the adult.

Two articulating surfaces (labels 10 and 18) are visible on the medial aspect of the os coxa. The upper one is the **sacrum articulating surface,** which interfaces with the sacrum; the lower one is the **symphysis pubis articulating surface,** which joins with the other os coxa to form the symphysis pubis.

The line of juncture between the ilium and sacrum is the **sacroiliac joint.**

The **ilium** is the yellow portion of the bone. On the greater portion of its medial surface is a large concavity called the **iliac fossa.** The **arcuate line** (label 14) is a ridge of demarcation below the iliac fossa.

The upper margin of the ilium, which is called the **iliac crest,** extends from the **anterior superior spine** (label 16) to the **posterior superior spine** (label 2). Just below the latter process is the **posterior inferior spine.** An **anterior inferior spine** is seen on the opposite margin below the anterior superior spine.

The reddish colored portion of the os coxa is the **ischium.** Note that it has two distinct processes: a small eminence, the **ischial spine,** and a larger one, the **tuberosity of the ischium,** which makes up the lower bulk of the bone. It is on this tuberosity that one sits. Just below the ischial spine is a depression, the **lesser sciatic notch.** The larger depression superior to it is the **greater sciatic notch.**

The orange colored bone is the **pubis.** The opening surrounded by the pubis and ischium is the **obturator foramen.** Note that the **inferior ramus of the ischium** and **inferior ramus of the pubis** form the lower bony arch around this foramen.

Assignment:

Label figure 13.4.

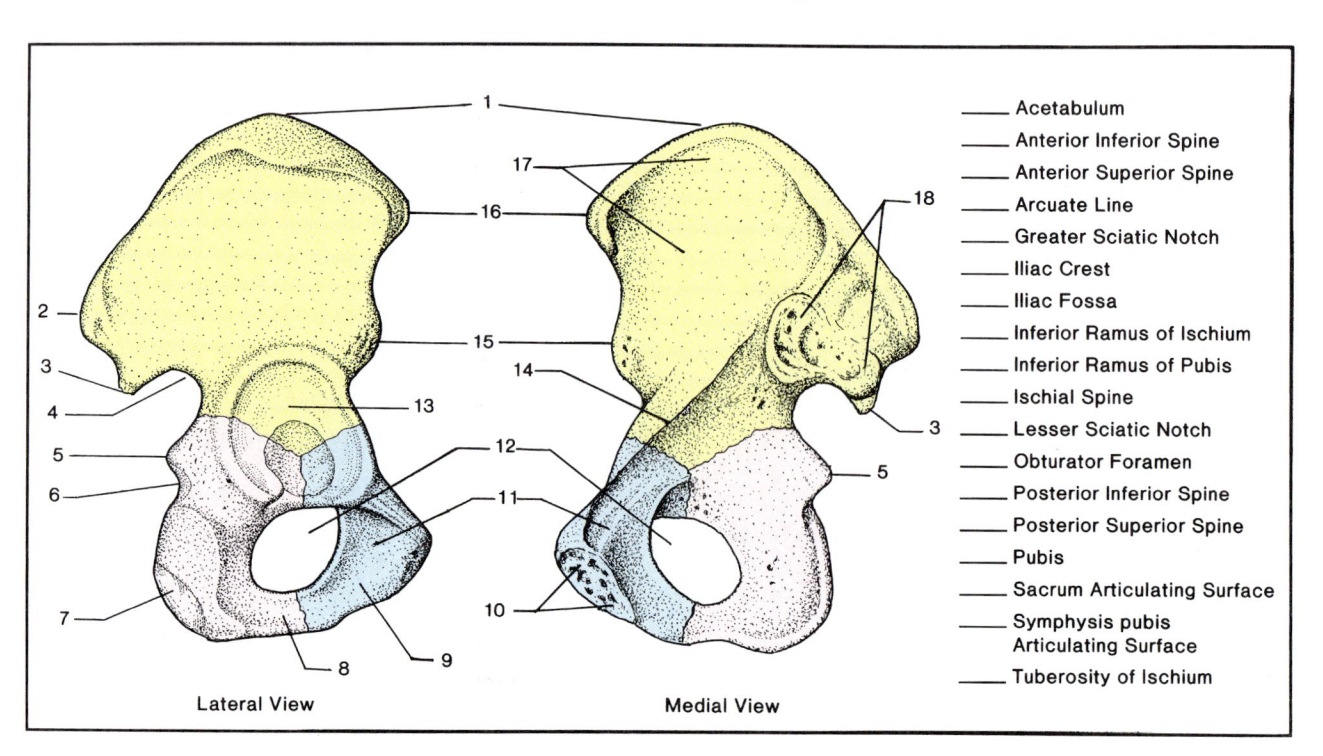

_____ Acetabulum
_____ Anterior Inferior Spine
_____ Anterior Superior Spine
_____ Arcuate Line
_____ Greater Sciatic Notch
_____ Iliac Crest
_____ Iliac Fossa
_____ Inferior Ramus of Ischium
_____ Inferior Ramus of Pubis
_____ Ischial Spine
_____ Lesser Sciatic Notch
_____ Obturator Foramen
_____ Posterior Inferior Spine
_____ Posterior Superior Spine
_____ Pubis
_____ Sacrum Articulating Surface
_____ Symphysis pubis Articulating Surface
_____ Tuberosity of Ischium

Lateral View   Medial View

Figure 13.4 The os coxa.

Compare a male pelvis with a female pelvis and answer questions on the Laboratory Report that pertain to their anatomical differences.

Upper Leg   Skeletal support of the thigh is achieved with one bone, the **femur.** Its upper end consists of a hemispherical **head,** a **neck,** and two eminences, the greater and lesser trochanters. The **greater trochanter** is the large process on the lateral surface. The **lesser trochanter** is located further down on the medial surface. A ridge, the **intertrochanteric line,** lies obliquely between the two trochanters on the anterior surface. The ridge between these two trochanters on the posterior surface of the femur is the **intertrochanteric crest.** A pronounced ridge extends longitudinally along the posterior surface of the shaft of the femur. Its upper portion is called the **gluteal tuberosity** and the remainder is known as the **linea aspera.** Several muscles are attached to this prominence.

The lower extremity of a femur is larger than the upper end and is divided into two condyles: the **lateral** and **medial condyles.**

Assignment:

Label figure 13.5.

Lower Leg   Figure 13.6 on the next page reveals the skeletal structure of the lower leg. It consists of the tibia, fibula, and foot bones.

Of the two long bones, the **tibia** is the stronger one. Its upper portion is expanded to form two condyles and a tuberosity: a **medial condyle** (label 7), a **lateral condyle** on the opposite side, and a **tibial tuberosity** inferior to the two condyles. Projecting upward between the condyles are two projections that constitute the **intercondylar eminence.**

The distal extremity of the tibia is smaller than the upper portion. A strong process, the **medial malleolus,** forms the inner prominence of the ankle. Locate this process on your own leg. Note that the triangular cross section of the tibia results in a sharp ridge, the **anterior crest,** being present on its anterior surface.

The **fibula** is lateral to the tibia and parallel to it. The upper extremity, or **head,** articulates with the tibia, but it does not form a part of the knee joint. Below the head is the **neck** of the fibula. The lower extremity of the fibula terminates in a pointed process, the **lateral malleolus,** which lies just under the skin forming the outer ankle bone. Locate this process on your own leg. Like the tibia, the fibula has an **anterior crest** extending down its anterior surface.

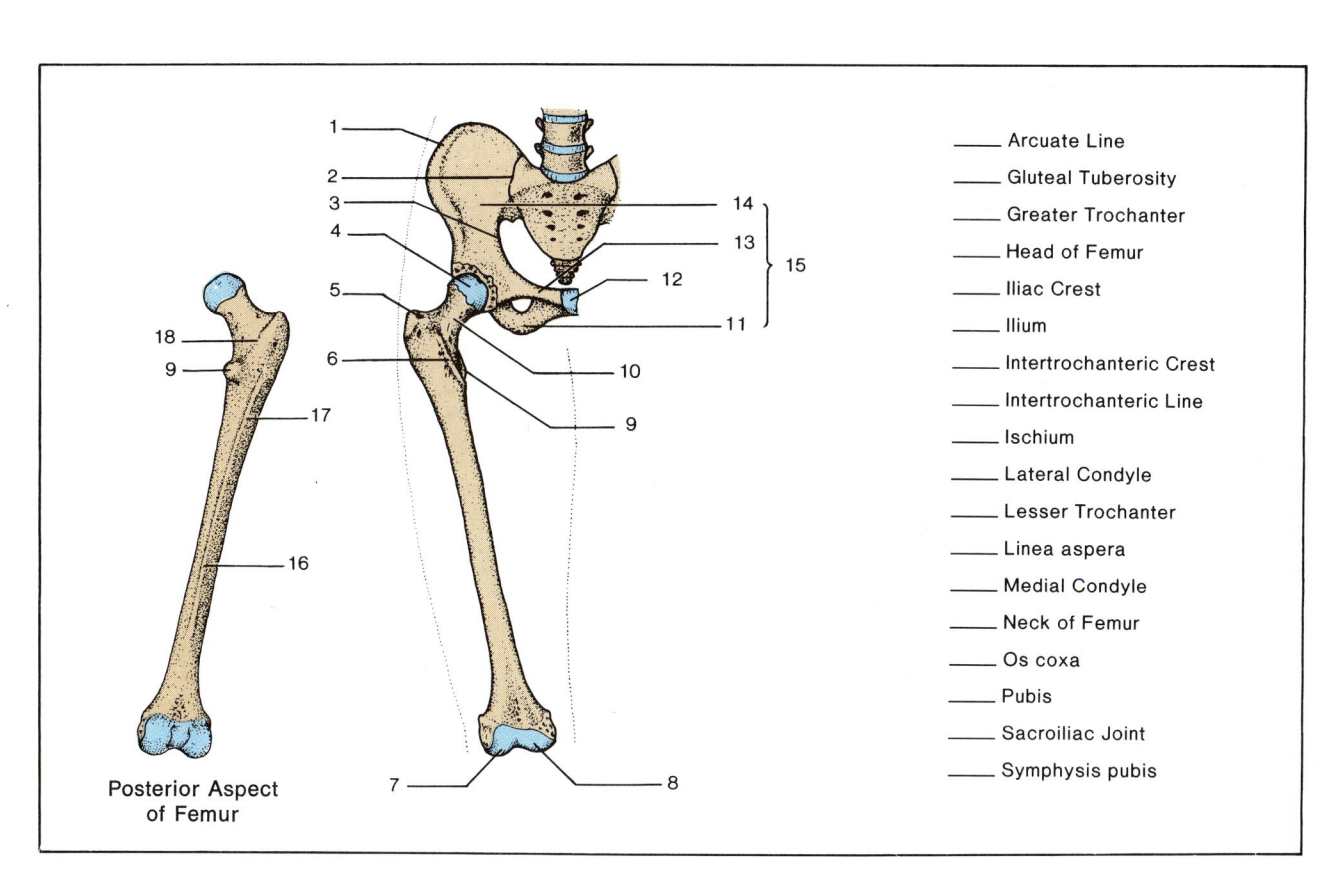

_____ Arcuate Line

_____ Gluteal Tuberosity

_____ Greater Trochanter

_____ Head of Femur

_____ Iliac Crest

_____ Ilium

_____ Intertrochanteric Crest

_____ Intertrochanteric Line

_____ Ischium

_____ Lateral Condyle

_____ Lesser Trochanter

_____ Linea aspera

_____ Medial Condyle

_____ Neck of Femur

_____ Os coxa

_____ Pubis

_____ Sacroiliac Joint

_____ Symphysis pubis

Posterior Aspect of Femur

Figure 13.5   The upper leg.

Foot Superior and lateral views of the skeleton of the foot are seen in figure 13.6. It consists of the ankle, instep, and toes.

The **tarsus,** or ankle of the foot, consists of seven tarsal bones: the calcaneous, talus, cuboid, navicular, and three cuneiforms. The **calcaneous,** or heel bone, is the largest tarsal bone. It forms a strong lever for muscles of the calf of the leg. The **talus** occupies the uppermost central position of the tarsus. It articulates with the tibia. In front of the talus on the medial side of the foot is the **navicular.** The **cuboid** is on the lateral side of the foot in front of the calcaneous. The three **cuneiform** bones are anterior to the navicular. They are numbered one, two, and three, number one being on the medial side of the foot.

The **metatarsus** forms the anterior portion of the instep of the foot. It consists of five elongated **metatarsal** bones. They are numbered one through five, number one being on the medial side of the foot.

The **phalanges** that make up the toes resemble the phalanges of the hand in general shape and number: two in the great toe and three in each of the other toes.

Assignment:

Label figure 13.6.

Complete the Laboratory Report for this exercise.

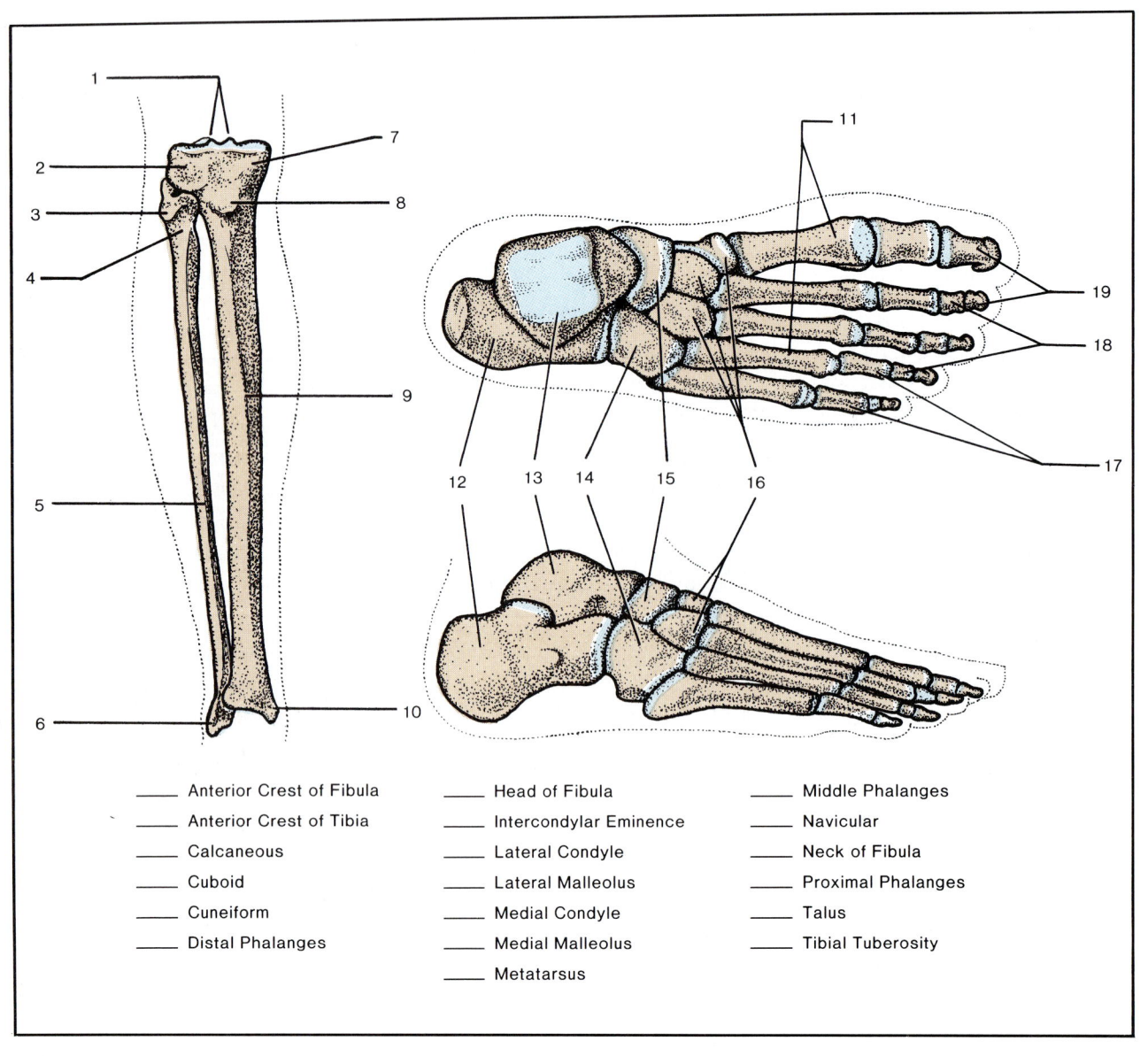

___ Anterior Crest of Fibula	___ Head of Fibula	___ Middle Phalanges
___ Anterior Crest of Tibia	___ Intercondylar Eminence	___ Navicular
___ Calcaneous	___ Lateral Condyle	___ Neck of Fibula
___ Cuboid	___ Lateral Malleolus	___ Proximal Phalanges
___ Cuneiform	___ Medial Condyle	___ Talus
___ Distal Phalanges	___ Medial Malleolus	___ Tibial Tuberosity
	___ Metatarsus	

Figure 13.6 The lower leg.

During this laboratory period we will study the basic characteristics of three types of joints, and the specifics of the shoulder, hip, and knee joints.

Materials:

> fresh knee joint of cow or lamb, sawed through longitudinally

The Basic Types

All joints in the body fall into one of the three categories illustrated in figure 14.1. Note that classification is based on the degree of movement.

Immovable Joints

The lack of movement in these *synarthrotic* joints is due to the bonding effect of fibrous connective tissue or cartilage. Two types exist: sutures and synchondroses.

Sutures These irregular joints that exist between the flat bones of the cranium are held together by **fibrous connective tissue.** This tissue is continuous with the **periosteum** (label 2) on the external surface of the bone and the **dura mater** on the inner surface.

Synchondroses This type of immovable joint utilizes cartilage instead of fibrous tissue as the bonding tissue. The metaphyses of long bones in children are joints of this type. As was noted in Exercise 10, these growth areas in children consist of hyaline cartilage during the growing years.

Slightly Movable Joints

Slightly movable, or *amphiarthrotic,* joints are either symphyses or syndesmoses.

Symphyses Slightly movable joints that have a pad of fibrocartilage between the bones fall into this category. The intervertebral joints and symphysis pubis are representative.

Note in the intervertebral joint of illustration B that the bony surfaces are covered with **articular cartilage** (hyaline type). A pad of **fibrocartilage** (label 6) provides a cushion. These joints are held together with a fibroelastic **capsule.**

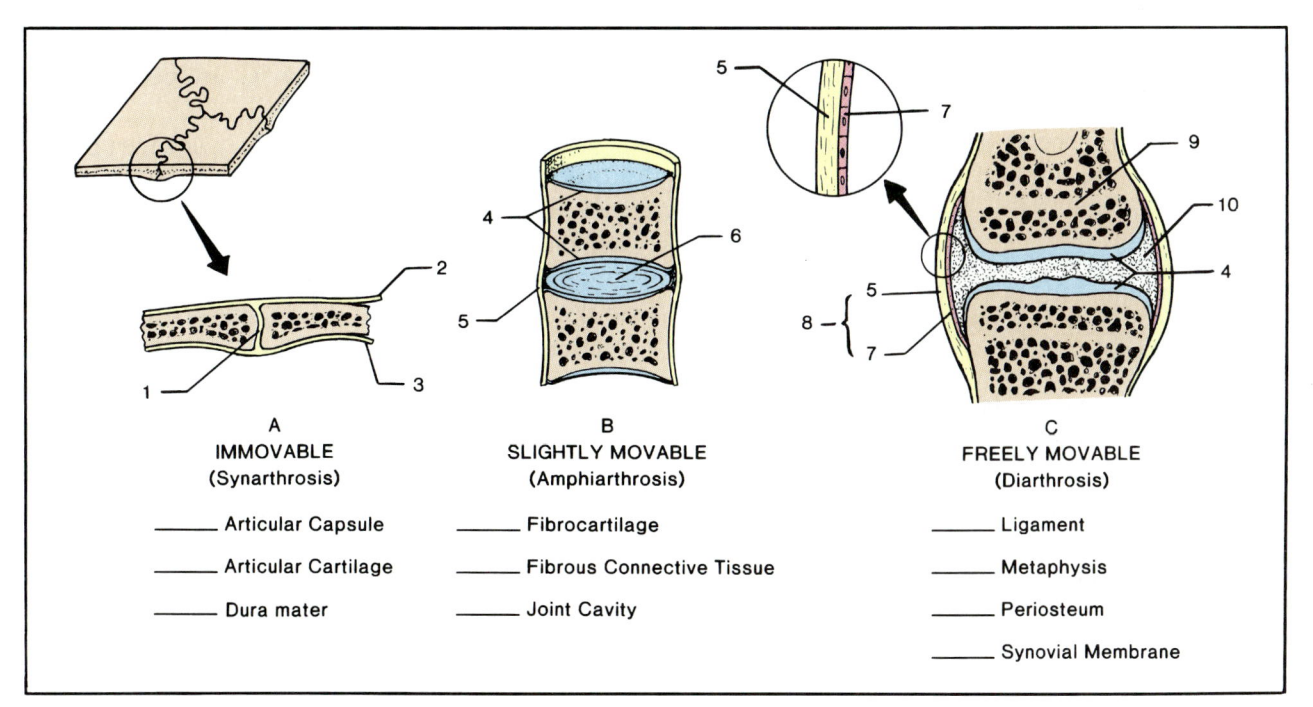

A IMMOVABLE (Synarthrosis)	B SLIGHTLY MOVABLE (Amphiarthrosis)	C FREELY MOVABLE (Diarthrosis)
_____ Articular Capsule	_____ Fibrocartilage	_____ Ligament
_____ Articular Cartilage	_____ Fibrous Connective Tissue	_____ Metaphysis
_____ Dura mater	_____ Joint Cavity	_____ Periosteum
		_____ Synovial Membrane

Figure 14.1 Types of articulations.

Syndesmoses Slightly movable joints that lack fibrocartilage and are held together by an interosseus ligament are of this type. A good example is the attachment of the fibula to the tibia, as seen in figure 14.4.

Freely Movable Joints

Articulations that move easily are designated as *diarthrotic,* or *synovial,* joints. Note in illustration C (figure 14.1) that the bone ends are covered with smooth **articular cartilage.** Holding the joint together is a fibrous **articular capsule** that consists of an outer layer of **ligaments** and an inner lining of **synovial membrane.** The latter membrane produces a viscous fluid, *synovium,* which lubricates the joint. These joints also contain sacs, or **bursae,** of synovial tissue. Fibrocartilaginous pads may also be present. Six different kinds of synovial joints are present in the body.

Gliding Joints The articular surfaces in these joints are nearly flat or slightly convex. Bones that exhibit gliding action are seen in between carpal bones of the wrist, and tarsals of the ankle.

Hinge Joints Joints such as the elbow, ankle, and knee that move in one direction only are of this type. Movement between the occipital condyles of the skull and the atlas is also hingelike.

Condyloid Joints Joints consisting of an oval-shaped head, or condyle, that moves in an elliptical cavity can move in two directions. The wrist is a typical condyloid joint.

Saddle Joints Like the condyloid joints, these joints allow movement in two directions. The bones' ends differ, however, in that each bone end is convex in one direction and concave in the other direction. The joint between the thumb metacarpal and trapezium is of this type.

Pivot Joints A joint in which movement is rotational around an axis is a pivot type. Rotation of the atlas around the odontoid process of the axis is a good example.

Ball and Socket Joints These joints have angular movement in all directions. The shoulder and hip joints are representative.

Assignment:

Label figure 14.1.

The Shoulder Joint

The shoulder joint is the most freely movable articulation of the body. Its structure is revealed in

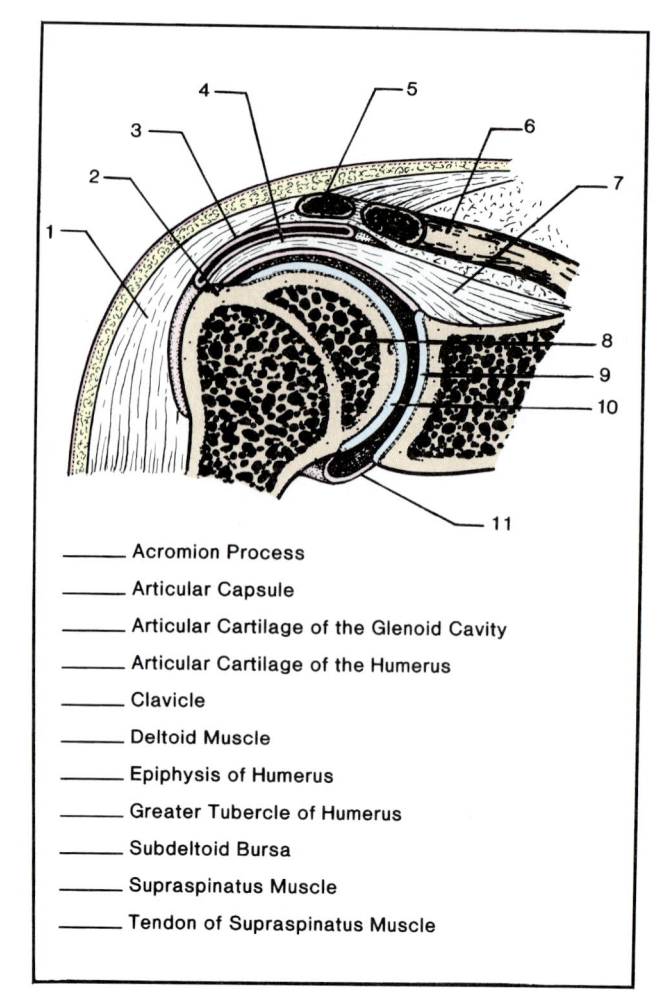

_____ Acromion Process
_____ Articular Capsule
_____ Articular Cartilage of the Glenoid Cavity
_____ Articular Cartilage of the Humerus
_____ Clavicle
_____ Deltoid Muscle
_____ Epiphysis of Humerus
_____ Greater Tubercle of Humerus
_____ Subdeltoid Bursa
_____ Supraspinatus Muscle
_____ Tendon of Supraspinatus Muscle

Figure 14.2 The shoulder joint.

figure 14.2. Note that the articulating surfaces of the humerus and glenoid cavity are covered with **articular cartilage.**

Although there are usually six or seven bursae in the neighborhood of this joint, only the **subdeltoid bursa** is shown in figure 14.2. Note that the **tendon of the supraspinatus muscle** inserts on the **greater tubercle of the humerus.** Bony sections seen in the upper portion of this illustration are the **acromion process** (label 5) and a portion of the **clavicle.** The membranous fold beneath the head of the humerus is a portion of the **articular capsule.**

Assignment:

Label figure 14.2.

The Hip Joint

The hip joint, another ball and socket joint, is shown in figure 14.3. The rounded head of the femur is confined in the acetabulum of the os coxa by the acetabular labrum and the transverse acetabular ligament. The **acetabular labrum** (label 8) is a fibrocartilaginous rim attached to the margin of the acetabulum. The **transverse acetabular ligament** (label 11) is an extension of the acetabular labrum. Note in the sectional view that a structure, the **ligamentum teres femoris,** is attached to the middle of the curved condylar surface of the femur. The other end of this ligament is attached to the surface of the acetabulum. This structure adds nothing to the strength of the joint; instead, it contributes to nourishment of the head of the femur and supplies synovial fluid to the joint.

The entire joint, including the preceding three structures, is enclosed in an **articular capsule.** This capsule consists of longitudinal and circular fibers surrounded by three external accessory ligaments. The three accessory ligaments are the iliofemoral, pubocapsular, and ischiocapsular. The **iliofemoral ligament** (label 7) is a broad band on the anterior surface of the joint. This ligament is attached to the **anterior inferior iliac spine** at its upper margin and the **intertrochanteric line** on its lower margin. Adjacent and medial to the iliofemoral ligament lies the **pubocapsular ligament.** The posterior surface of the capsule is reinforced by the **ischiocapsular ligament.** Lining the inside of the capsule is the **synovial membrane** which provides the lubricant for the joint.

Movements of flexion, extension, abduction, adduction, rotation, and circumduction of the thigh are readily achieved through this joint. This is made possible by the unique angle of the neck of the femur and the relationship of the condyle to the acetabulum. Excessive backward movement of the body at the joint is controlled to a great extent by the iliofemoral ligament, taking some of the strain from certain muscles.

Assignment:

Label figure 14.3.

The Knee Joint

Two views and a sagittal section of the knee are shown in figure 14.4. Although the action of this joint has been described earlier as being essentially hingelike, it is by no means a simple hinge. The curved surfaces of the condyles of the femur allow rolling and gliding movements within the joint. There is also some rotary movement due to the nature of hip and foot alignment.

The knee joint is probably the most highly stressed joint in the body. To absorb some of this stress are two *semilunar cartilages,* or *menisci,* in each joint. As revealed in the sagittal section, these fibrocartilaginous pads are thick at the periphery and thin in the center of the joint, providing a deep recess for the condyles. The **lateral meniscus** lies between the lateral condyle of the femur and the tibia; the **medial meniscus** is between the medial condyle and the tibia. These menisci are best seen in the anterior and posterior views of figure 14.4. Anteriorly and peripherally, they are connected by a **transverse ligament.**

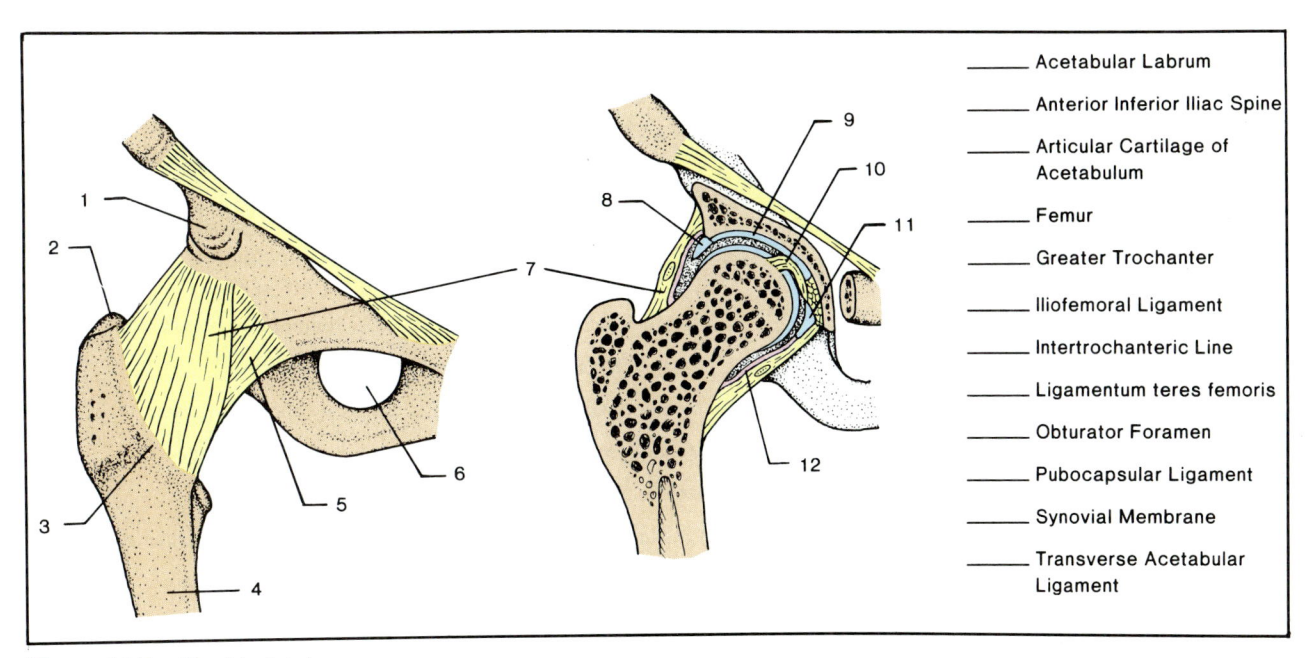

_____	Acetabular Labrum
_____	Anterior Inferior Iliac Spine
_____	Articular Cartilage of Acetabulum
_____	Femur
_____	Greater Trochanter
_____	Iliofemoral Ligament
_____	Intertrochanteric Line
_____	Ligamentum teres femoris
_____	Obturator Foramen
_____	Pubocapsular Ligament
_____	Synovial Membrane
_____	Transverse Acetabular Ligament

Figure 14.3 The hip joint.

The entire joint is held together by several layers of ligaments. Innermost are the two cruciate and two collateral ligaments. The **posterior** and **anterior cruciate ligaments** form an X on the median line of the posterior surface, with the posterior cruciate ligament being outermost. The anterior cruciate ligament is the outermost one seen on the anterior surface when the leg is flexed. The **fibular collateral ligament** is on the lateral surface, extending from the lateral epicondyle of the femur to the head of the fibula. The **tibial collateral ligament** extends from the medial epicondyle of the femur to the upper medial surface of the tibia. In addition to these four ligaments are the *oblique* and *arcuate popliteal ligaments* on the posterior surface. These are not shown in figure 14.4.

Encompassing the entire joint is the *fibrous capsule*. It is a complicated structure of special ligaments united with strong expansions of the muscle tendons that pass over the joint.

Observe in the sagittal section that the kneecap is held in place by an upper **quadriceps tendon** and a lower **patellar ligament.** The inner surfaces of these latter structures are lined with **synovial membrane.** The space between the synovial membrane and femur is the **suprapatellar bursa.**

It is significant that although this joint is capable of sustaining considerable stress, it lacks bony reinforcement to prevent dislocations in almost any direction. It relies almost entirely on soft tissues to hold the bones in place. It is because of this fact that knee injuries are so commonplace today among the general populace, as well as professional athletes. It is a vulnerable joint particularly to lateral and rotational forces. An understanding of its anatomy should alert one to its limitations.

Assignment:

Label figure 14.4.

Laboratory Assignment

Animal Joint Study Examine the knee joint of a cow or lamb that has been sawed through longitudinally. Identify as many of the structures as possible that are shown in figure 14.4.

Laboratory Report Complete the Laboratory Report for this exercise.

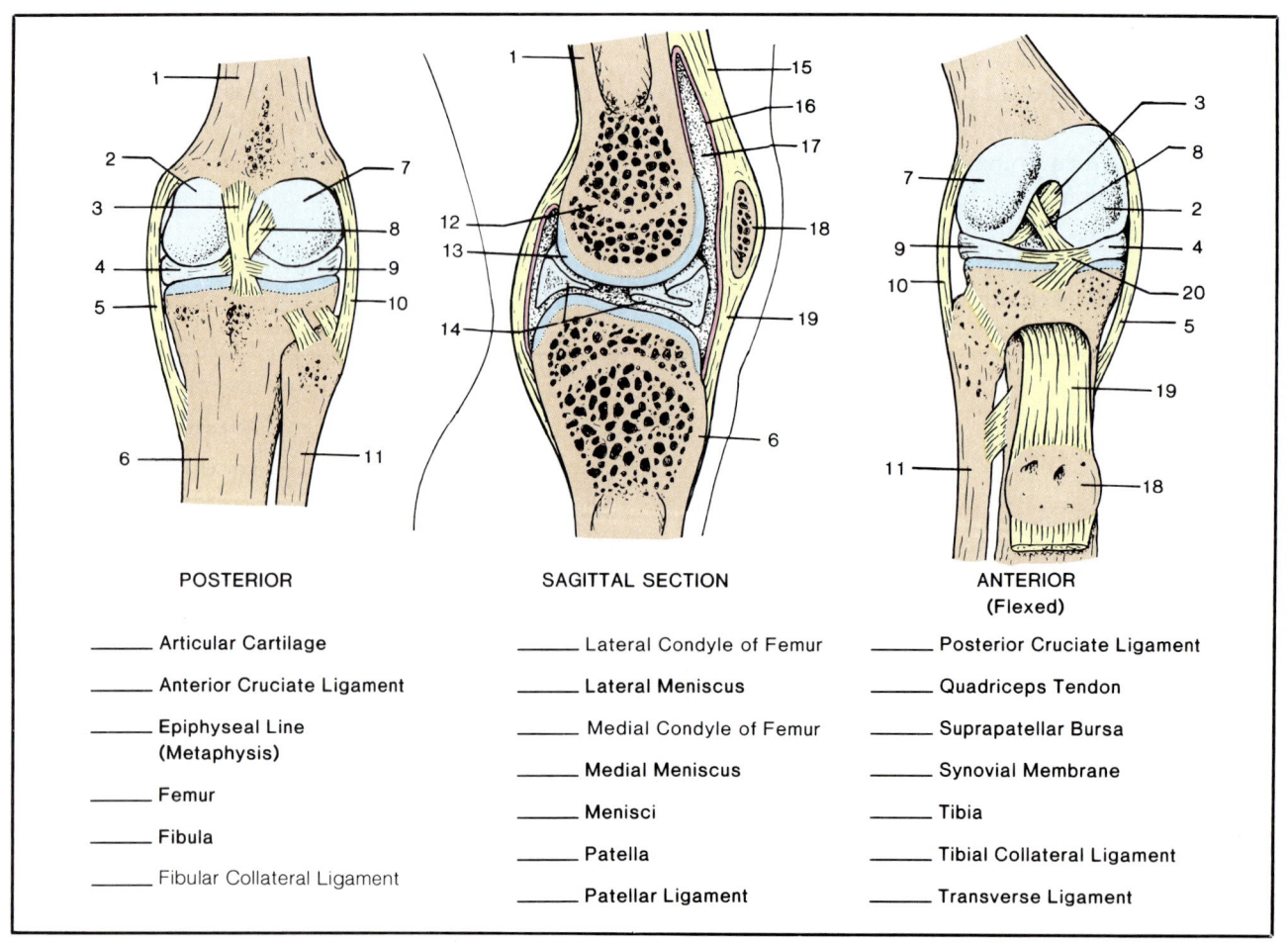

POSTERIOR   SAGITTAL SECTION   ANTERIOR (Flexed)

_____ Articular Cartilage	_____ Lateral Condyle of Femur	_____ Posterior Cruciate Ligament
_____ Anterior Cruciate Ligament	_____ Lateral Meniscus	_____ Quadriceps Tendon
_____ Epiphyseal Line (Metaphysis)	_____ Medial Condyle of Femur	_____ Suprapatellar Bursa
_____ Femur	_____ Medial Meniscus	_____ Synovial Membrane
_____ Fibula	_____ Menisci	_____ Tibia
_____ Fibular Collateral Ligament	_____ Patella	_____ Tibial Collateral Ligament
	_____ Patellar Ligament	_____ Transverse Ligament

Figure 14.4 The knee joint.

Part 4 The Major Skeletal Muscles

The nine exercises of this unit include around 105 skeletal muscles of the human body. Although this is not a complete listing of all the muscles, it does include all the surface muscles and most of the deeper ones. If time does not permit the study of all these muscles, the instructor will indicate which ones the student should know.

This is the first unit in which the cat will be used for dissection. Prior to studying cat muscles, it is recommended that the human musculature be studied first by labeling the illustrations. Although cat musculature differs to some extent from the human, the similarities far outweigh the differences.

One thing to keep in mind about the cat dissection is that we are not concerned about the cat muscles from a comparative standpoint. The fact that the cat may have certain muscles that are lacking in humans is really irrelevant. Our principal concern is to reinforce our knowledge of the human muscles by studying the similarities rather than the differences.

15 Muscle Tissue

All muscle tissue fibers in the body have one characteristic in common: the ability to contract when properly stimulated. This property is made possible by the presence of contractile protein fibers within the cells.

As noted previously, there are three kinds of muscle fibers in the body: skeletal, smooth, and cardiac. Although most of the exercises in this unit (Part 4) pertain to skeletal muscles, an opportunity will be provided here to do a microscopic study to compare all three types.

On the basis of cytoplasmic differences, there are two categories of muscle fibers: striated and smooth. *Striated muscle* is characterized by regularly spaced transverse bands called **striae.** *Smooth muscle* lacks these transverse bands and has other distinctions to set them apart.

Striated muscle cells are further subdivided into skeletal and cardiac muscle. *Skeletal muscle* cells are multinucleated, or *syncytial*. Attached primarily to the skeleton, they are responsible for voluntary body movements. *Cardiac muscle* cells, which make up the muscle of the heart wall, are not syncytial and have less prominent striations than skeletal muscle.

Smooth Muscle

Smooth muscle fibers are long, spindle-shaped cells as illustrated in figure 15.1. Each cell has a single elongated nucleus that usually has two or more nucleoli. When studied with electron microscopy, the cytoplasm reveals the presence of fine linear filaments of the same protein composition that are seen in striated muscle.

Smooth muscle cells are found in the walls of blood vessels, walls of organs of the digestive tract, the urinary bladder, and other internal organs. They are innervated by the autonomic nervous system and, thus, are under *involuntary nervous control*.

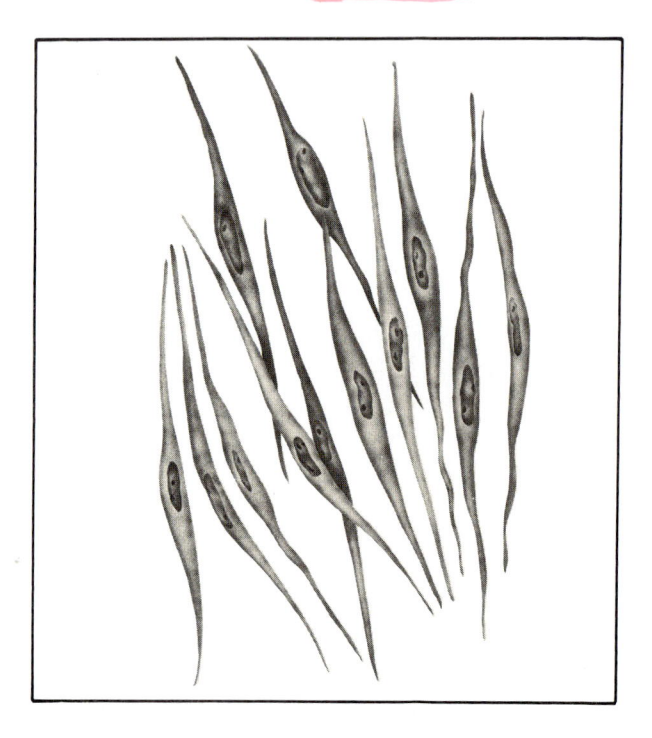

Figure 15.1   Smooth muscle fibers, teased.

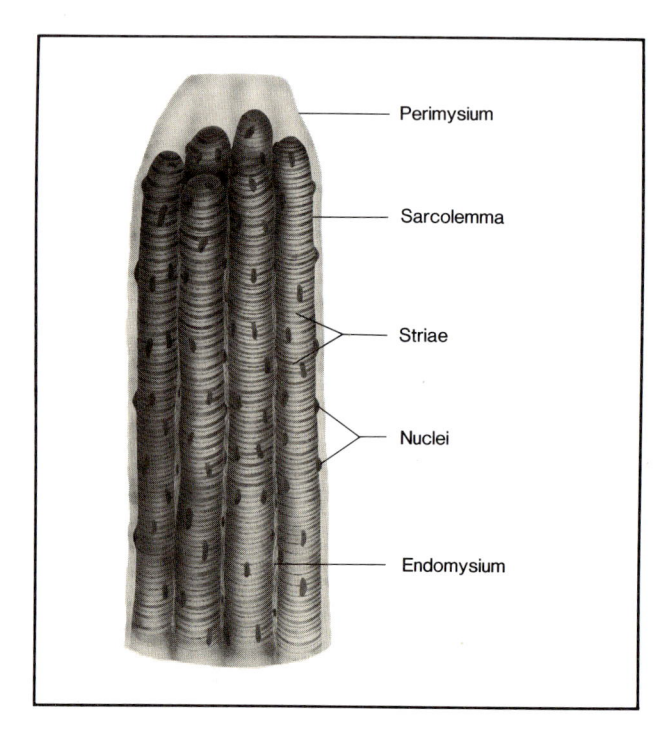

Figure 15.2   A fascicle of skeletal muscle fibers.

Skeletal Muscle

Muscle fibers of this type are long, cylindrical, and multinucleated. Note in figure 15.2 that these fibers are grouped together into bundles called **fasciculi.** Note, also, that between the cells is a thin layer of connective tissue called **endomysium,** that enables each cell to respond independently to nerve stimuli.

Examination of the **sarcoplasm** (cytoplasm) with a light microscope reveals distinct dark and light **striae** (cross stripes). Note in figure 15.2 that each cell has many nuclei positioned just beneath the **sarcolemma** (plasma membrane).

Although striated muscle is usually thought of as being under voluntary control and always attached to the skeleton, there are exceptions: (1) striated muscles of the tongue may not be attached to bone; and (2) striated muscles of the pharynx and upper esophagus have no skeletal attachment and are not voluntarily controlled.

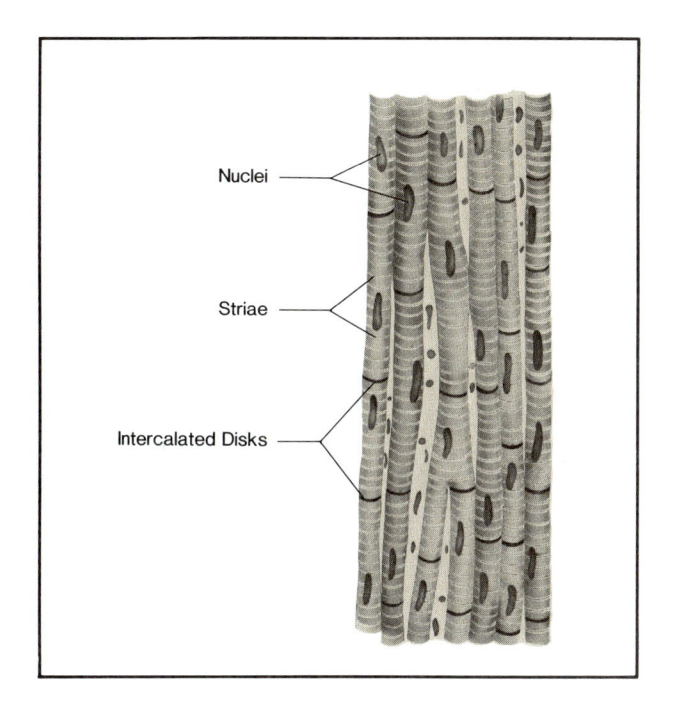

Figure 15.3 Cardiac muscle fibers.

Cardiac Muscle

Muscle cells of this type (figure 15.3) are found in the wall of the heart (myocardium) and in the walls of the vena cavae where they enter the right atrium of the heart. This muscle tissue is unique in its ability to contract rhythmically and continuously as a result of intrinsic cellular activity. Four significant distinguishing characteristics of cardiac muscle are:

- Instead of being anatomically syncytial, cardiac muscle is made up of individual cellular units separated by **intercalated disks** (cell membranes).
- Some cardiac muscle fibers are bifurcated to form a branching, three-dimensional network.
- The nucleus of a cardiac fiber lies deep within the cell, not near the surface as in skeletal fibers.
- Cardiac muscle, unlike skeletal muscle, is not normally subject to voluntary control.

Laboratory Assignment

After answering the questions on the Laboratory Report that pertain to muscle structure and physiology, examine microscope slides of the various types of muscle tissue, using the Histology Atlas for reference.

Materials:

prepared slides of
striated muscle (H3.11 and H3.13)
smooth muscle (H3.21 and H3.22)
heart muscle (H3.31, H3.32, H3.33)

Skeletal Muscle: Scan a slide of striated muscle tissue with low power to find a muscle fiber with the most pronounced striae. Increase the magnification to 1000× (oil immersion) and see if you can differentiate the *A* and *I bands.* Use figure HA-7 for reference. Look, also, for the **endomysium** in a cross-section of striated muscle tissue.

Cardiac Muscle: Scan a slide of this tissue with low power, looking for pronounced *striae* and *intercalated disks.* Look also for evidence of bifurcation of the fibers. Consult illustration A, figure HA-8 of the Histology Atlas.

Smooth Muscle: Study slides of this type of muscle tissue in the same manner as above. Finding individual fibers on teased tissue (H3.21) is not always as easy as it might seem. Compare your observations to illustrations B and C in figure HA-8.

Laboratory Report

Answer the questions on the first portion of Laboratory Report 15-17.

16 Skeletal Muscle Structure

The movement of limbs and other structures by skeletal muscles is a function of the contractility of muscle fibers and the manner of attachment of the muscles to the skeleton. In this exercise our concern will be with the detailed structure of whole muscles and their mode of attachment to the skeleton.

Figure 16.1 reveals a portion of the arm and shoulder girdle with only two muscles shown. Several other muscles of the upper arm have been omitted that would obscure the points of attachment of these muscles. The longer muscle which is attached to the scapula and humerus at its upper end is the **triceps brachii.** The shorter muscle on the anterior aspect of the humerus is the **brachialis.**

Muscle Attachments

Each muscle of the body is said to have an origin and insertion. The **origin** of the muscle is the immovable end. The **insertion** is the other end, which moves during contraction. Contraction of the muscle results in shortening of the distance between the origin and insertion, causing movement at the insertion end.

Muscles may be attached to bone in three different ways: (1) directly to the periosteum, (2) by means of a tendon, or (3) with an aponeurosis. The upper end of the brachialis (the origin) is attached by the first method, i.e., directly to the periosteum. The insertion end of this muscle, however, does have a short tendon for attachment. A **tendon** is a band or cord of white fibrous tissue that provides a durable connection to the skeleton. The tendon of the triceps insertion is much longer and larger due to the fact that this muscle exerts a greater force in moving the forearm. An example of the aponeurosis type of attachment is seen in figure 22.1, page 108. Label 5 in this figure is the aponeurosis of the external oblique muscle. An **aponeurosis** is a broad flat sheet of glistening pearly-white fibrous connective tissue that attaches a muscle to the skeleton or another muscle.

Although most muscles attach directly to the skeleton there are many that attach to other muscles or soft structures (skin) such as the lips and eyelids. In Exercises 19 through 23 the precise origins and insertions of various muscles will be identified.

Microscopic Structure

Illustrations B and C in figure 16.1 reveal the microscopic structure of a portion of the brachialis muscle. Note that the muscle is made up of bundles, or **fasciculi,** of skeletal muscle cells. A single fasciculus is shown, enlarged, in illustration C. Protruding upward from the upper cut surface of the fasciculus is a portion of an individual muscle cell, or **muscle fiber.** Note that between the individual muscle fibers of each fascicle is a thin layer of connective tissue, the **endomysium.** This connective tissue enables each muscle fiber to react independently of the others when stimulated by nerve impulses. Surrounding each fascicle is a tough sheath of fibrous connective tissue, the **perimysium.**

Surrounding the fasciculi of the muscle is another layer of coarser connective tissue that is called the **epimysium.** Exterior to the epimysium is the **deep fascia,** which covers the entire muscle. Since this muscle lies close to the skin, the deep fascia of this muscle would have fibers that intermesh with the *superficial fascia* that lies between the muscle and the skin. The connective tissue fibers of the deep fascia are also continuous with the tissue in the tendons, ligaments, and periosteum. Illustration A reveals the continuity of the connective tissue of the endomysium, perimysium, and epimysium. A fasciculus of muscle fibers is shown bracketed in this illustration.

Laboratory Assignment

Label figure 16.1.

Examine some muscles in a freshly killed or embalmed animal, identifying as many of the aforementioned structures as possible.

Complete the middle portion of combined Laboratory Report 15-17.

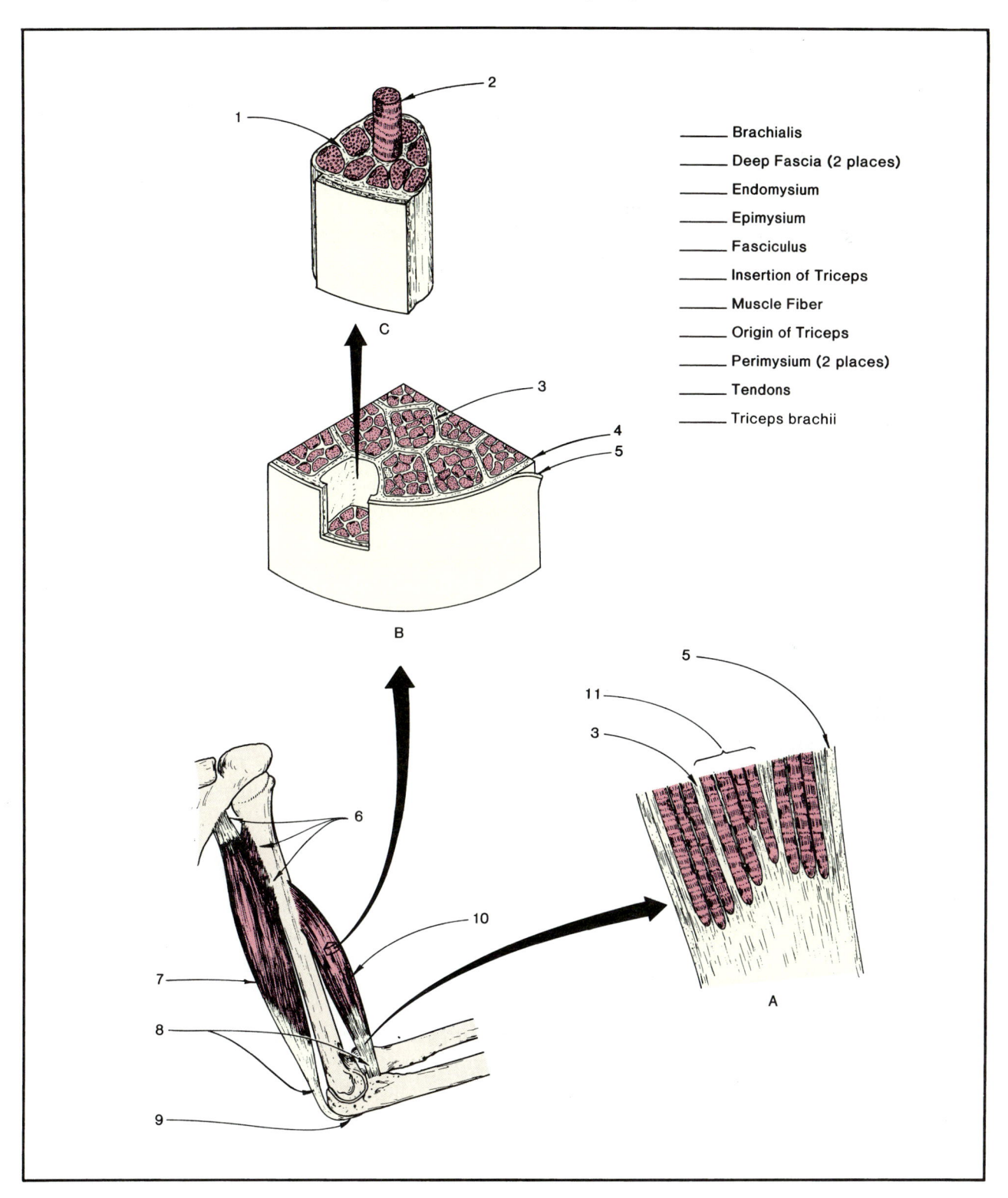

_____ Brachialis

_____ Deep Fascia (2 places)

_____ Endomysium

_____ Epimysium

_____ Fasciculus

_____ Insertion of Triceps

_____ Muscle Fiber

_____ Origin of Triceps

_____ Perimysium (2 places)

_____ Tendons

_____ Triceps brachii

Figure 16.1 Muscle anatomy and attachment.

17 Body Movements

The action of muscles through diarthrotic joints results in a variety of types of movement. The nature of movement is dependent on the construction of the individual joint and the position of the muscle. Muscles working through hinge joints result in movements that are primarily in one plane. Ball and socket joints, on the other hand, will have many axes through which movement can occur; thus, movement through these joints is in many planes. The different types of movement are as follows.

Flexion When the angle between two parts of a limb is decreased the limb is said to be *flexed*. Flexion of the arm takes place at the elbow when the antebrachium is moved toward the brachium. The term *flexion* may also be applied to movement of the head against the chest and the thigh against the abdomen.

When the foot is flexed upward, the flexion is designated as being **dorsiflexion.** Movement of the sole of the foot downward, or flexion of the toes, is called **plantar flexion.**

Extension Increasing the angle between two portions of a limb or two parts of the body is *extension*. Straightening the arm from a flexed position is an example of extension. Extension of the foot at the ankle is essentially the same as plantar flexion. When extension goes beyond the normal posture, as in leaning backward, the term **hyperextension** is used.

Abduction and Adduction The movement of a limb away from the median line of the body is called *abduction*. When the limb moves toward the median line, *adduction* occurs. These terms may also be applied to parts of a limb, such as the fingers and toes, by using the longitudinal axes of the limbs as points of reference.

Rotation and Circumduction The movement of a bone or limb around its longitudinal axis without lateral displacement is *rotation*. Rotation of the arm occurs through the shoulder joint. The head can be rotated through movement in the cervical vertebrae. If the rotational movement of a limb through a freely movable joint describes a circle at its terminus, the movement is called *circumduction*. The arm, leg, and fingers can be circumducted.

Supination and Pronation Rotation of the antebrachium at the elbow affects the position of the palm. When the palm is raised upward from a downward facing position, *supination* occurs. When the rotation is reversed so that the palm is returned to a downward position, *pronation* takes place.

Inversion and Eversion These two terms apply to foot movements. When the sole of the foot is turned inward or toward the median line, *inversion* occurs. When the sole is turned outward, *eversion* takes place.

Sphincter Action Circular muscles such as those around the lips (*orbicularis oris*) and the eye (*orbicularis oculi*) are called sphincter muscles. When their fibers shorten they close the opening.

Muscle Grouping

For reasons of simplicity, muscles are often studied individually, as in figure 17.1. It should be kept in mind, however, that seldom, if ever, do they act singly. Rather, muscles are arranged in groups with specific functions to perform, i.e., flexion and extension, abduction and adduction, supination and pronation.

The flexors are the prime movers, or **agonists.** The opposing muscles, or **antagonists,** contribute to smooth movements by their power to maintain tone and give way to movement by the flexor group. Variance in the tension of the flexor muscles results in a reverse reaction in the extensor muscles.

Muscles that assist the agonists to reduce undesired action or unnecessary movement are called **synergists.** Other groups of muscles that hold structures in position for action are called **fixation muscles.**

Laboratory Report

Identify the types of movement in figure 17.1 and complete the last portion of Laboratory Report 15-17.

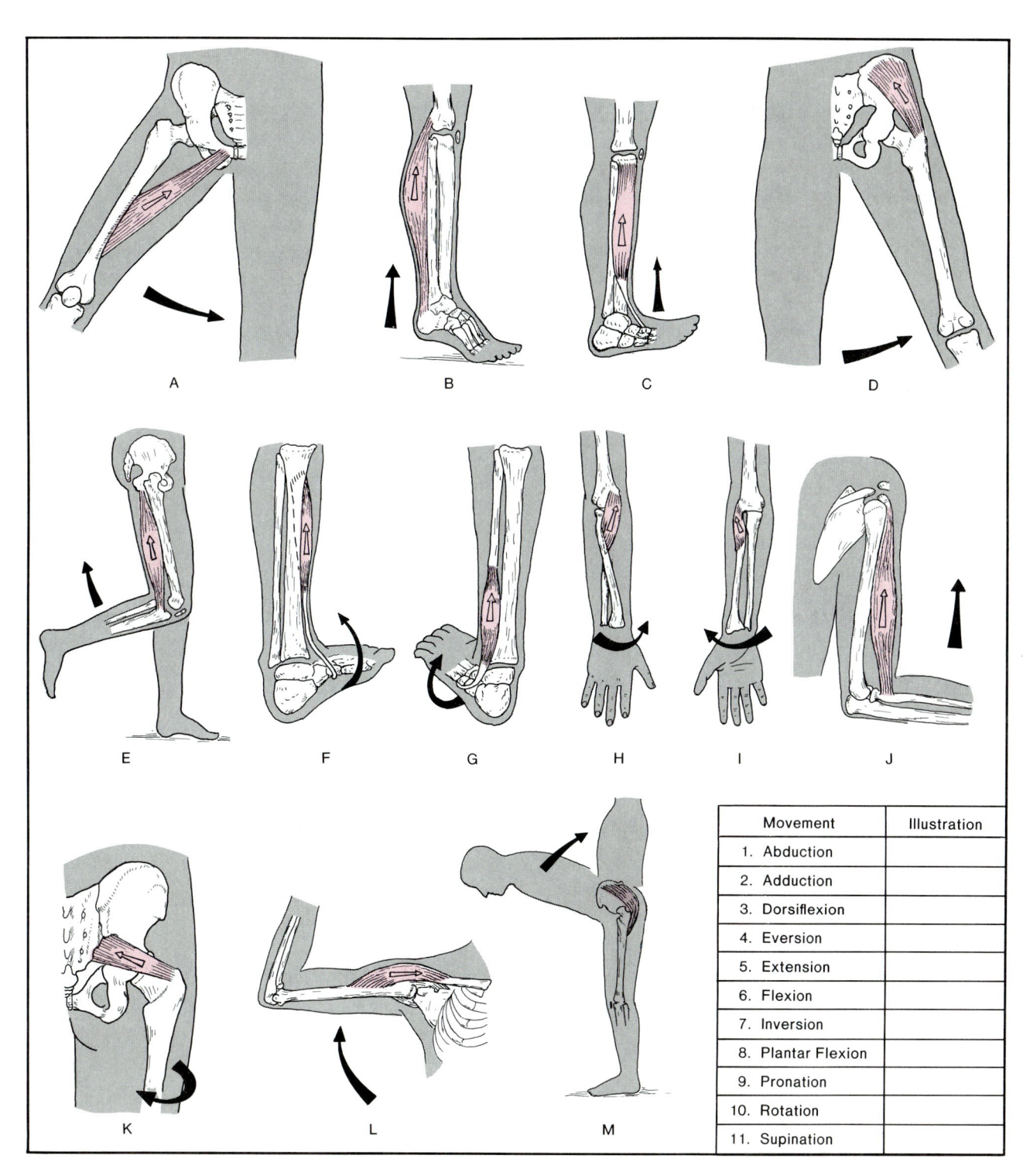

Movement	Illustration
1. Abduction	
2. Adduction	
3. Dorsiflexion	
4. Eversion	
5. Extension	
6. Flexion	
7. Inversion	
8. Plantar Flexion	
9. Pronation	
10. Rotation	
11. Supination	

Figure 17.1 Body movements.

18 Cat Dissection: Skin Removal

In preparation for the muscle studies in the next few exercises it will be necessary to remove the skin from your cat. Once removed, the skin will be used as a wrap for the carcass to prevent dehydration.

Laboratory cats are preserved with a mixture of alcohol and formaldehyde that is unpleasant to the nose, eyes, and skin; yet, this preservative is essential in preventing bacterial deterioration of the specimen. Protection of the hands is best achieved with rubber gloves. If gloves are not used, a protective cream, such as *Protek,* affords some protection to the skin. The latter is rubbed into the pores of the skin before dissection begins.

Students will work in pairs to dissect their cat. At the end of each laboratory period the specimen will be packed away in a plastic bag and sealed tightly with a name tag tied to one end. Under no circumstances should a student use any other student's cat for dissection.

When the dissection is completed, your specimen should look like the one illustrated in figure 18.1. Proceed as follows:

Materials:

    cat (preserved and injected)
    dissecting board or tray
    dissecting instruments
    plastic bag for cat
    rubber gloves or Protek
    hand lotion

1. Place the cat ventral side down on a dissecting board. Make a short incision on the midline of the neck region with a sharp scalpel, as illustrated in figure 18.2. Cut only through the skin, which is about ⅛ inch thick here. Avoid cutting into the muscles beneath the skin.
2. With a pair of scissors or scalpel continue the incision along the back midline all the way to the tail. See figure 18.3.

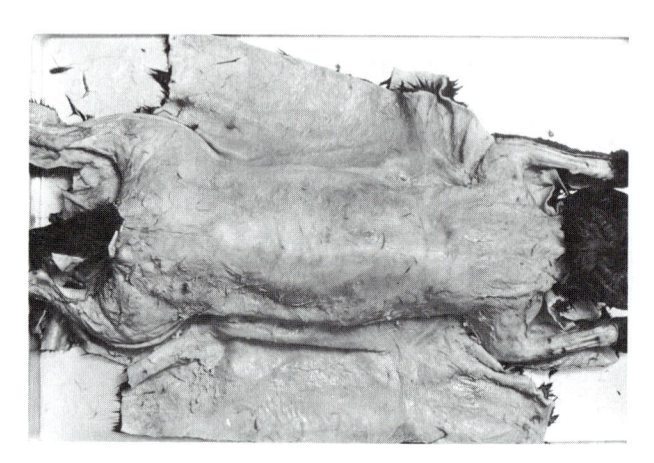

Figure 18.1 Cat with skin removed.

3. As illustrated in figures 18.4 and 18.5, separate the skin from the body muscles by pulling on it and severing the superficial fascia with a scalpel.
4. From the tail, make incisions down each hind leg to the ankles and cut all around each ankle. See figure 18.6.
5. As shown in figure 18.7, cut the skin around the neck and down each foreleg to the wrists. Cut the skin around each wrist.
6. Now, gripping the skin with your fingers, gently pull it away from the body. If your specimen is a female, look for the **mammary glands** on the underside of the abdomen and thorax. Remove glands and discard.
7. If laboratory time is still available, proceed to the next exercise to study the neck muscles of your cat.
8. If no more time is available, clean your instruments and tray with soap and water and scrub down your desktop to get rid of any debris. Your table should be left as clean as it was when you entered the room. Wrap the specimen in the skin and seal it in the plastic bag. Attach a label with your names. Place the cat in the assigned storage bin.
9. After washing your hands with soap and water, apply hand lotion.

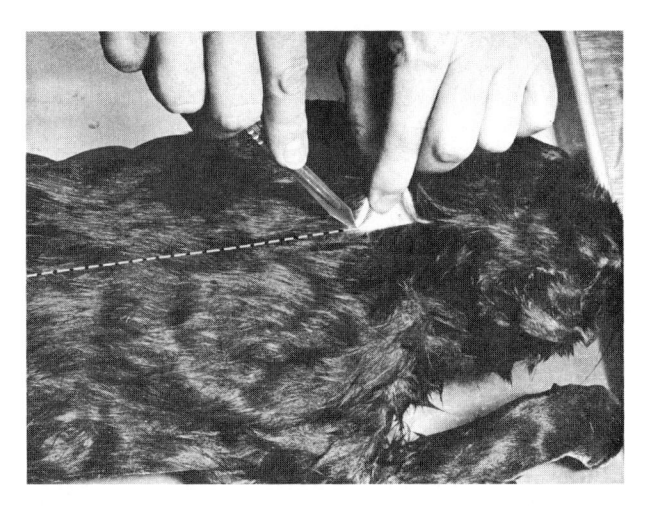

Figure 18.2 Make the first cut in neck region with a sharp scalpel. Be careful to cut only through the skin, not into the muscles.

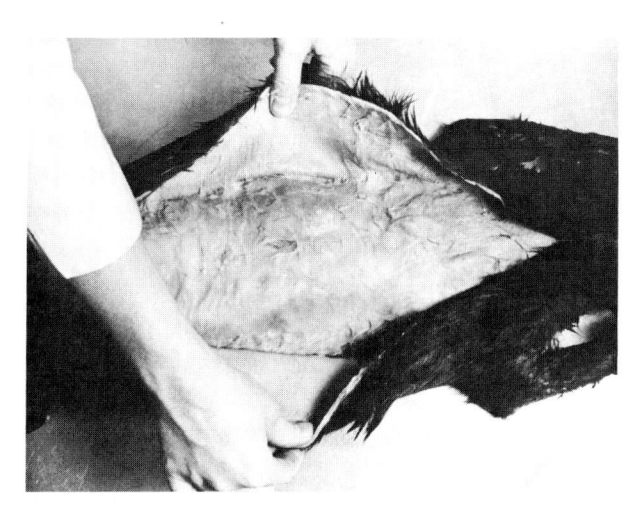

Figure 18.5 Separate as much of the skin as possible from the muscles of the body before proceeding to the next step.

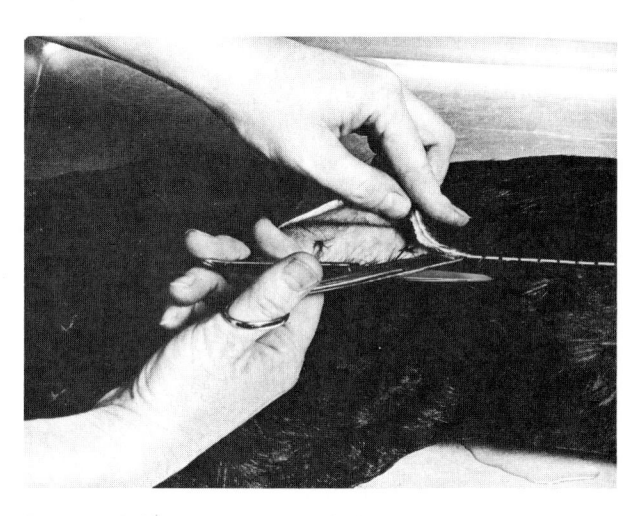

Figure 18.3 With a pair of sharp scissors (or a very sharp scalpel) cut the skin along the back from the neck to the tail region.

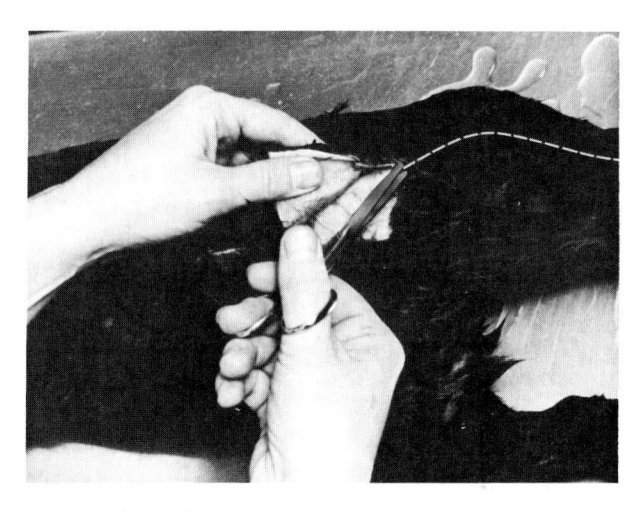

Figure 18.6 With scissors cut the skin around the tail and down each of the hind legs to the ankles. Cut around each ankle.

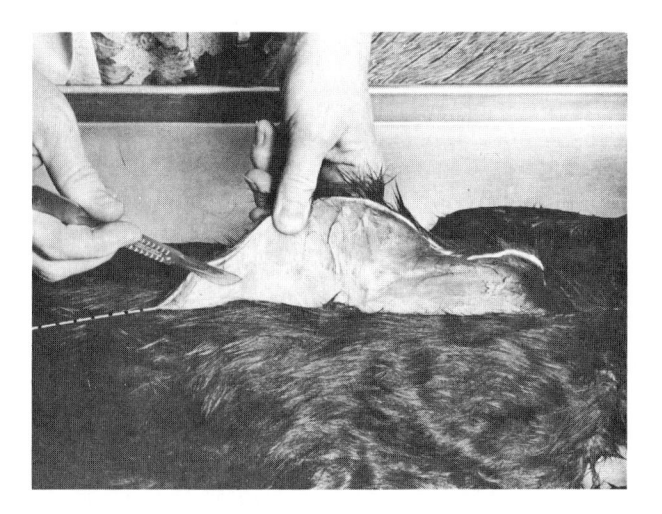

Figure 18.4 Pull the skin away from the muscles, using the scalpel to separate the superficial fascia from the muscles.

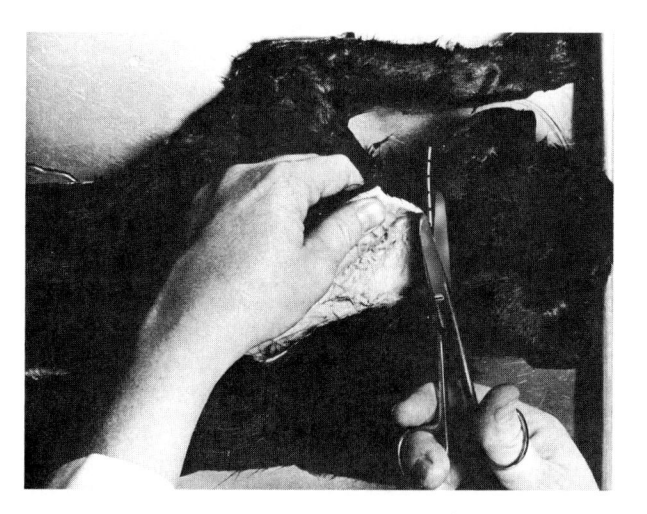

Figure 18.7 With scissors cut the skin around the neck and down each side of the front legs to the wrists. Cut around wrists.

19 Head and Neck Muscles

The principal muscles of the head and neck will be studied in this exercise. Depending on the availability of materials, muscle manikins, cadavers, or cat dissection may be used for laboratory studies. The head muscles are grouped here according to their functions.

Scalp Movements

Removal of the scalp reveals an underlying muscle known as the **epicranial.** It consists of the **frontalis** in the forehead region, an **occipitalis** in the occiput region, and an aponeurosis extending between these two over the top of the skull.

The occipitalis has its *origin* on the mastoid process and occipital bone; its *insertion* is on the aponeurosis. The frontalis takes its *origin* on the aponeurosis and its *insertion* on the soft tissue of the eyebrows.

Action: Contraction of the frontalis causes horizontal wrinkling of the forehead and elevation of the eyebrows. Action of the occipitalis causes the scalp to be pulled backward.

Sphincter Action

Circular muscles that close openings are called *sphincters.* The eyes and mouth are surrounded by muscles of this type.

Orbicularis oris This circular muscle lies just under the skin of the lips. It takes its *origin* in various facial muscles, the maxilla, mandible, and septum of the nose. Its *insertion* is on the lips.

Action: It closes the lips in various ways: by compression over the teeth, or by pouting and pursing them; utilized in kissing.

Orbicularis oculi Each eye is surrounded by one of these sphincters. Each muscle *arises* from the nasal portion of the frontal bone, the frontal process of the maxilla, and the medial palpebral ligament. It *inserts* within the tissues of the eyelids (palpebrae).

Action: Blinking and squinting.

Facial Expressions

Emotions such as pleasure, sadness, fear, and anger are expressed by certain muscles of the face. The following five muscles play different roles in facial expressions.

Zygomaticus This muscle extends diagonally from the zygomatic bone to the corner of the mouth. Its *origin* is on the zygomatic; its *insertion* is on the edge of the orbicularis oris.

Action: Contraction of these muscles draws the angles of the mouth upward and backward as in smiling and laughing.

Quadratus labii superioris This thin muscle, consisting of three heads, lies between the eye and upper lip. Its *origin* is on the upper part of the maxilla and part of the zygomatic bone. Its *insertion* is mainly on the superior margin of the orbicularis oris, and partially on the alar region of the nose.

Action: Furrowing of the upper lip occurs when the entire muscle contracts; result: expression of disdain or contempt. Expression of sadness occurs if only the infraorbital head contracts.

Quadratus labii inferioris This small muscle extends from the lower lip to the mandible. Its *origin* is on the mandible, and its *insertion* is on the lower margin of the orbicularis oris.

Action: It pulls the lower lip down in irony.

Triangularis This muscle is lateral to the quadratus labii inferioris. Its *origin* is on the mandible. Its *insertion* is on the orbicularis oris.

Action: Since it is an antagonist of the zygomaticus, it depresses the corner of the mouth.

Platysma This broad sheetlike muscle extends from the mandible over the side of the neck. Only a portion of it is seen in figure 19.1. Figure 19.2 (label 3) reveals its entirety. Since its *insertion* is on the mandible and muscles around the mouth, it profoundly affects facial expressions. Contraction causes the lower lip to move backward and downward, expressing horror.

Masticatory Movements

The chewing of food (mastication) involves five pairs of muscles. Four pairs move the mandible and one pair helps to hold the food in place. All of these muscles are revealed in illustrations A and B, figure 19.1.

Masseter Of the four muscles that move the mandible, the masseter is most powerful. It extends from the angle of the mandible to the zygomatic. Only the lower portion of this muscle is seen in illustration A; its entirety is seen on the large illustration. Its *origin* is on the zygomatic arch, and it *inserts* on the mandible.

Action: It raises the mandible.

Temporalis The large fan-shaped muscle on the side of the skull is the temporalis. It *arises* on portions of the frontal, parietal, and temporal bones and is *inserted* on the coronoid process of the mandible.

Action: It acts synergistically with the masseter to raise the mandible. It can also cause retraction of the mandible when only the posterior fibers of the muscle are activated.

Pterygoideus internus (*Internal pterygoid*) The position of this muscle has led some to refer to it as the "internal masseter." It lies on the medial surface of the ramus, taking its *origin* on the maxilla, sphenoid, and palatine bones. Its *insertion* is on the medial surface of the mandible between the mylohyoid line and the angle. See illustration B, figure 19.1.

Action: It works synergistically with the masseter and temporalis to raise the mandible.

Pterygoideus externus (*External pterygoid*) This muscle is the uppermost one in illustration B. It *arises* on the sphenoid bone and *inserts* on the neck of the mandibular condyle and the articular disk of the joint.

Action: Acting together, the two external pterygoids can cause the mandible to move forward (protrusion), and downward. Individually, they can move the mandible, laterally, to the right or left.

Buccinator The horizontal muscle that partially obscures the teeth in illustration B is the buccinator. It is situated in the cheeks (*buccae*) on each side of the mouth. It *arises* on the maxilla, mandible, and a ligament, the **pterygomandibular raphé** (figure 19.1, label 17). This ligament joins the buccinator to the **constrictor pharyngis superioris.** The buccinator *inserts* on the orbicularis oris.

Action: It compresses the cheek to hold food between the teeth during chewing.

Assignment:

Locate all these muscles on a muscle manikin or cadaver.

Label figure 19.1.

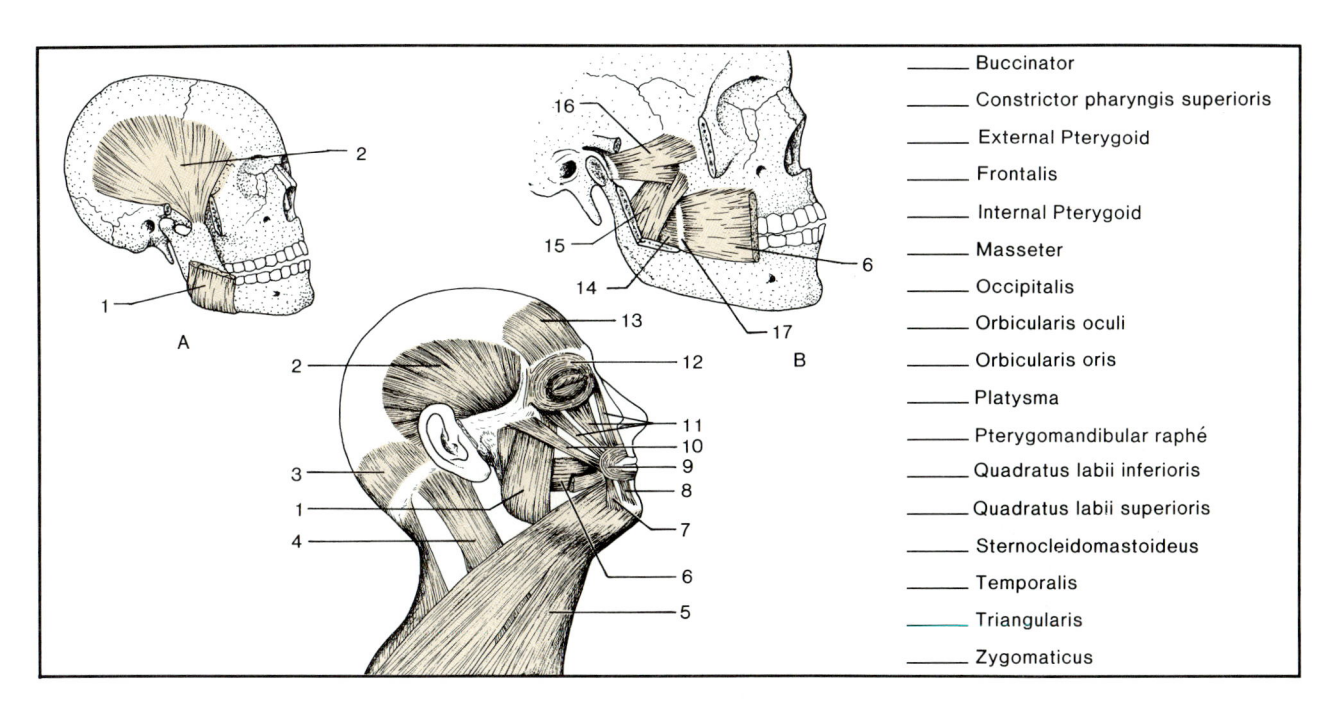

	Buccinator
	Constrictor pharyngis superioris
	External Pterygoid
	Frontalis
	Internal Pterygoid
	Masseter
	Occipitalis
	Orbicularis oculi
	Orbicularis oris
	Platysma
	Pterygomandibular raphé
	Quadratus labii inferioris
	Quadratus labii superioris
	Sternocleidomastoideus
	Temporalis
	Triangularis
	Zygomaticus

Figure 19.1   Head muscles.

Neck Muscles

Figure 19.2 and 19.3 illustrate a majority of the major muscles of the neck region. While figure 19.2 is primarily of surface and posterior deep muscles, figure 19.3 reveals the deeper anterior muscles.

Surface Muscles

The principal surface muscles of the neck are the platysma on the anterolateral surfaces, and the trapezius on the back of the neck.

Platysma It was noted on page 86 that this muscle takes its *insertion* on the mandible and the muscles around the mouth. Its *origin* is primarily the fascia that covers the pectoralis and deltoideus muscles of the shoulder region.

> *Action:* Primarily to draw the lower lip backward and downward; assists to some extent in opening the jaws.

Trapezius This large triangular muscle occupies the upper shoulder region of the back. Only its upper portion functions as a neck muscle. It *arises* on the occipital bone, the ligamentum nuchae, and the spinous processes of the seventh cervical and all thoracic vertebrae. The **ligamentum nuchae** is a ligament that extends from the occipital bone to the seventh cervical vertebra, uniting the spinous processes of all the cervical vertebrae. The *insertion* of this muscle is on the spine and acromion of the scapula and the outer third of the clavicle.

Action: Pulls the scapula toward the median line (adduction); raises the scapula, as in shrugging the shoulder, and draws the head backward (hyperextension), if the shoulders are fixed.

Deeper Neck Muscles, Posterior

Illustration C, figure 19.2, reveals three posterior muscles of the neck as seen when the trapezius is removed. Another prominent muscle, the levator scapulae, has been omitted here for clarity. It will be studied in the next exercise.

Splenius capitis This muscle lies just beneath the trapezius and medial to the levator scapulae. Only the left splenius is shown in illustration C. Its *origin* is on the ligamentum nuchae and the spinous processes of the seventh cervical and upper three thoracic vertebrae. Its *insertion* is on the mastoid process.

> *Action:* Hyperextension of the head if both muscles act together; however, if only one muscle contracts, the head is inclined and rotated toward the contracting muscle.

Semispinalis capitis This muscle is the larger of two muscles shown on the right side of the neck. Its *origin* consists of the transverse processes of the upper six thoracic vertebrae and the articular processes of the lower four cervical vertebrae. The *insertion* is on the occipital bone.

> *Action:* Same as splenius capitis.

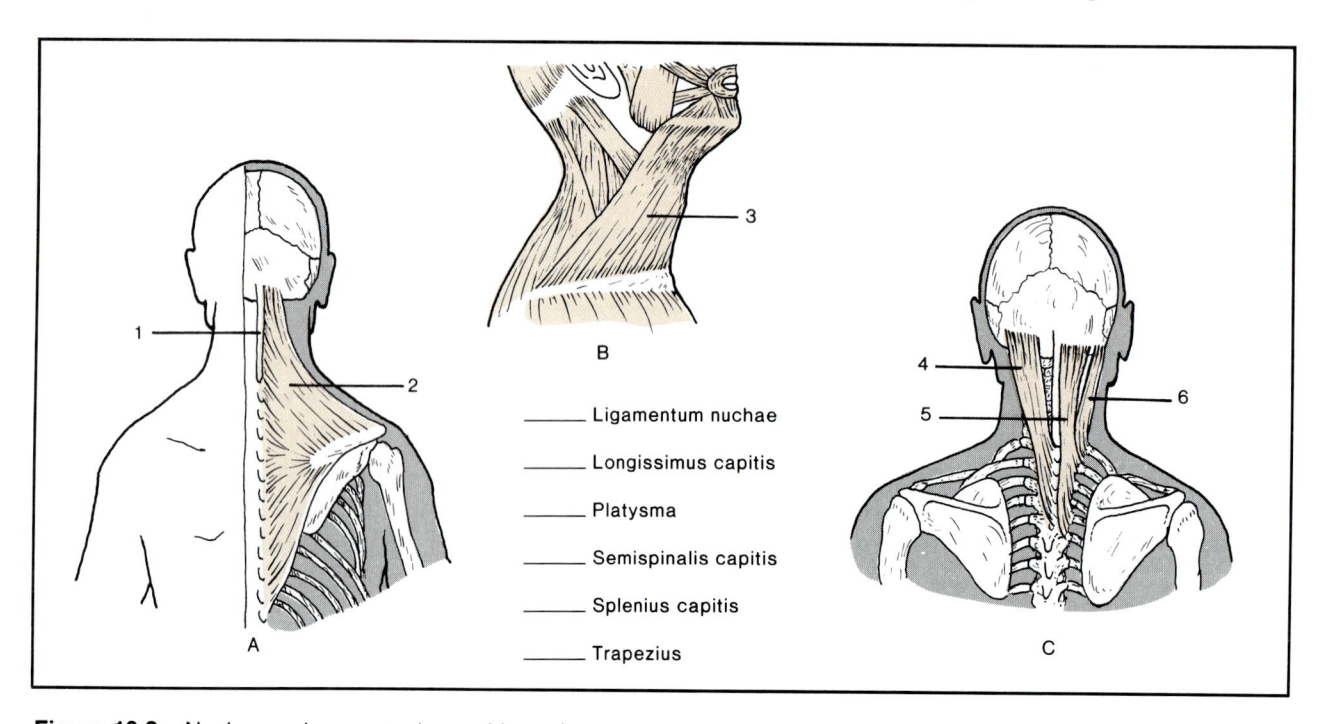

_____ Ligamentum nuchae

_____ Longissimus capitis

_____ Platysma

_____ Semispinalis capitis

_____ Splenius capitis

_____ Trapezius

Figure 19.2 Neck muscles, posterior and lateral.

Longissimus capitis This muscle is lateral and slightly anterior to the semispinalis capitis. The *origin* of this muscle is on the transverse processes of the first three thoracic vertebrae and the articular processes of the lower four cervical vertebrae. The *insertion* is on the mastoid process.

Action: Same as the above two muscles.

Deeper Neck Muscles, Anterior

Refer to figure 19.3 to identify the anterior muscles that are seen when the two platysma muscles are removed from the neck.

Sternocleidomastoideus This large neck muscle derives its name from the skeletal components that provide its anchorage. Its *origin* is located on the manubrium of the sternum and the sternal (medial) end of the clavicle. The *insertion* is on the mastoid process.

Action: Simultaneous contraction of both sternocleidomastoids causes the head to be flexed forward and downward on the chest. Independently, each muscle draws the head down toward the shoulder on the same side as the muscle.

Sternohyoideus This long muscle extends from the hyoid bone to the sternum and clavicle. The left sternohyoid is exposed in illustration D by the removal of the lower portion of the left sternocleidomastoid. The sternohyoid *arises* on a portion of the manubrium and clavicle. It *inserts* on the lower border of the hyoid bone.

Action: Draws the hyoid bone downward.

Sternothyroideus This muscle is somewhat shorter than the sternohyoideus. It *originates* on the posterior surface of the manubrium and *inserts* on the inferior edge of the thyroid cartilage of the larynx.

Action: Draws the thyroid cartilage of the larynx downward.

Omohyoideus The long curving muscle that is seen on the left side of the neck that extends from the hyoid bone into the shoulder region is the omohyoid. It *arises* from the upper surface of the scapula and *inserts* on the hyoid bone, lateral to the sternohyoid.

Action: Draws the hyoid bone downward.

Digastricus Two of these narrow V-shaped muscles are visible under the mandible in figure 36.3. Each muscle consists of anterior and posterior bellies with the central portion attached to the hyoid bone by a fibrous loop.

The posterior belly *arises* from the medial side of the mastoid process of the temporal bone. The anterior belly *arises* on the inner surface of the body of the mandible near the symphysis. The point of *insertion* is the fibrous loop on the hyoid bone.

Action: Raises the hyoid bone and assists in lowering the mandible. Acting independently, the anterior belly can pull the hyoid bone forward; the posterior belly can pull it backward.

Mylohyoideus The two mylohyoids extend from the medial surfaces of the mandible to the median line of the head to form the floor of the mouth. They

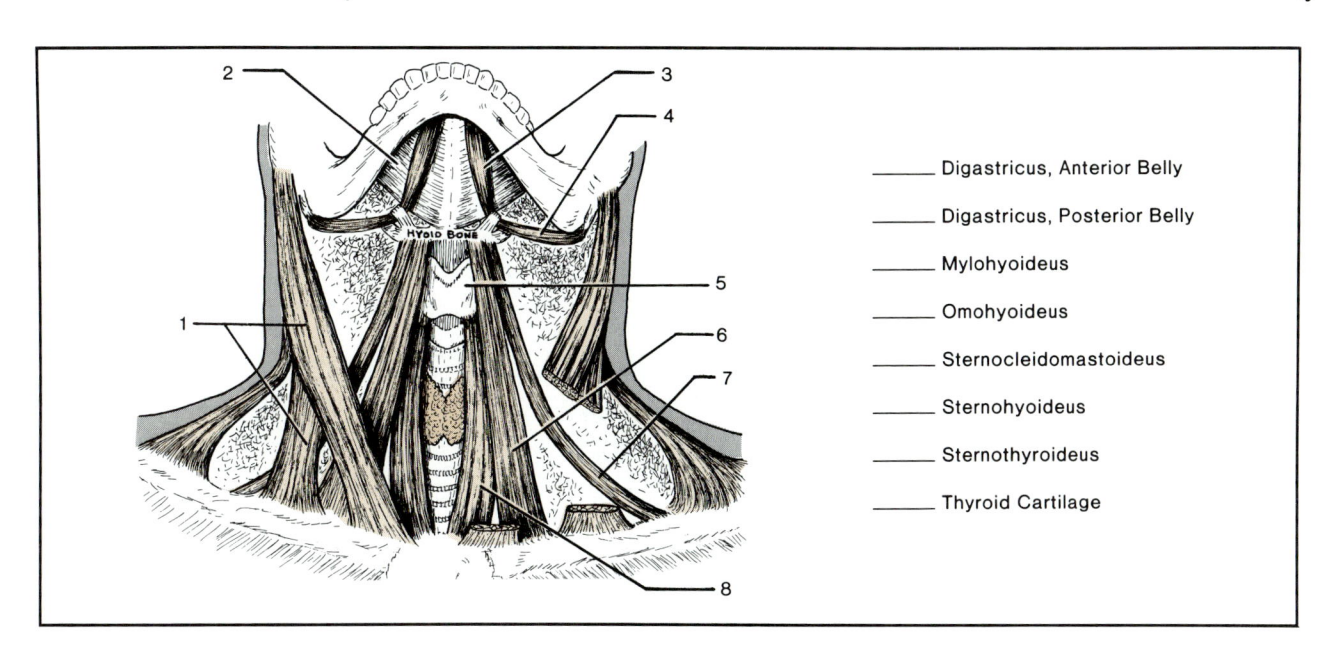

_____ Digastricus, Anterior Belly

_____ Digastricus, Posterior Belly

_____ Mylohyoideus

_____ Omohyoideus

_____ Sternocleidomastoideus

_____ Sternohyoideus

_____ Sternothyroideus

_____ Thyroid Cartilage

Figure 19.3 Neck muscles, anterior view (platysma removed).

lie just superior to the anterior bellies of the digastric muscles. Each mylohyoid *arises* along the mylohyoid line of the mandible and *inserts* on a median fibrous raphé that extends from the symphysis menti of the mandible to the hyoid bone.

Action: Raises the hyoid bone and tongue.

Assignment:

Label figures 19.2 and 19.3 and proceed to cat dissection of neck muscles.

Cat Dissection

Once the skin has been removed from the cat, place the animal ventral side up on a dissecting tray and identify the neck muscles by referring to figures 19.4 and 19.5. Since an embalming incision, which destroys several muscles, has been made along one

side of the neck, perform your studies on the side of the neck opposite to the incision. As you read through these instructions, you will encounter three key words, that are defined as follows:

Dissect: To dissect a muscle in this laboratory means to use a probe to free the muscle from adjacent muscles, exposing its full length. The muscle is not to be cut up.

Transect: Transection involves cutting the muscle transversally with a scalpel or scissors.

Reflect: Once a muscle has been transected its cut ends can be lifted out of the way, or reflected, to expose deeper muscles.

It is important that the muscles on your specimen not be mutilated or accidentally removed, unless directed to do so. Muscle dissection should be methodical and careful. A good way to keep

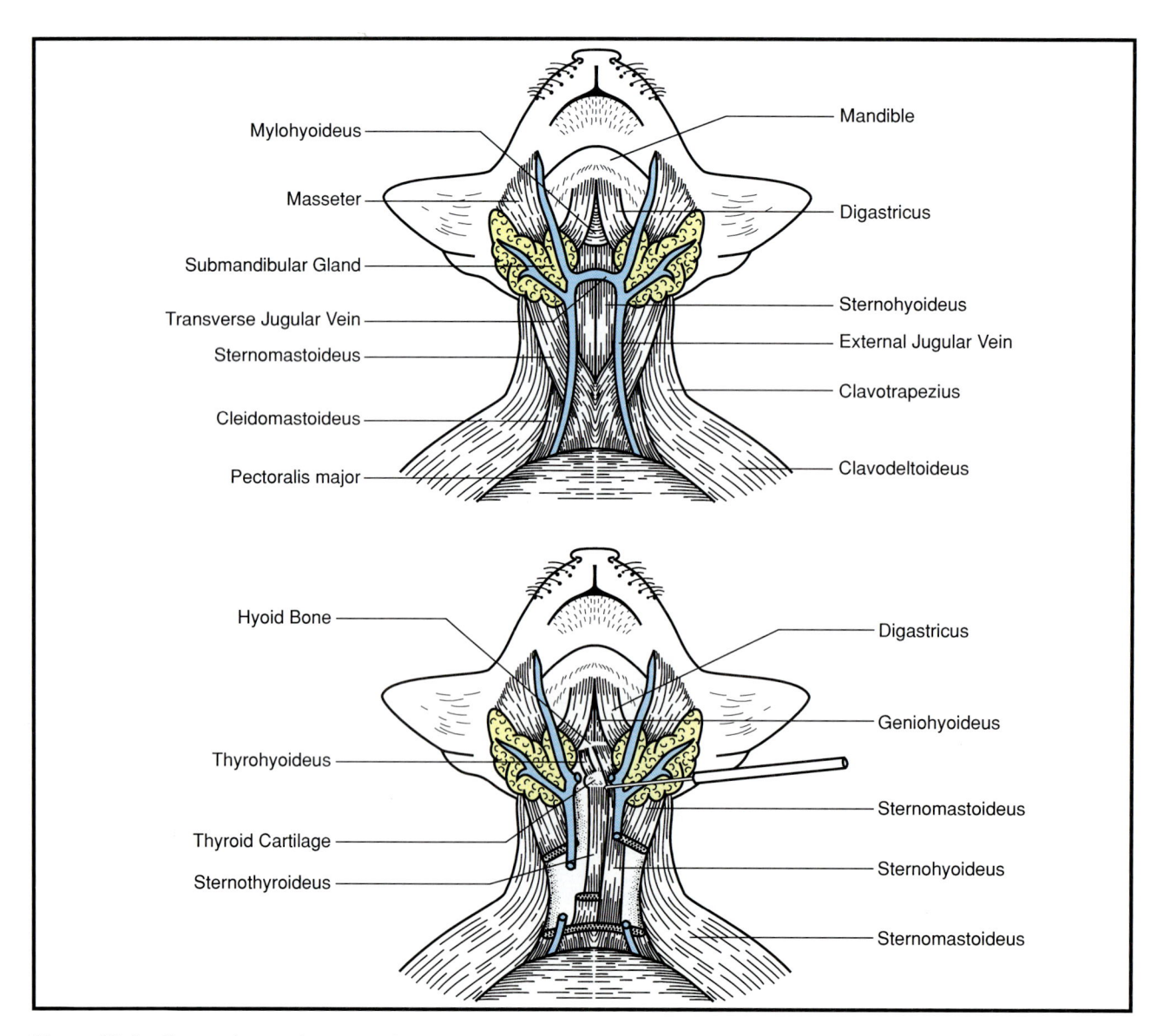

Figure 19.4 Cat neck muscles, superficial and deep.

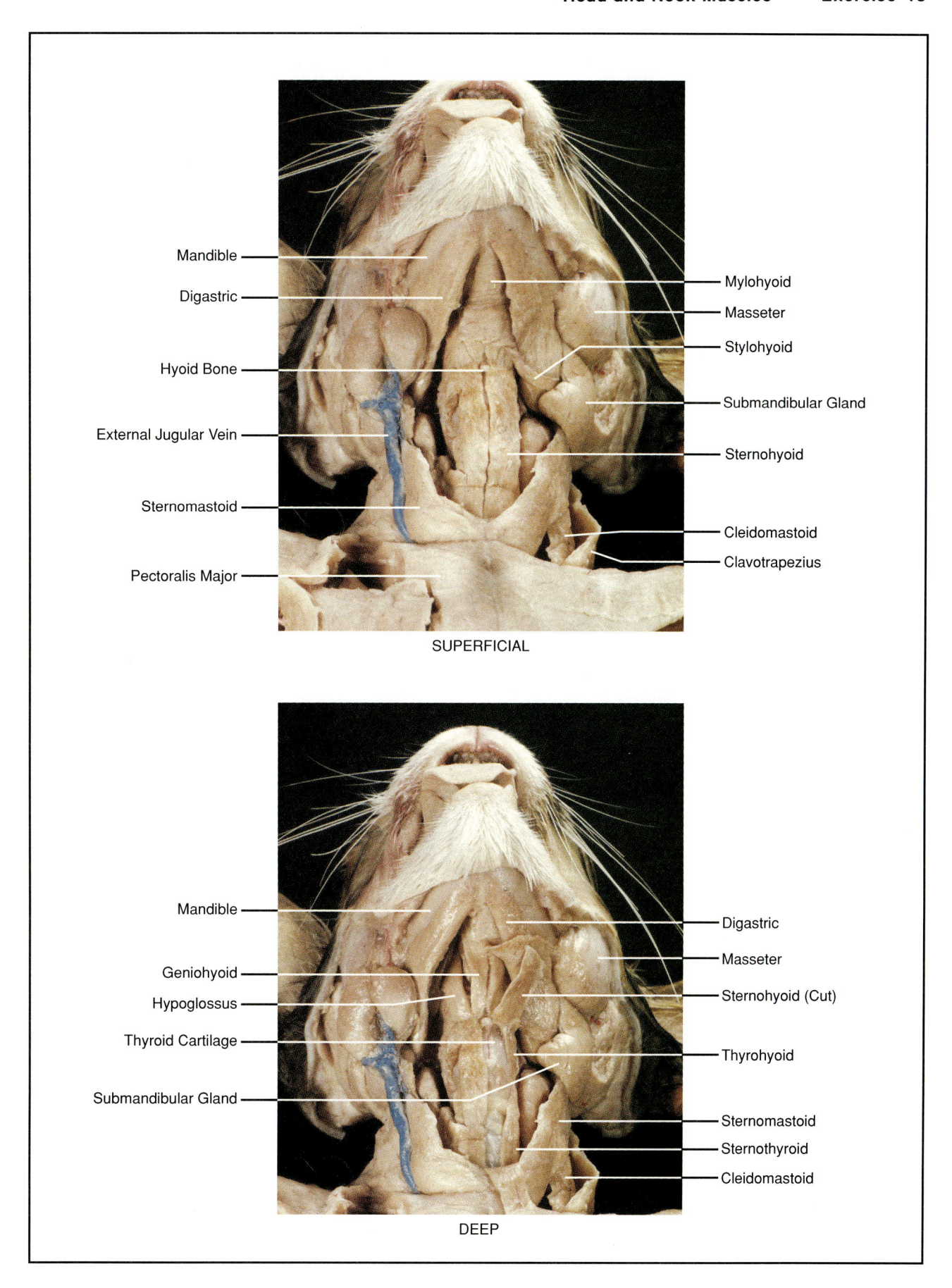

Mandible

Digastric

Hyoid Bone

External Jugular Vein

Sternomastoid

Pectoralis Major

Mylohyoid

Masseter

Stylohyoid

Submandibular Gland

Sternohyoid

Cleidomastoid

Clavotrapezius

SUPERFICIAL

Mandible

Geniohyoid

Hypoglossus

Thyroid Cartilage

Submandibular Gland

Digastric

Masseter

Sternohyoid (Cut)

Thyrohyoid

Sternomastoid

Sternothyroid

Cleidomastoid

DEEP

Figure 19.5   Cat neck muscles, superficial and deep.

track of muscles as they are identified is to color each of the muscles on the diagrams with different colored pencils. This procedure may also be helpful for review purposes.

Digastric Like the human digastric, this superficial muscle has two portions, an anterior belly and a posterior belly. The anterior belly is attached to the mandible and the posterior belly is attached to the mastoid process of the skull.

Mylohyoid This thin, flat muscle with fibers that course horizontally below the mandible, lies deep to the anterior belly of the diagastric. Pull the anterior bellies of the diagastric muscles laterally to see the full extent of the mylohyoid.

Sternomastoid This bandlike muscle extends from the manubrium of the sternum to the mastoid portion of the temporal bone, and lies deep to the external jugular vein.

Note that the right and left sternomastoid muscles fuse in the midline. Cut through this point of fusion in the caudal direction to the manubrium. _Dissect_ the sternomastoid that is on the side opposite to the embalming incision.

Cleidomastoid Note that this narrow band of muscle is located between the sternomastoid and clavotrapezius. _Dissect_. What muscle in the human takes the place of these last two muscles?

Sternohyoid This straight, narrow muscle extends from the manubrium to the hyoid bone, covering the larynx and trachea. _Dissect_. It will be necessary to cut away the transverse jugular vein at this time.

Sternothyroid This narrow band of muscle is lateral and dorsal to the sternohyoid. It extends from the manubrium to the thyroid cartilage of the larynx. To expose the sternothyroid, it will be necessary to lift up the sternohyoid and push it to one side. _Dissect_.

Thyrohyoid Cranial to the sternothyroid, and extending between the hyoid bone and the lateral portion of the thyroid cartilage, is a very small muscle, the thyrohyoid.

Masseter This most powerful muscle of mastication is seen as a large, rounded muscle in the cheek region. Its origin is on the zygomatic arch and its insertion is on the lateral surface of the mandible.

Laboratory Report

Complete the Laboratory Report for this exercise.

Trunk and Shoulder Muscles 20

In this study of the trunk and shoulder muscles, all of the surface and a majority of the deeper muscles will be studied. These muscles function primarily to move the shoulders, upper arms, spine, and head. Some of them assist in respiration.

Anterior Muscles

Removal of the skin and subcutaneous fat from the body will reveal muscles as shown in figure 20.1.

Surface Muscles

Pectoralis major This muscle is the thick fan-shaped one that occupies the upper quadrant of the chest. Its *origin* is on the clavicle, sternum, costal cartilages, and the aponeurosis of the external oblique. It *inserts* in the groove between the greater and lesser tubercles of the humerus.

Action: Adducts, flexes, and rotates the humerus medially.

Deltoideus This muscle is the principal muscle of the shoulder. It *originates* on the lateral third of the clavicle, the acromion, and the spine of the scapula. It *inserts* on the deltoid tuberosity of the humerus.

Action: Abduction of the arm when the entire muscle is activated; flexion, extension, and rotation (medial and lateral) take place when only certain parts of the muscle are activated.

Serratus anterior The upper and lateral surfaces of the rib cage are covered by this muscle. It takes its *origin* on the upper eight or nine ribs and *inserts* on the anterior surface of the scapula near the vertebral border.

Action: Pulls the scapula forward, downward, and inward toward the chest wall.

Deeper Muscles

Pectoralis minor This muscle lies beneath the pectoralis major and is completely obscured by the

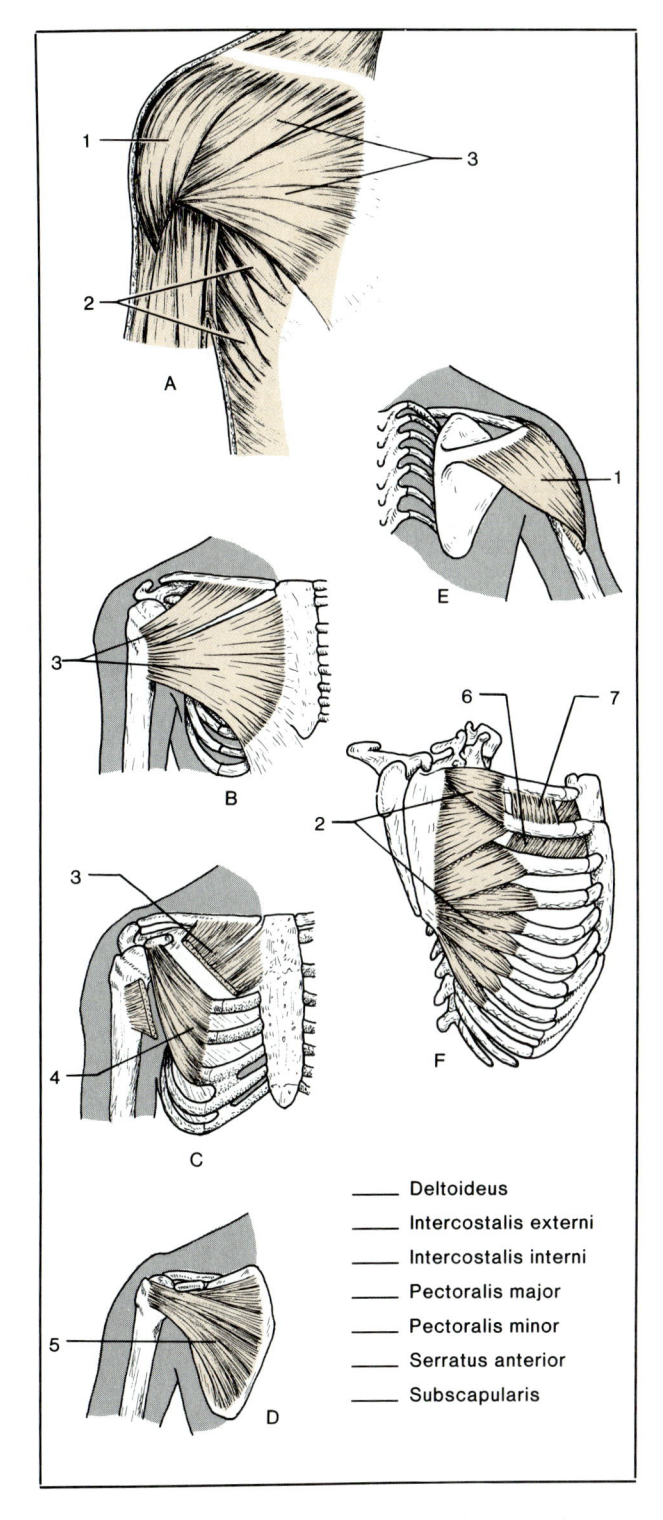

_____ Deltoideus
_____ Intercostalis externi
_____ Intercostalis interni
_____ Pectoralis major
_____ Pectoralis minor
_____ Serratus anterior
_____ Subscapularis

Figure 20.1   Shoulder and trunk muscles, anterior.

latter. It *arises* on the third, fourth, and fifth ribs, and *inserts* on the coracoid process of the scapula.

>Action: Draws the scapula forward and downward with some rotation.

Intercostalis externi (*External intercostals*) Between the ribs on both sides are eleven pairs of short muscles, the external intercostals. The *origin* of each of these muscles is on the lower outer border of the upper rib; the *insertion* is on the upper outer border of the lower rib. Their fibers are directed obliquely forward on the front of the ribs. Label 7 in figure 20.1 illustrates one of these muscles.

>Action: They pull the ribs closer to each other, causing them to be raised. Raising the ribs increases the volume of the thorax to cause inspiration of air in breathing.

Intercostalis interni (*Internal intercostals*) These antagonists of the external intercostals lie on the internal surface of the rib cage. The complete rib cage is lined with these muscles.

Each internal intercostal *arises* from the lower inner margin of the upper rib and *inserts* on the upper inner margin of the rib below. The fibers of these muscles are oriented in a direction that is opposite to the fibers of the external intercostals.

>Action: Draw adjacent ribs closer together. This action has the effect of lowering the ribs and decreasing the volume of the thoracic cavity. Expiration of air from the lungs results.

Subscapularis The anterior surface of the scapula is almost completely covered by this muscle. It takes its *origin* on the axillary border of the scapula and on an aponeurosis which separates the muscle from the teres major and long head of the triceps brachii. Its *insertion* is on the lesser tubercle of the humerus and the anterior portion of the joint capsule.

>Action: Rotates the arm medially; assists in other directional movements of the arm, depending on position of the arm.

Assignment:

Label figure 20.1.

Posterior Muscles

The muscles of the upper back region that are revealed when the skin is removed are shown in illustration A, figure 20.2. The deeper muscles of the back and shoulder are shown in illustrations B, C, and D of figure 20.2.

Latissimus dorsi This large muscle of the back covers the lumbar area. It takes its *origin* in a broad aponeurosis that is attached to thoracic and lumbar vertebrae, the spine of the sacrum, iliac crest, and the lower ribs. Its *insertion* is on the intertubercular groove of the humerus.

>Action: Extends, adducts, and rotates the arm medially; draws the shoulder downward and backward.

Infraspinatus This muscle derives its name from its position. It is attached to the inferior margin of the scapular spine. Although a portion of it can be seen in illustration A, its complete structure cannot be seen unless the deltoideus and trapezius are removed as in illustration C. Its *origin* occupies the infraspinous fossa. Its *insertion* is the middle facet of the greater tubercle of the humerus.

>Action: Rotates the humerus laterally.

Teres major Of the three muscles that cover most of the scapula in illustration C, the teres major is the most inferior one. Note that, although the latissimus dorsi obscures part of it, a greater portion of it is visible in illustration A. It *originates* near the inferior angle of the scapula and *inserts* into the crest of the lesser tubercle of the humerus.

>Action: Rotates the humerus medially and weakly adducts it.

Teres minor This small muscle lies between the infraspinatus and teres major. Only a small portion of it is visible in illustration A. It takes its *origin* from the lateral margin of the scapula and its *insertion* is on the lowest facet of the greater tubercle of the humerus.

>Action: Rotates the arm laterally and weakly adducts it.

Levator scapulae This muscle lies under the trapezius in the neck region. It takes its *origin* on the transverse processes of the first four cervical vertebrae. Its *insertion* is on the upper portion of the vertebral border of the scapula.

>Action: Raises the scapula and draws it medially. With the scapula in a fixed position, it can bend the neck laterally.

Supraspinatus This muscle is completely covered by the trapezius and deltoideus; thus, it cannot be seen in illustration A. It *arises* from the fossa above the scapular spine and *inserts* on the greater tubercle of the humerus.

>Action: Assists the deltoid in abduction of the humerus.

Rhomboideus major and minor These two muscles lie beneath the trapezius. They are flat muscles that extend from the vertebral border of the scapula to the spine (see illustration C).

The rhomboideus minor is the smaller one. It occupies a position between the levator scapulae and the rhomboideus major. It *arises* from the lower part of the ligamentum nuchae and the first thoracic vertebra. It *inserts* on that part of the scapular vertebral margin where the scapular spine originates.

The rhomboideus major *arises* from the spinous processes of the second, third, fourth, and fifth thoracic vertebrae. It *inserts* below the rhomboideus minor on the vertebral border of the scapula.

Action: These two muscles act together to pull the scapula medially and slightly upward. The lower part of the major rotates the scapula to depress the lateral angle, assisting in adduction of the arm.

Sacrospinalis (*Erector spinae*) This long muscle extends over the back from the sacral region to the midshoulder region (see illustration B, figure 20.2). It consists of three portions: a lateral **iliocostalis,** an intermediate **longissimus,** and a medial **spinalis.** It *arises* from the lower and posterior portion of the sacrum, the iliac crest, and the lower two thoracic vertebrae. *Insertion* of the muscle is on the ribs and transverse processes of the vertebrae.

Action: This muscle is an extensor, pulling backward on the ribs and vertebrae to maintain erectness.

Assignment:

Label figure 20.2.

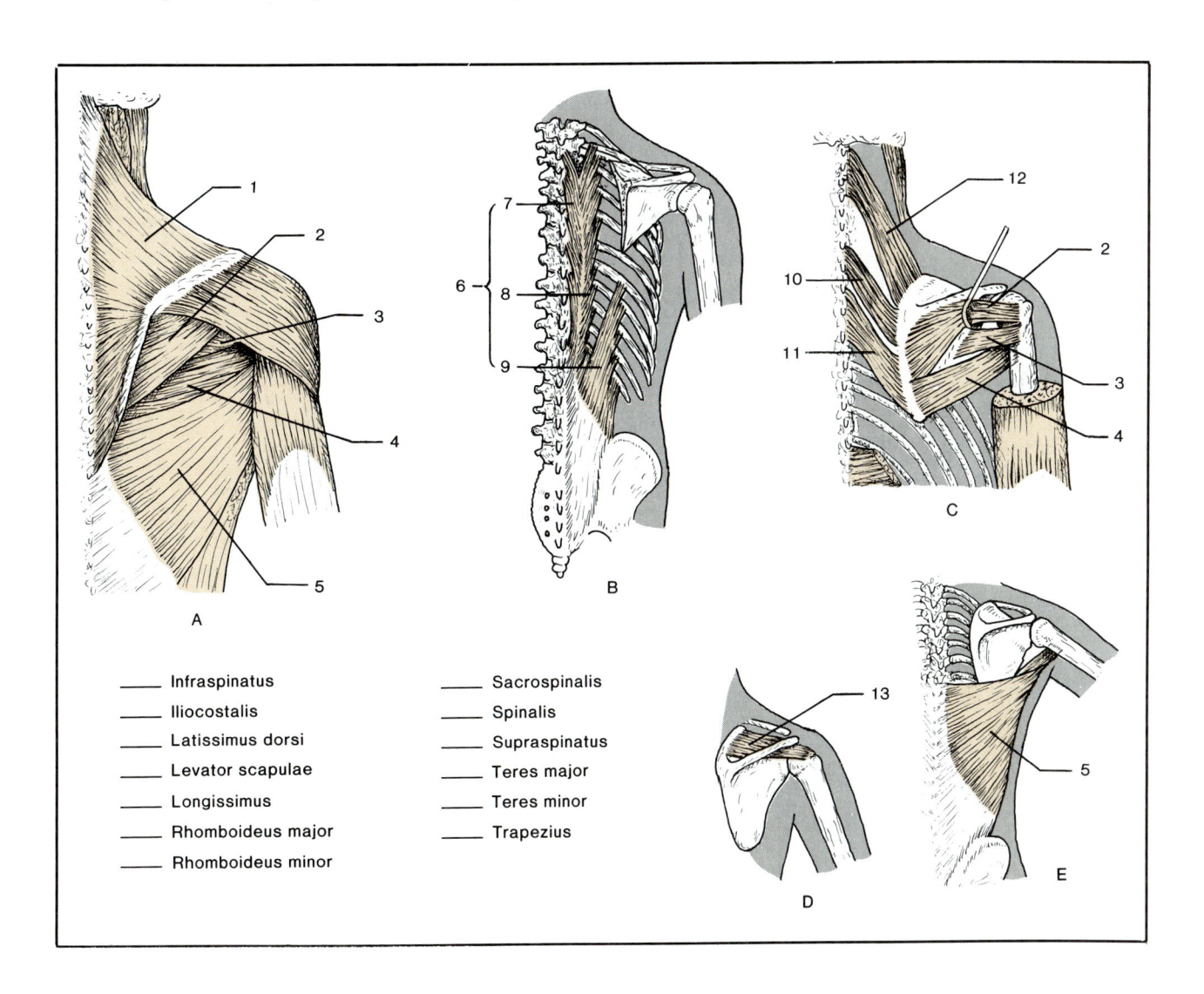

_____ Infraspinatus	_____ Sacrospinalis
_____ Iliocostalis	_____ Spinalis
_____ Latissimus dorsi	_____ Supraspinatus
_____ Levator scapulae	_____ Teres major
_____ Longissimus	_____ Teres minor
_____ Rhomboideus major	_____ Trapezius
_____ Rhomboideus minor	

Figure 20.2 Shoulder and back muscles.

Cat Thorax and Shoulder Muscles
(*Superficial*)

Cat muscles of the thorax fall in three categories: the pectoralis, trapezius, and deltoideus groups. Identify the superficial muscles first, using figures 20.3, 20.4 and 20.5 for reference. Only those muscles that have human homologs will be studied in detail.

Pectoralis Group

Pectoantebrachialis A narrow ribbonlike muscle about 1 cm. wide that extends from the upper sternum to the forearm fascia. Since there is no homolog in humans, transect and remove this muscle.

Pectoralis major A muscle about 5 cm. wide that lies deep to the pectoantebrachialis. With a blunt probe separate it from the clavodeltoid and pectoralis minor. *Dissect.*

Pectoralis minor Note that this muscle is larger than the pectoralis major. It arises from the sternum, passes diagonally craniad and laterad beneath the pectoralis major to insert on both the scapula and humerus. Note that in humans, this muscle inserts only on the scapula. *Transect* and *reflect.*

Xiphihumeralis The most caudal muscle of the pectoral group. Its fibers run parallel to the pectoralis minor and eventually pass deep to the pectoralis minor to insert on the humerus. There is no human homolog. Remove this muscle.

Trapezius Group

The trapezius muscle in humans is represented by three separate muscles in the cat. Use figure 20.4 and 20.5 to identify them on your specimen.

Clavotrapezius The most cranial trapezius muscle on the cat; covers the dorsal surface of the neck. It inserts on the clavicle and unites with the clavodeltoid to form a single muscle, the ***brachiocephalicus.*** This muscle is homologous to the portion of the human trapezius that inserts on the clavicle.

Acromiotrapezius This muscle lies caudad to the clavotrapezius. It is comparable to that part of the human trapezius that inserts on the acromion. *Dissect, transect* by cutting through the tendon of origin on the mid-dorsal line, and *reflect.*

Spinotrapezius This muscle is caudad to the acromiotrapezius and superficial to the cranial border of the latissimus dorsi. That part of the human trapezius that inserts on the spine of the scapula is comparable to this muscle. *Dissect, transect,* and *reflect.*

Deltoid Group

The cat has three deltoid muscles that are homologs of the single human deltoid. Locate each of the following muscles.

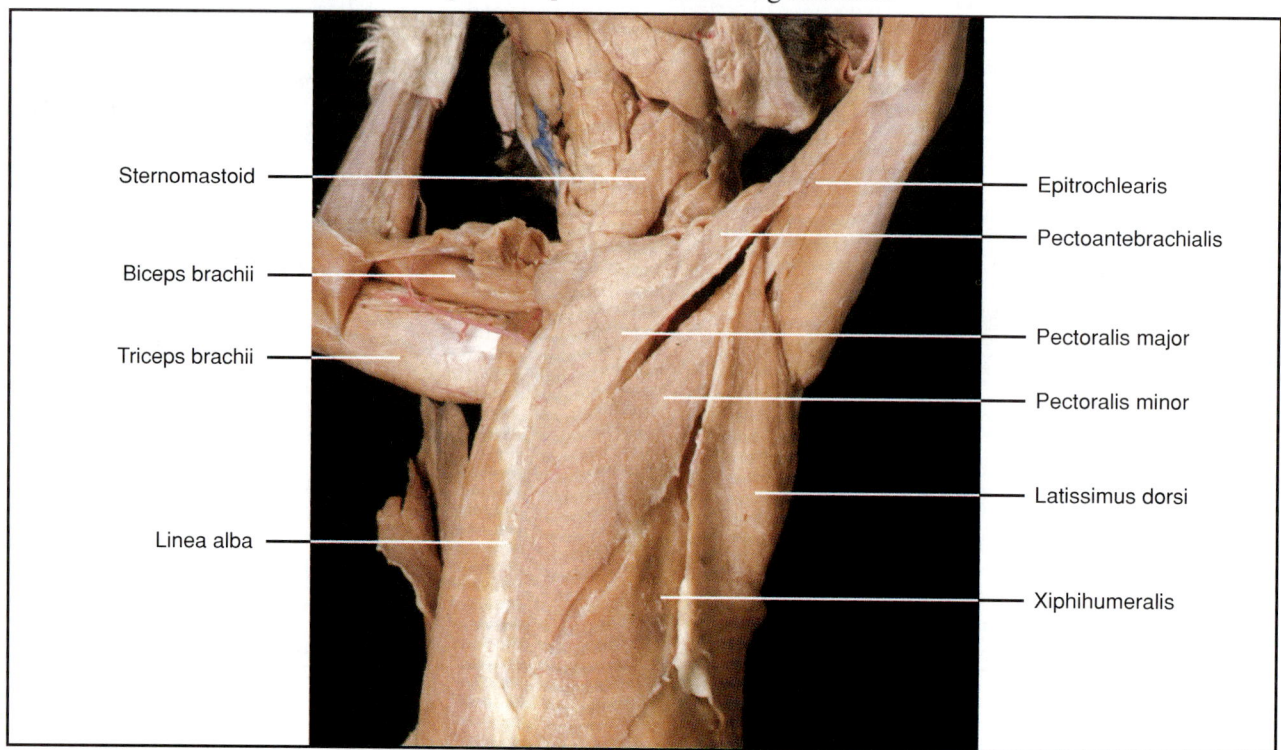

Sternomastoid

Biceps brachii

Triceps brachii

Linea alba

Epitrochlearis

Pectoantebrachialis

Pectoralis major

Pectoralis minor

Latissimus dorsi

Xiphihumeralis

Figure 20.3 Ventrolateral aspect of superficial thorax muscles of the cat.

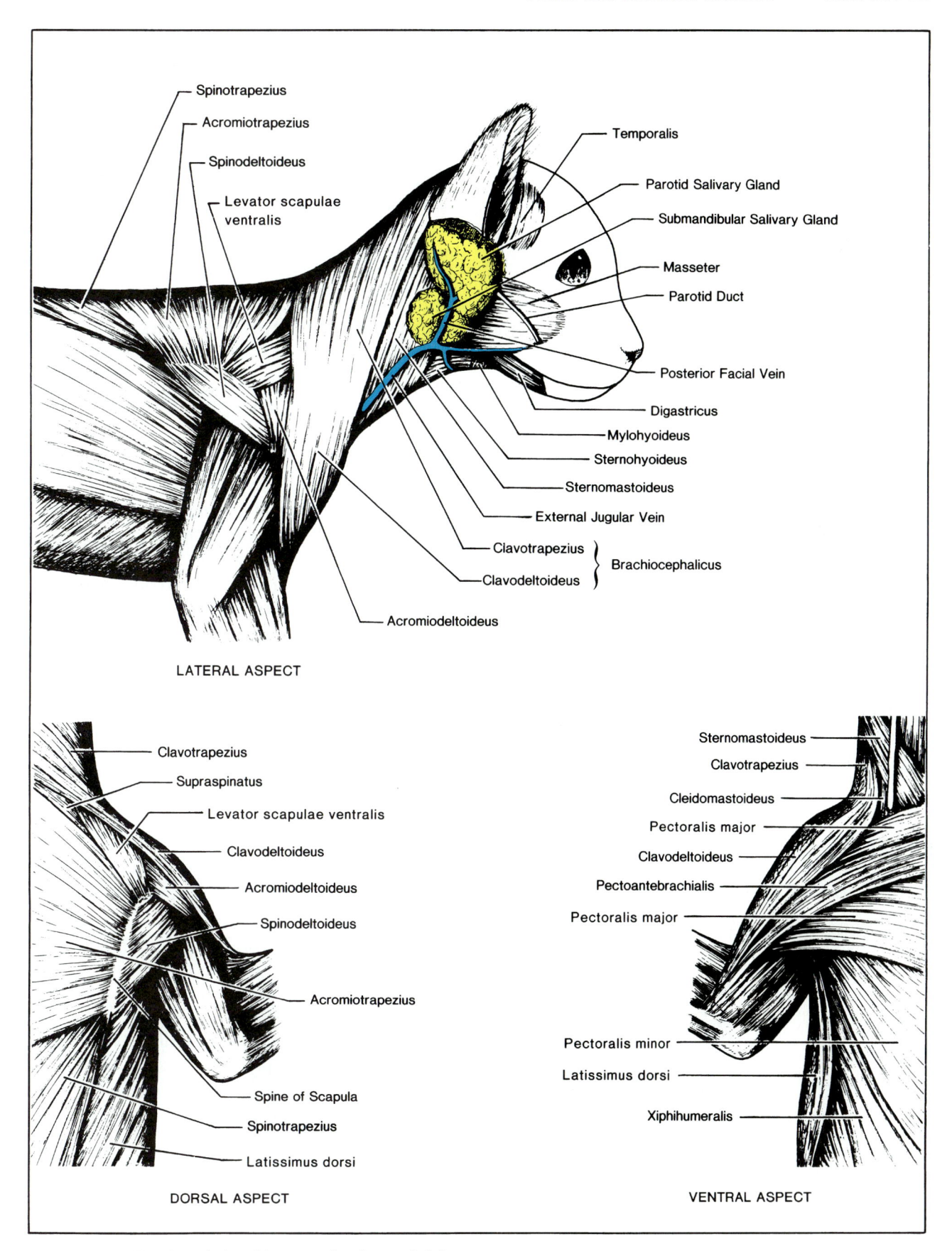

Spinotrapezius
Acromiotrapezius
Spinodeltoideus
Levator scapulae ventralis
Temporalis
Parotid Salivary Gland
Submandibular Salivary Gland
Masseter
Parotid Duct
Posterior Facial Vein
Digastricus
Mylohyoideus
Sternohyoideus
Sternomastoideus
External Jugular Vein
Clavotrapezius
Clavodeltoideus
} Brachiocephalicus
Acromiodeltoideus

LATERAL ASPECT

Clavotrapezius
Supraspinatus
Levator scapulae ventralis
Clavodeltoideus
Acromiodeltoideus
Spinodeltoideus
Acromiotrapezius
Spine of Scapula
Spinotrapezius
Latissimus dorsi

DORSAL ASPECT

Sternomastoideus
Clavotrapezius
Cleidomastoideus
Pectoralis major
Clavodeltoideus
Pectoantebrachialis
Pectoralis major
Pectoralis minor
Latissimus dorsi
Xiphihumeralis

VENTRAL ASPECT

Figure 20.4   Trunk and shoulder muscles (superficial).

Clavodeltoid (*Clavobrachialis*) The position of this muscle is best seen on the ventral view, figure 20.4, and on figure 20.5. This muscle is an extension of the clavotrapezius. It originates on the clavicle and inserts, primarily, on the proximal end of the ulna; some of its fibers, however, merge with the pectoantebrachialis to insert in the fascia of the forearm. *Dissect.*

Acromiodeltoid This muscle is comparable to the acromial portion of the human deltoid. *Dissect.* Although freeing up this muscle is difficult, at least the cranial and caudal borders need to be clearly separated from adjacent muscles.

Spinodeltoid This thick muscle lies caudad to the acromiodeltoid and arises from the spine of the scapula. Use the dorsal view, figure 20.4 and figure 20.5 for reference. *Dissect, transect,* and *reflect.*

Other Superficial Thorax Muscles

Levator scapulae ventralis The location of this muscle is shown in the lateral and dorsal views, figure 20.4. Note that this muscle is caudad of the clavotrapezius and passes beneath the clavotrapezius. It joins the craniolateral edge of the acromiotrapezius and inserts on the acromial part of the scapular spine. It arises from the transverse process of the atlas and the occipital bone.

Since it has no human homolog, identify it and move on to the next muscle.

Latissimus dorsi A broad, flat, triangular muscle that has an extensive origin on the spines of the last six thoracic vertebrae, the lumbar vertebrae, the sacrum, and the iliac crest. The lumbodorsal fascia, an aponeurosis, contains the fibers of this origin. The muscle inserts on the proximal portion of the humerus. *Dissect, transect,* and *reflect.*

Deeper Muscles of the Thorax

Examine the following deeper muscles of the thorax using figures 20.6, 20.7 and 20.8 for reference.

Serratus ventralis Pull the scapula away from the body wall and rotate it dorsad. Clean off the fascia from the body wall. Note the serrate margin of this muscle due to the origin by digitations from the upper eight or nine ribs.

This muscle, which extends to the vertebral border of the scapula, is homologous to two human muscles: the cranial portion is homologous to the human *levator scapulae* and the caudal portion is homologous to the *serratus anterior. Dissect.*

Subscapularis This large, flat muscle fills the subscapular fossa of the scapula. It inserts on the lesser tubercle of the humerus. Locate this muscle but *do not attempt to pass a probe between the muscle and the scapula.*

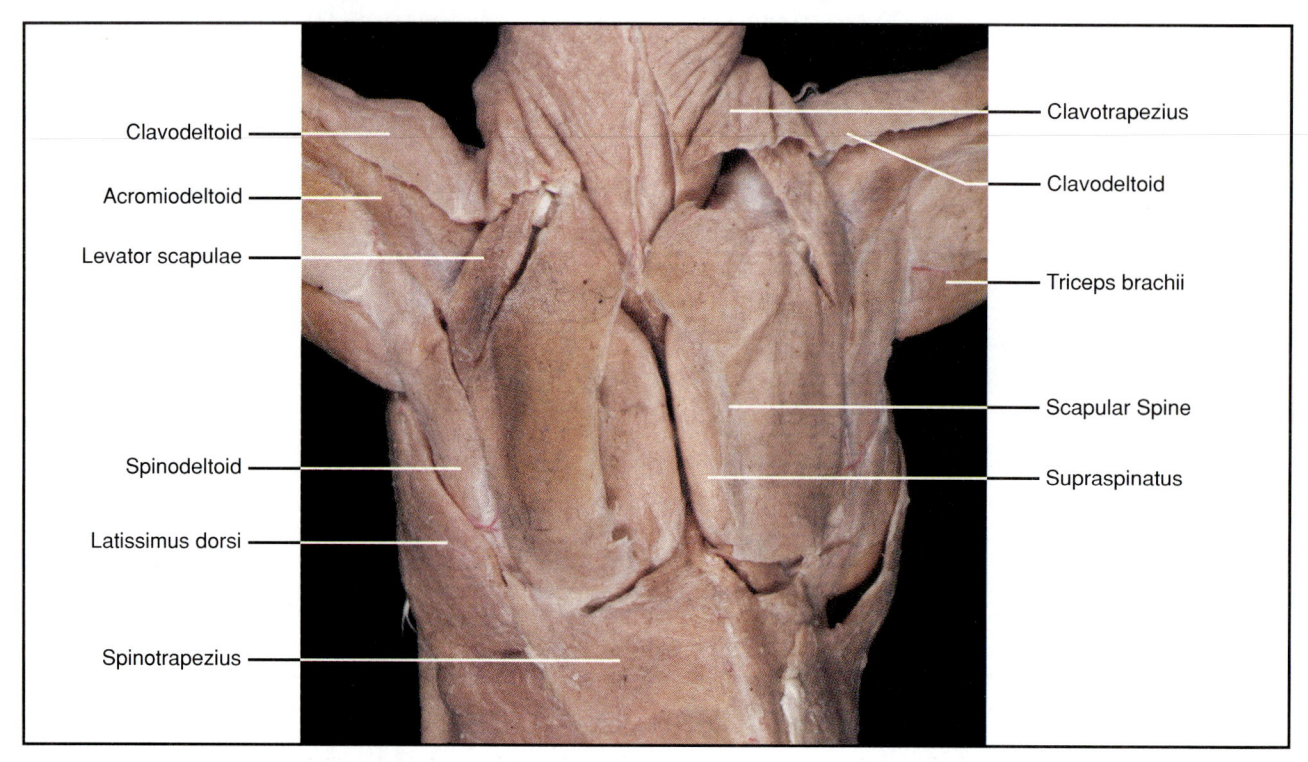

Figure 20.5 Dorsal aspect of superficial thorax muscles.

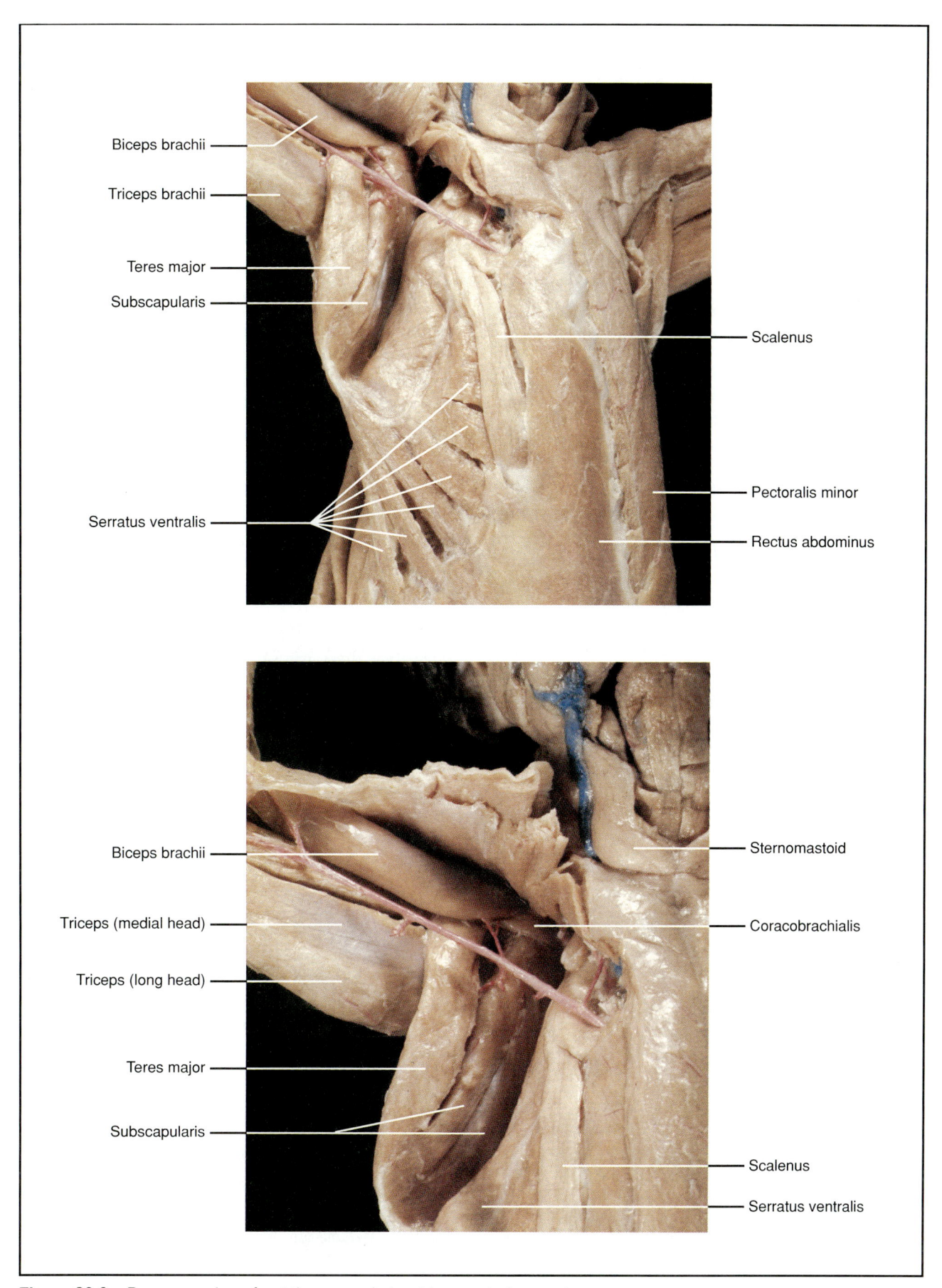

Biceps brachii

Triceps brachii

Teres major

Subscapularis

Scalenus

Serratus ventralis

Pectoralis minor

Rectus abdominus

Biceps brachii

Sternomastoid

Triceps (medial head)

Coracobrachialis

Triceps (long head)

Teres major

Subscapularis

Scalenus

Serratus ventralis

Figure 20.6   Deep muscles of cat thorax and shoulder, ventral aspect.

Rhomboideus Lies deep to the acromiotrapezius and spinotrapezius, which should have been transected previously. Pull the two forelegs together on the ventral side of the cat. This will abduct the scapulae so that you can see the full extent of the rhomboids.

The rhomboideus extends from the spines of the upper thoracic vertebrae to the vertebral border of the scapula. The cranial (and larger) part of this muscle is homologous to the *rhomboideus minor* muscle in humans, and the caudal (smaller) part is homologous to the *rhomboideus major.* The rhomboideus major is larger than the rhomboideus minor in the human.

Levator scapulae This is not a separate muscle, but a cranial continuation of the serratus ventralis. Its origin is from the transverse processes of the caudal five cervical vertebrae, and it inserts on the vertebral border of the scapula ventral to the insertion of the rhomboideus.

In the human, the insertion of the levator scapulae is comparable to that of the cat, but the origin (transverse processes of C_1 to C_4) is roughly comparable to the origin of the cat's levator scapulae ventralis.

Supraspinatus With the acromiotrapezius fully reflected, this muscle can be seen filling the supraspinous fossa of the scapula. From its origin in the supraspinous fossa it passes to the greater tubercle of the humerus.

Infraspinatus Reflect the transected spinodeltoid. The infraspinatus can now be observed extending from its origin in the infraspinous fossa of the scapula to the greater tubercle of the humerus.

Teres major This thick band of muscle is located caudad to the infraspinatus muscle and covers the axillary border of the scapula. It extends forward to insert on the proximal end of the humerus. *Dissect.* Reflect the latissimus dorsi to expose the full extent of this muscle.

Teres minor This small muscle is positioned between the infraspinatus and the long head of the triceps brachii. Since it is not labeled on any of the illustrations in this manual, you will have to look for it by reflecting the spinodeltoid. The muscle extends from the axillary border of the scapula to the humerus.

Laboratory Report

Complete the Laboratory Report for this exercise.

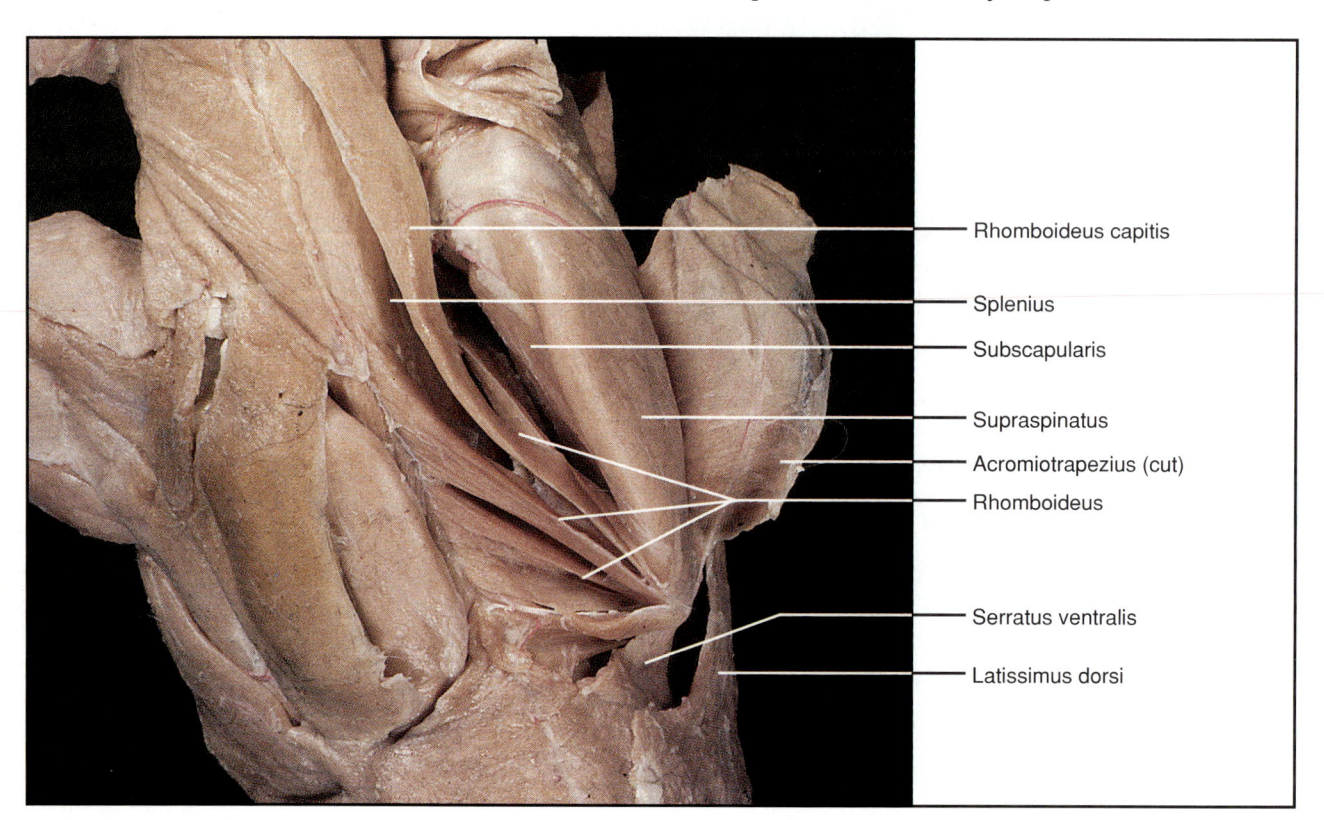

Rhomboideus capitis

Splenius

Subscapularis

Supraspinatus

Acromiotrapezius (cut)

Rhomboideus

Serratus ventralis

Latissimus dorsi

Figure 20.7 Deep muscles of cat's shoulder and back, dorsal aspect.

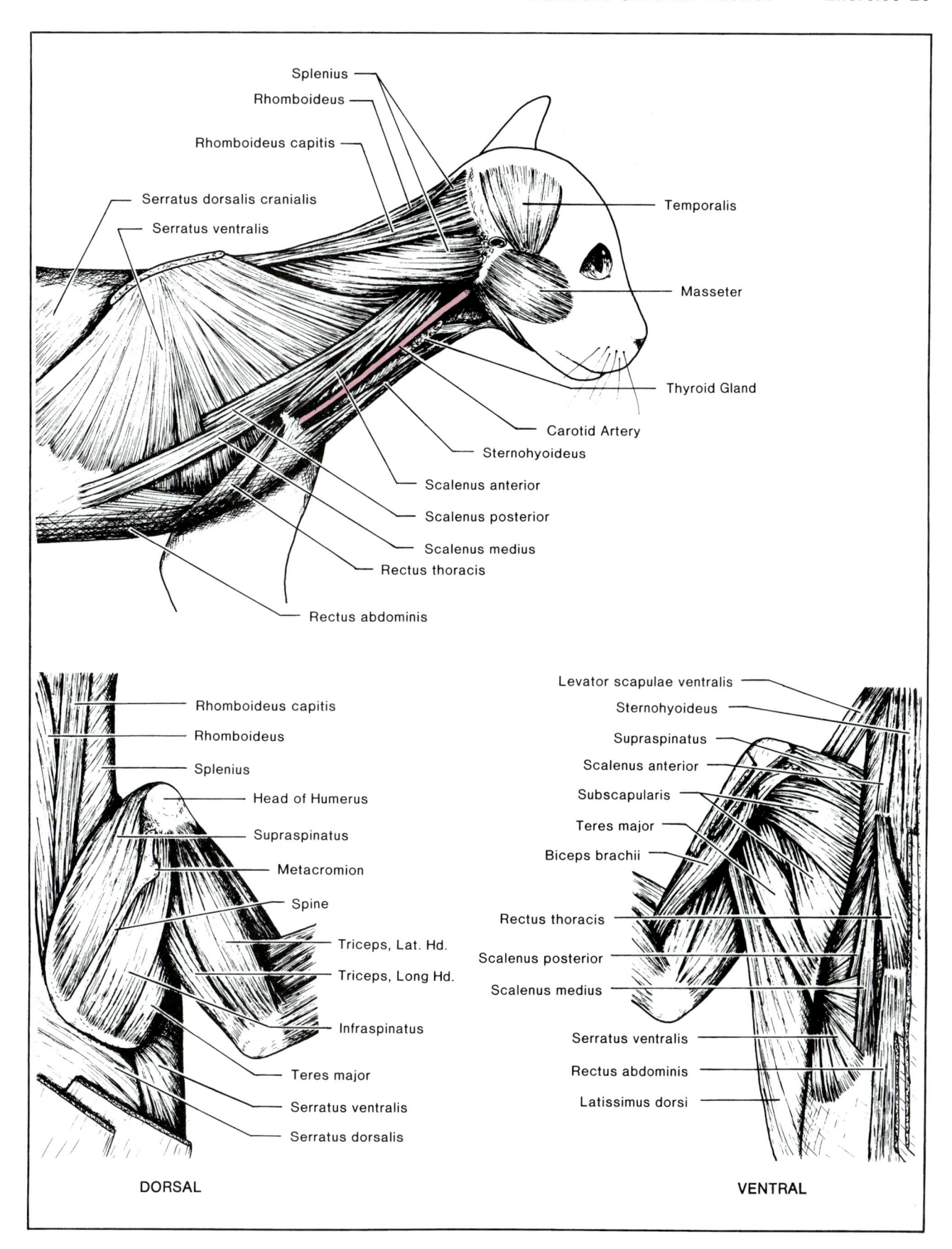

Figure 20.8   Deep trunk, shoulder, and neck muscles.

21 Upper Extremity Muscles

Muscles that move the brachium are primarily muscles of the shoulder and trunk, which were studied in the last exercise. In this exercise the muscles of the brachium that control movements of the forearm will be studied. One muscle, however, that was not mentioned in the last exercise that does move the upper arm is the **coracobrachialis.** It is a muscle of the upper arm and is illustrated in figure 21.1.

Coracobrachialis This muscle covers a portion of the upper medial surface of the humerus. It takes its *origin* on the apex of the coracoid process of the scapula. Its *insertion* is in the middle of the medial surface of the humerus.

> *Action:* Carries the arm forward in flexion and adducts the arm.

Forearm Movements

The principal movers of the forearm are the *biceps brachii, brachialis, brachioradialis,* and *triceps brachii.* These muscles are also illustrated in figure 21.1. Note that incorporated into all the names of these upper arm muscles is the Latin term for the upper arm: *brachium.*

Biceps brachii This is the large muscle on the anterior surface of the upper arm that bulges when the forearm is flexed. Its *origin* consists of two tendinous heads: a medial tendon which is attached to the coracoid process, and a lateral tendon that fits into the intertubercular groove on the humerus. The latter tendon is attached to the supraglenoid tubercle of the scapula. At the lower end of the muscle the two heads unite to form a single tendinous *insertion* on the radial tuberosity of the radius.

> *Action:* Flexion of the forearm; also, rolls the radius outward to supinate the hand.

Brachialis Immediately under the biceps brachii on the distal anterior portion of the humerus lies the brachialis. Its *origin* occupies the lower half of the humerus. Its *insertion* is attached to the front surface of the coronoid process of the ulna.

> *Action:* Flexion of the forearm.

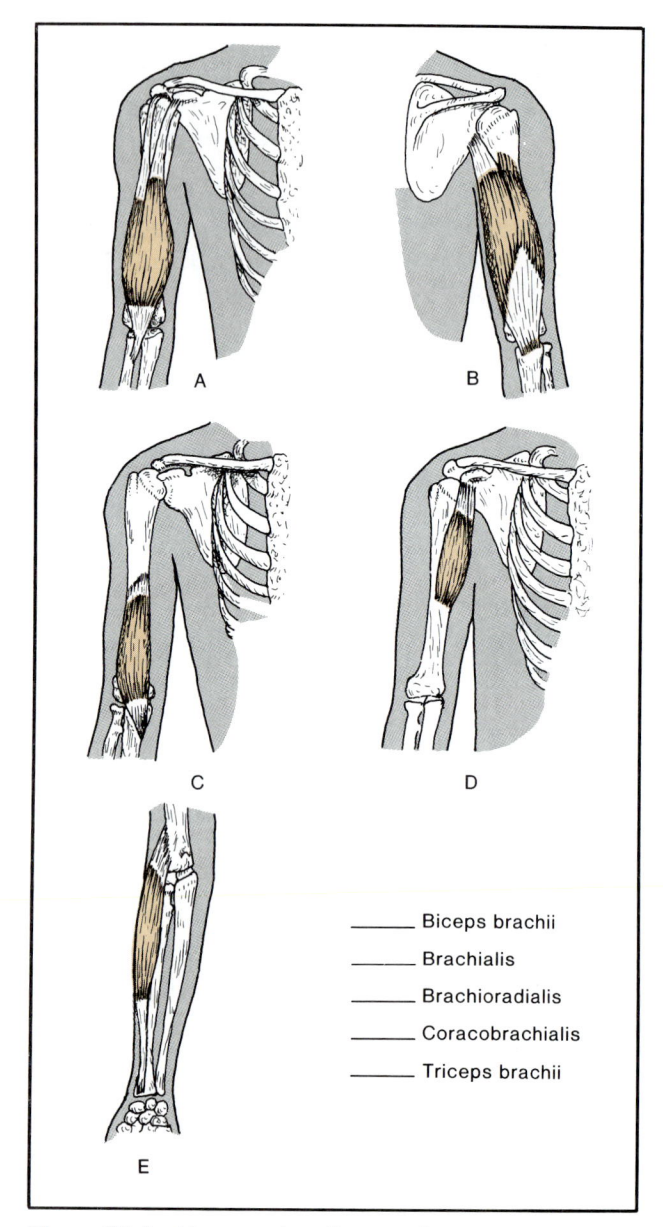

Figure 21.1   Upper extremity muscles.

_____ Biceps brachii
_____ Brachialis
_____ Brachioradialis
_____ Coracobrachialis
_____ Triceps brachii

Brachioradialis This muscle is the most superficial muscle on the lateral (radial) side of the forearm. It *originates* above the lateral epicondyle of the humerus and *inserts* on the lateral surface of the radius slightly above the styloid process.

> *Action:* Flexion of the forearm.

Triceps brachii The entire back surface of the upper arm is covered by this muscle. It has three heads of *origin*. A long head arises from the scapula, a lateral head from the posterior surface of the humerus, and a medial head from the surface below the radial groove. The tendinous *insertion* of the muscle is attached to the olecranon process of the ulna.

Action: Extension of the forearm; antagonist of the brachialis.

Assignment:

Identify the muscles in figure 21.1 by placing the correct letter in front of each name in the legend.

Hand Movements

Muscles of the arm that cause hand movements are illustrated in figures 21.2 and 21.3. All illustrations are of the right arm; thus, if the thumb points to the left side of the page the anterior aspect is being viewed; when pointing to the right, the posterior view is observed. Keeping this in mind will facilitate understanding the descriptions that follow.

Supination and Pronation

Two muscles can cause supination: the biceps brachii and the supinator.

The **supinator** is a short muscle near the elbow that *arises* from the lateral epicondyle of the humerus and the ridge of the ulna. It curves around the upper portion of the radius and *inserts* on the lateral edge of the radial tuberosity and the oblique line of the radius.

Pronation is achieved by the pronator teres and the pronator quadratus. The **pronator teres** is the upper one in illustration B, figure 21.2. It *arises* on the medial epicondyle of the humerus and *inserts* on the upper lateral surface of the radius.

The **pronator quadratus** is located in the wrist region. It *originates* on the distal portion of the ulna and *inserts* on the distal lateral portion of the radius.

Flexion of the Hand

Two muscles that flex the hand are shown in illustration C, figure 21.2.

The muscle that extends diagonally across the forearm is the **flexor carpi radialis.** It *arises* on the medial epicondyle of the humerus and *inserts* on the proximal portions of the second and third metacarpals.

The other muscle in illustration C is the **flexor carpi ulnaris.** Its *origin* is on the medial epicondyle of the humerus and the posterior surface (olecranon process) of the ulna. Its *insertion* consists of a tendon that attaches to the base of the fifth metacarpal.

While both muscles flex the hand, the radialis muscle causes abduction and the ulnaris muscle causes adduction of the hand.

Flexion of Fingers of the Hand

Three muscles (see illus. D, fig. 21.2, and illus. A, fig. 21.3) flex the fingers.

The broad muscle in illustration D that flexes all fingers except the thumb is the **flexor digitorum**

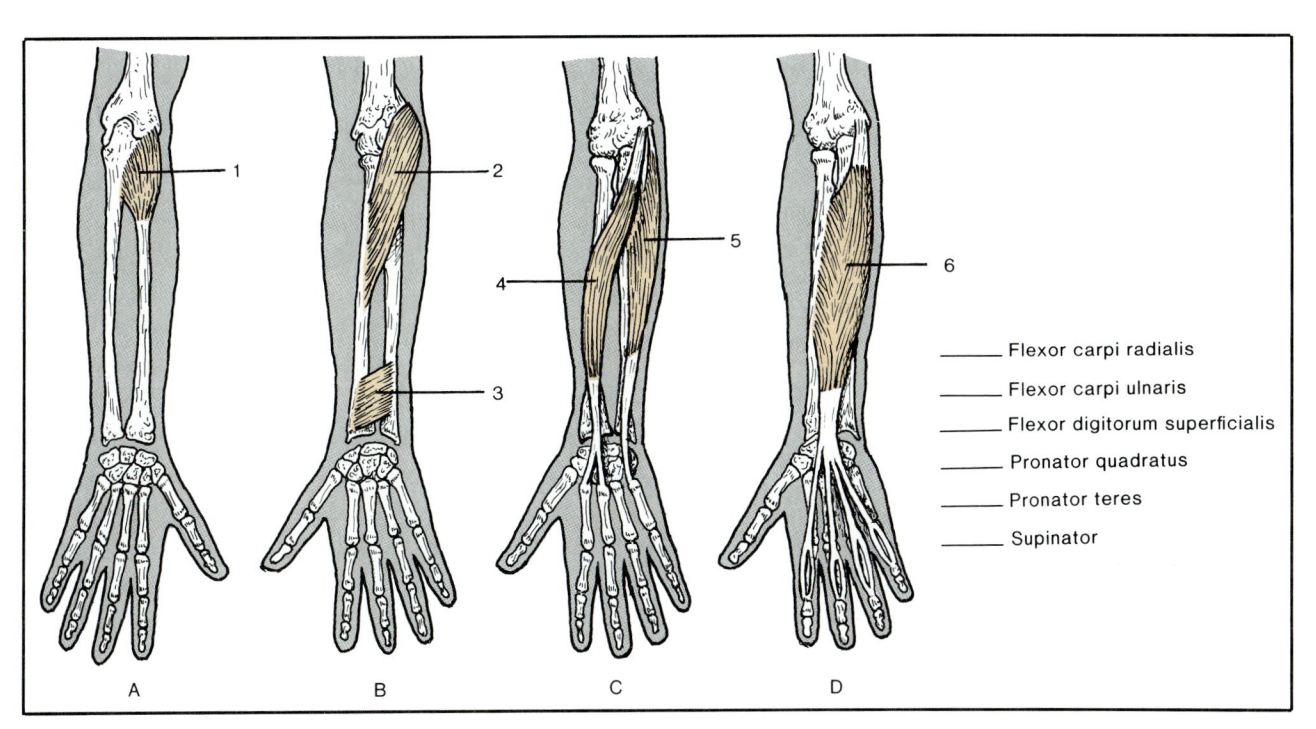

Legend:
_____ Flexor carpi radialis
_____ Flexor carpi ulnaris
_____ Flexor digitorum superficialis
_____ Pronator quadratus
_____ Pronator teres
_____ Supinator

Figure 21.2 Forearm muscles.

superficialis. It *arises* on the humerus, ulna, and radius. Its *insertion* consists of tendons that are attached to the middle phalanges of the second, third, fourth, and fifth fingers.

The second muscle that flexes fingers is the **flexor digitorum profundus.** It is the larger muscle in illustration A, figure 21.3. It lies directly under the flexor digitorum superficialis. It *originates* on the ulna and the interosseous membrane between the radius and ulna. It *inserts* with four tendons on the distal phalanges of the second, third, fourth, and fifth fingers. This muscle flexes the distal portions of the fingers.

The **flexor pollicis longus** (Latin: *pollex,* thumb) is the smaller muscle in illustration A. Note that it *arises* on the radius, ulna, and interosseous membrane. Its *insertion* consists of a tendon that is anchored to the distal phalanx of the thumb. It flexes only the thumb.

Extension of Wrist and Hand

Three muscles extend the hand at the wrist. Illustrations B and D reveal them.

The **extensor carpi radialis longus** and **brevis** are shown in illustration B. The brevis muscle is medial to the longus. Both muscles *originate* on the humerus, with the longus taking a more proximal position. The longus *inserts* on the second metacarpal; the brevis on the middle metacarpal.

The **extensor carpi ulnaris** is the third muscle involved in extending the hand. It is the muscle on the medial edge of the arm in illustration D. It *arises* on the lateral epicondyle of the humerus and part of the ulna. It *inserts* on the fifth metacarpal.

Extension and Abduction of Fingers

Three muscles cause extension of the fingers; one abducts the thumb.

The **extensor digitorum communis** lies alongside the extensor carpi ulnaris; it is shown in illustration D. It *arises* from the lateral epicondyle of the humerus and *inserts* on the distal phalanges of fingers two through five. It extends all fingers except the thumb.

The **extensor pollicis longus, extensor pollicis brevis,** and **abductor pollicis** move the thumb. The longus muscle is the lower one in illustration C. It *arises* on both the ulna and radius. It *inserts* on the distal phalanx of the thumb. The brevis muscle, which lies superior to it, is not shown in illustration C. It inserts on the proximal phalanx of the thumb, and assists the longus in extending the thumb.

The abductor pollicis is the superior muscle shown in illustration C. It takes its *origin* on the interosseous membrane, and it *inserts* on the lateral portion of the first metacarpal and trapezium. Its only action is to abduct the thumb.

Assignment:

Label figures 21.2 and 21.3, and complete the Laboratory Report for this exercise.

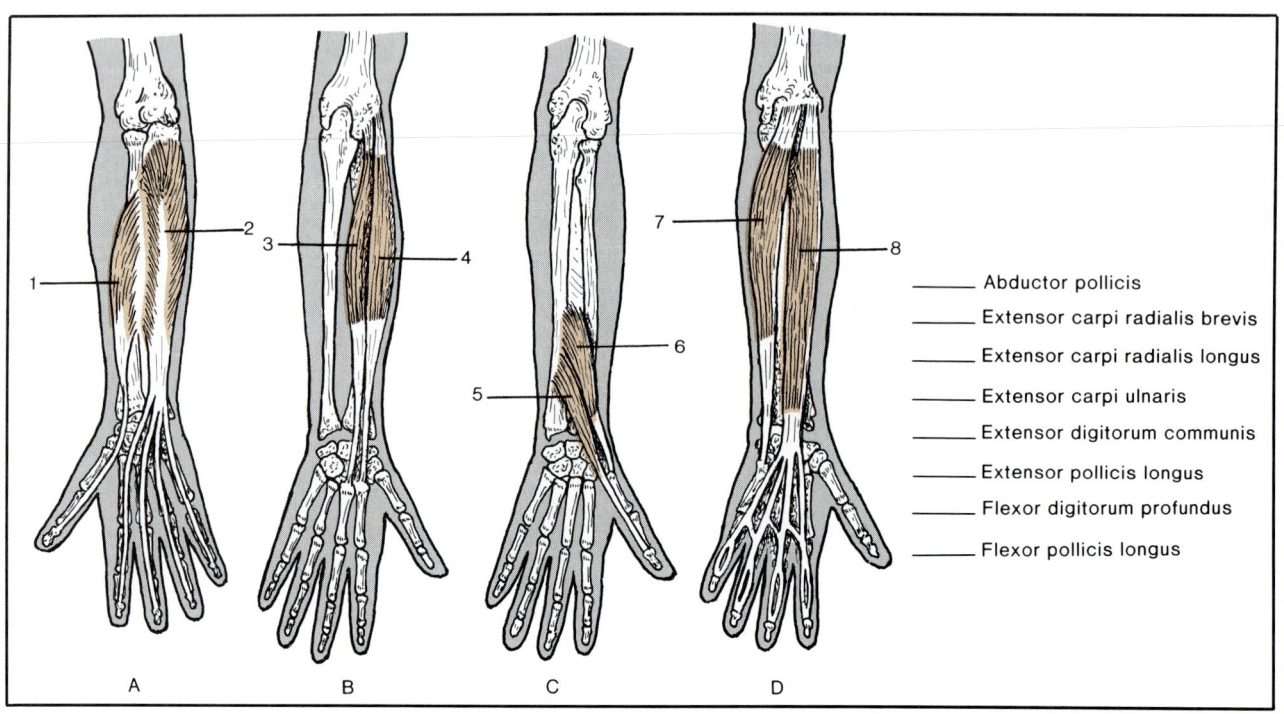

_____ Abductor pollicis

_____ Extensor carpi radialis brevis

_____ Extensor carpi radialis longus

_____ Extensor carpi ulnaris

_____ Extensor digitorum communis

_____ Extensor pollicis longus

_____ Flexor digitorum profundus

_____ Flexor pollicis longus

Figure 21.3 Forearm muscles.

Cat Dissection
(*Forelimb*)

Muscles of the Brachium

Six homologs of the human brachium are seen in the cat. Except for the anconeus, all the human muscles were identified on pages 102 and 103.

One muscle of the cat's brachium, the *epitrochlearis,* has no homolog in the human, and should be removed prior to studying the six homologs. It is a flat, thin, superficial muscle on the medial side of the brachium, and can be seen in figure 21.5. It arises from the latissimus dorsi and is continuous, distally, with the fascia of the forearm. After removing this muscle, proceed to identify and free up with a probe the six homologs in the following order:

Triceps brachii This muscle has three heads of origin, which merge to insert by a common tendon on the olecranon process of the ulna. The long head, located on the caudal surface of the arm, is the largest. The lateral head covers much of the lateral surface of the arm. *Dissect.* To reveal the medial head, which is between the long and lateral heads, *transect* and *reflect* the lateral head (see figure 21.6). Only the long head arises from the scapula.

Biceps brachii In the cat this muscle lies deep to the pectoral muscles, just medial to their humeral insertions. This muscle is, therefore, located on the ventromedial surface of the arm (see figure 21.4). It inserts on the radius. *Dissect.*

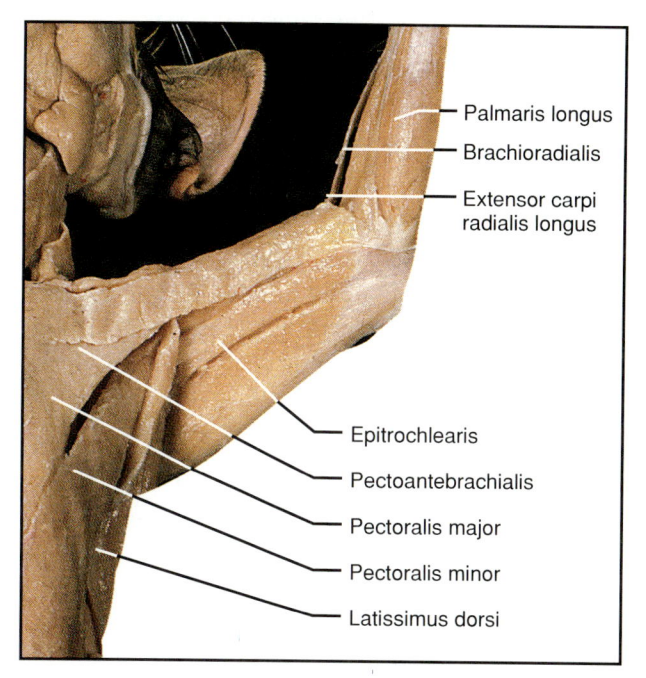

Figure 21.5 Superficial forelimb muscles of cat.

Brachialis This muscle is located on the ventrolateral surface of the arm, craniad to the lateral head of the triceps brachii. Refer to figure 21.6.

The insertion of the pectoralis major separates the biceps brachii and brachialis. Since this muscle arises from the lateral surface of the humerus, you will not be able to run a probe underneath it from its origin to its insertion on the ulna.

Brachioradialis In the cat this muscle (figures 21.4 and 21.8) is a narrow ribbon, which may have been

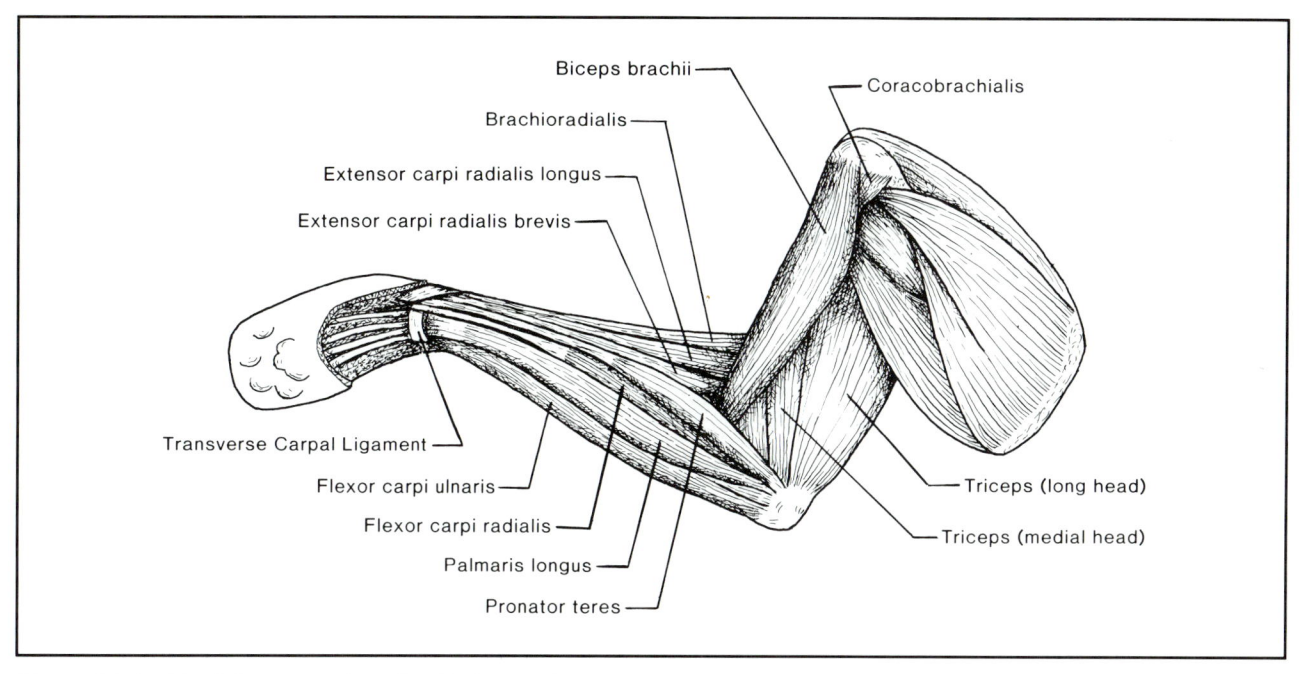

Figure 21.4 Medial aspect of cat forelimb muscles.

removed with the superficial fascia. It arises on the lateral side of the humerus and passes along the radial side of the forearm to insert on the styloid process of the radius. *Dissect.*

Coracobrachialis Use figures 21.4 and 21.7 to locate this small muscle. Note that it is on the medial side of the scapula caudad of the proximal (origin) end of the biceps brachii. This muscle is almost impossible to locate if the pectoralis major and minor muscles have not been previously transected and reflected.

Anconeus This small muscle is shown in figure 21.6. It consists of short superficial fibers that originate near the lateral epicondyle of the humerus, and inserts near the olecranon. It assists the triceps in both the cat and human to extend the forearm.

Muscles of the Antebrachium

Eight muscles of the cat's forearm will be identified. As on the brachium homologs, free up each muscle with a probe. They are as follows:

Pronator teres This muscle extends from the medial epicondyle of the humerus to the middle third of the radius. Use figure 21.4 for reference. *Dissect.*

Palmaris longus Note in figure 21.4 that this muscle is a large, flat, broad muscle near the center of the medial surface of the forearm. It arises from the medial epicondyle of the humerus and inserts by means of four tendons on the digits. Note that

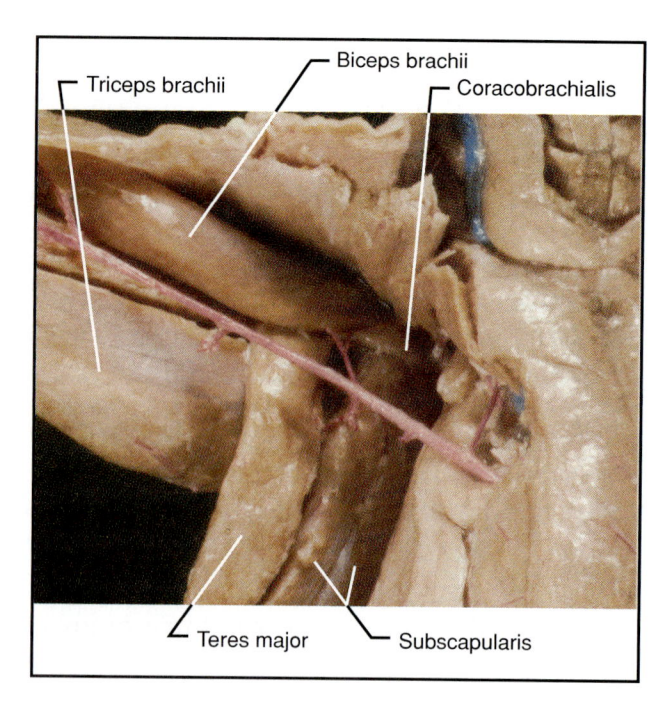

Figure 21.7 Brachium and shoulder muscles of cat.

at its distal end the four insertion tendons pass under a *transverse carpal ligament*. This muscle is not found in about 10 percent of humans. *Dissect.*

Flexor carpi radialis As illustrated in figure 21.4, this long, spindle-shaped muscle lies between the palmaris longus and the pronator teres. It arises from the medial epicondyle of the humerus and inserts at the base of the second and third metacarpals.

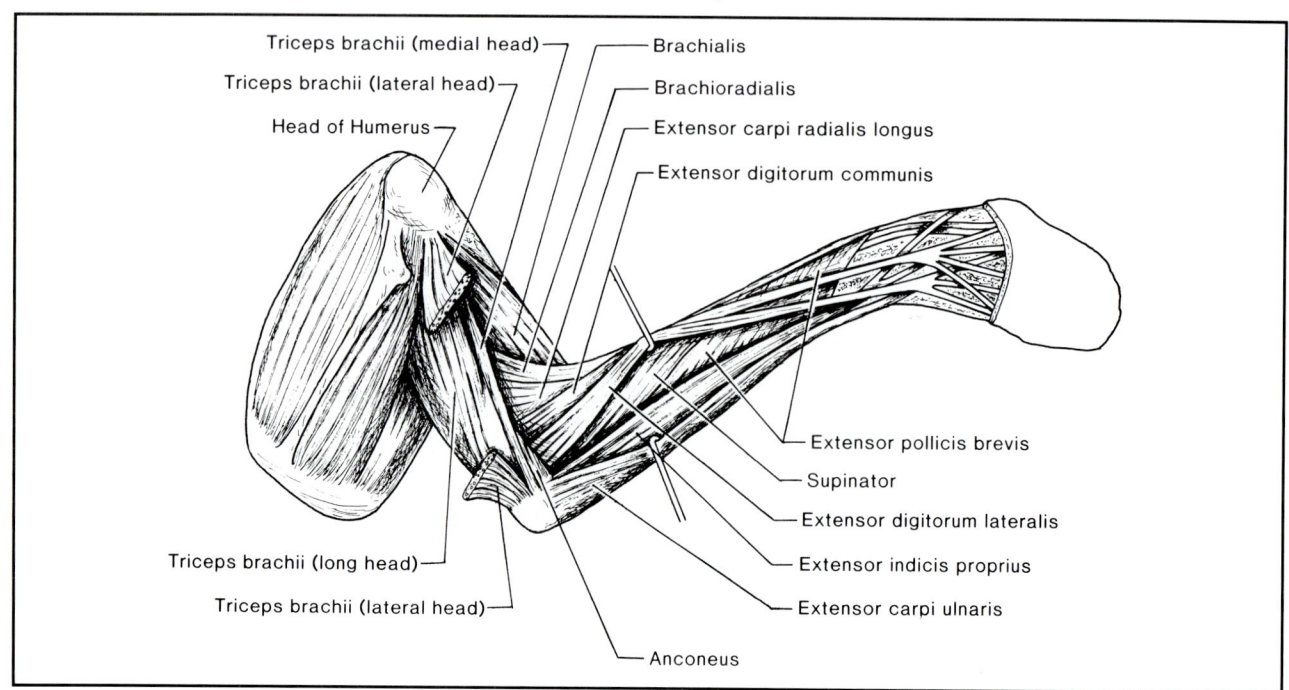

Figure 21.6 Cat forelimb muscles, lateral aspect.

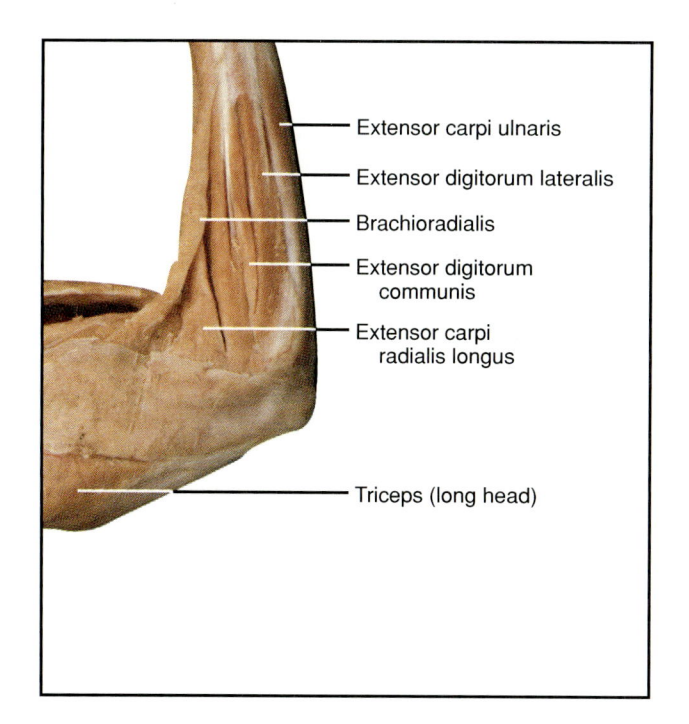

Figure 21.8 Superficial muscles of forearm, lateral aspect.

Flexor carpi ulnaris Figure 21.4 shows the location of this muscle. What appears to be two muscles is actually two heads of origin: one originates from the medial epicondyle of the humerus and the other from the olecranon. About the middle of the ulna, the two heads join to form a single band of muscle fibers that inserts on the pisiform and hamate bones. *Dissect.*

Extensor carpi ulnaris This muscle, shown in figures 21.6 and 21.8, arises from the lateral epicondyle of the humerus and inserts on the base of the fifth metacarpal. *Dissect.*

Extensor digitorum communis Use figure 21.6 to locate this muscle. It arises from the lateral epicondyle of the humerus and extends to the wrist where it divides into four tendons that insert on the second phalanges of digits 2–5. Note that these four tendons lie superficial to the three tendons of the extensor digitorum lateralis. *Dissect.*

Extensor carpi radialis longus Use figure 21.8 to identify this muscle, which lies adjacent to the brachioradialis. Its origin is on the lateral supracondylar ridge of the humerus and it inserts at the base of the second metacarpal. *Dissect.*

Supinator This muscle can be exposed by reflecting the extensor digitorum lateralis as shown in figure 21.6. This muscle originates from ligaments on the elbow. It inserts on the proximal end of the radius and acts as a lateral rotator of the radius (supination).

Complete exposure of the supinator would require transection and reflection of the overlying muscles. To avoid irreversible mutilation of your cat, do not do this.

Laboratory Report

Complete the Laboratory Report for this exercise.

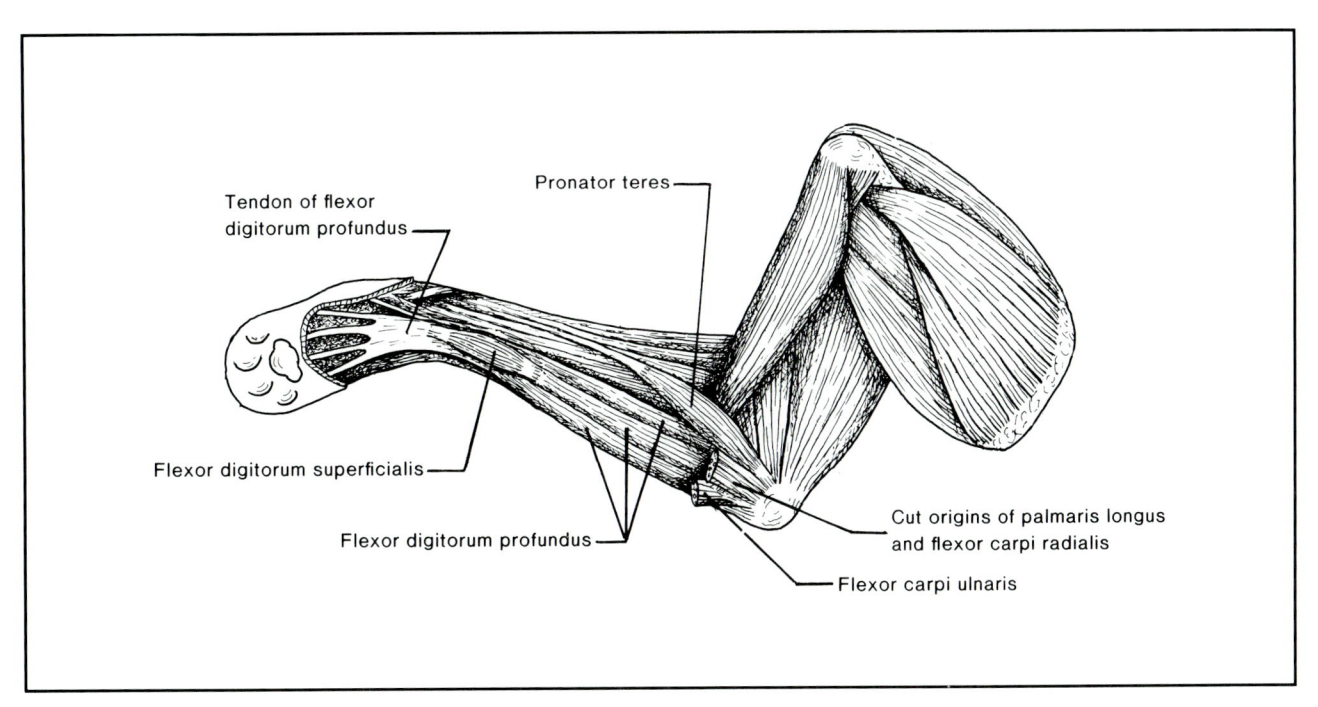

Figure 21.9 Deep muscles of cat's forearm, medial aspect.

Abdominal, Pelvic, and Intercostal Muscles

The muscles of the abdominal wall and pelvis will be studied in this exercise. Cat dissection will be utilized for this muscle study.

Abdominal Muscles

The abdominal wall consists of four pairs of thin muscles. The human illustration in figure 22.1 has portions of the right abdominal wall removed to reveal the nature of the laminations. Identify the following muscles in this illustration:

Obliquus externus (*external oblique*) This muscle is the most superficial layer on the abdominal wall. It is ensheathed by the **aponeurosis of the obliquus externus,** which terminates at the linea alba and inguinal ligament.

The muscle takes its *origin* on the external surfaces of the lower eight ribs. Although it appears to insert on the linea semilunaris, its actual *insertion* is the **linea alba** (white line), where fibers of the left and right aponeuroses interlace on the midline of the abdomen.

The lower border of each aponeurosis forms the **inguinal ligament,** which extends from the anterior spine of the ilium to the pubic tubercle. Label 5, figure 22.3 is of this ligament.

Obliquus internus (*internal oblique*) This muscle lies immediately under the external oblique, i.e., between the external oblique and the transversus abdominis. Its *origin* is on the lateral half of the inguinal ligament, the anterior two-thirds of the iliac crest, and the thoracolumbar fascia. Its *insertion* is on the costal cartilages of the lower three ribs, the linea alba, and the crest of the pubis.

Transversus abdominis The innermost muscle of the abdominal wall is the transversus abdominis. It *arises* on the inguinal ligament, the iliac crest, the costal cartilages of the lower six ribs, and the thoracolumbar fascia. It *inserts* into the linea alba and the crest of the pubis.

Rectus abdominis The right rectus abdominis is the long, narrow, segmented muscle running from the rib cage to the pubic bone. It is enclosed in a fibrous

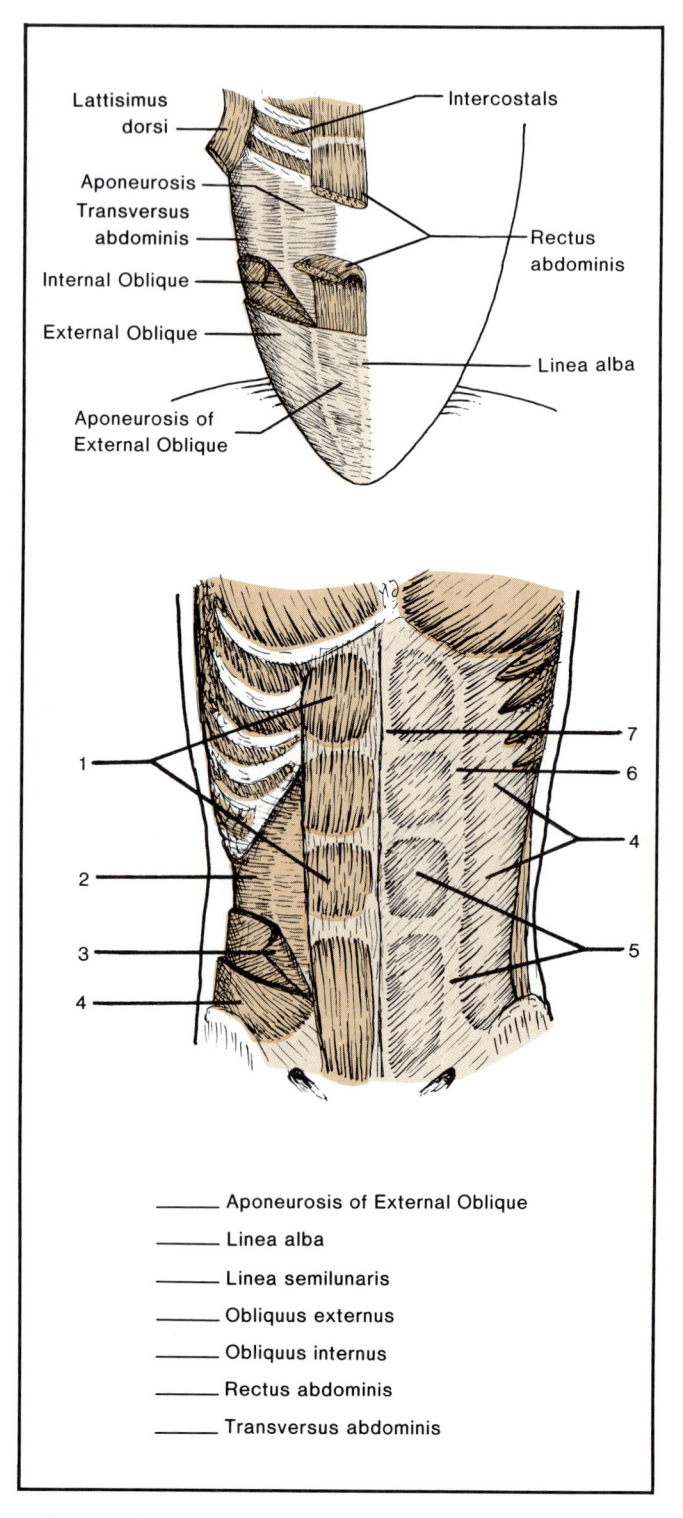

Labels on upper figure: Lattisimus dorsi, Intercostals, Aponeurosis Transversus abdominis, Rectus abdominis, Internal Oblique, External Oblique, Linea alba, Aponeurosis of External Oblique

Lower figure labels: 1, 2, 3, 4 (left); 7, 6, 4, 5 (right)

_____ Aponeurosis of External Oblique
_____ Linea alba
_____ Linea semilunaris
_____ Obliquus externus
_____ Obliquus internus
_____ Rectus abdominis
_____ Transversus abdominis

Figure 22.1 Abdominal muscles, cat and human.

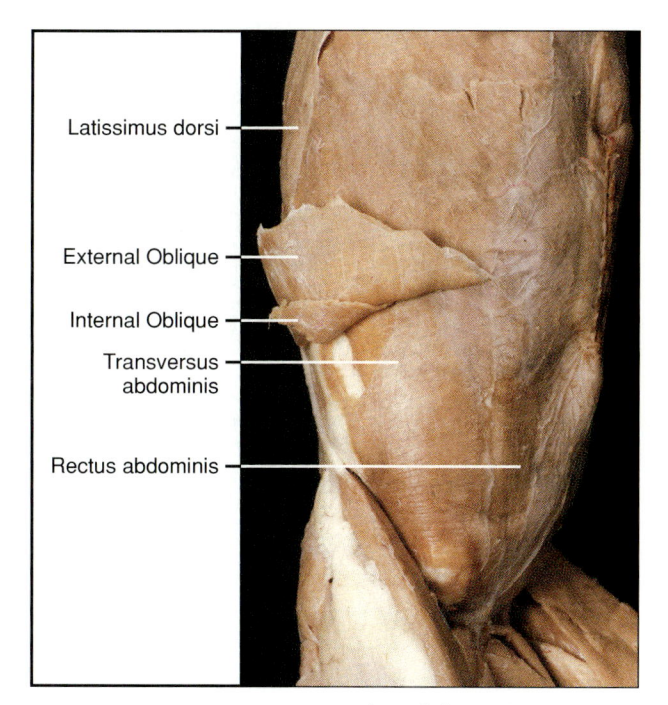

Latissimus dorsi

External Oblique

Internal Oblique

Transversus
abdominis

Rectus abdominis

Figure 22.2   Abdominal muscles of the cat.

sheath formed by the aponeuroses of the above three muscles.

Its *origin* is on the pubic bone. Its *insertion* is on the cartilages of the fifth, sixth, and seventh ribs. The linea alba lies between the pair of muscles. Contraction of the rectus abdominis muscles aids in flexion of the spine in the lumbar region.

Collective Action

The above four abdominal muscles keep the abdominal organs compressed and assist in maintaining intraabdominal pressure.

They act as antagonists to the diaphragm. When the latter contracts, they relax. When the diaphragm relaxes, they contract to effect expiration of air from the lungs. They also assist in defecation, micturition, parturition, and vomiting. Flexion of the body at the lumbar region is also achieved by them.

Assignment:

Label figure 22.1.

Cat Dissection

Abdominal Wall

As shown in the upper illustration of figure 22.1 and figure 22.2, the abdominal wall of the cat has the same four muscles as seen in humans. As you separate each muscle layer, pay particular attention to the direction of the fibers. Body wall strength is greatly enhanced by the different directions of the fibers in each layer.

External Oblique This outer muscle of the body wall arises from the external surface of the lower nine ribs. Note how the cranial portion of this muscle interdigitates with the origin of the serratus ventralis. Insertion is on the iliac crest and by an aponeurosis which fuses with that of the opposite side to form the *linea alba*.

Loosen the cranial border of the muscle with a blunt probe and slide the probe underneath the muscle in a caudal direction. *Transect* alongside of the probe and *reflect*. (Remember, when you transect a muscle, your cut should be through the midbelly half way between the origin and insertion).

Internal Oblique To expose this muscle it will be necessary to make a shallow incision on the right side through the external oblique from the ribs to the pelvis. *Reflect* the external oblique. Since the external oblique is very thin, take care not to cut too deep. Note that, in general, the fibers of this muscle layer course at approximately right angles to those of the external oblique. Note, also, where the muscle fibers end and become continuous with the aponeurosis.

Transversus abdominis This innermost muscle layer of the ventrolateral abdominal wall is very difficult to separate from the internal oblique; therefore, only a small "window" should be cut to expose the transversus abdominis.

Try to slide the tip of a blunt probe underneath either a small area of the aponeurosis or the muscle fibers of the internal oblique. Make a cut to create a small opening and note the general transverse direction of the muscle of this muscle.

Rectus abdominis This muscle extends from the pubis to the sternum on each side of the linea alba. It extends farther craniad in the cat than in the human. The cranial two-thirds of the aponeurosis of the internal oblique splits at the lateral border of the rectus abdominis, creating a dorsal leaf that passes dorsal, and a ventral leaf that passes ventral to the rectus abdominis. The dorsal and ventral leaves unite at the medial border of the rectus abdominis to help form the linea alba.

Because the rectus abdominis is "wrapped" in the aponeurosis in this manner, it is difficult to pass a probe under this muscle from its origin to the insertion.

Intercostal Muscles

These muscles of respiration in the cat are essentially the same as in humans except that there are twelve sets in the cat and eleven sets in humans. Proceed to dissect these muscles as follows:

External Intercostals Reflect the external oblique to expose the lateral aspect of the rib cage. The external intercostal muscles can be seen occupying the intercostal spaces. Note that the direction of the fibers is forward and downward from the caudal border of one rib to the cranial border of the next rib caudad. Note that the external intercostals do not reach the sternum, and that the internal intercostals can be seen in the interval.

Internal Intercostals These muscles are immediately deep to the external intercostals. Cut a small window through an external intercostal between two ribs to expose one of these muscles. Note that the fibers course at approximately right angles to the fibers of the external muscle as they pass from the cranial border of the rib to the caudal border of the next rib craniad.

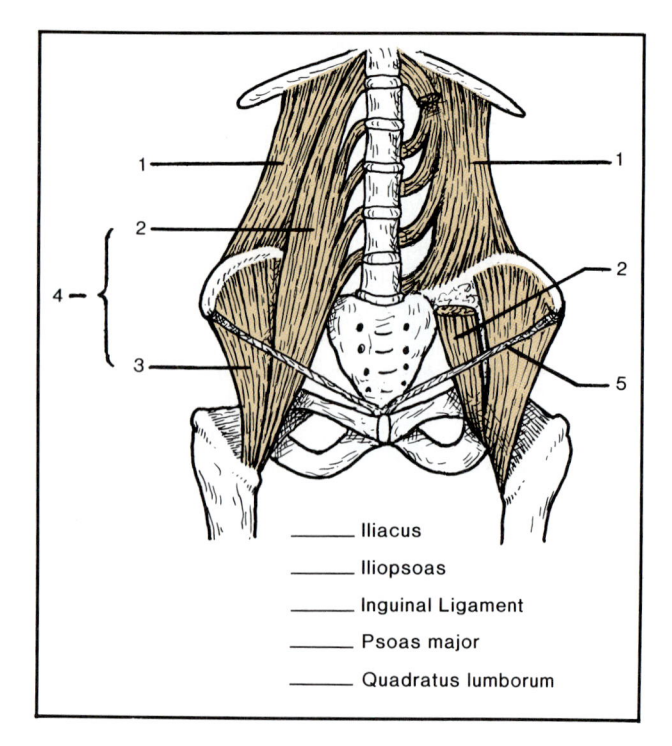

_____ Iliacus

_____ Iliopsoas

_____ Inguinal Ligament

_____ Psoas major

_____ Quadratus lumborum

Figure 22.3 Pelvic muscles.

Pelvic Muscles

The principal muscles of the pelvic region are shown in figure 22.3. They are the quadratus lumborum, psoas major, and iliacus. Muscles in this region of the cat will be dissected in Exercise 23.

Quadratus lumborum The muscle that extends from the iliac crest of the os coxa to the lowest rib in figure 22.3 is this muscle. Its *origin* is on the iliac crest, the iliolumbar ligament, and the transverse processes of the lower four lumbar vertebrae. Its *insertion* is on the inferior margin of the last rib and the transverse processes of the upper four lumbar vertebrae.

Acting together, these two muscles extend the spine at the lumbar vertebrae. Lateral flexion or abduction results when one acts independently of the other.

Psoas major This is the long muscle shown on the right side of the pelvic cavity in figure 22.3. Only the cut ends of the left muscle are shown in this illustration.

The psoas major *arises* from the sides of the bodies and transverse processes of the lumbar vertebrae. It *inserts* with the iliacus on the lesser trochanter of the femur.

The two psoas majors work synergistically with the rectus abdominis muscles to flex the lumbar region of the vertebral column.

Iliacus This muscle extends from the iliac crest to the proximal end of the femur. Its *origin* is the whole iliac fossa. Its *insertion* is the lesser trochanter of the femur. The psoas major and iliacus are jointly referred to as the **iliopsoas** because of their intimate relationship at their insertion.

The iliacus works synergistically with the psoas major to flex the femur on the trunk.

Laboratory Report

After labeling figure 22.3, answer the questions on combined Laboratory Report 22,23 that pertain to the muscles studied in this exercise.

Lower Extremity Muscles 23

Twenty-seven muscles of the leg will be studied in this exercise. As in the case of the upper extremity muscles they are grouped according to type of movement.

Thigh Movements

Seven muscles that move the femur are shown in figure 23.1. All originate on a part of the pelvis.

Gluteus maximus This muscle of the buttock region is covered by a deep fascia, the *fascia lata,* that completely invests the thigh muscles. Emerging downward from the fascia lata is a broad tendon, the **iliotibial tract,** which is attached to the tibia.

This muscle *arises* on the ilium, sacrum, and coccyx; it *inserts* on the iliotibial tract and the posterior part of the femur. It causes extension and outward rotation of the femur.

Gluteus medius This muscle lies immediately under the gluteus maximus, covering a good portion of the ilium. Its *origin* is on the ilium and its *insertion* is on the lateral part of the greater trochanter. It causes abduction and medial rotation of the femur.

Gluteus minimus This is the smallest of the three gluteal muscles, and is located immediately under the gluteus medius. It, too, *arises* on the ilium; it *inserts* on the anterior border of the greater trochanter. The femur is abducted, rotated inward, and slightly flexed by this muscle.

Piriformis This small muscle takes its *origin* on the anterior surface of the sacrum and *inserts* on the upper border of the greater trochanter. It causes outward rotation, some abduction, and extension of the femur.

Adductor longus and Adductor brevis These two muscles are shown in illustration E. The adductor longus *originates* on the front of the pubis and *inserts* on the linea aspera of the femur.

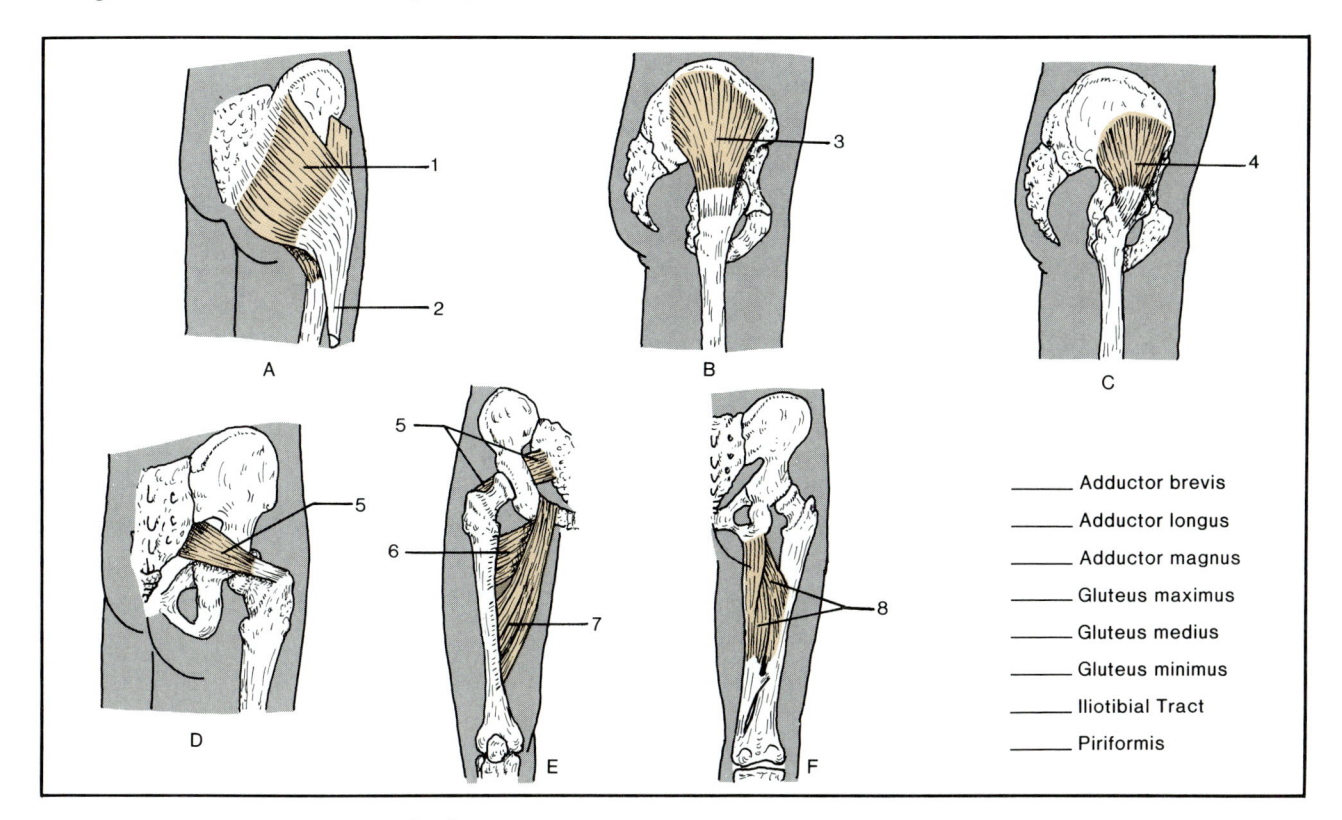

Figure 23.1 Muscles that move the femur.

Adductor brevis
Adductor longus
Adductor magnus
Gluteus maximus
Gluteus medius
Gluteus minimus
Iliotibial Tract
Piriformis

The adductor brevis *arises* on the posterior side of the pubis and *inserts* on the femur above the longus muscle. In addition to adduction, these muscles flex and rotate (medially) the femur.

Adductor magnus This muscle is the strongest of the three adductors. It *arises* on the ischium and part of the pubis. It *inserts* on the linea aspera of the femur in the same region as the other two adductors. Its action is synergistic with the longus and brevis adductors.

Assignment:

Label figure 23.1.

Thigh and Lower Leg Movements

The muscles illustrated in figure 23.2 are primarily concerned with flexion and extension of the lower part of the leg. Most of them are anchored to some part of the os coxa.

Hamstrings Three muscles, the *biceps femoris, semitendinosus,* and *semimembranosus,* constitute a group of muscles on the back of the thigh known as hamstrings. They are grouped together in illustration A.

Biceps femoris This muscle occupies the most lateral position of the three hamstrings. It has two heads: one long, and the other short. The long head, which obscures the short one, *arises* on the ischial tuberosity. The short head *originates* on the linea aspera of the femur. *Insertion* of the muscle is on the head of the fibula and the lateral condyle of the tibia.

Semitendinosus Medial to the biceps femoris is this muscle, which *arises* on the ischial tuberosity and *inserts* on the upper end of the shaft of the tibia.

Semimembranosus This muscle occupies the most medial position of the three hamstrings. Its *origin* consists of a thick semimembranous tendon attached to the ischial tuberosity. Its *insertion* is primarily on the posterior medial part of the medial condyle of the tibia.

Collective Action: All of these muscles flex the calf upon the thigh. They also extend and rotate the thigh. Rotation by the biceps is outward; the other two muscles cause inward rotation.

Quadriceps femoris The large muscle that makes up the anterior portion of the thigh is the quadriceps femoris. It consists of four parts, which are shown in illustrations C and D, figure 23.2. Note that all of them are united into a common tendon that passes over the patella to *insert* on the tibia.

Rectus femoris This portion of the quadriceps occupies a superficial central position. It *arises* by two tendons: one from the anterior inferior iliac spine and the other from a groove just above the acetabulum. The lower portion of the muscle is a broad aponeurosis that terminates in the tendon of **insertion.**

Vastus lateralis This is the largest and lateral portion of the quadriceps femoris. It *arises* from the lateral lip of the linea aspera.

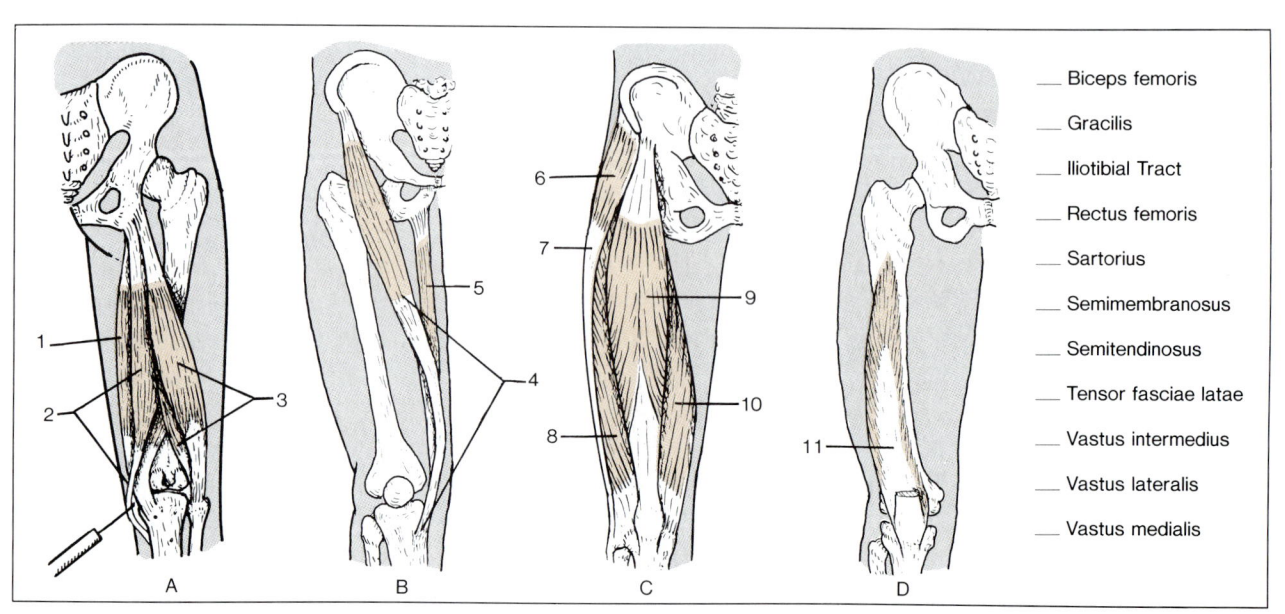

___ Biceps femoris

___ Gracilis

___ Iliotibial Tract

___ Rectus femoris

___ Sartorius

___ Semimembranosus

___ Semitendinosus

___ Tensor fasciae latae

___ Vastus intermedius

___ Vastus lateralis

___ Vastus medialis

Figure 23.2 Muscles that move the tibia and fibula.

Vastus medialis This muscle occupies the medial position on the thigh. It *arises* from the linea aspera.

Vastus intermedius Since this muscle is completely obscured by the other three muscles, it is shown separately in illustration D. Its *origin* is on the front and lateral surfaces of the femur.

Collective Action: The entire quadriceps femoris extends (straightens) the leg. Flexion of the thigh, however, is achieved by the rectus femoris.

Sartorius This is the longest muscle shown in illustration B. It *arises* from the anterior superior spine of the ilium and *inserts* on the medial surface of the tibia. It flexes the calf on the thigh, the thigh upon the pelvis, and rotates the leg laterally.

Tensor fasciae latae This muscle is shown in illustration C, figure 23.2. It *arises* from the anterior outer lip of the iliac crest, the anterior superior spine, and from the deep surface of the fascia lata. It is *inserted* between the two layers of the iliotibial tract at about the junction of the middle and upper thirds of the thigh. It flexes and slightly rotates the thigh.

Gracilis This muscle is located on the medial surface of the thigh. It *arises* from the lower margin of the pubic bone and *inserts* on the medial surface of the tibia near the insertion of the sartorius. It adducts, flexes, and rotates the thigh medially.

Assignment:

Label figure 23.3.

Lower Leg and Foot Movements

Figures 23.3 and 23.4 illustrate most of the muscles of the lower leg that cause flexion and foot movements.

Triceps surae The large superficial muscle that covers the calf of the leg is the triceps surae. It consists of two parts that are shown in illustrations A and B, figure 23.3. They are united by a common **tendon of Achilles** that *inserts* on the calcaneous of the foot. Collectively, the two muscles cause plantar flexion (standing on tiptoe).

Gastrocnemius This outer portion of the triceps surae has two heads that *arise* from the posterior surfaces of the medial and lateral condyles of the femur. In addition to plantar flexion, this muscle can, independently, flex the calf on the thigh.

Soleus This inner portion *arises* on the heads of the fibula and tibia.

Tibialis anterior The anterior lateral portion of the tibia is covered by this muscle. It *arises* from the lateral condyle and upper two-thirds of the tibia. Its distal end is shaped into a long tendon that passes over the tarsus and *inserts* on the inferior surface of the first cuneiform and first metatarsal bones. It causes dorsiflexion and inversion of the foot.

Tibialis posterior This muscle is a deep one that lies on the posterior surfaces of the tibia and fibula. It *arises* from both these bones and the interosseous membrane that extends between them. It *inserts* on the inferior surfaces of the navicular, the

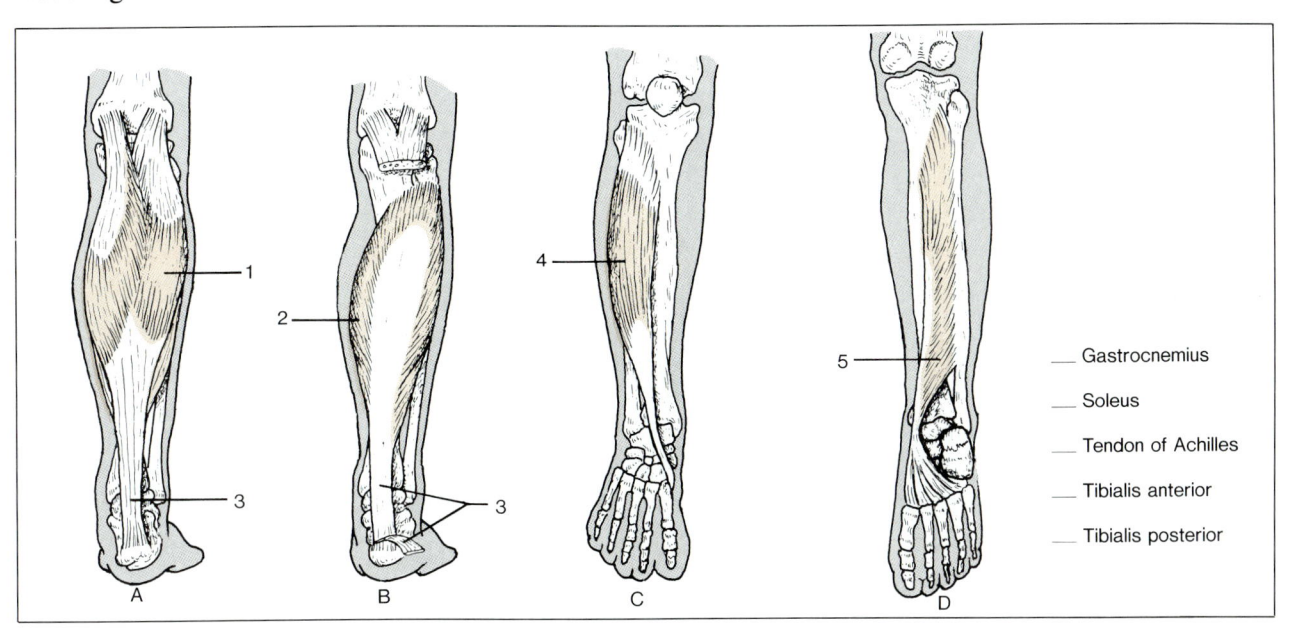

Figure 23.3 Lower leg muscles.

cunciforms, the cuboid, and the second, third, and fourth metatarsals. It causes plantar flexion and inversion of the foot. It assists in maintenance of the longitudinal and transverse arches of the foot.

The Peroneus Muscles (Latin: *peroneus,* fibula) Three peroneus muscles are shown in illustrations A and B, figure 23.4. Note that all three of them *originate* on the fibula. The **peroneus longus** is the longest one and takes its origin on the head and upper two-thirds of the fibula. The **peroneus tertius** is the smallest one, and the **peroneus brevis** is the one of in-between size. Note that the longus *inserts* on the first metatarsal and second cuneiform bones. The brevis and tertius muscles *insert* at different points on the fifth metatarsal bone. The longus and brevis muscles cause plantar flexion and eversion of the foot. The peroneus tertius causes dorsiflexion and eversion of the foot.

Flexor Muscles Two flexor muscles of the foot are shown in illustration C, figure 23.4. The **flexor hallucis longus** (Latin: *hallux,* big toe) has its *origin* on the fibula and intermuscular septa. Its long distal tendon *inserts* on the distal phalanx of the great toe. It flexes the great toe.

The **flexor digitorum longus** is the longer muscle shown in illustration C that *originates* on the tibia and the fascia that covers the tibialis posterior. Its distal end divides into four tendons that *insert* on the bases of the distal phalanges of the second, third, fourth, and fifth toes. It flexes the distal phalanges of the four smaller toes.

Extensor Muscles Two extensors of the foot are shown in illustration D, figure 23.4. The **extensor digitorum longus** is the longer one that takes its *origin* on the lateral condyle of the tibia, part of the fibula, and part of the interosseous membrane. Its tendon of insertion divides into four parts that *insert* on the superior surfaces of the second and third phalanges of the four smaller toes. It extends the proximal phalanges of the four smaller toes. It also flexes and inverts the foot.

The **extensor hallucis longus** is the other extensor in illustration D. It takes its *origin* on the fibula and interosseous membrane. Its distal tendon *inserts* at the base of the distal phalanx of the great toe. This muscle extends the proximal phalanx of the great toe and aids in dorsiflexion of the foot.

Assignment:

Label figures 23.3 and 23.4.

Cat Dissection

Hip Muscles

Remove the superficial fat and fascia that encase the muscles of the hip and thigh so that muscle fiber direction can be determined. Take care not to remove the fascia lata and iliotibial tract. The latter is a white, tendinous band on the lateral side of the thigh. Although the sartorious muscle is usually considered as a muscle of the thigh, it will be dissected here first to expose the full extent of the tensor fasciae latae.

Sartorius This broad straplike muscle occupies the cranial half of the medial side of the thigh. See figures 23.5 and 23.8. *Dissect, transect,* and *reflect.*

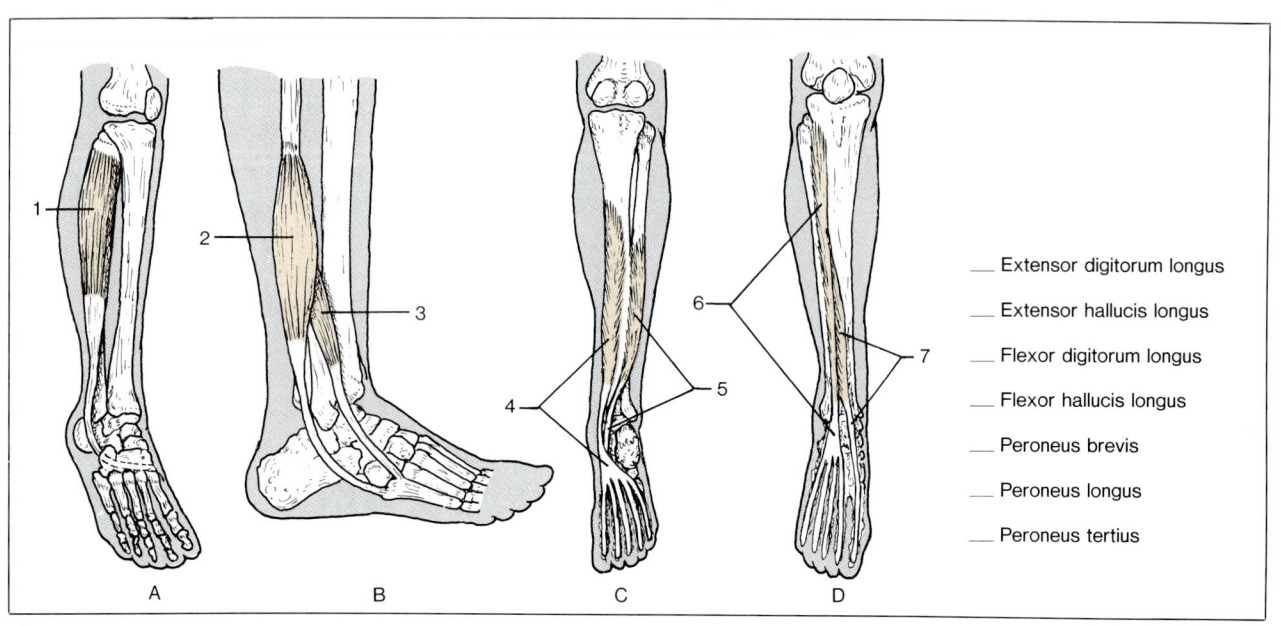

_____ Extensor digitorum longus

_____ Extensor hallucis longus

_____ Flexor digitorum longus

_____ Flexor hallucis longus

_____ Peroneus brevis

_____ Peroneus longus

_____ Peroneus tertius

Figure 23.4 Lower leg muscles.

Tensor fasciae latae This fan-shaped muscle is located on the anterolateral side of the hip region somewhat ventral to the other muscles in this group. Refer to figures 23.5 and 23.6. It arises from the lateral ilium and inserts in the iliotial tract portion of the fascia lata. The *fascia lata* is a tough layer of connective tissue that can be seen covering the vastus lateralis muscle.

Slide a blunt probe underneath the fascia lata to separate it from the vastus lateralis and *transect* the fascia lata so that you can completely *reflect* the tensor fascial latae. (The tensor muscle usually fuses somewhat with the gluteus maximus. This connection should be cut).

Gluteus medius With the tensor fasciae latae fully reflected, you can see the full extent of the gluteus medius. This thick muscle arises from the lateral surface of the ilium and inserts on the greater trochanter. In the cat this muscle is much larger than the gluteus maximus and will be found craniad of the latter.

Gluteus maximus This small hip muscle lies just caudad to the gluteus medius. It arises from the last sacral and first caudal vertebrae and inserts on the greater trochanter; therefore, the origin and insertion in the cat are far less extensive than in the human. *Dissect.*

Caudofemoralis This small muscle lies just caudad to the gluteus maximus. See figure 23.6. It is difficult to see because it is "hiding" below the cranial

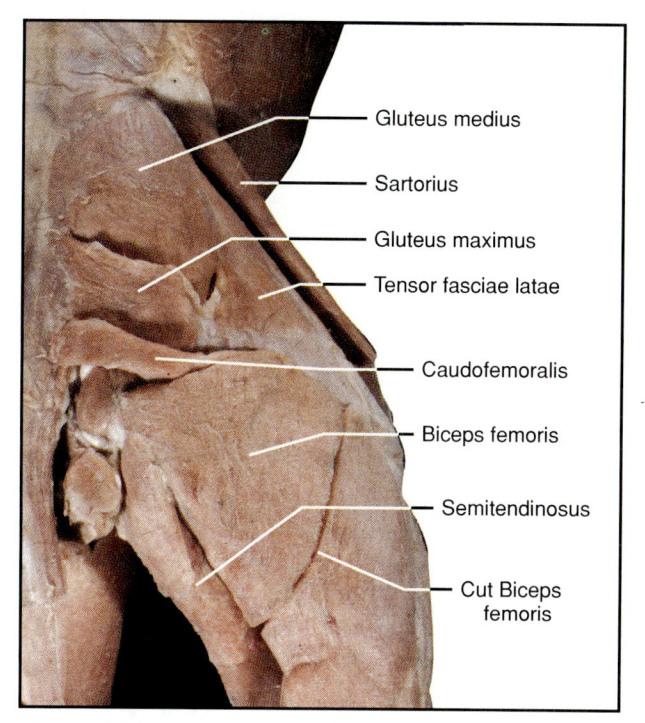

Figure 23.6 Hip muscles of the cat.

border of the biceps femoris. It arises on the caudal vertebrae and inserts by a very thin tendon on the patella.

This muscle is not present in humans; however, in the cat the caudofemoralis and the gluteus maximus together are more comparable to the human gluteus maximus than is the cat's gluteus maximus alone. *Dissect.*

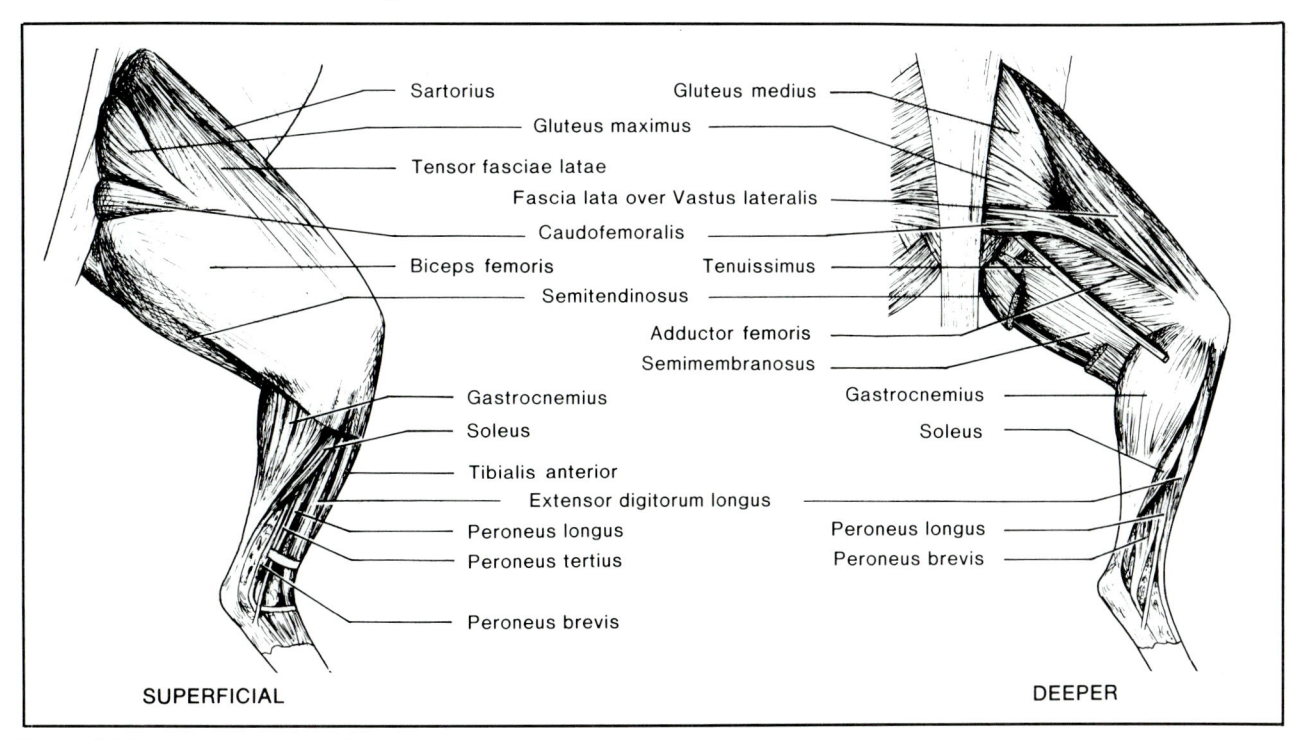

Figure 23.5 Lateral aspect of hindlimb.

Thigh Muscles

Thirteen muscles make up the musculature of the cat's thigh. Identify them in the following order:

Sartorius Previously dissected (see page 114).

Gracilis Wide (2–3 cm), flat muscle covering most of the caudal portion of the medial side of the thigh. Refer to figures 23.7 and 23.9. At the insertion the fibers end in a very thin flat tendon, part of which becomes continuous with the fascia covering the distal portion of the leg. *Dissect, transect,* and *reflect.*

The Hamstrings The cat has the same group of three muscles that are designated as hamstrings in humans:

Semimembranosus This is a large, thick muscle seen just beneath the gracilis; therefore, the latter must be reflected to see the full extent of this muscle. Dorsal to this muscle is seen the adductor femoris and ventral to this muscle is the semitendinosus.

Dissect by separating this muscle from the adductor femoris and semitendinosus. While the human homolog inserts only on the tibia, this muscle in the cat inserts on both the femur and tibia.

Semitendinosus Large band of muscle on the ventral border of the thigh between the semimembranosus and the biceps femoris. It inserts on the tibia. *Dissect.*

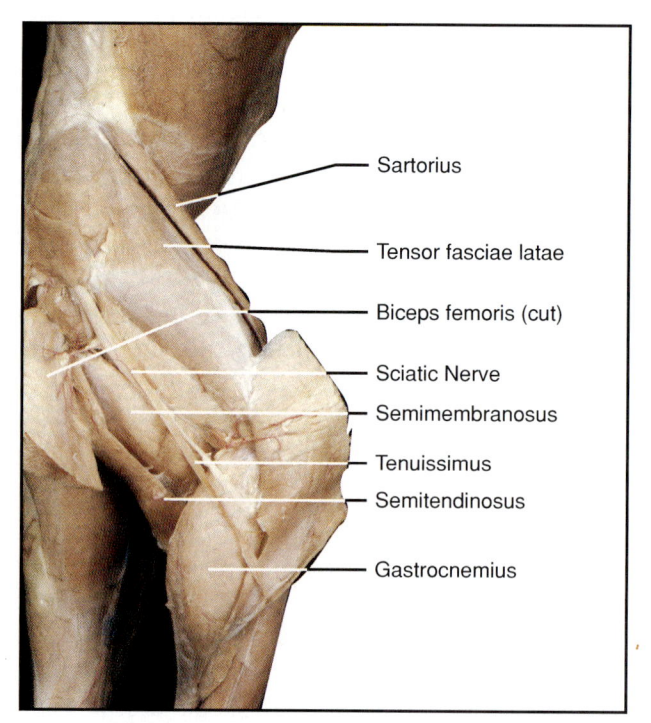

Figure 23.8 Deep muscles of thigh, lateral aspect.

Labels: Sartorius, Tensor fasciae latae, Biceps femoris (cut), Sciatic Nerve, Semimembranosus, Tenuissimus, Semitendinosus, Gastrocnemius

Biceps femoris This large broad muscle covers most of the lateral surface of the thigh. *Dissect, transect,* and *reflect.* When the muscle is transected, be careful not to cut the caudofemoralis and sciatic nerve. The nerve, shown in figure 23.8, appears as a white cord just beneath the biceps femoris.

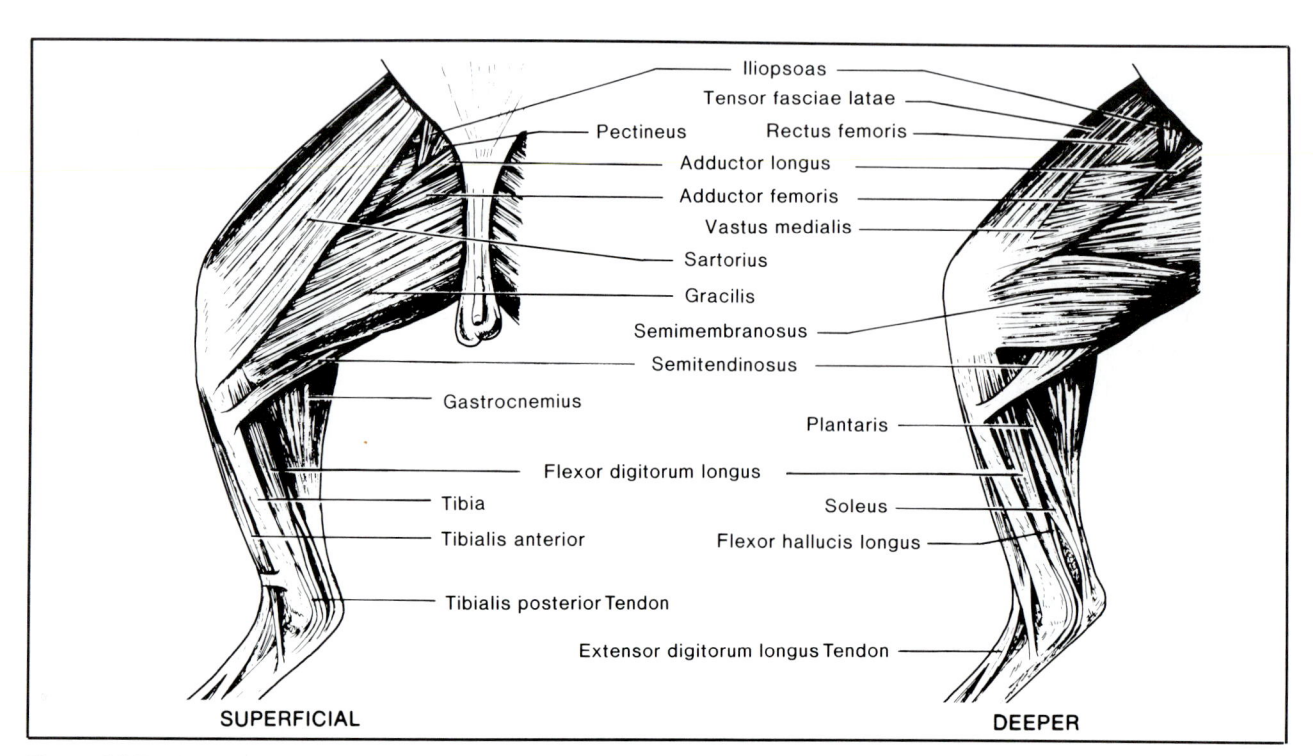

Labels: Iliopsoas, Tensor fasciae latae, Pectineus, Rectus femoris, Adductor longus, Adductor femoris, Vastus medialis, Sartorius, Gracilis, Semimembranosus, Semitendinosus, Gastrocnemius, Plantaris, Flexor digitorum longus, Tibia, Soleus, Tibialis anterior, Flexor hallucis longus, Tibialis posterior Tendon, Extensor digitorum longus Tendon, SUPERFICIAL, DEEPER

Figure 23.7 Medial aspect of hindlimb.

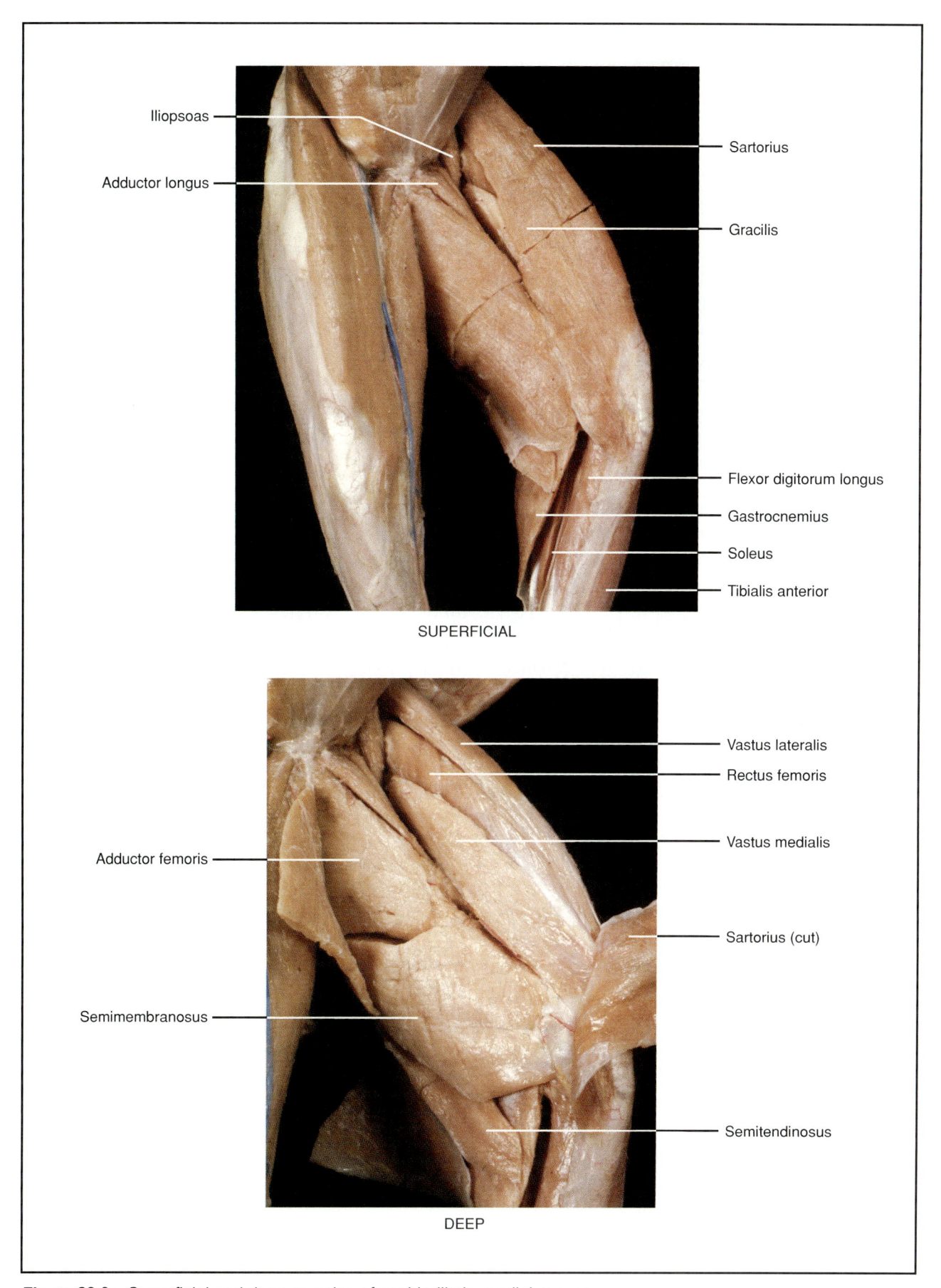

Figure 23.9 Superficial and deep muscles of cat hindlimb, medial aspect.

Adductor femoris This muscle lies deep to the gracilis and dorsal to the semimembranosus. It originates on the hip bone and inserts on the femur. The adductor femoris corresponds to the adductor magnus and adductor brevis of the human. *Dissect.*

Adductor longus This thin muscle lies along the cranial border of the adductor femoris, and extends from the hip bone to the femur.

Pectineus A very small triangular muscle (see figure 23.7) that lies cranial to the adductor longus and extends from the hip bone to the proximal end of the femur.

Iliopsoas This is actually two muscles, the *iliacus* and the *psoas major*. They are referred to as a single muscle because they join at their distal ends and have a common insertion on the lesser trochanter. Only the distal (insertion) end will be observed at this time.

Note that the muscle fibers of the iliopsoas are oriented almost perpendicular to the fibers of the pectineus and adductor longus.

Quadriceps femoris As in humans, the cat has a quadriceps femoris that consists of four muscles. This great extensor muscle of the knee joint has a common insertion by a large tendon that extends to the patella, attaches around the patella, and passes to the tibial tuberosity to insert.

Vastus lateralis Large muscle deep to the tensor fascia latae that occupies the craniolateral surface of the thigh.

Vastus medialis Large muscle deep to the sartorius that occupies the craniomedial surface of the thigh.

Rectus femoris A cigar-shaped muscle bordered laterally and medially by the vastus medialis. *Dissect, transect,* and *reflect.*

Vastus intermedius A flat muscle deep to the rectus femoris and attached to the anterior surface of the femur. The rectus femoris must be reflected to see the full extent of this muscle. Try to separate the vastus intermedius from the vastus lateralis and vastus medialis.

Leg and Foot Muscles

Five muscles of the leg and foot of the cat will be identified here.

Gastrocnemius This muscle on the dorsal side of the leg has two heads of origin: a lateral head from the lateral epicondyle of the femur and a medial head from the medial epicondyle of the femur. The muscle inserts by way of the calcaneal (*Achilles*) tendon on to the calcaneous.

In the cat a large **plantaris** (figure 23.7) muscle can be seen between the two heads of the gastrocnemius. In humans the plantaris is a small fusiform muscle of little importance. *Dissect.*

Soleus Deep to the lateral head of the gastrocnemius lies the soleus muscle. Note that this muscle inserts with the gastrocnemius on the calcaneous bone by way of the calcaneous tendon.

Tibialis anterior This tapered band of muscle is situated on the anterolateral (ventrolateral) aspect of the tibia. Follow the tendon of insertion of this muscle as it crosses the ankle obliquely to reach the medial surface of the foot.

Extensor digitorum longus This muscle is covered throughout most of its length by the tibialis anterior. Separate these two muscles and follow the tendon of insertion as it crosses the ankle ventrally and divides into four tendons that are distributed to the digits. *Dissect.*

Peroneus muscles Like in the human, the cat has three peroneus muscles: *peroneus longus, peroneus brevis,* and *peroneus tertius.* These muscles are found on the lateral side of the leg between the extensor digitorum longus and the soleus.

The positions of the tendons of insertion in relation to the lateral malleolus in the cat differ from those in humans; also, the insertion points are somewhat different. Therefore, you should identify these muscles as a "group" and not try to distinguish which muscle is which.

Surface Muscles Review

Figure 23.10 has been included here in this exercise to summarize our study of the muscles of the body as a whole. Only the surface muscles are shown. To determine your present understanding of the human musculature, attempt to label these diagrams first by *not referring back* to previous illustrations. This type of self-testing will determine what additional study is needed.

Laboratory Report

Complete the last portion of combined Laboratory Report 22,23.

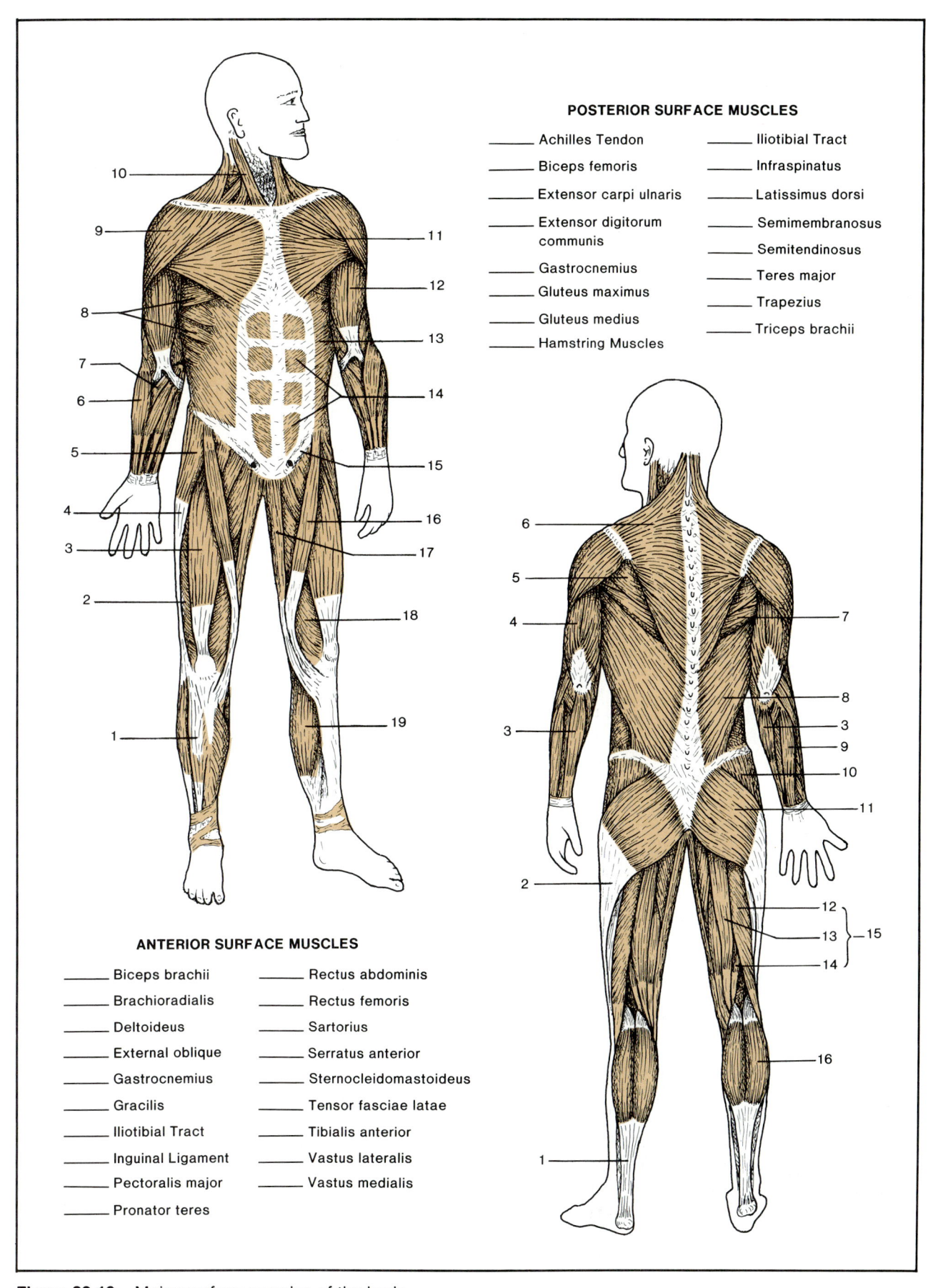

POSTERIOR SURFACE MUSCLES

_____ Achilles Tendon
_____ Biceps femoris
_____ Extensor carpi ulnaris
_____ Extensor digitorum communis
_____ Gastrocnemius
_____ Gluteus maximus
_____ Gluteus medius
_____ Hamstring Muscles

_____ Iliotibial Tract
_____ Infraspinatus
_____ Latissimus dorsi
_____ Semimembranosus
_____ Semitendinosus
_____ Teres major
_____ Trapezius
_____ Triceps brachii

ANTERIOR SURFACE MUSCLES

_____ Biceps brachii
_____ Brachioradialis
_____ Deltoideus
_____ External oblique
_____ Gastrocnemius
_____ Gracilis
_____ Iliotibial Tract
_____ Inguinal Ligament
_____ Pectoralis major
_____ Pronator teres

_____ Rectus abdominis
_____ Rectus femoris
_____ Sartorius
_____ Serratus anterior
_____ Sternocleidomastoideus
_____ Tensor fasciae latae
_____ Tibialis anterior
_____ Vastus lateralis
_____ Vastus medialis

Figure 23.10   Major surface muscles of the body.

Part 5 The Nervous System

The nervous system consists of an intricate maze of neurons and receptors that functions to coordinate various physiological activities of the body. It includes the brain and spinal cord of the *central nervous system* and all the cranial and spinal nerves of the *peripheral nervous system.* It is divided functionally into the *somatic* (voluntary) and *autonomic* (involuntary) systems. It includes the sense organs of sight, hearing, smell, and taste.

This unit is divided into six exercises. Exercise 24 is a survey of the different types of nerve cells that make up the entire nervous system. Exercise 25 pertains to the spinal cord, spinal nerves, and the reflex arcs of both the somatic and autonomic types. The external and internal anatomy of the brain is studied in the next two exercises. The sheep brain will be used here for dissection; preserved human brains will be used for observation, not dissection. The eye and ear are studied in the last two exercises of this unit. Some receptors, such as the taste buds of the tongue, will be studied later.

24 Nerve Tissue

The nervous system is composed of two kinds of cells: neurons and neuroglia. **Neurons** are the functional units of the nervous system in that they transmit nerve impulses. **Neuroglial cells,** or **glia,** are connective, supportive, and nutritive; nerve impulse transmission is not one of their characteristics. Although our prime concern here is with neurons, both kinds of cells will be studied in this exercise.

The first portion of this exercise is descriptive and should be completed prior to laboratory studies. The laboratory work will involve an indepth study of the different kinds of neurons seen in the spinal cord and brain.

As you study the neurons illustrated in figure 24.1 keep in mind that not all the structures shown in the illustration will be visible with your laboratory microscope; however, once you start studying microscope slides of spinal cord and brain tissues, you will find that most of the cellular structures are visible to some extent.

Neuron Structure

Because neurons perform different roles in different parts of the nervous system, they exist in a variety of sizes and configurations. In spite of this diversity, all neurons have much in common. Figure 24.1 illustrates most structures that all neurons have in common.

The Cell Body and its Processes

The large peripheral neurons illustrated in figure 24.1 are the principal neurons associated with skeletal muscle physiology. The cross-section through the spinal cord illustrates the relationship of these neurons to the spinal cord and to each other. Three kinds of neurons are shown: the sensory neuron, the motor neuron, and the interneuron. These three neurons, together with the receptor and effector, compose a reflex arc, which is described more in detail in the next exercise.

The cell body of a neuron is called a **perikaryon.** It usually contains a rather large nucleus surrounded by Nissl bodies and neurofibrils in the cytoplasm. **Nissl bodies** are dense aggregations of rough endoplasmic reticulum. They stain readily with basic aniline dyes such as toluidine blue or cresyl violet. They represent sites of protein synthesis. Some Nissl bodies are shown in the perikaryon of the motor neuron in figure 24.1.

Neurofibrils are slender protein filaments that extend throughout the cytoplasm parallel to the long axis. They resemble roadways that circumvent the Nissl bodies. It is significant that these minute fibers converge into the axon to form the core of the nerve fiber.

The most remarkable features of neurons are their cytoplasmic processes: the axons and dendrites. Traditional terminology once categorized these processes purely from a morphological sense; however, numerous exceptions require more accurate and universal definitions which emphasize their functional attributes. A **dendrite,** or **dendritic zone,** functions in receiving signals from receptors or other neurons and plays an important part in integration of information. An **axon,** on the other hand, is a single elongated extension of the cytoplasm that has the specialized function of transmitting impulses away from the dendritic zone. The cell body can be located at any position along the conduction pathway. In the motor neuron of figure 24.1 the dendrites are the short branching processes of the perikaryon; the axon is the long single process. Although a neuron will usually have several dendrites, there will be only one axon. Some neurons, however, such as the *amacrine cells* of the retina, have no axon at all.

Fiber Construction

The neural fibers of all peripheral neurons are enclosed by a covering of **neurolemmocytes** (Schwann cells). This covering extends from the perikaryon to the peripheral termination of the fiber. In the larger peripheral neurons, such as those seen in figure 24.1, the neurolemmocytes are wrapped around the axon in a unique manner to form a **myelin sheath** of lipoprotein. The outer portion of

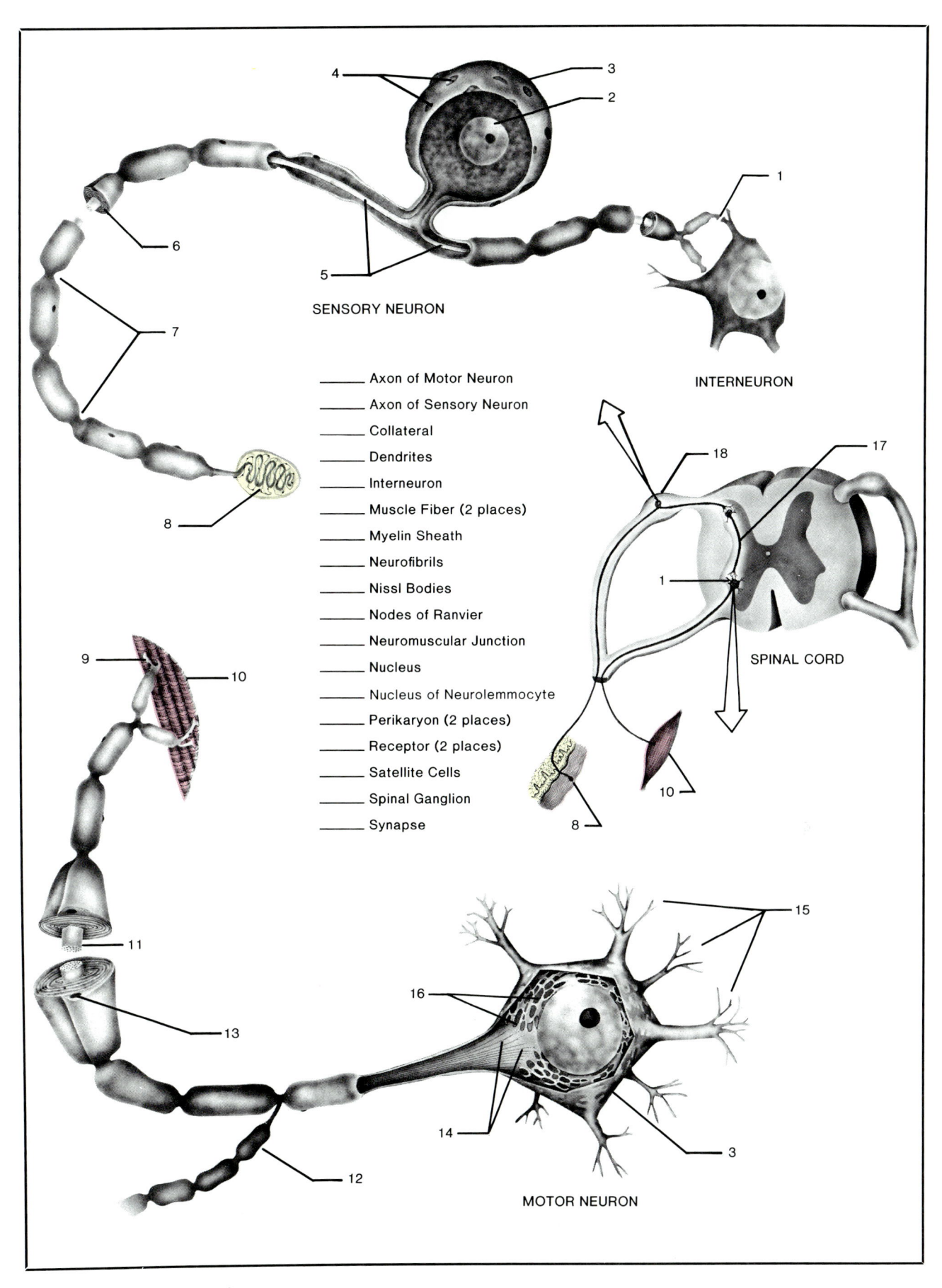

SENSORY NEURON

INTERNEURON

_____ Axon of Motor Neuron
_____ Axon of Sensory Neuron
_____ Collateral
_____ Dendrites
_____ Interneuron
_____ Muscle Fiber (2 places)
_____ Myelin Sheath
_____ Neurofibrils
_____ Nissl Bodies
_____ Nodes of Ranvier
_____ Neuromuscular Junction
_____ Nucleus
_____ Nucleus of Neurolemmocyte
_____ Perikaryon (2 places)
_____ Receptor (2 places)
_____ Satellite Cells
_____ Spinal Ganglion
_____ Synapse

SPINAL CORD

MOTOR NEURON

Figure 24.1 Sensory and motor neurons.

the neurolemmocytes that contain nuclei and cytoplasm make up the **neurolemma** (neurolemmal sheath). Those axons that have a thick myelin sheath with a neurolemma are designated as being *myelinated*. The smaller peripheral neurons that have fibers enclosed in neurolemmocytes, but lack the myelin sheath, are said to have *unmyelinated* fibers. One of the most important functions of neurolemmocytes is to facilitate the regeneration of damaged fibers. When a fiber is damaged, regeneration occurs along the pathway formed by the neurolemmocytes.

The myelin sheath and neurolemma are formed during embryological development by the folding of the neurolemmocytes around the axons. The axon of the motor neuron in figure 24.1 reveals an enlarged cross-section of the lipoprotein sheath and neurolemma.

The myelin sheath and neurolemma are interrupted at regular intervals by **nodes of Ranvier,** which are points of discontinuity between successive neurolemmocytes; each internode consists of a single neurolemmocyte. Each node of Ranvier represents a place where the exposed axon lacks the myelin and neurolemma. The nodes of Ranvier play a significant role in facilitating the speed of nerve impulse transmission through a nerve fiber.

Types of Neurons

The variability in size, shape, and arborization of neurons is considerable. Neurons may be multipolar, bipolar, unipolar, or pseudounipolar. Some of them have perikarya as small as 4 micrometers; others may be as large as 150 micrometers. Some neurons have perikarya that are encapsulated with satellite cells; others are not encapsulated. Many have myelinated fibers; others do not. More detailed structural features of spinal cord and brain neurons follows.

Neurons of the Spinal Cord

The principal neurons of the spinal cord are motor neurons, sensory neurons, and interneurons. Each type has unique characteristics.

Motor Neurons As indicated in figure 24.1, these *multipolar* neurons have their perikarya located in the gray matter of the central nervous system (CNS). They are also referred to as *efferent neurons* since they carry nerve impulses away from the CNS. The axons of these neurons are myelinated and terminate in skeletal muscle fibers. They function in the maintenance of voluntary control over skeletal muscles.

The perikarya of these neurons are somewhat angular or star-shaped rather than oval. The cytoplasm in a properly stained perikaryon reveals a nucleus, many Nissl bodies, and neurofibils. Many short branching dendrites are present that make synaptic connections with axons of interneurons or sensory neurons. Illustrations C and D of figure HA-12 in the Histology Atlas reveal the appearance of these cells when observed under oil immersion optics.

The myelinated axons of these neurons often have **collaterals** emanating at right angles from a node of Ranvier. Collaterals are branches that provide innervation to additional muscle fibers, other neurons, and even the same neuron in some instances.

Sensory Neurons These neurons are also called *ganglion cells* because their perikarya are located in ganglia outside the CNS. Since they carry nerve impulses from the receptor toward the CNS, they are also often referred to as *afferent neurons*.

As illustrated in figure 24.1, the perikaryon of a sensory neuron is ovoid in shape and is covered with a capsule of **satellite cells.** These cells are continuous with neurolemmocytes and have the same relationship to those neurons that certain neuroglia (oligodendrocytes) have to cells of the CNS. Satellite cells are not neuroglia, however, since they have a different embryological origin. Illustration E, figure HA-12 of the Histology Atlas, reveals what satellite cells look like in a sectioned sensory ganglion.

Although sensory neurons appear to be unipolar, histologists classify them as *pseudounipolar* on the basis of their embryological development. Note that the entire fiber is myelinated from the *receptor* in the skin to the *synaptic connection* (synapse) in the spinal cord. The entire myelinated fiber is designated as an **axon** even though part of it functions like a dendrite in carrying nerve impulses toward the cell body.

Interneurons (*Associated* or *Internuncial*) These multipolar unmyelinated neurons exist in large numbers in the gray matter of the CNS. They are essentially the integrator cells between sensory and motor neurons. Most reflexes involve one or more interneurons between the sensory and motor neurons. However, some automatic responses, such as the knee jerk reflex, are monosynaptic in that they lack interneurons.

Assignment:

Before going on to the study of brain cells, label figure 24.1.

Neurons of the Brain

Four different types of neurons that are found in various parts of the brain are shown in figure 24.2. They are pyramidal, Purkinje, stellate, and basket cells.

Pyramidal Cells These multipolar neurons are the principal cells of the cortex of the cerebrum. The upper neuron in figure 24.2 is of this type. Figure HA-13 of the Histology Atlas reveals actual photomicrographs of these cells.

The perikarya of these neurons are somewhat triangular to impart a pyramidlike shape. A unique characteristic of these cells is that they have two separate sets of dendrites: (1) a long dendritic trunklike structure with many branches that ascends vertically in the cortex, and (2) several basal branching dendrites that extend outward from the surfaces of the perikaryon. The axon of each of these neurons can be differentiated from the dendrites by its smoother surface.

Purkinje Cells The large multipolar neuron in the lower left-hand corner of figure 24.2 is a Purkinje cell. The perikarya of these neurons are located deep within the molecular layer of the cerebellum (see figure HA-14, Histology Atlas). The large branching dendritic processes of these cells fill up most of the space in the molecular layer. The axons of these neurons extend inward into the granule cell layer of the brain.

Stellate Cells (*Golgi Type II*) These small neurons are found in both the cerebrum and cerebellum, where they act as linkage (association) cells for the pyramidal cells of the cerebrum and the Purkinje cells of the cerebellum. Both multipolar and bipolar types exist. See figures 24.2, HA-13, and HA-14.

Basket Cells These multipolar neurons are a variety of large stellate cells that are located deep in the molecular layer of the cerebellum in close association with the Purkinje cells (figures 24.2 and HA-14). They have short, thick, branching dendrites and a long axon. The axons of these neurons usually have five or six collaterals that make synaptic connections with dendrites of the Purkinje cells. Like the stellate cells, these cells function as association neurons.

Neuroglia

Numerically, the neuroglial cells of the nervous system exceed neurons by a ratio of approximately

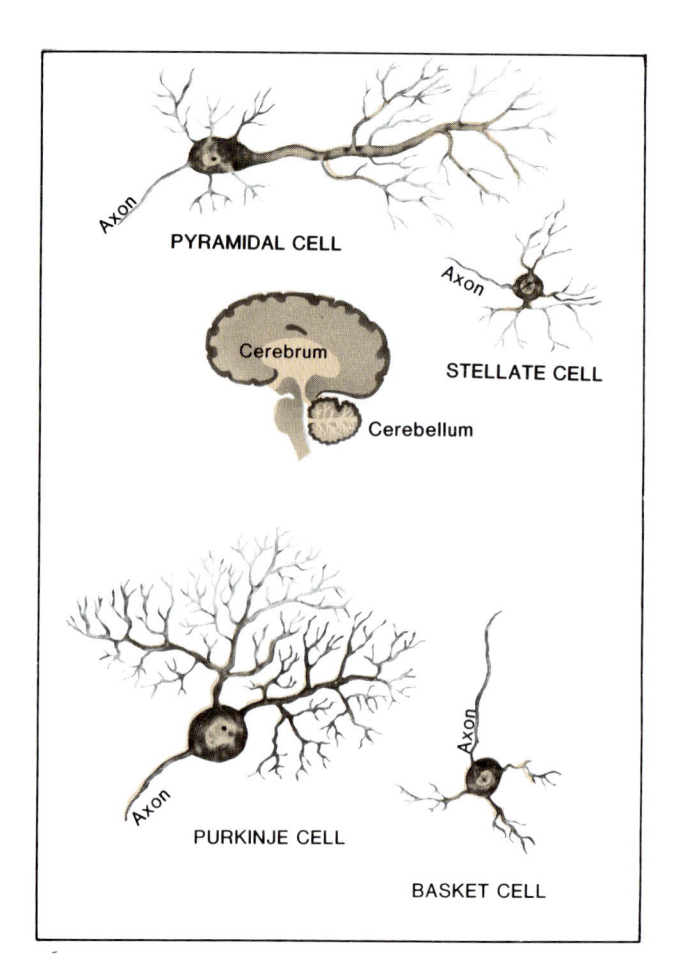

Figure 24.2   Neurons of the brain.

5:1. The term *neuroglia* (nerve glue) is applied to the ependyma, which lines the ventricles of the brain and spinal cord, and to the neuroglial cells, which intermesh with neurons of the nervous system and retina. The satellite and neurolemmocytes, which function much like neuroglial cells but have a different origin, are often referred to as *peripheral neuroglia* to set them apart.

Although neuroglial cells do not carry nerve impulses, they do perform many important functions within the CNS. First, during embryological development, they provide a framework in the CNS for young developing neurocytes. As the nervous system develops, the neuroglial cells also seem to act as barriers to the formation of synaptic connections so that they control the development of functional reflex patterns in the CNS. They appear to play a role as mediators for the normal metabolism of neurons, and they are involved in the degeneration and regeneration of nerve fibers. They are also the chief source of tumors of the CNS.

The neuroglia are divided into three distinct morphological categories: astrocytes, oligodendro-

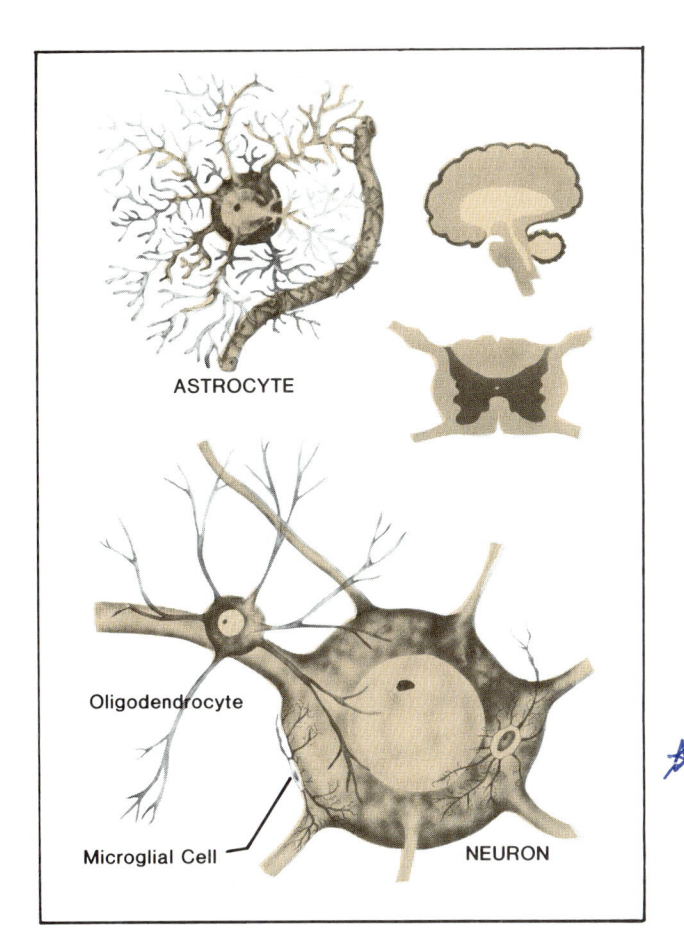

Figure 24.3 Neuroglial cells.

cytes, and microglia. Representatives of each group are illustrated in figure 24.3.

Astrocytes These neuroglial cells have large cell bodies with numerous processes radiating out in all directions. There are two types: protoplasmic and fibrous astrocytes. The one shown in figure 24.3 is of the protoplasmic variety. These cells may be attached to blood vessels (figure 24.3), pia mater, or neurons, much like satellite cells.

Oligodendrocytes These cells have much in common with neurolemmocytes since they develop in rows along nerve fibers and produce myelin within the CNS. These cells are large like the astrocytes and together with astrocytes are often referred to as *macroglia*. In tissue culture, these cells exhibit rhythmic pulsatile movements, which are not well understood.

Microglia These cells are much smaller than macroglial cells. Two of them are seen attached to the perikaryon of a neuron in figure 24.3. The cytoplasmic processes on these cells are more twisted than the processes on astrocytes and oligodendrocytes. Microglia are scattered throughout the brain and spinal cord. They appear to function as CNS phagocytes.

Microscopic Studies

After answering the questions on the Laboratory Report that pertain to cells of the nervous system, examine prepared slides of the nervous system using oil immersion optics whenever necessary. The following procedure will involve most of the cells discussed in this exercise.

Materials:

> prepared slides: x.s. spinal cord (H10.341 or H10.342), spinal cord smear (H4.11), spinal ganglion (H4.25), cerebral cortex (H10.11 or H10.12), and cerebellum (H10.23)

Spinal Cord Examine the cross section of a rat spinal cord under low power and identify the structures labeled in figure HA-12. Study several of the large *motor neurons* in the gray matter with the high-dry objective.

Also, study a smear ox spinal cord tissue and compare the cells with the photomicrograph in illustration D, figure HA-12.

Ganglion Cells Study a slide of a section through a spinal ganglion and look for *satellite cells* that surround the sensory neurons. Refer to illustration E, figure HA-12.

Cerebral Cortex Examine a slide of the cerebral cortex. Look for *pyramidal* and *stellate cells.* Refer to figure HA-13. Try to differentiate dendrites from axons on the pyramidal cells.

Note the presence of spiny processes called "gemmules" that are seen on the branches of the dendrites. These processes greatly increase the surface area of the dendrites, allowing large neurons to receive as many as 100,000 separate axon terminals or synapses.

Cerebellum Examine a slide of the cerebellum and look for *Purkinje cells, stellate cells,* and *basket cells.* Refer to figure HA-14.

Laboratory Report

Complete the Laboratory for this exercise.

25 The Spinal Cord, Spinal Nerves, and Reflex Arcs

In this exercise we will study a portion of the central nervous system (the spinal cord) and the origins of the various spinal nerves, which are parts of the peripheral nervous system. Incorporated into this study will be a comparison of the differences in the reflex arcs of two divisions of the nervous system. There will be no dissection at this time pertaining to the study of the spinal cord and nerves. As the dissection progresses on the cat in subsequent exercises, many of these nerves will be encountered. At this time our principal concern is to understand the relationship of the spinal cord to the spinal nerves.

The Spinal Cord

The spinal cord is a downward extension of the medulla oblongata of the brain. Figure 25.1 reveals its gross structure, as seen posteriorly. To expose it, the posterior portions of the vertebrae and sacrum have been removed.

The spinal cord starts at the upper border of the atlas and terminates as the **conus medullaris** at the lower border of the first lumbar vertebra. In fetal life the spinal cord occupies the entire length of the vertebral canal (spinal cavity), but as the vertebral column continues to elongate, the spinal cord fails to lengthen with it; thus, the vertebral canal extends downward beyond the end of the spinal cord.

Extending downward from the conus medullaris is an aggregate of fibers called the **cauda equina** (horse's tail), which fills the lower vertebral canal. The innermost fiber of the cauda equina, which is located on the median line, is called the **filum terminale interna.** This delicate median prolongation of the conus medullaris becomes the **filum terminale externa** after it passes through the dural sac. The **dural sac** (dura mater) is continuous with the dura mater that surrounds the brain. Only a portion of it (label 25) is shown in figure 25.1. The remainder of the dura mater has been left out of this illustration for clarity.

The Spinal Nerves

The spinal nerves emerge from the spinal cord in pairs through the intervertebral foramina on each side of the spinal cavity. There are eight cervical, twelve thoracic, five lumbar, and five sacral pairs. These thirty pairs of nerves, plus one pair of coccygeal nerves, make a total of thirty-one pairs of spinal nerves.

Reference to the sectional view of the spinal cord in figure 25.1 reveals that each spinal nerve is connected to the spinal cord by structures called **anterior** and **posterior roots.** Note that the posterior root (label 21) has an enlargement, the **spinal ganglion,** that contains cell bodies of sensory neurons. Neuronal fibers from these roots pass through the outer **white matter** of the spinal cord into the inner **gray matter** where neuronal connections *(synapses)* are made.

Cervical Nerves The first cervical nerve (C_1) emerges from the spinal cord in the space between the base of the skull and the atlas. The eighth cervical nerve (C_8) emerges between the seventh cervical and first thoracic vertebrae. Note that the first four cervical nerves are united in the neck region to form a network called the **cervical plexus.** The remaining cervical nerves (C_5, C_6, C_7, and C_8) and the first thoracic nerve unite to form the **brachial plexus** in the shoulder region.

Thoracic (*Intercostal*) Nerves The first thoracic nerve (T_1) emerges through the intervertebral foramen between the first and second thoracic vertebrae. The twelfth thoracic nerve (T_{12}) emerges through the foramen between the twelfth thoracic and first lumbar vertebrae. Each of these nerves lies adjacent to the lower margin of the rib above it.

Lumbar Nerves The first lumbar nerve (L_1) emerges from the intervertebral foramen between the first and second lumbar vertebrae. Close to where the nerve emerges from the spinal cavity, it divides to

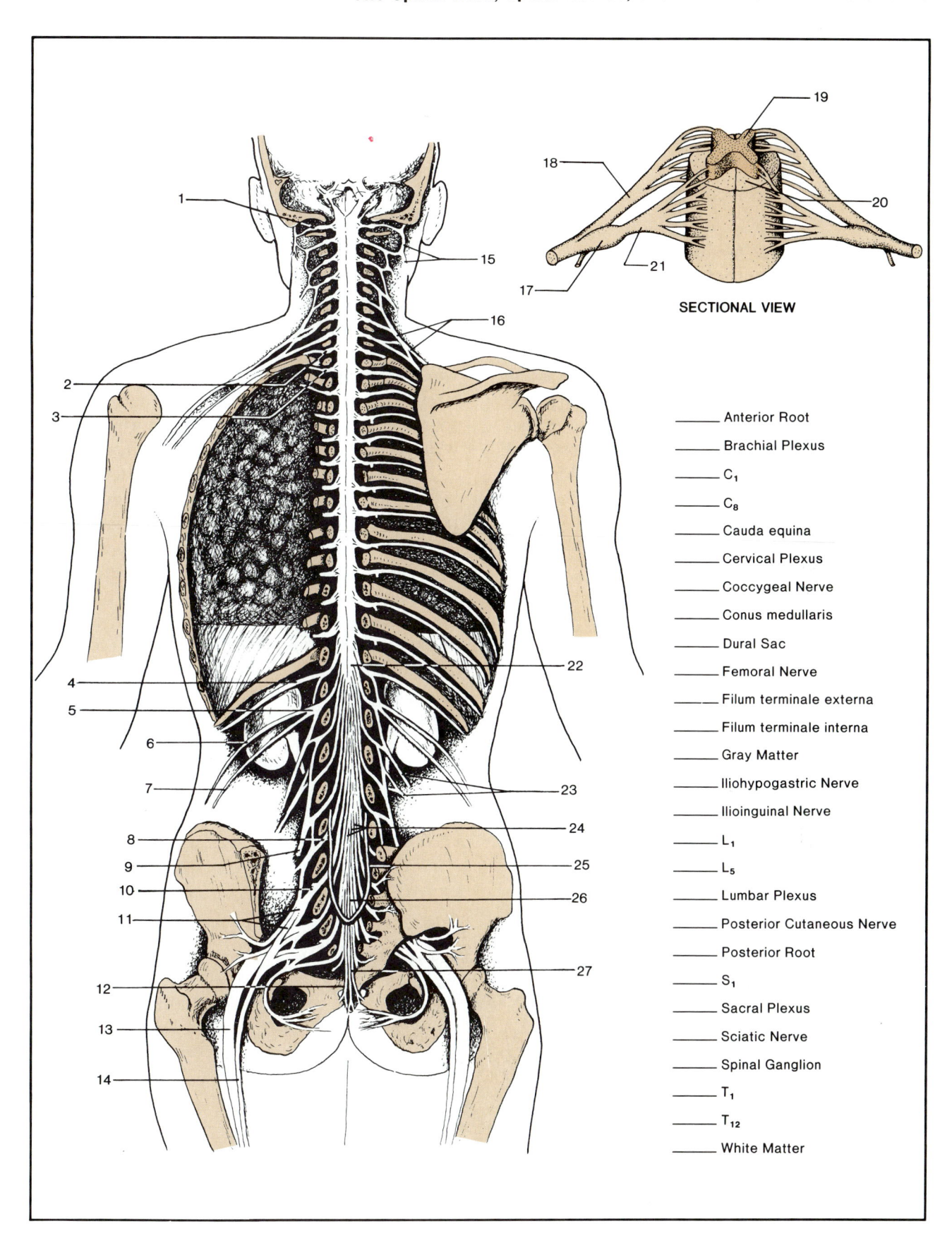

SECTIONAL VIEW

_____ Anterior Root
_____ Brachial Plexus
_____ C₁
_____ C₈
_____ Cauda equina
_____ Cervical Plexus
_____ Coccygeal Nerve
_____ Conus medullaris
_____ Dural Sac
_____ Femoral Nerve
_____ Filum terminale externa
_____ Filum terminale interna
_____ Gray Matter
_____ Iliohypogastric Nerve
_____ Ilioinguinal Nerve
_____ L₁
_____ L₅
_____ Lumbar Plexus
_____ Posterior Cutaneous Nerve
_____ Posterior Root
_____ S₁
_____ Sacral Plexus
_____ Sciatic Nerve
_____ Spinal Ganglion
_____ T₁
_____ T₁₂
_____ White Matter

Figure 25.1 The spinal cord and spinal nerves.

form an upper **iliohypogastric nerve** and a lower **ilioinguinal nerve.**

Note in figure 25.1 that L_1, L_2, L_3, and most of L_4 are united to form the **lumbar plexus** (label 23). The largest trunk emanating from this plexus is the **femoral nerve,** which innervates part of the leg. In reality, the femoral is formed by the union of L_2, L_3, and L_4.

Sacral and Coccygeal Nerves The remaining nerves of the cauda equina include five pairs of sacral and one pair of coccygeal nerves. A **sacral plexus** (label 11) is formed by the union of roots of L_4, L_5, and the first three sacral nerves (S_1, S_2, and S_3). The largest nerve that emerges from this plexus is the **sciatic nerve,** which passes down into the leg. The smaller nerve that parallels the sciatic is the **posterior cutaneous nerve** of the leg. The **coccygeal nerve** (label 12) contains nerve fibers from the fourth and fifth sacral nerves (S_4 and S_5).

Assignment:

Label figure 25.1.

Spinal Cord and Nerve Protection

Injury to the spinal cord is medically grave in that once the spinal cord is traumatized or severed the damage is permanent. Fortunately, the bony protection of the spinal cavity and the tissues around the spinal cord afford considerable protection. The presence of areolar connective tissue, meninges, and cerebrospinal fluid act as a combined shock absorber to protect the vulnerable cord. The cross-sectional view shown in figure 25.2 illustrates how the cord and spinal nerves are surrounded by these protective layers.

Cord Structure Before examining the surrounding tissues, identify the following structures on the cord in figure 25.2. The most noticeable characteristic of the spinal cord is the pattern of the **gray matter,** which resembles the configuration of the outstretched wings of a swallow-tailed butterfly. Surrounding this darker material is the **white matter,** which consists primarily of myelinated nerve fibers.

Along its median line the spinal cord is divided by a septum and a fissure. Note that the dorsal portion of the cord is bisected by a **posterior median septum** of neuroglial tissue that extends deep into the white matter. On the ventral surface of the cord is an **anterior median fissure**. In the gray matter on the median line lies a tiny **central canal,** evidence of the tubular nature of the spinal cord. This canal is continuous with the ventricles of the brain and extends into the filum terminale. It is lined with ciliated ependymal cells.

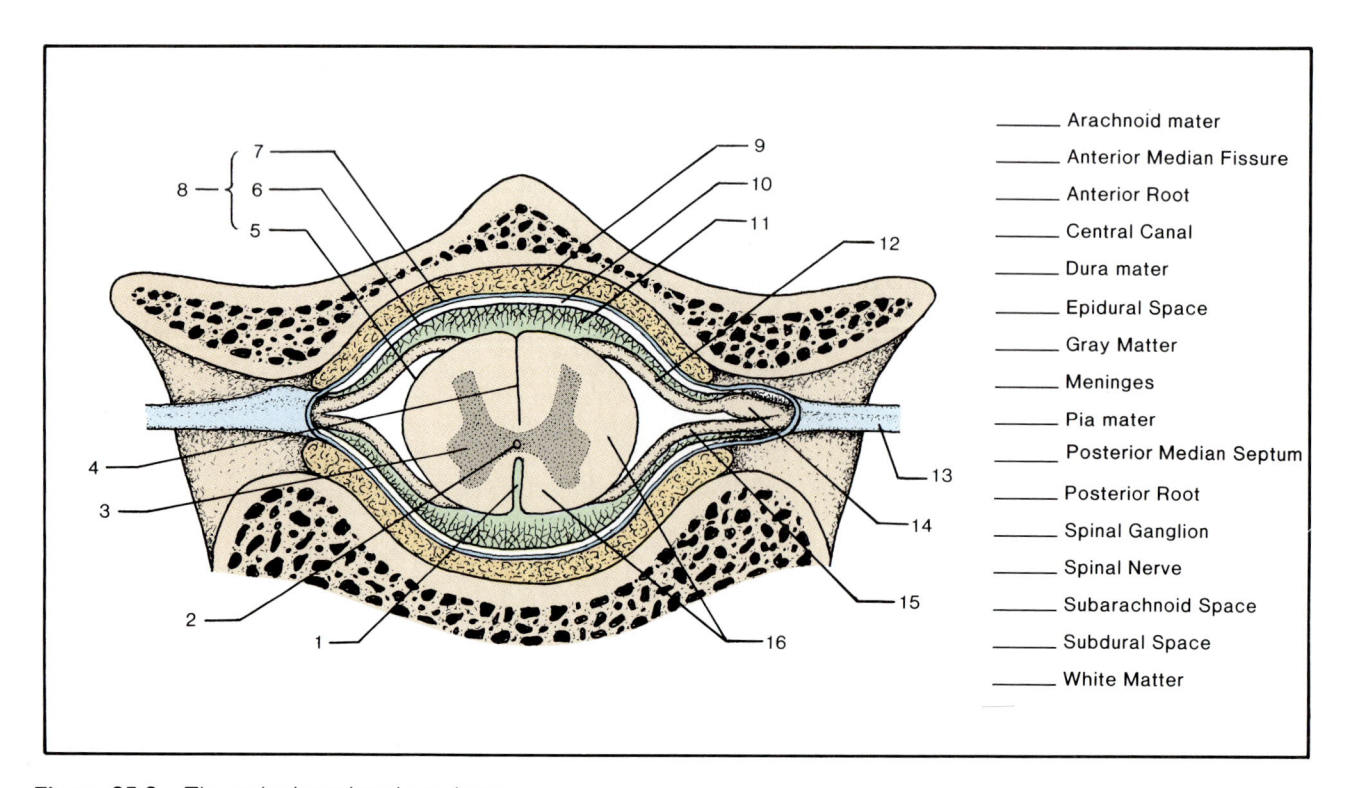

_____ Arachnoid mater
_____ Anterior Median Fissure
_____ Anterior Root
_____ Central Canal
_____ Dura mater
_____ Epidural Space
_____ Gray Matter
_____ Meninges
_____ Pia mater
_____ Posterior Median Septum
_____ Posterior Root
_____ Spinal Ganglion
_____ Spinal Nerve
_____ Subarachnoid Space
_____ Subdural Space
_____ White Matter

Figure 25.2 The spinal cord and meninges.

Spinal Nerves Note how the spinal nerves (label 13) emerge from the vertebrae on each side of the spinal column. Identify the **posterior root** with its **spinal ganglion** and the **anterior root.**

The Meninges Surrounding the spinal cord (and brain) are three meninges (*meninx,* singular). The outermost membrane is the **dura mater** (label 7), which also forms a covering for the spinal nerves. A cutaway portion of the dura on each side in figure 25.2 reveals the inner spinal nerve roots. The dura mater is the toughest of the three meninges, consisting of fibrous connective tissue. Between the dura and the bony vertebrae is an **epidural space,** which contains areolar connective tissue and blood vessels.

The innermost meninx is the **pia mater.** It is a thin delicate membrane that is actually the outer surface of the spinal cord. Between the pia mater and dura mater is the third meninx, the **arachnoid mater.** Note that the outer surface of the arachnoid mater lies adjacent to the dura mater. The space between the dura and arachnoid mater is actually a potential cavity that is called the **subdural space.** The inner surface of the arachnoid mater has a delicate fibrous texture that forms a netlike support around the spinal cord. The space between the arachnoid mater and the pia mater is the **subarachnoid space.** This space is filled with cerebrospinal fluid that provides a protective fluid cushion around the spinal cord.

Assignment:

Label figure 25.2.

The Somatic Reflex Arc

A brief mention of the somatic reflex arc was made in Exercise 24. In that exercise our prime concern was with the structure of neuronal elements that make up the circuit. Figure 25.3 is very similar to figure 24.1, although figure 25.3 is simpler.

The principal components of this type of reflex arc are: (1) a **receptor,** such as a neuromuscular spindle or a cutaneous endorgan that receives the stimulus; (2) a **sensory** (afferent) **neuron,** which carries impulses through a peripheral nerve and posterior root to the spinal cord; (3) an **interneuron** (association neuron), which forms synaptic connections between the sensory and motor neurons in the gray matter of the spinal cord; (4) a **motor** (efferent) **neuron,** which carries nerve impulses from the central nervous system through the ventral root to the effector via a peripheral nerve; and (5) an **effector** (muscle tissue), which responds to the stimulus by contracting.

Reflex arcs may have more than one interneuron, or may be completely lacking in interneurons. If no interneuron is present, as is true of the "knee-jerk" reflex, the reflex arc is said to be *monosynaptic.* When one or more interneurons exist, the reflex arc is classified as being *polysynaptic.*

The Visceral Reflex Arc

Muscular and glandular responses of the viscera to internal environmental changes are controlled by the **autonomic nervous system.** The reflexes of this system follow a different pathway in the nervous

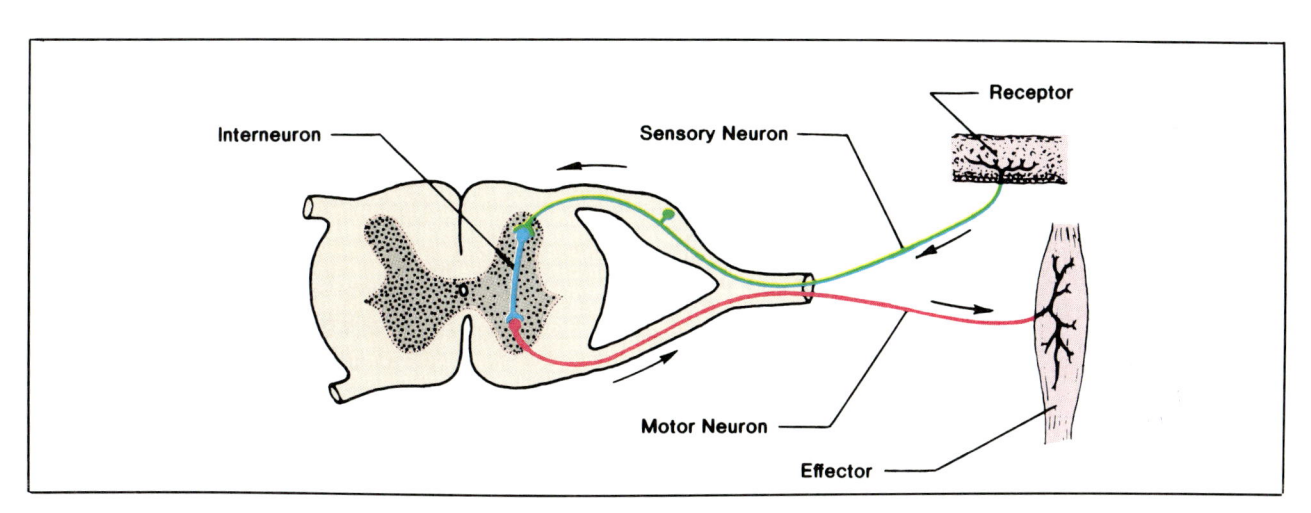

Figure 25.3 The somatic reflex arc.

system. Figure 25.4 illustrates the components of a visceral reflex arc.

The principal anatomical difference between somatic and visceral reflex arcs is that the latter type has two efferent neurons instead of one. These two neurons synapse outside of the central nervous system in an autonomic ganglion.

Two types of autonomic ganglia are shown in figure 25.4: vertebral and collateral. The **vertebral autonomic ganglia** are united to form a chain that lies along the vertebral column. The **collateral ganglia** are located further away from the central nervous system.

A visceral reflex originates with a stimulus acting on a receptor in the viscera. Impulses pass along the dendrite of a **visceral afferent neuron.** Note that the cell bodies of these neurons are located in the **spinal ganglion.** The axon of the visceral afferent neuron forms a synapse with the **preganglionic efferent neuron** in the spinal cord. Impulses in this neuron are conveyed to the **postganglionic efferent neuron** at synaptic connections in either type of autonomic ganglion (note the short

portions of cut-off postganglionic efferent neurons in the vertebral autonomic ganglia). From these ganglia the postganglionic efferent neuron carries the impulses to the organ innervated.

In this brief mention of the autonomic nervous system, the student is reminded that the system consists of two parts: the sympathetic and parasympathetic divisions. The *sympathetic* (thoracolumbar) *division* involves the spinal nerves of the thoracic and lumbar regions. The *parasympathetic* (craniosacral) *division* incorporates the cranial and sacral nerves. Most viscera of the body are innervated by nerves from both of these systems. This form of double innervation enables an organ to be stimulated by one system and inhibited by the other.

Assignment:

Label figure 25.4.

Laboratory Report

Complete the Laboratory Report for this exercise.

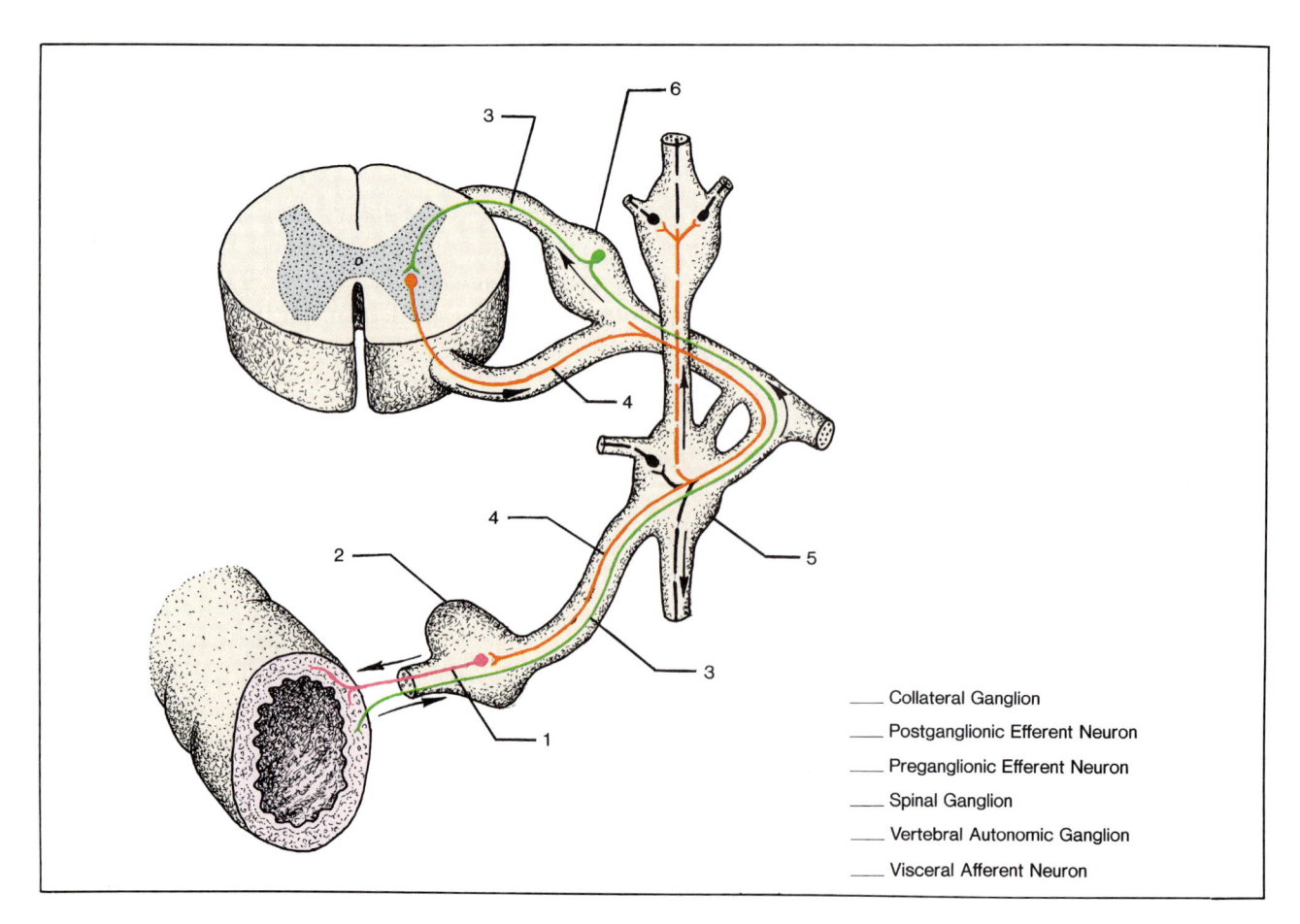

_____ Collateral Ganglion
_____ Postganglionic Efferent Neuron
_____ Preganglionic Efferent Neuron
_____ Spinal Ganglion
_____ Vertebral Autonomic Ganglion
_____ Visceral Afferent Neuron

Figure 25.4 The visceral reflex arc.

Brain Anatomy: External

This study of the human brain will be done in conjunction with dissection of the sheep brain. The ample size and availability of sheep brains make them preferable to brains of most other animals; also, the anatomical similarities that exist between the human and sheep brains are considerably greater than their differences.

Preserved human brains will also be available for study in this laboratory period. Dissection, however, will be confined to the sheep brain. A discussion of the meninges will precede the sheep brain dissection.

The Meninges

It was observed in Exercise 25 that the spinal cord, as well as the brain, is surrounded by three membranes called *meninges.* Due to the importance of these protective structures it will be necessary to reemphasize certain anatomical characteristics of these membranes.

Dura mater The outermost meninx is the *dura mater,* which is a thick tough membrane made up of fibrous connective tissue. The lateral view of the opened skull in figure 26.1 reveals the dura mater lifted away from the exposed brain. On the median line of the skull it forms a large **sagittal sinus** (label 6) that collects blood from the surface of the brain. Note that a large number of cerebral veins empty into this sinus.

Extending downward between the two halves of the cerebrum is an extension of the dura mater, the **falx cerebri.** This structure can also be seen in the frontal section. At its anterior end, the falx cerebri is attached to the crista galli of the ethmoid bone.

Arachnoid mater Inferior to the dura mater lies the second meninx, the *arachnoid mater* (label 8). Between this delicate netlike membrane and the surface of the brain is the **subarachnoid space,** which contains cerebrospinal fluid. Note that the arachnoid mater has small projections of tissue, the **arachnoid granulations,** which extend up into the

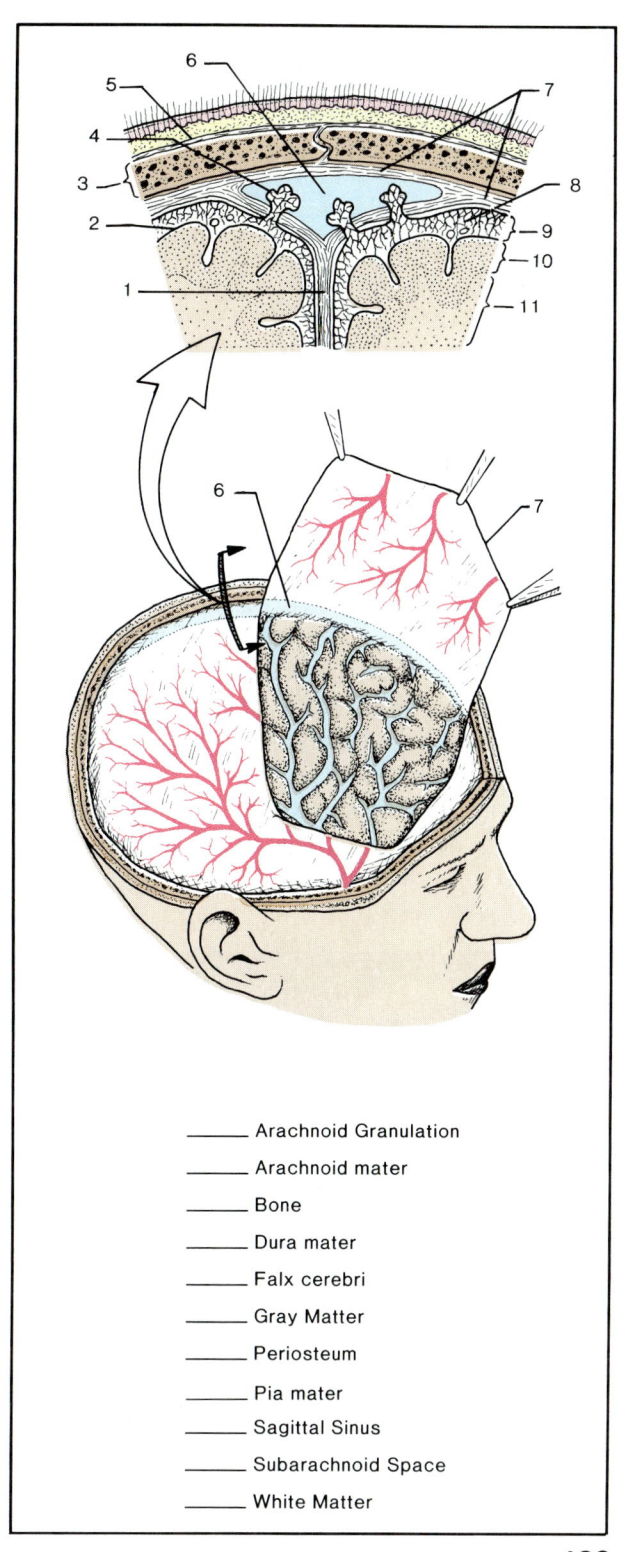

_____ Arachnoid Granulation

_____ Arachnoid mater

_____ Bone

_____ Dura mater

_____ Falx cerebri

_____ Gray Matter

_____ Periosteum

_____ Pia mater

_____ Sagittal Sinus

_____ Subarachnoid Space

_____ White Matter

Figure 26.1   The meninges.

sagittal sinus. These granulations allow cerebrospinal fluid to diffuse from the subarachnoid space into the venous blood of the sagittal sinus.

Pia mater The surface of the brain is covered by the third meninx, the *pia mater.* This membrane is very thin. Note that the surface of the brain has grooves, or **sulci,** which increase the surface of the **gray matter** (label 10). As in the case of the spinal cord, the gray matter is darker than the inner **white matter** because it contains cell bodies of neurons. The white matter consists of neuron fibers that extend from the gray matter to other parts of the brain and spinal cord.

Assignment:

Label figure 26.1.

Sheep Brain Dissection

Two procedures are provided here for this sheep brain study: (1) an *in situ* study of fresh brain material, and (2) the dissection of a preserved, formalin-hardened sheep brain. In the *in situ* dissection, the brain can be observed as it appears, undisturbed, in the skull. To get to the brain it is necessary to remove the top of the skull with an autopsy saw. This type of dissection enables one to see many things that cannot be seen in a preserved specimen that has already been removed from the skull. The value of the second dissection is that the formalin-hardened tissue will reveal structures that are usually destroyed when trying to remove the

fresh brain from the skull. If time restrictions prevent doing both dissections, the second dissection is preferred.

Sheep Head Dissection

To examine the sheep's brain within the cranium it will be necessary to remove the top of the skull with an autopsy saw, as illustrated in figures 26.3 through 26.5. The blade of this type of saw cuts through bone with a reciprocating action. Since it does not have a rotary action, it is a relatively safe tool to use; however, care must be exercised to avoid accidents. It will be necessary for one person to hold the sheep's head while someone does the cutting. *At no time should the holder's hands be in the cutting path of the saw blade.*

If only one or two saws are available, it will not be possible for everyone to start cutting at the same time. Since it takes five to ten minutes to remove the top of the skull, some students will have to be working on other parts of this exercise until a saw is available. Proceed as follows:

Materials:

fresh sheep head
autopsy saw
screwdriver (8″ long)
dissecting kit
black felt pen

1. With a black felt pen, mark a line on the skull across the forehead between the eyes, around the sides of the skull, and over the occipital condyles. Refer to figure 26.2.

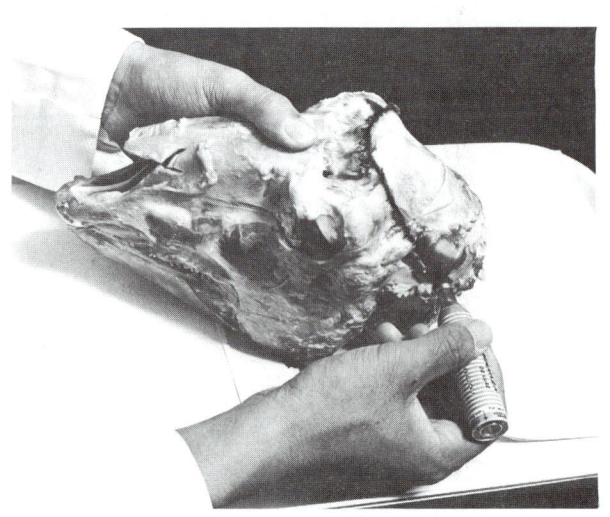

Figure 26.2 The skull is marked with a felt pen to indicate the line of cut.

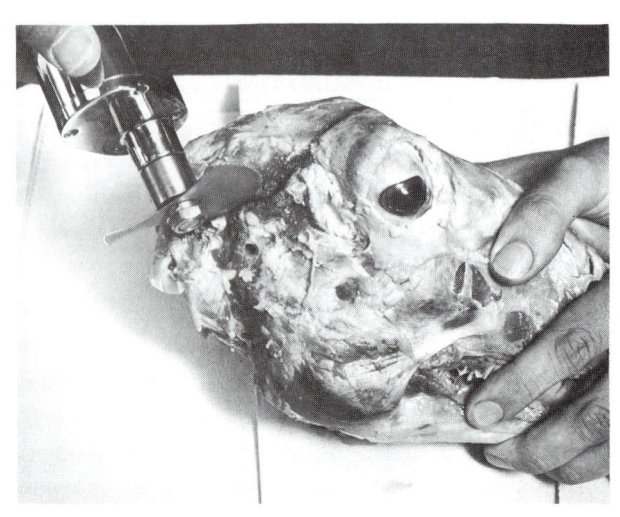

Figure 26.3 While the head is held securely by an assistant, the cut is made with an autopsy saw.

2. While you hold the saw securely with both hands, cut around the skull following the marked line. Brace your hands against the table for support. Don't try to "free hand" it. Use the large cutting edge for straight cuts; the small cutting edge for sharp curves.

   Be sure that the head is held securely by your laboratory partner. Cut only deep enough to get through the bone. Try not to damage the brain. Rest your hands after cutting an inch or two. To avoid accidents, do not allow your wrists to get too tired. As mentioned above, watch out for your partner's hands!

3. After cutting all the way around the skull, place the end of a screwdriver into the saw cut (figure 26.4) and pry upward to loosen the bony plate. Cut free any remaining portions.

4. Gently lift the bone section off the top of the skull. Note how fragments of the **dura mater** prevent you from completely removing the cap. Use a sharp scalpel or scissors to cut the dura mater loose as the skull cap is lifted off.

5. Examine the inside surface of the removed bone and study the dura mater. Note how thick and tough it is. Its toughness is due to the presence of collagenous fibers.

6. Locate the **sagittal sinus.** Open it with a scalpel or scissors and see if you can see any evidence of the **arachnoid granulations.**

7. Examine the surface of the brain. Observe that it is covered with convolutions called **gyri** (*gyrus,* singular). Between the gyri are the grooves, or **sulci.**

8. Locate the middle meninx, or **arachnoid mater,** on the surface of the brain. This meninx is a very thin, net-like membrane that appears to be closely attached to the brain. In actuality, there is a thin space, the **subarachnoid space,** between the arachnoid mater and the surface of the brain. This space contains **cerebrospinal fluid.** Probe into a sulcus with a blunt probe, pressing down on the arachnoid mater. Can you detect the presence of the cerebrospinal fluid immediately under the arachnoid mater?

9. Gently force your second, third, and fourth fingers under the anterior portion of the brain, lifting the brain from the floor of the cranial cavity. Take care not to damage the brain. Locate the **olfactory bulbs** (see figure 26.6). Note that they are attached to the forepart of the skull. From these bulbs pass olfactory nerves through the cribriform plate into the nasal cavity.

10. Free the olfactory bulbs from the skull with your scalpel.

11. Raise the brain further to expose the **optic chiasma** (see figure 26.6). Note how the optic nerves coming through the skull are continuous with this structure. It is in the optic chiasma where some of the neurons from the retina of each eye cross over.

12. Sever the optic nerves as close to the skull as possible with your scalpel and raise the brain further to expose the two **internal carotid arteries** that supply the brain with blood. Do you remember from your study of the skull what openings of the skull allow these vessels to pass through?

13. Sever the internal carotid arteries and raise the brain a little more to expose the **infundibulum**

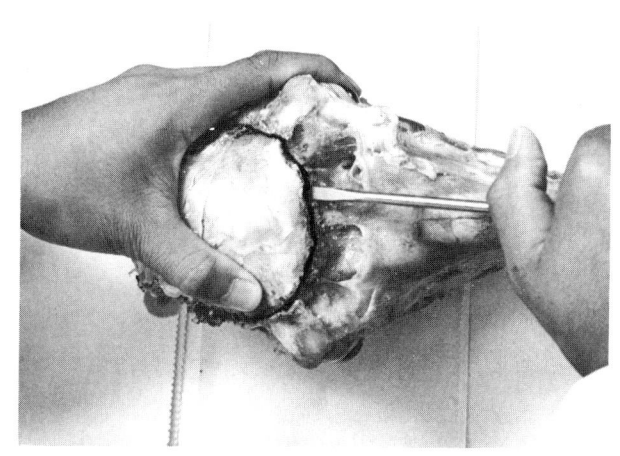

Figure 26.4 A large screwdriver is used to pry the cut section off the head.

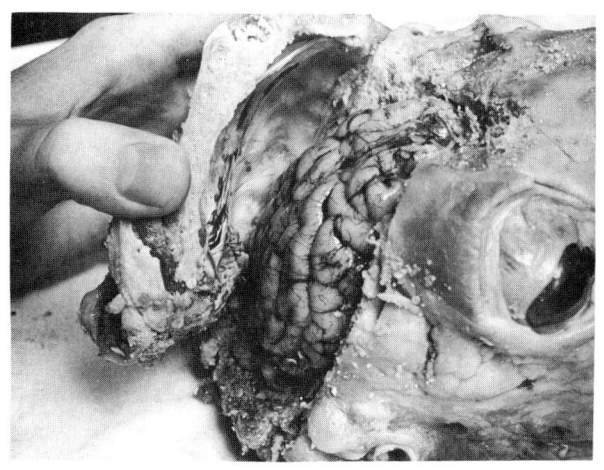

Figure 26.5 The intact brain is exposed by lifting off the cut portion.

that connects with the hypophysis. Figure 26.9 illustrates the relationship of the infundibulum to the hypophysis.

14. Carefully dissect the **hypophysis** out of the sella turcica without severing the infundibulum.

15. Continue lifting the brain to identify as many cranial nerves as you can. Refer to figures 26.6 and 26.9 to identify these nerves.

16. Remove the brain completely from the cranium. Section the brain, frontally, to expose the inner material. Note how distinct the gray matter is from the white matter.

17. Dispose of the remains in the proper waste receptacle and proceed to the next dissection, which will utilize preserved material.

Preserved Sheep Brain Dissection

This portion of our brain study concerns the finer details of its external and internal structure. Constant comparisons will be made with the human brain. Once you have located a structure on the sheep brain, try to find a comparable structure on the human brain; in some instances, however, direct comparisons are not always possible.

Materials:

> preserved sheep brains
> preserved human brains
> human brain models
> dissecting instruments
> dissecting trays

Place a sheep brain on a dissecting tray and, by comparing it to figures 26.6 and 26.9, identify the **cerebrum, cerebellum, pons Varolii, midbrain,** and **medulla oblongata.** Study each of these five major divisions to identify the fissures, grooves, ridges, and other structures as follows:

Cerebral Hemispheres In both the sheep and man, the cerebrum is the predominant portion of the brain. Note that when observed from the dorsal or ventral aspect, the cerebrum is divided along the median line to form two *cerebral hemispheres* by the **longitudinal cerebral fissure.**

Observe that the surface of the cerebrum is covered with ridges and furrows of variable depth. The deeper furrows are called **fissures,** and the shallow ones, **sulci.** The ridges or convolutions are called **gyri.** The frontal section in figure 26.1 reveals how this infolding of the cerebral surface greatly increases the amount of gray matter of the brain.

The principal fissures of the human cerebrum are the **central sulcus** (fissure of Rolando), **lateral cerebral fissure** (fissure of Sylvius), and the **parieto-occipital fissure.** In figure 26.9 the central sulcus is label 14; the lateral cerebral fissure is label 12. The greater portion of the parieto-

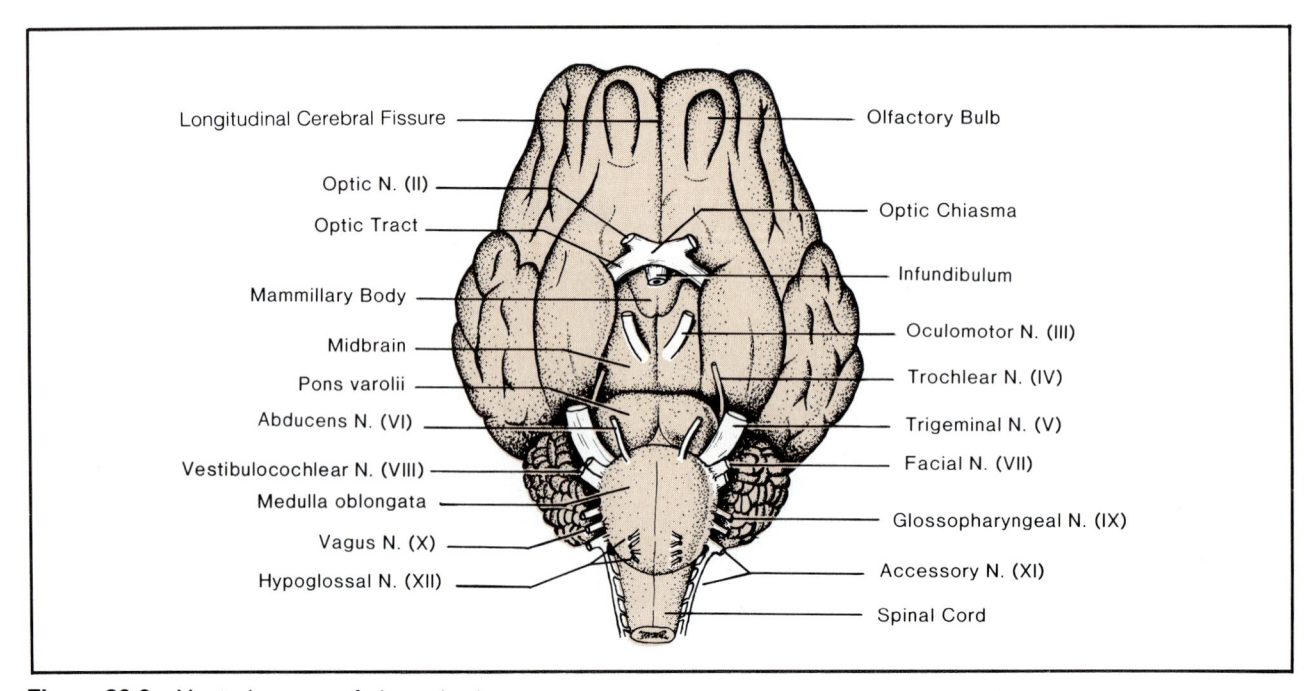

Figure 26.6 Ventral aspect of sheep brain.

occipital fissure is seen on the medial surface of the cerebrum (label 1, figure 27.2). If the lateral cerebral fissure is retracted as shown in the lower illustration of figure 26.9, an area called the **island of Reil** (*insula*) is exposed.

Each half of the human cerebrum is divided into four lobes. The **frontal lobe** is the most anterior portion. Its posterior margin falls on the central sulcus and its inferior border consists of the lateral cerebral fissure. The **occipital lobe** is the most posterior lobe of the brain. The anterior margin of this lobe falls on the parieto-occipital fissure. Because most of this fissure is seen on the medial face of the cerebrum, an imaginary dotted line in figure 26.9 reveals its position. The **temporal lobe** lies inferior to the lateral cerebral fissure and extends back to the parieto-occipital fissure. An imaginary horizontal dotted line provides a border between the temporal and **parietal lobes.** Labels 1, 4, 8, and 10 are for these four lobes.

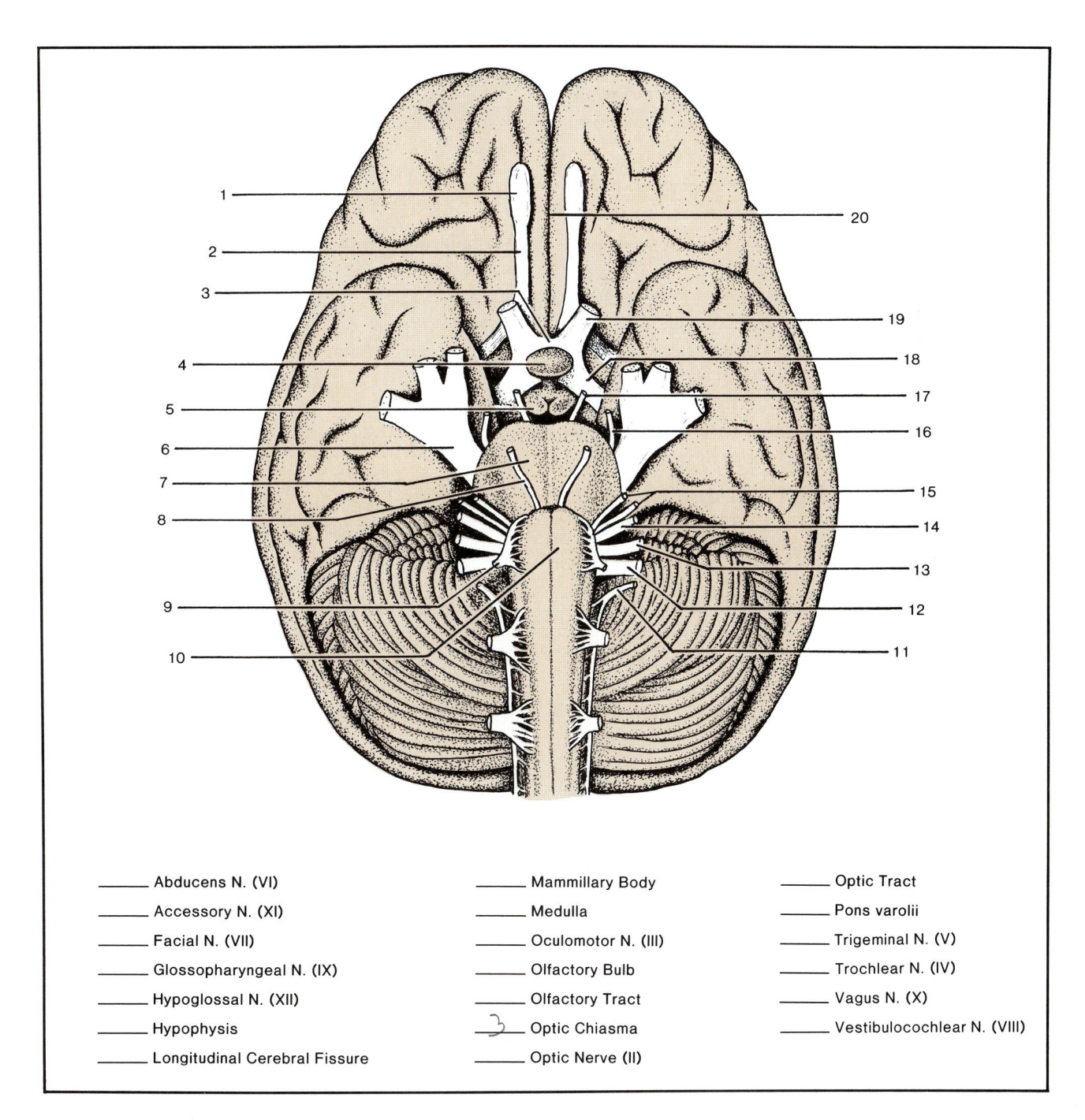

_____ Abducens N. (VI)	_____ Mammillary Body	_____ Optic Tract
_____ Accessory N. (XI)	_____ Medulla	_____ Pons varolii
_____ Facial N. (VII)	_____ Oculomotor N. (III)	_____ Trigeminal N. (V)
_____ Glossopharyngeal N. (IX)	_____ Olfactory Bulb	_____ Trochlear N. (IV)
_____ Hypoglossal N. (XII)	_____ Olfactory Tract	_____ Vagus N. (X)
_____ Hypophysis	_3_ Optic Chiasma	_____ Vestibulocochlear N. (VIII)
_____ Longitudinal Cerebral Fissure	_____ Optic Nerve (II)	

Figure 26.7 Inferior aspect of human brain.

Cerebellum Examine the surface of the sheep cerebellum. Note that its surface is furrowed with sulci. How do these sulci differ from those of the cerebrum? The human cerebellum is constricted in the middle to form right and left hemispheres. Can the same be said for the sheep's cerebellum? This part of the brain plays an important part in the maintenance of posture and the coordination of complex muscular movements.

The Brain Stem

The remaining structures to be observed are components of what is called the "brain stem." This axial portion of the brain includes the midbrain, diencephalon, pons Varolii, and medulla oblongata; it excludes the cerebrum and cerebellum.

Midbrain Since the midbrain lies concealed under the cerebellum and cerebrum, expose its dorsal surface by forcing the cerebellum downward with the thumb as illustrated in figure 26.8. In doing so, you have also exposed the *corpora quadrigemina,* which consist of two **superior colliculi** and two smaller **inferior colliculi.** In some animals the superior colliculi are called optic lobes because of their close association with the optic tracts. In animals the colliculi are important analytical centers concerned with brightness and sound discrimination.

Diencephalon (*Interbrain*) The **pineal gland,** which is exposed in figure 26.8, is a portion of the diencephalon. From an evolutionary point of view, there are indications that this gland is a remnant of the third eye that exists in certain reptiles. The hormone *melatonin,* which inhibits the estrus cycle in lower animals, is produced by the gland. The exact role of melatonin in humans is not completely understood at this time. It is probably significant that this structure is, histologically, glandular until puberty, and then becomes fibrous after puberty.

The diencephalon is a difficult area to observe because it is dorsal and anterior to the midbrain, and lies ventral to the cerebrum. In addition to the pineal gland the diencephalon includes the thalamus, hypothalamus, and mammillary bodies, which will be discussed more in detail on page 142.

Pons Varolii Locate this portion of the sheep's brain by examining its ventral surface and comparing it with figures 26.6 and 26.7. This part of the brain stem contains fibers that connect parts of the cerebellum and the medulla with the cerebrum. It also contains nuclei of the fifth, sixth, seventh, and eighth cranial nerves.

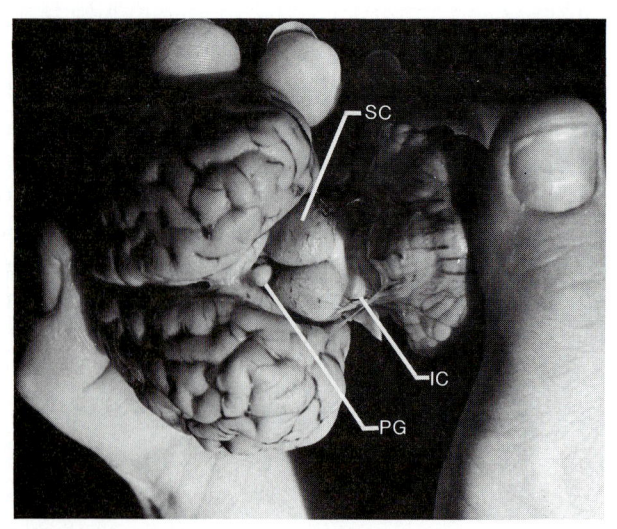

Figure 26.8 Exposing structures of the diencephalon and midbrain: SC—superior colliculus; IC—inferior colliculus; PG—pineal gland.

Medulla oblongata This portion of the brain stem is also known as the *spinal bulb.* It contains centers of gray matter that control the heart, respiration, and vasomotor reactions. The last four cranial nerves emerge from the medulla.

Assignment:

Label figure 26.9.

The Cranial Nerves

There are twelve pairs of nerves that emerge from various parts of the brain and pass through foramina of the skull to innervate parts of the head and trunk. Each pair has a name as well as a position number. Although most of these nerves contain both motor and sensory fibers (*mixed nerves*), a few contain only sensory fibers (*sensory nerves*). The sensory fibers have their cell bodies in ganglia outside of the brain; the cell bodies of the motor neurons, on the other hand, are situated within *nuclei* of the brain.

Compare your sheep brain with figures 26.6 and 26.9 to assist you in identifying each pair of nerves. As you proceed with the following study, avoid damaging the brain tissue with dissecting instruments. Keep in mind, also, that once a nerve is broken off it is difficult to determine where it was.

I Olfactory Nerve This cranial nerve contains sensory fibers for the sense of smell. Since it extends from the mucous membranes in the nose through the ethmoid bone to the olfactory bulb, it cannot be seen on your specimen. In the **olfactory bulb** synapses are made with fibers that extend inward

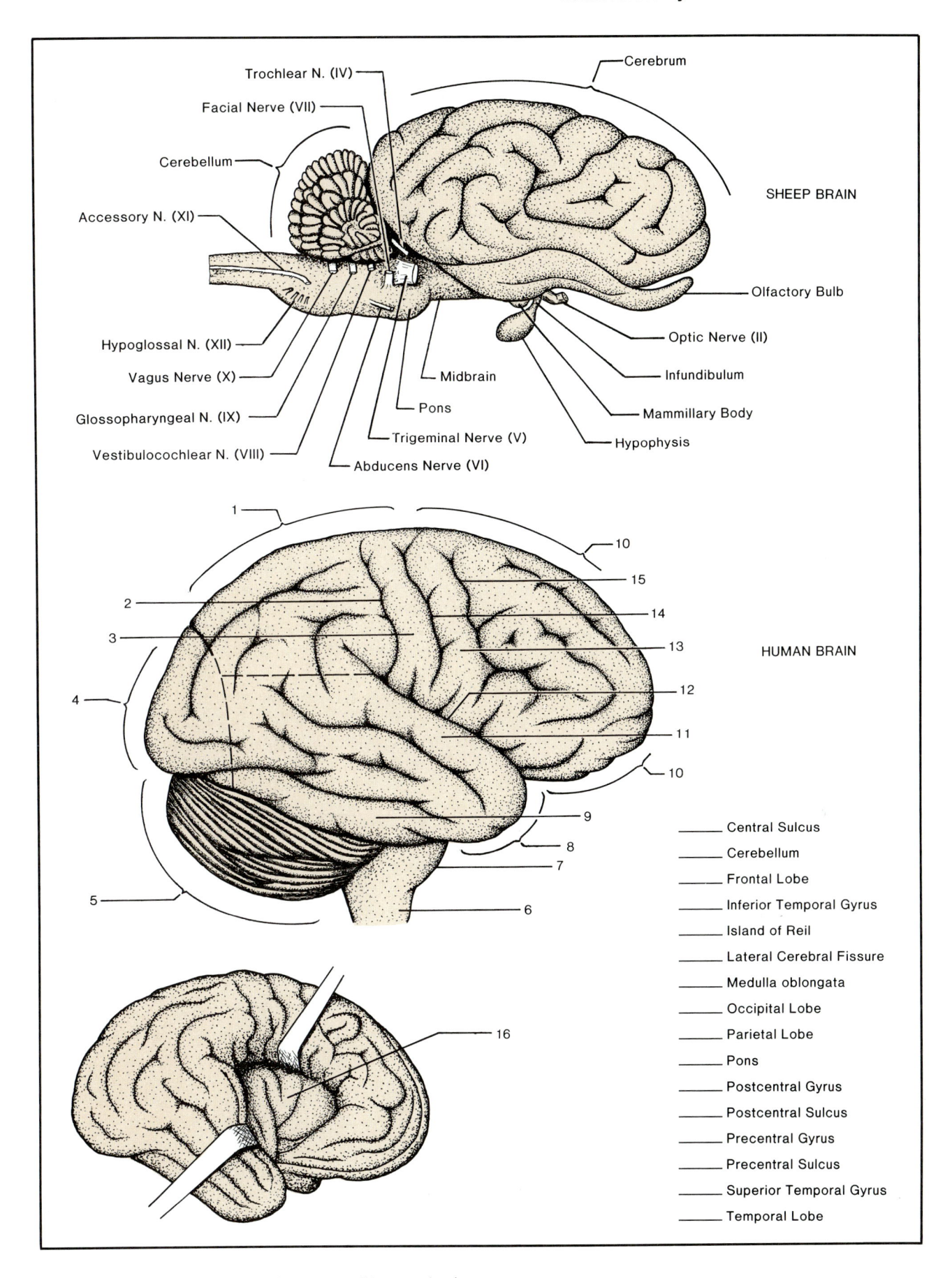

Figure 26.9 Lateral aspects of sheep and human brains.

to olfactory areas in the cerebrum. Note that on the human brain an **olfactory tract** (label 2) extends between the bulb and the brain.

II Optic Nerve This sensory nerve functions in vision. It contains axon fibers from ganglion cells of the retina of the eye. Part of the fibers from each optic nerve cross over to the other side of the brain as they pass through the **optic chiasma.** From the optic chiasma the fibers pass through the **optic tracts** to the thalamus and finally to the visual areas of the cerebrum. Identify these structures on the sheep brain.

III Oculomotor Nerve This nerve emerges from the midbrain and supplies somatic nerve fibers to the *levator palpebrae* (eyelid muscle) and four of the extrinsic ocular muscles: *superior rectus, medial rectus, inferior rectus,* and *inferior oblique.* (The superior oblique and lateral rectus muscles are innervated by IV and VI, respectively.)

The oculomotor nerve also supplies parasympathetic fibers to the *constrictor pupillaris* of the iris and the *ciliaris muscle* of the ciliary body. These fibers constrict the iris and change the lens shape as needed in accommodation (focusing).

If the oculomotor nerves are not visible on your sheep brain, it may be that they are obscured by the hypophysis (pituitary gland). The sheep brain illustrated in figure 26.6 lacks this structure. To remove the hypophysis without damaging other structures, lift it up with a pair of forceps and cut the infundibulum with a scalpel or a pair of scissors.

IV Trochlear Nerve This nerve provides muscle sense and motor stimulation of the *superior oblique* muscle of the eye. As in the case of the oculomotor, this nerve also emerges from the midbrain. Because of its small diameter it is one of the more difficult nerves to locate.

V Trigeminal Nerve Just posterior to the trochlear nerve lies the largest cranial nerve, the trigeminal. Although it is a mixed nerve, its sensory functions are much more extensive than its motor functions. Because of its extensive innervation of parts of the mouth and face, it is described in detail on pages 143 through 145.

VI Abducens Nerve This small nerve provides innervation of the *lateral rectus* muscle of the eye. It is a mixed nerve in that it provides muscle sense as well as muscular contraction. On the human brain

it emerges from the lower part of the pons near the medulla.

VII Facial Nerve This nerve consists of motor and sensory divisions. Label 15, figure 26.7, reveals the double nature of this nerve on the human brain. It innervates muscles of the face, salivary glands, and taste buds of the anterior two-thirds of the tongue.

VIII Vestibulocochlear (*Auditory*) **Nerve** This nerve goes to the inner ear. It has two branches: the *vestibular division,* which innervates the semicircular canals, and the *cochlear division,* which innervates the cochlea. The former branch functions in maintaining equilibrium; the cochlear portion is auditory in function. The vestibulocochlear nerve emerges just posterior to the facial nerve on the human brain.

IX Glossopharyngeal Nerve This mixed nerve emerges from the medulla posterior to the vestibulocochlear. It functions in reflexes of the heart, taste, and swallowing. Taste buds on the back of the tongue are innervated by some of its fibers. Efferent fibers innervate muscles of the pharynx (swallowing) and the parotid salivary glands (secretion).

X Vagus Nerve This cranial nerve, which originates on the medulla, exceeds all of the other cranial nerves in its extensive ramifications. In addition to supplying parts of the head and neck with nerves, it has branches that extend down into the chest and abdomen. It is a mixed nerve. Sensory fibers in this nerve go to the heart, external acoustic meatus, pharynx, larynx, and thoracic and abdominal viscera. Motor fibers pass to the pharynx, base of the tongue, larynx, and to the autonomic ganglia of thoracic and abdominal viscera. Many references will be made to this nerve in subsequent discussions of the physiology of the lungs, heart, and digestive organs.

XI Accessory Nerve Since this nerve emerges from both the brain and spinal cord it is sometimes called the *spinal accessory* nerve. Note that on both the sheep and human brains it parallels the lower part of the medulla and the spinal cord with branches going into both structures. On the human brain it appears to occupy a more posterior position than the twelfth nerve. Afferent and efferent spinal components innervate the sternocleidomastoid and trapezius muscles. The cranial portion of the nerve innervates the pharynx, upper larynx, uvula, and palate.

XII Hypoglossal Nerve This nerve emerges from the medulla to innervate several muscles of the tongue. It contains both afferent and efferent fibers. On the human brain in figure 26.7, it has the appearance of a cut-off tree trunk with roots extending into the medulla.

The Hypothalamus

The ventral portion of the brain that includes the mammillary bodies, infundibulum, and part of the hypophysis is collectively called the *hypothalamus.* This portion of the brain is a part of the diencephalon that lies between the cerebral hemispheres and the midbrain. The entire diencephalon, including the hypothalamus, will be studied more in detail in the next exercise when the internal parts of the brain are revealed by dissection.

Mammillary Bodies This part of the hypothalamus lies superior to the hypophysis. Although it appears as a single body on the sheep, it consists of a pair of rounded eminences just posterior to the infundibulum on the human. The mammillary bodies receive fibers from the olfactory areas of the brain and ascending pathways; fibers exit from it to the thalamus and other brain nuclei.

Hypophysis This structure, which is also called the *pituitary gland,* is attached to the base of the brain by a stalk, the **infundibulum.** It consists of two distinctly different parts: an anterior adenohypophysis and a posterior neurohypophysis. Only the neurohypophysis and infundibulum are considered to be part of the hypothalamus because they both have the same embryological origin as the brain. The adenohypophysis originates as an outpouching of the ectodermal stomodeum (mouth cavity) and is quite different histologically from the neurohypophysis. A close functional relationship exists between the hypothalamus, hypophysis, and the autonomic nervous system.

Assignment:

Label figure 26.7.

The remainder of this exercise pertains to the labeling of figures 26.10 and 26.11 and does not pertain to sheep brain dissection. To continue the sheep brain study, proceed to Exercise 27.

Functional Localization of the Cerebrum

Extensive experimental studies on monkeys, apes, and humans have resulted in considerable knowledge of the functional areas of the cerebrum. Figure 26.10 shows the positions of these various centers. Before attempting to identify each of these areas be sure you know the boundaries (sulci and fissures) of the cerebral lobes (figure 26.9).

Somatomotor Area This area occupies the surface of the precentral gyrus of the frontal lobe. Electrical stimulation of this portion of the cerebral cortex in a conscious human results in movement of specific muscular groups.

Premotor Area The large area anterior to the somatomotor area is the premotor area. It exerts control over the motor area.

Somatosensory Area This area is located on the postcentral gyrus of the parietal lobe. It functions to localize very precisely those points on the body where sensations of light touch and pressure originate. It also assists in determining organ position. Other sensations, such as aching pain, crude touch, warmth, and cold are localized by the thalamus rather than this area.

Motor Speech Area This area is located in the frontal lobe just above the lateral cerebral fissure, anterior to the somatomotor area. It exerts control over the muscles of the larynx and tongue that produce speech.

Visual Area This area is located on the occipital lobe. Note that only a small portion of it is seen on the lateral aspect; the greater portion of this area is on the medial surface of the cerebrum. On this surface it extends anteriorly to the parieto-occipital fissure, becoming narrower as it approaches the fissure. This area receives impulses from the retina via the thalamus. Destruction of this region causes blindness, although light and dark are still discernible.

Auditory Area This area receives nerve impulses from the cochlea of the inner ear via the thalamus. It is responsible for hearing and speech understanding. It is located on the superior temporal gyrus, which borders on the lateral cerebral fissure.

Olfactory Area This area is located on the medial surface of the temporal lobe. The recognition of various odors occurs here. Tumors in this area cause individuals to experience nonexistent odors of various kinds, both pleasant and unpleasant.

Association Areas Adjacent to the somatosensory, visual, and auditory areas are association areas that lend meaning to what is felt, seen, or heard. These areas are lined regions in figure 26.10.

Common Integrative Area The integration of information from the above three association areas and the olfactory and taste centers is achieved by a small area which is called the common integrative or *gnostic area*. This area is located on the **angular gyrus,** which is positioned approximately midway between the three association areas.

Assignment:

Label figure 26.10.

The Trigeminal Nerve

Although a detailed study of all cranial nerves is precluded in an elementary anatomy course, the trigeminal nerve has been singled out for a thorough study here. This fifth cranial nerve is the largest one that innervates the head and is of particular medical-dental significance.

Figure 26.11 illustrates the distribution of this nerve. You will note that it has branches that supply the teeth, tongue, gums, forehead, eyes, nose, and lips. The following description identifies the various ganglia and branches.

On the left margin of the diagram is the severed end of the nerve at a point where it emerges from the brain. Between this cut end and the three main branches is an enlarged portion, the **Gasserian ganglion.** This ganglion contains the nerve cell bodies of the sensory fibers in the nerve. The three branches that extend from this ganglion are the *ophthalmic, maxillary,* and *mandibular nerves.* Locate the bony portion of the skull in figure 26.11 through which these three branches pass.

Ophthalmic Nerve The ophthalmic nerve is the upper branch that passes out of the cranium through the *superior orbital fissure.* It has three branches that innervate the lacrimal gland; the upper eyelid, and the skin of the nose, forehead, and scalp. One of the branches also supplies parts of the eye such as the *cornea, iris,* and the *ciliary body* (muscle attached to the lens of the eye). Superior to the lower branch of the ophthalmic is the **ciliary ganglion,** which contains nerve cell bodies

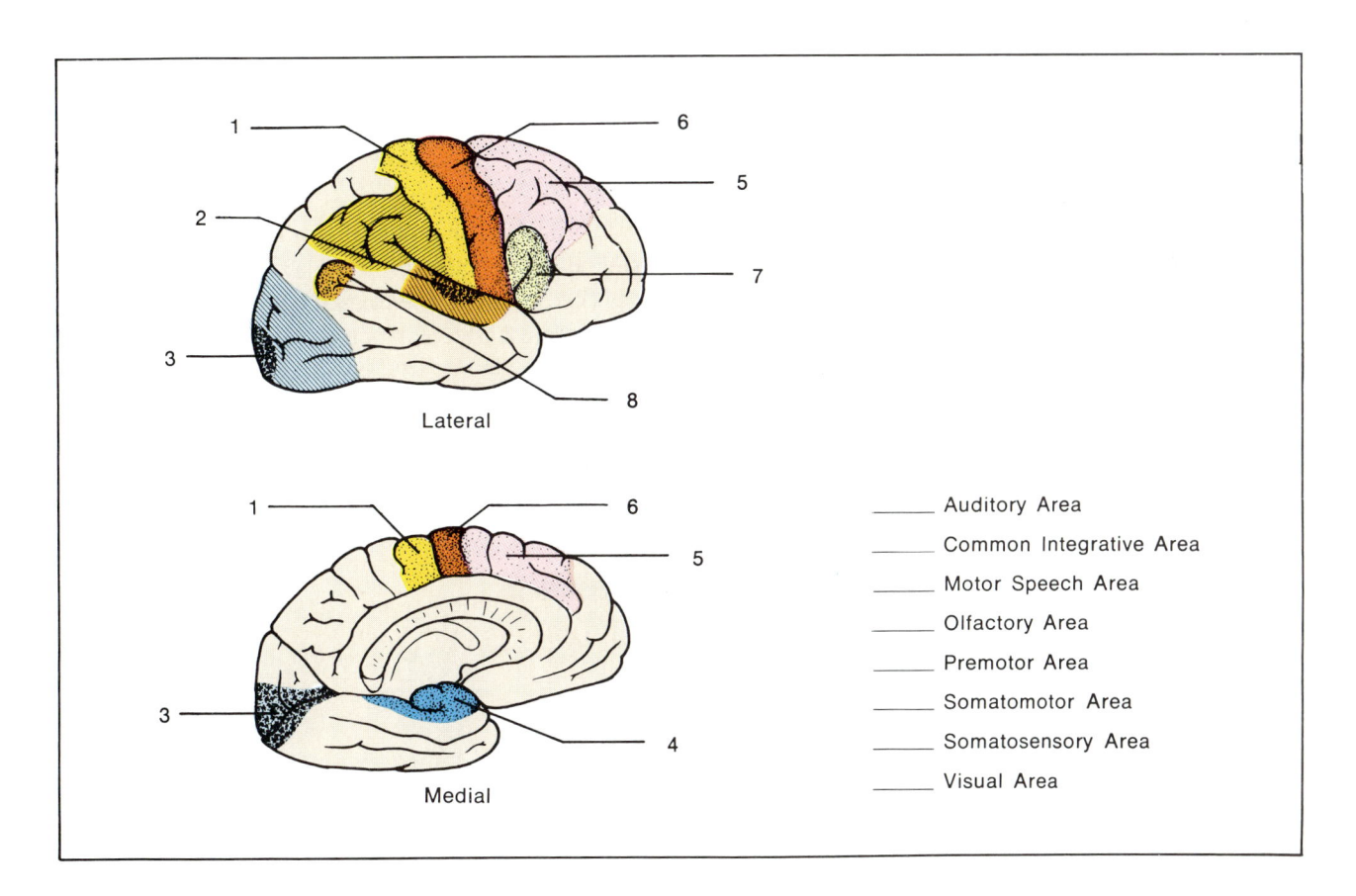

Lateral

Medial

_____ Auditory Area

_____ Common Integrative Area

_____ Motor Speech Area

_____ Olfactory Area

_____ Premotor Area

_____ Somatomotor Area

_____ Somatosensory Area

_____ Visual Area

Figure 26.10 Functional areas of human brain.

that are incorporated into reflexes controlling the ciliary body. The ophthalmic nerve and its branches are not involved in dental anesthesia.

Maxillary Nerve This nerve, also known as the *second division* of the trigeminal nerve, is a sensory nerve that provides innervation to the nose, upper lip, palate, maxillary sinus, and upper teeth. It is the branch that comes off just inferior to the ophthalmic nerve.

Note that the maxillary nerve has two short branches that extend downward to an oval body, the **sphenopalatine ganglion.** The major portion of the maxillary nerve becomes the **infraorbital nerve,** which passes through the *infraorbital nerve canal* of the maxilla. This canal is shown with dotted lines in figure 26.11. This nerve emerges from the maxilla through the **infraorbital foramen** to innervate the tissues of the nose and upper lip.

The upper teeth are innervated by three superior alveolar nerves. The **posterior superior alveolar nerve** is a branch of the maxillary nerve that enters the posterior surface of the upper jaw and innervates the molars. The **anterior superior alveolar nerve** is a branch of the infraorbital nerve that supplies the anterior teeth and bicuspids with nerve fibers. The anterior superior alveolar nerve forms a loop with the **middle superior alveolar nerve.** This latter nerve is shown clearly where a portion of the maxilla has been cut away. It contains fibers that pass to the bicuspids and first molar.

To desensitize all of the upper teeth on one side of the maxilla, a dentist can inject anesthetic near either the maxillary nerve or the sphenopalatine ganglion. Desensitization of the maxillary nerve is called a *second division nerve block.* This type of nerve block will affect the palate as well as the teeth because it involves fibers of the **anterior palatine nerve.** This latter nerve extends downward from the sphenopalatine ganglion to the soft tissues of the palate through the *greater palatine foramen.*

Mandibular Nerve The mandibular nerve, or *third division* of the trigeminal nerve, is the most inferior branch of this nerve. It innervates the teeth and gums of the mandible, the muscles of mastication, the anterior part of the tongue, the lower part of the face, and some skin areas on the side of the head.

Moving downward from the Gasserian ganglion, the first branch of the mandibular nerve that we encounter is the **nerve to the muscles of mastication.** This nerve has five branches with small identifying letters near their cut ends (**T** for temporalis, **M** for masseter, **EP** for external pterygoid, **B** for buccinator, and **IP** for internal pterygoid). The fibers in these nerves control the motor activities of these five muscles.

The largest branch of the mandibular nerve is the **inferior alveolar nerve,** which enters the ramus of the mandible through the **mandibular foramen** and supplies branches to all the teeth on one side of the mandible. At the mental foramen the inferior alveolar nerve becomes the **incisive nerve,** which innervates the anterior teeth. Emerging from the **mental foramen** is the **mental nerve,** which supplies the soft tissues of the chin and lower lip.

Desensitization of the mandibular teeth is generally achieved by injecting anesthetic near the mandibular foramen. This type of injection, called a *lower nerve block* or *third division nerve block,* is widely used in dentistry because the external and internal alveolar plates of the mandibular alveolar process are too dense to facilitate anesthesia by infiltration of the solid bone. The lower nerve block of one side of the mandible desensitizes all of the teeth on one side except for the anterior teeth. The fact that the anterior teeth receive nerve fibers from both the left and right incisive nerves prevents complete desensitization.

A branch of the mandibular nerve that emerges just above the inferior alveolar nerve and innervates the tongue is the **lingual nerve.** As in the case of the inferior alveolar nerve, it is sensory in function.

The **long buccal nerve** is another sensory branch of the mandibular nerve that innervates the buccal gum tissues of the molars and bicuspids. This nerve arises from a point that is just superior to the lingual nerve.

Assignment:

Label figure 26.11.

Laboratory Report

Complete the Laboratory Report for this exercise.

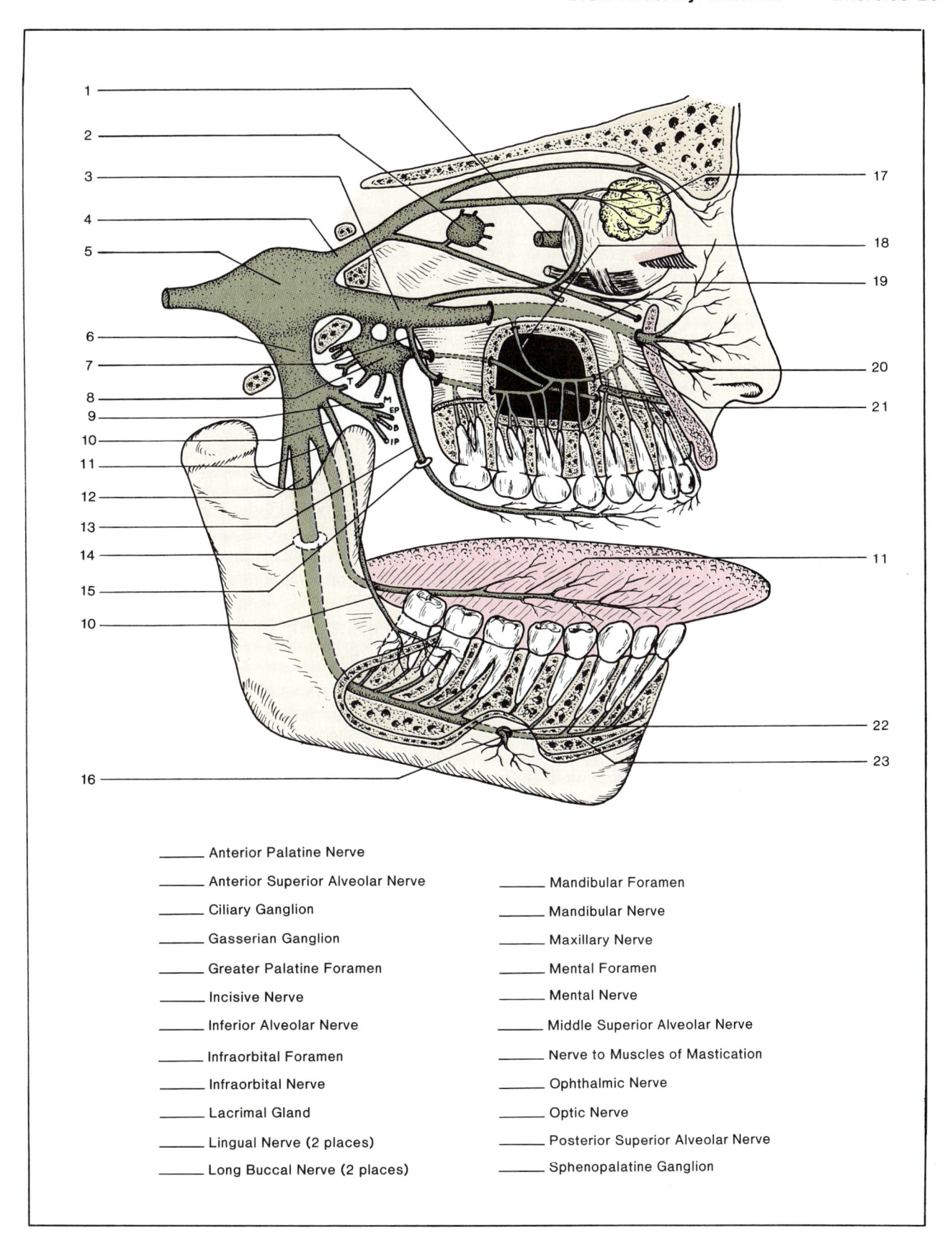

Figure 26.11 The trigeminal nerve.

___ Anterior Palatine Nerve

___ Anterior Superior Alveolar Nerve

___ Ciliary Ganglion

___ Gasserian Ganglion

___ Greater Palatine Foramen

___ Incisive Nerve

___ Inferior Alveolar Nerve

___ Infraorbital Foramen

___ Infraorbital Nerve

___ Lacrimal Gland

___ Lingual Nerve (2 places)

___ Long Buccal Nerve (2 places)

___ Mandibular Foramen

___ Mandibular Nerve

___ Maxillary Nerve

___ Mental Foramen

___ Mental Nerve

___ Middle Superior Alveolar Nerve

___ Nerve to Muscles of Mastication

___ Ophthalmic Nerve

___ Optic Nerve

___ Posterior Superior Alveolar Nerve

___ Sphenopalatine Ganglion

27 Brain Anatomy: Internal

The interrelations of the various divisions of the brain can be seen only by studying sections such as those in figures 27.1 and 27.2. Bundles of interconnecting fibers unite the cerebral hemispheres, cerebellum, pons, and medulla to each other in a manner that enables the brain to function as an integrated whole. In this part of our brain study we will identify those important fiber tracts as well as brain cavities, meningeal spaces, and other related parts.

Materials:

    preserved sheep brains
    preserved human brains
    human brain models
    dissecting instruments
    long sharp knife
    dissecting tray

Midsagittal Section

With the preserved sheep brain resting ventral side down on a dissecting tray, place a long sharp meat-cutting knife (butcher knife) in the longitudinal cerebral fissure. Carefully slice through the tissue, cutting the brain into right and left halves on the midline. If only a scalpel is available, attempt to cut the tissue as smoothly as possible. Proceed to identify the structures on the sheep brain and their counterparts on the human brain as follows.

If the brain has been cut exactly on the midline, the only portion of the cerebrum that is cut is the **corpus callosum.** Locate this long band of white matter on the sheep brain by referring to figure 27.1. Also, compare your specimen with the human brain in figure 27.2. The corpus callosum is a commissural tract of fibers that connects the right and left cerebral hemispheres, correlating their functions. Note that the corpus callosum on the human brain is significantly thicker.

The Diencephalon

Between the corpus callosum of the cerebral hemisphere and the midbrain exists a section called the *diencephalon* or *interbrain.* This region includes the fornix, third ventricle, thalamus, intermediate mass, and hypothalamus.

Fornix Locate this structure on the sheep brain. This body contains fibers that are an integral part

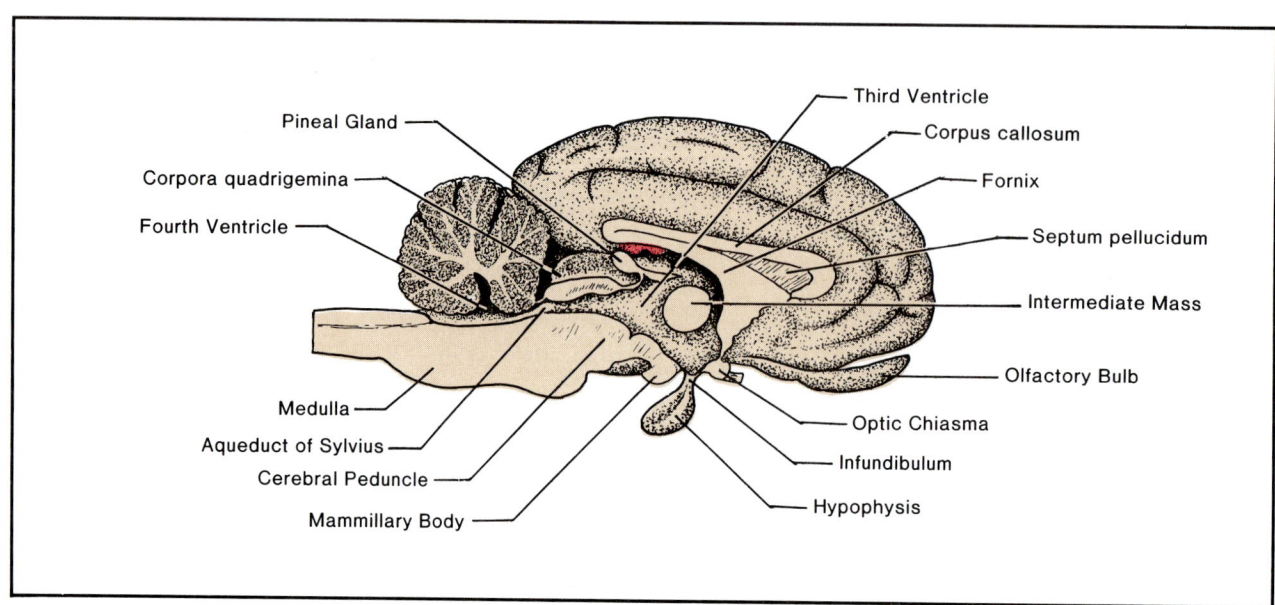

Figure 27.1 Midsagittal section of sheep brain.

of the olfactory mechanism of the brain, the *rhinencephalon*. Note how much larger, proportionately, it is on the sheep than on the human.

Intermediate Mass This oval area in the midsection of the diencephalon is the only part of the thalamus that can be seen in the midsagittal section. The *thalamus* is a large ovoid structure on the lateral walls of the third ventricle. It is an important relay station in which sensory pathways of the spinal cord and brain form synapses on their way to the cerebral cortex. The intermediate mass contains fibers that pass through the third ventricle, uniting both sides of the thalamus.

Hypothalamus This portion of the diencephalon extends about two centimeters up into the brain from the ventral surface. It has many nuclei that control various physiological functions of the body (temperature regulation, hypophysis control, coordination of the autonomic nervous system). The only part of the hypothalamus that is labeled in figure 27.2 is the left **mammillary body** (label 7).

Inferior and anterior to the mammillary body in figure 27.2 lies the **infundibulum** and **hypophysis.**

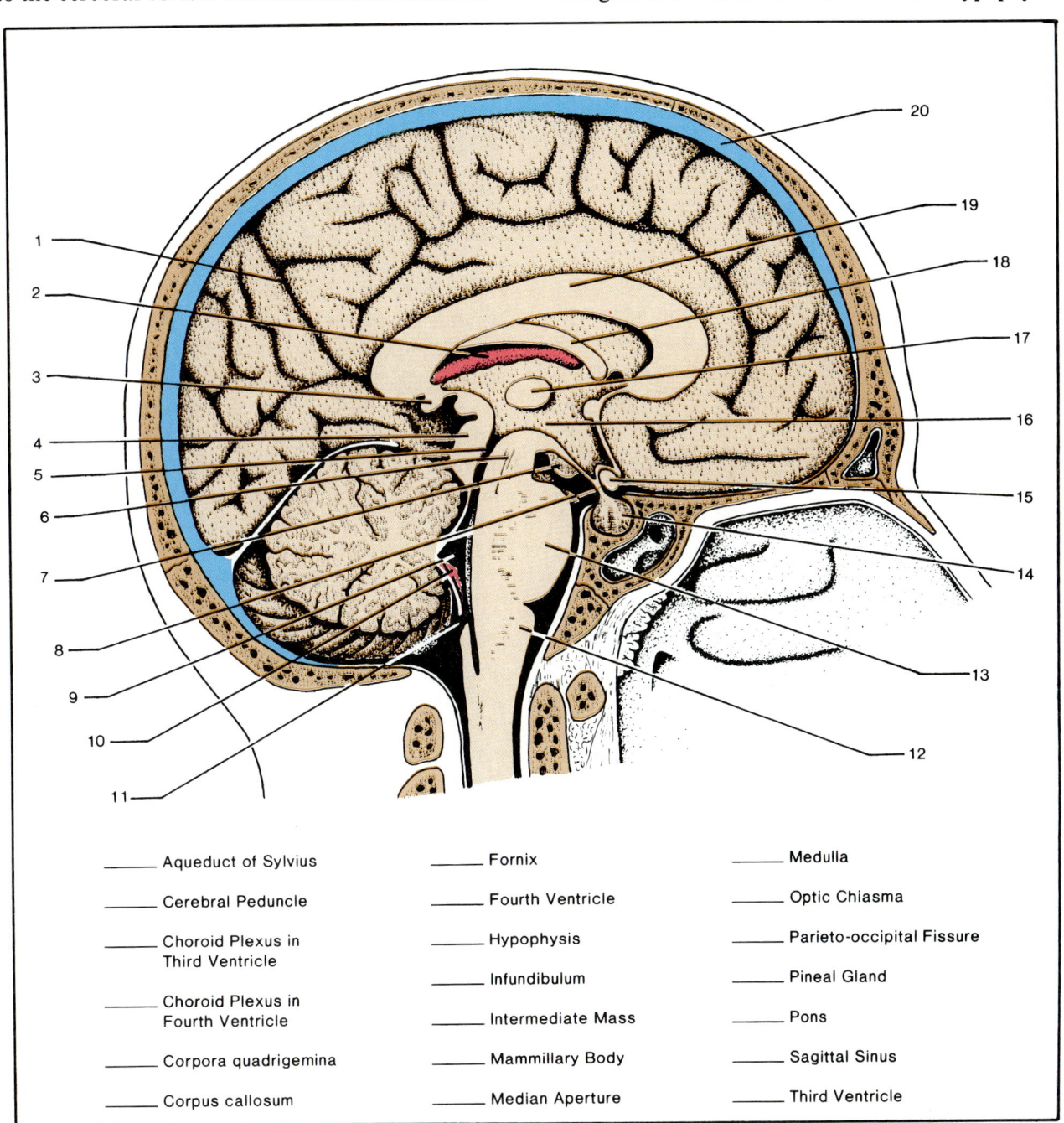

_____ Aqueduct of Sylvius	_____ Fornix	_____ Medulla
_____ Cerebral Peduncle	_____ Fourth Ventricle	_____ Optic Chiasma
_____ Choroid Plexus in Third Ventricle	_____ Hypophysis	_____ Parieto-occipital Fissure
_____ Choroid Plexus in Fourth Ventricle	_____ Infundibulum	_____ Pineal Gland
_____ Corpora quadrigemina	_____ Intermediate Mass	_____ Pons
_____ Corpus callosum	_____ Mammillary Body	_____ Sagittal Sinus
	_____ Median Aperture	_____ Third Ventricle

Figure 27.2 Midsagittal section of human brain.

Note how the latter lies encased in the bony recess of the *sella turcica.* The **optic chiasma** is the small round body just above the hypophysis, anterior to the infundibulum.

The Diencephalon and Midbrain

Locate the following structures on the sheep's midbrain and diencephalon: **corpora quadrigemina, cerebral peduncle, aqueduct of Sylvius,** and **pineal gland.**

The *cerebral peduncles* of the midbrain consist of a pair of cylindrical bodies made up largely of ascending and descending fiber tracts that connect the cerebrum with the other brain divisions.

The *aqueduct of Sylvius* is a duct that runs longitudinally through the midbrain, connecting the third and fourth ventricles.

The Cerebellum

Examine the cut surface of the cerebellum and note that gray matter exists near the outer surface. The cerebellum receives nerve impulses along cerebellar peduncles from motor and visual centers of the brain, the semicircular canals of the inner ears, and muscles of the body. Nerve impulses pass from this region to all the motor centers of the body wall to maintain posture, equilibrium, and muscle tonus. None of the activities of the cerebellum are of a conscious nature. It is significant that each hemisphere controls the muscles on its side of the body.

The Pons and Medulla

These two parts make up the greater portion of the brain stem. The pons is that portion of the brain stem between the midbrain and medulla. Note that it consists primarily of white matter (fiber tracts). Locate the pons and medulla on both the sheep and human brains.

Within the brain stem is a complex interlacement of nuclei and white fibers (gray and white matter) that constitutes the *reticular formation.* Nuclei of this formation generate a continuous flow of impulses to other parts of the brain to keep the cerebrum in a state of alert consciousness.

The Ventricles and Cerebrospinal Fluid

The brain has four cavities, or **ventricles,** which contain cerebrospinal fluid. There are two **lateral ventricles** situated in the lower medial portions of each cerebral hemisphere. Although they are not visible in a midsagittal section, the **septum pellucidum,** a thin membrane may be seen that separates these two cavities. A frontal section of the brain, such as the one in figure 27.4, shows the position of the lateral ventricles (label 5). The **third** and **fourth ventricles,** however, are readily visible in figures 27.1 and 27.2. Note that the intermediate mass passes through the third ventricle. Within this ventricle is seen a **choroid plexus** (label 2, figure 27.2), which secretes cerebrospinal fluid. Each ventricle has its own choroid plexus.

Cerebrospinal Fluid Pathway The path of cerebrospinal fluid is indicated in figure 27.3. From the lateral ventricles the fluid enters the third ventricle through the **foramen of Monro.** Note in figure 27.3 that this foramen lies anterior to the fornix and choroid plexus of the third ventricle.

From the third ventricle the cerebrospinal fluid passes into the **aqueduct of Sylvius.** This duct conveys the cerebrospinal fluid to the fourth ventricle. The **choroid plexus of the fourth ventricle** lies on the posterior wall of this cavity.

From the fourth ventricle the cerebrospinal fluid exits into the subarachnoid space that surrounds the cerebellum through three foramina: one median aperture (foramen of Magendie), and two lateral apertures (foramina of Luschka).

In figure 27.3, the **median aperture** is the lower opening, which has two arrows leading from it. That part of the subarachnoid space that it empties into is the **cisterna cerebellomedullaris.** Since the **lateral apertures** are located on the lateral walls of the fourth ventricle, only one is shown in figure 27.3.

From the cisterna cerebello-medullaris the cerebrospinal fluid moves up into the **cisterna superior** (above the cerebellum) and finally into the subarachnoid space around the cerebral hemispheres. From the subarachnoid space this fluid escapes into the blood of the sagittal sinus through the **arachnoid granulations.** The cerebrospinal fluid passes down the subarachnoid space of the spinal cord on the posterior side and up along its anterior surface.

Assignment:

After identifying all the structures of the sheep brain, label figure 27.2.

Label figure 27.3.

Frontal Sections

To get a better understanding of the special relationships of the thalamus, ventricles, and other parts of the brain, it is necessary to study frontal sections of the brain. Once frontal sections of the sheep brain are studied, a frontal section of the human brain is relatively easy to understand. Two frontal sections of a sheep brain and one of the human brain are shown in figure 27.4.

Infundibular Section (Sheep Brain)

Place a whole sheep brain on a dissecting tray with the dorsal side down. Cut a frontal section with a long knife by starting at the point of the infundibulum. Cut through perpendicularly to the tray and to the longitudinal axis of the brain. Then, make a second cut parallel to the first cut ¼ inch further back. The latter cut should be through the center of the hypophysis.

Place this slice, *with the first cut upward,* on a piece of paper toweling for study. Illustration A, figure 27.4, is of this surface. Proceed to identify the following structures. You may need to refer back to figure 27.1 for reference.

Note the pattern of the **gray matter** of the cerebral cortex. Force a probe down into a sulcus. What meninx do you break through as the probe moves inward? What is the average thickness of the gray matter in the sulci of the dorsal part of the brain?

Locate the two triangular **lateral ventricles.** Probe into one of the ventricles to see if you can locate the **choroid plexus.** What is its function? Identify the **corpus callosum** and **fornix.**

Identify the **third ventricle,** which is situated on the median line under the fornix. Also, identify the **thalamus** and **intermediate mass.** Does the thalamus appear to consist of white or gray matter? What is the function of the white matter between the thalamus and cerebral cortex?

Hypophyseal Section (Sheep Brain)

Produce a section of the brain by cutting another ¼ inch slice off the posterior portion of the brain. Place this slice, with its *anterior face upward,* on paper toweling. This section through the hypophysis should look like illustration B, figure 27.4. Identify the structures in illustration B that are labeled.

Infundibular Section (Human Brain)

Illustration C, figure 27.4, reveals the close similarities of sheep and human brains; yet differences are apparent. To complete this study of the brain, identify the following structures:

Locate first the two triangular **lateral ventricles** and the **third ventricle.** Note how the **longitudinal cerebral fissure** extends downward to the **corpus callosum,** which forms the upper wall of the lateral ventricles. Although no label exists for the *septum*

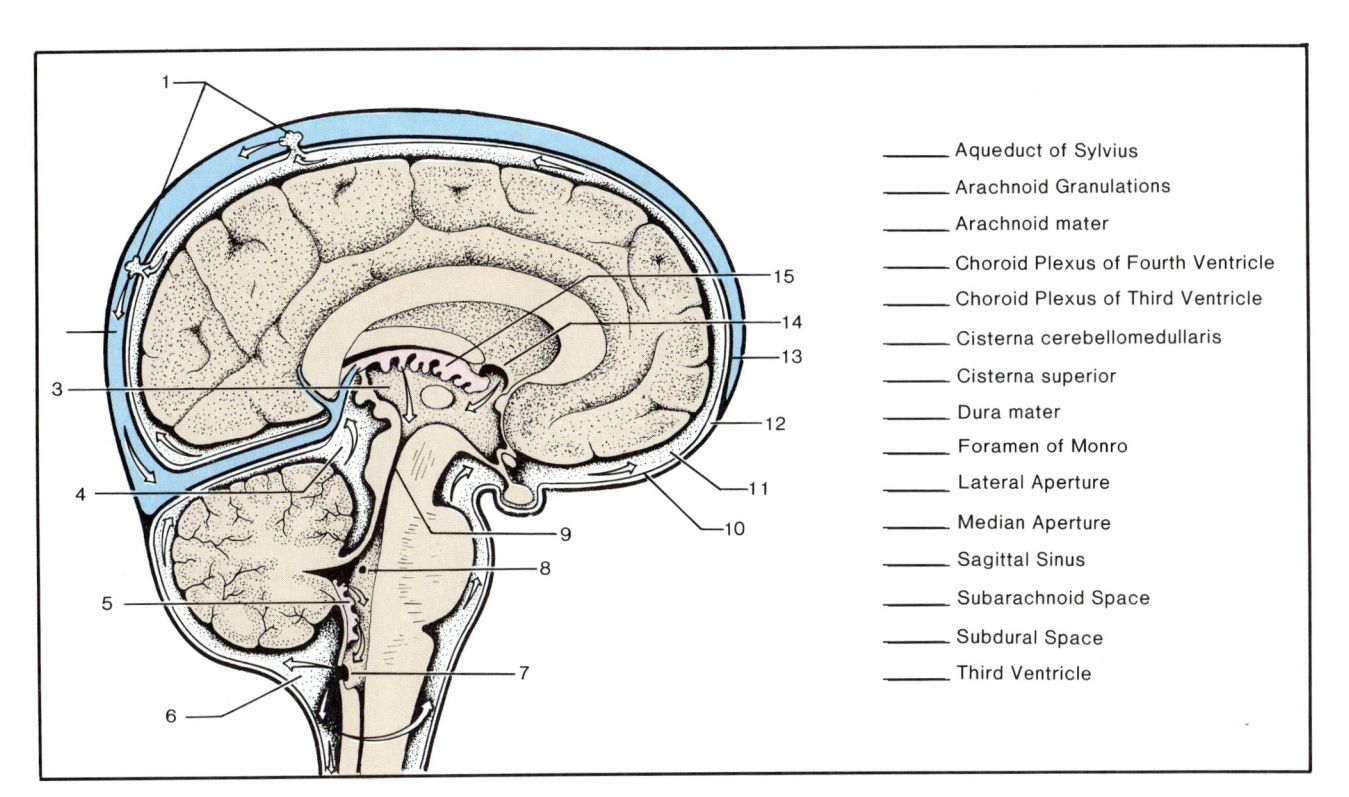

_____ Aqueduct of Sylvius
_____ Arachnoid Granulations
_____ Arachnoid mater
_____ Choroid Plexus of Fourth Ventricle
_____ Choroid Plexus of Third Ventricle
_____ Cisterna cerebellomedullaris
_____ Cisterna superior
_____ Dura mater
_____ Foramen of Monro
_____ Lateral Aperture
_____ Median Aperture
_____ Sagittal Sinus
_____ Subarachnoid Space
_____ Subdural Space
_____ Third Ventricle

Figure 27.3 Origin and circulation of cerebrospinal fluid.

pellucidum, can you find it? Identify the two masses of gray matter just below the septum pellucidum that constitute the **fornix.**

Identify the areas on each side of the third ventricle that make up the nuclei of the **hypothalamus.** Approximately eight separate masses of gray matter are seen here. What physiological functions are regulated by these nuclei?

Locate the two large areas on the walls of the lateral ventricles that constitute the **thalamus.** Note, also, how these two portions of the thalamus are united by the **intermediate mass** that passes through the third ventricle.

Labels 12, 13, 14, and 15 are masses of gray matter known collectively as the *basal ganglia.* The largest basal ganglia are the **putamen** and **globus pallidus** (labels 12 and 13). The latter is medial to the putamen. Together the putamen and globus

pallidus form a triangular mass, the **lentiform nucleus.** These two ganglia exert a steadying effect on voluntary muscular movements.

The **caudate nuclei** are smaller basal ganglia located in the walls of the lateral ventricles superior to the thalamus. These nuclei have something to do with muscular coordination, since surgically produced lesions in these centers can correct certain kinds of palsy.

Although some anatomists prefer to designate the thalamus and hypothalamus as basal ganglia, functionally, they differ considerably.

Assignment:

Label figure 27.4.

Laboratory Report

Complete the Laboratory Report for this exercise.

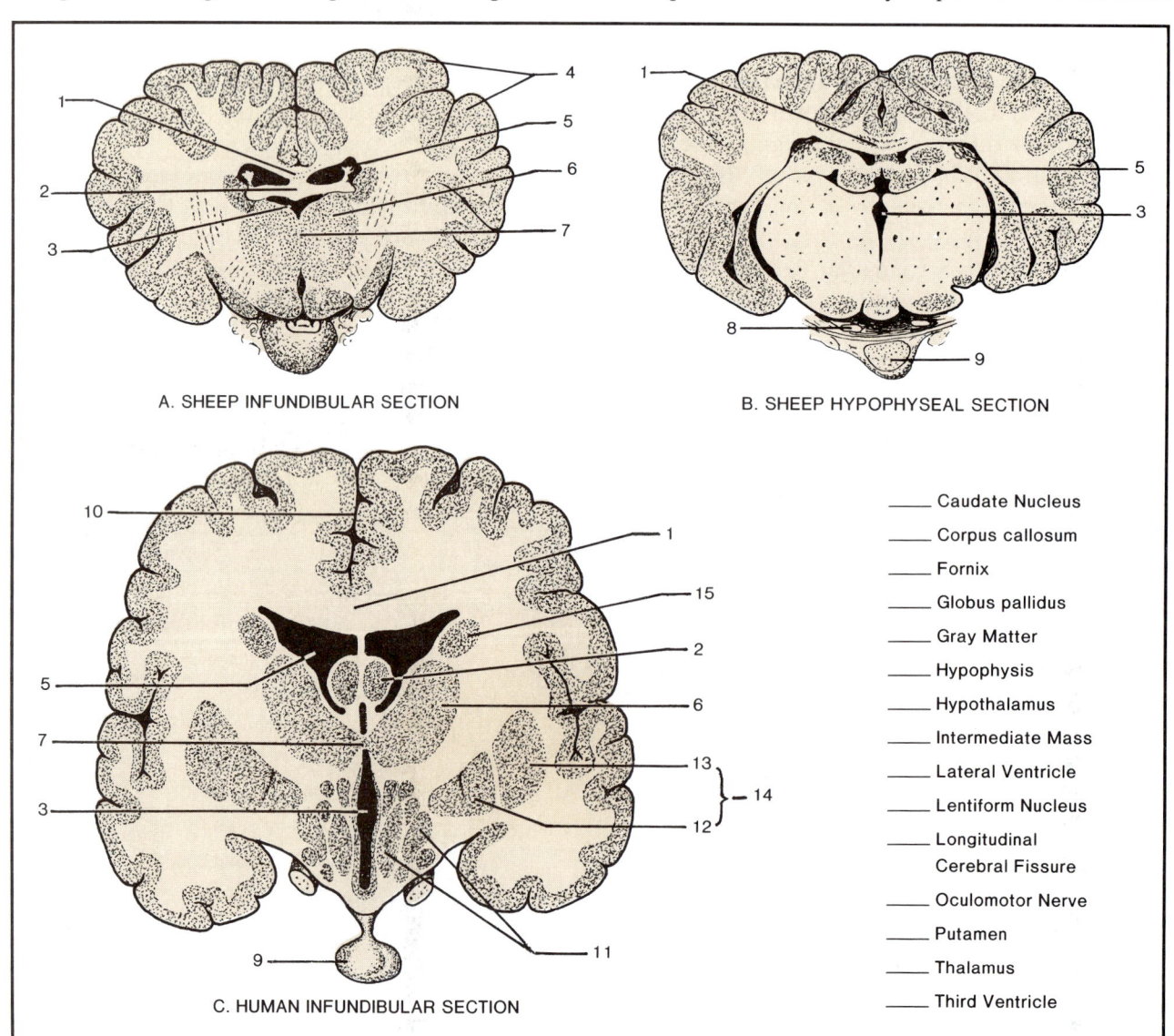

A. SHEEP INFUNDIBULAR SECTION

B. SHEEP HYPOPHYSEAL SECTION

C. HUMAN INFUNDIBULAR SECTION

_____ Caudate Nucleus
_____ Corpus callosum
_____ Fornix
_____ Globus pallidus
_____ Gray Matter
_____ Hypophysis
_____ Hypothalamus
_____ Intermediate Mass
_____ Lateral Ventricle
_____ Lentiform Nucleus
_____ Longitudinal Cerebral Fissure
_____ Oculomotor Nerve
_____ Putamen
_____ Thalamus
_____ Third Ventricle

Figure 27.4 Frontal sections of sheep and human brains.

The Eye 28

In this exercise we will study the anatomy of the eye through dissection and ophthalmoscopy. Before these laboratory experiments are performed, however, the illustrations in figures 28.1, 28.2 and 28.3 should be labeled. A fresh beef eye will be used for dissection. Its large size makes it an ideal dissection specimen. Ophthalmoscopy will be used to study the interior of the living eye to identify structures on the retina.

The Lacrimal Apparatus

Each eye lies protected in a bony recess of the skull and is covered externally by the *eyelids*. Lining the eyelids that cover the exposed surface of the eyeball is a thin membrane, the *conjunctiva*. The conjunctival surfaces are kept constantly moist by protective secretions of the *lacrimal gland,* which lies between the upper eyelid and the eyeball.

Figure 28.1 reveals the external anatomy of the right eye, with particular emphasis on the lacrimal apparatus. Note that the lacrimal gland consists of two portions: a large **superior lacrimal gland** and a smaller **inferior lacrimal gland.** Secretions from these glands pass through the conjunctiva of the eyelid via six to twelve small ducts.

The flow of fluid from these ducts moves across the eyeball to the *medial canthus* (angle) of the eye, where the fluid enters two small orifices, the **lacrimal puncta.** These openings lead into the **superior** and **inferior lacrimal ducts;** the superior one is in the upper eyelid, and the inferior one is in the lower eyelid. These two ducts empty directly into an enlarged cavity, the **lacrimal sac,** which, in turn, is drained by the **nasolacrimal duct.** The tears finally exit into the nasal cavity through the end of the nasolacrimal duct.

Two other structures, the caruncula and the plica semilunaris, are seen near the puncta in the medial canthus of the eye. The **caruncula** is a small red conical body that consists of a mound of skin containing sebaceous and sweat glands and a few small hairs. This structure produces a whitish secretion that constantly collects in this region. Lateral to the caruncula is a curved fold of conjunctiva, the **plica semilunaris.** This structure contains some smooth muscle fibers; in the cat and many other animals it is more highly developed and is often referred to as the "third eyelid."

Assignment:

Label figure 28.1.

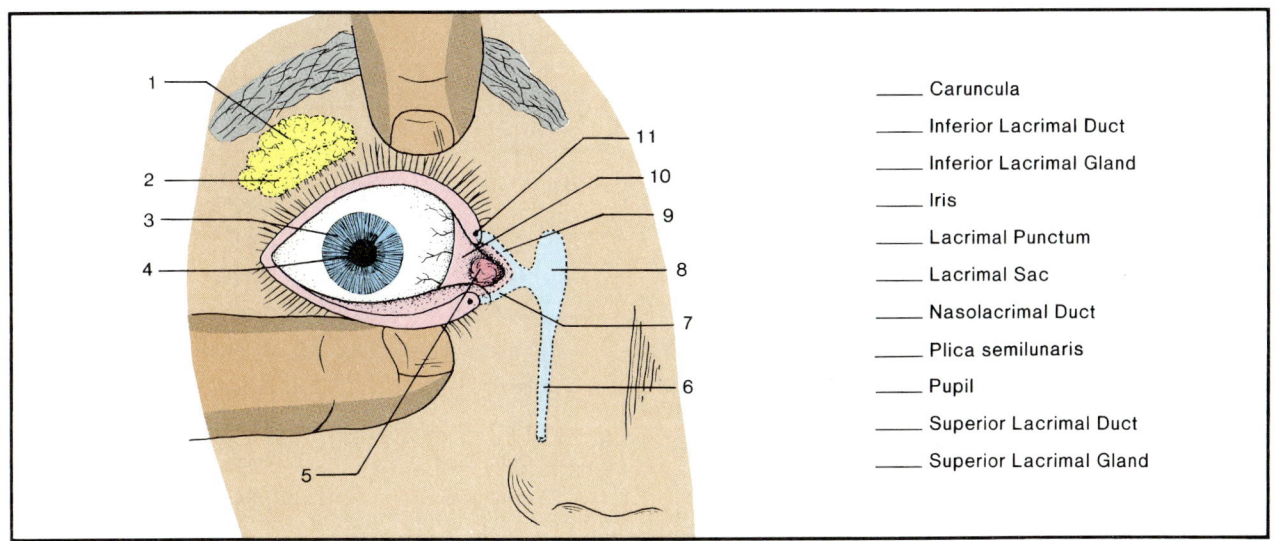

_____ Caruncula

_____ Inferior Lacrimal Duct

_____ Inferior Lacrimal Gland

_____ Iris

_____ Lacrimal Punctum

_____ Lacrimal Sac

_____ Nasolacrimal Duct

_____ Plica semilunaris

_____ Pupil

_____ Superior Lacrimal Duct

_____ Superior Lacrimal Gland

Figure 28.1   The lacrimal apparatus of the eye.

Internal Anatomy

Figure 28.2 is a horizontal section of the right eye as seen looking down upon it. Note that the wall of the eyeball consists of three layers: an outer **scleroid coat,** a middle **choroid coat,** and an inner **retina.** The continuity of the surface of the retina is interrupted only by two structures, the optic nerve and the fovea centralis.

The **optic nerve** (label 3) contains fibers leading from the rods and cones of the retina to the brain. That point on the retina where the optic nerve makes its entrance is lacking in rods and cones. The absence of light receptors at this spot makes it insensitive to light; thus, it is called the **blind spot.** It is also known as the **optic disk.**

Note that the optic nerve is wrapped in a sheath, the **dura mater** (an extension of the dura that surrounds the brain). To the right of the blind spot is a pit, the **fovea centralis,** which is the center of a round yellow spot, the *macula lutea.* The macula, which is only a half a millimeter in diameter, is composed entirely of cones and is that part of the eye where all critical vision occurs.

Light entering the eye is focused on the retina by the **lens,** an elliptical crystalline clear structure suspended in the eye by a **suspensory ligament.** Attached to this ligament is the **ciliary body,** a circular smooth muscle that can change the shape of the lens to focus on objects at different distances.

In front of the lens is a cavity that contains a watery fluid, the **aqueous humor.** Between the lens and the retina is a larger cavity that contains a more viscous, jellylike substance, the **vitreous body.** Immediately in front of the lens lies the circular colored portion of the eye, the **iris.** It consists of circular and radiating muscle fibers that can change the size of the **pupil** of the eye. The iris regulates the amount of light that enters the eye through the pupil.

Covering the anterior portion of the eye is the **cornea,** a clear, transparent structure that is an extension of the scleroid coat. It acts as a window to the eye, allowing light to enter.

Aqueous humor is constantly being renewed in the eye. The enlarged inset of the lens-iris area in figure 28.2 illustrates where the aqueous humor is produced (point A) and where it is reabsorbed (point B). At point A, which is in the **posterior chamber,** aqueous humor is produced by capillaries of the ciliary body. As this fluid is produced, it

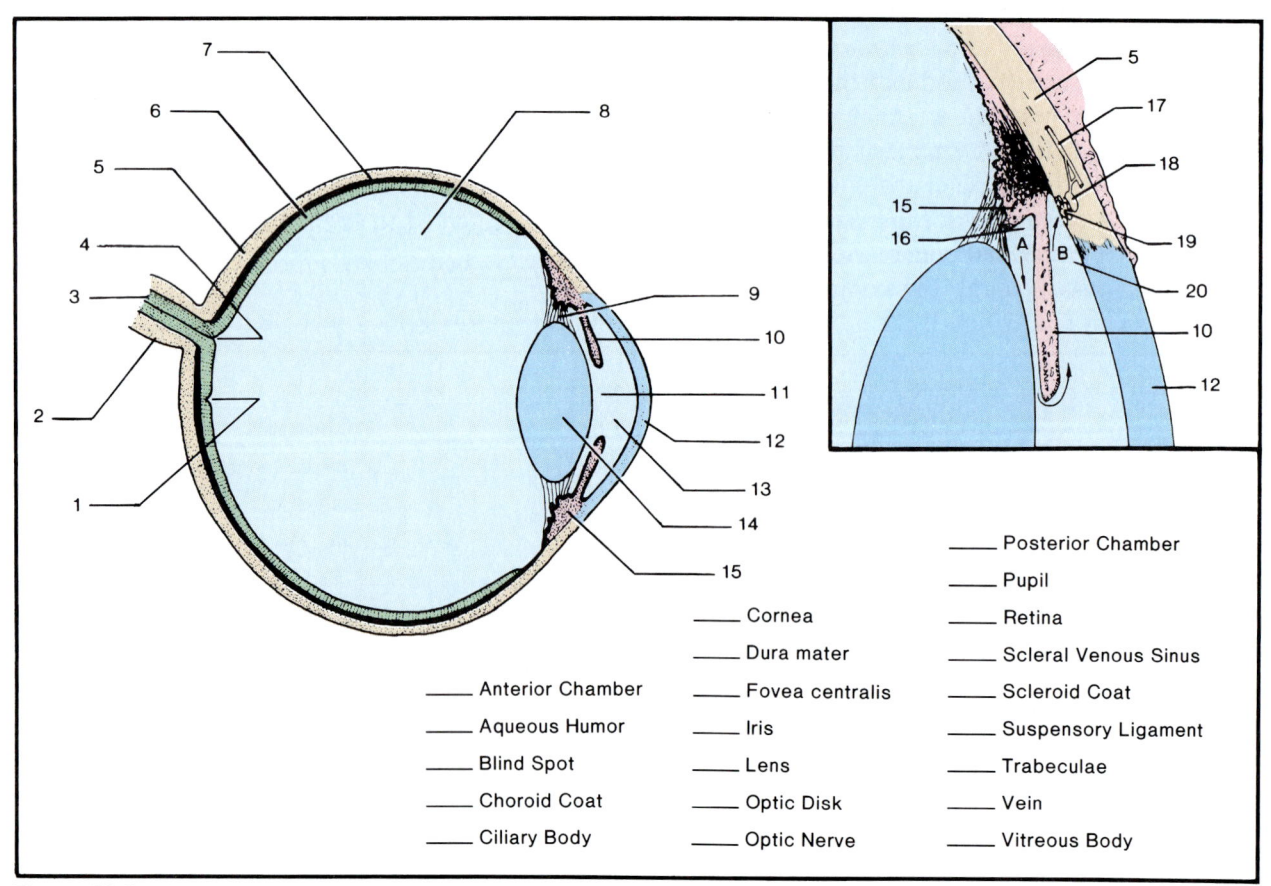

_____ Anterior Chamber

_____ Aqueous Humor

_____ Blind Spot

_____ Choroid Coat

_____ Ciliary Body

_____ Cornea

_____ Dura mater

_____ Fovea centralis

_____ Iris

_____ Lens

_____ Optic Disk

_____ Optic Nerve

_____ Posterior Chamber

_____ Pupil

_____ Retina

_____ Scleral Venous Sinus

_____ Scleroid Coat

_____ Suspensory Ligament

_____ Trabeculae

_____ Vein

_____ Vitreous Body

Figure 28.2   Internal anatomy of the eye.

passes through the pupil into the **anterior chamber** and is reabsorbed into minute spaces called **trabeculae** at the juncture of the cornea and the iris (point B). From the trabeculae the fluid passes to the **scleral venous sinus** (canal of Schlemm), which empties into the venous system.

Assignment:

Label figure 28.2.

The Ocular Muscles

The ability of each eye to be moved in all directions within its orbit is controlled by six *extrinsic* ocular muscles. Movement of the upper eyelid is controlled by a single muscle, the **superior levator palpebrae.**

Figure 28.3, which is a lateral view of the right eye, reveals the insertions of all seven of these muscles. The origins of these muscles are on various bony formations at the back of the eye orbit.

The muscle on the side of the eye that has a portion of it removed is the **lateral rectus.** Opposing it on the other side of the eye is the **medial rectus.** The muscle that inserts on top of the eye is the **superior rectus;** its antagonist on the bottom of the eye is the **inferior rectus.** Just above the stub of the lateral rectus is seen the insertion of the **superior oblique,** which passes through a cartilaginous loop, the **trochlea.** Opposing the superior oblique is the **inferior oblique,** of which only a portion of the insertion can be seen.

Assignment:

Label figure 28.3.

Beef Eye Dissection

The nature of the tissues of the eye can best be studied by actual dissection of an eye. A beef eye will be used for this study. Figure 28.4 illustrates various steps that will be followed.

Materials:

> beef eye, preferably fresh
> dissecting instruments
> dissecting tray

1. Examine the external surfaces of the eyeball. Identify the **optic nerve** and look for remnants of extrinsic muscles on the sides of the eyeball.
2. Note the shape of the **pupil.** Is it round or elliptical? Identify the **cornea.**
3. Holding the eyeball as shown in illustration 1, figure 28.4, make an incision into the scleroid coat with a sharp scalpel about one-quarter of an inch away from the cornea. Note how difficult it is to penetrate. Insert scissors into the incision and carefully cut all the way around the cornea, *taking care not to squeeze the fluid out of the eye.* Refer to illustration 2, figure 28.4.
4. Gently lift the front portion off the eye and place it on the tray with the inner surface upward. The lens usually remains attached to the vitreous body, as shown in illustration 3. If the eye is preserved (not fresh), the lens may remain in the anterior part of the eye.
5. Examine the inner surface of the anterior portion and identify the thickened, black circular **ciliary body.** What function does the black pigment perform?

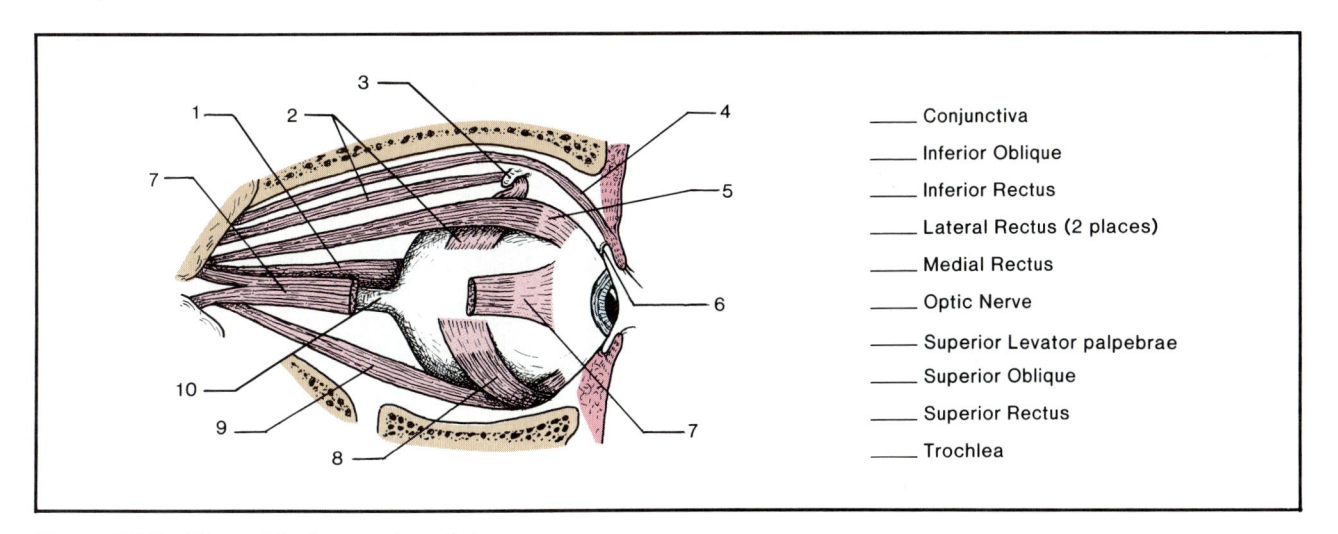

Conjunctiva
Inferior Oblique
Inferior Rectus
Lateral Rectus (2 places)
Medial Rectus
Optic Nerve
Superior Levator palpebrae
Superior Oblique
Superior Rectus
Trochlea

Figure 28.3 The extrinsic muscles of the eye.

6. Study the **iris** carefully. Can you distinguish **circular** and **radial** muscle fibers?

7. Is there any **aqueous humor** left between the cornea and iris? Compare its consistency with the **vitreous body.**

8. With a dissecting needle separate the lens from the vitreous body by working the needle around its perimeter as shown in illustration 3. Hold the lens up by its edge with a forceps and look through it at some distant object. What is unusual about the image?

9. Place the lens on printed matter. Are the letters magnified?

10. Compare the consistency of the lens at its center and near its circumference. Use a probe or forceps. Do you detect any differences?

11. Locate the **retina** at the back of the eye. It is a thin colorless inner coat which separates easily from the pigmented **choroid coat.** Now, locate the **blind spot.** This is the area where the retina is attached to the back of the eye.

12. Note the iridescent nature of a portion of the choroid coat. This reflective surface is the *tapetum lucidum.* It causes the eyes of animals to reflect light at night and appears to enhance night vision by reflecting some light back into the retina.

13. Answer all questions on the Laboratory Report that pertain to this dissection.

Ophthalmoscopy

Routine physical examinations invariably involve an examination of the *fundus,* or interior, of the eye. A careful examination of the fundus provides

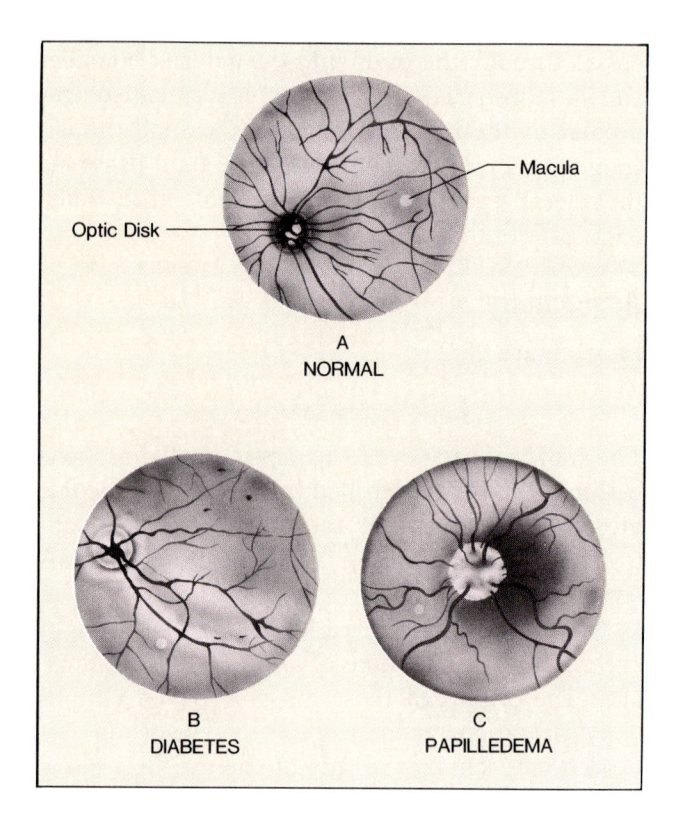

Figure 28.5 Normal and abnormal retinas as seen through an ophthalmoscope.

valid information about the general health of the patient. The retina of the eye is the only part of the body where relatively large blood vessels may be inspected without surgical intervention.

Figure 28.5 illustrates what one might expect to see in a normal eye (A); the eye of a diabetic (B); and the eye of one who has hypertension, a brain tumor, or meningitis (C). In *diabetic retinopathy* the peripheral vessels are generally irreg-

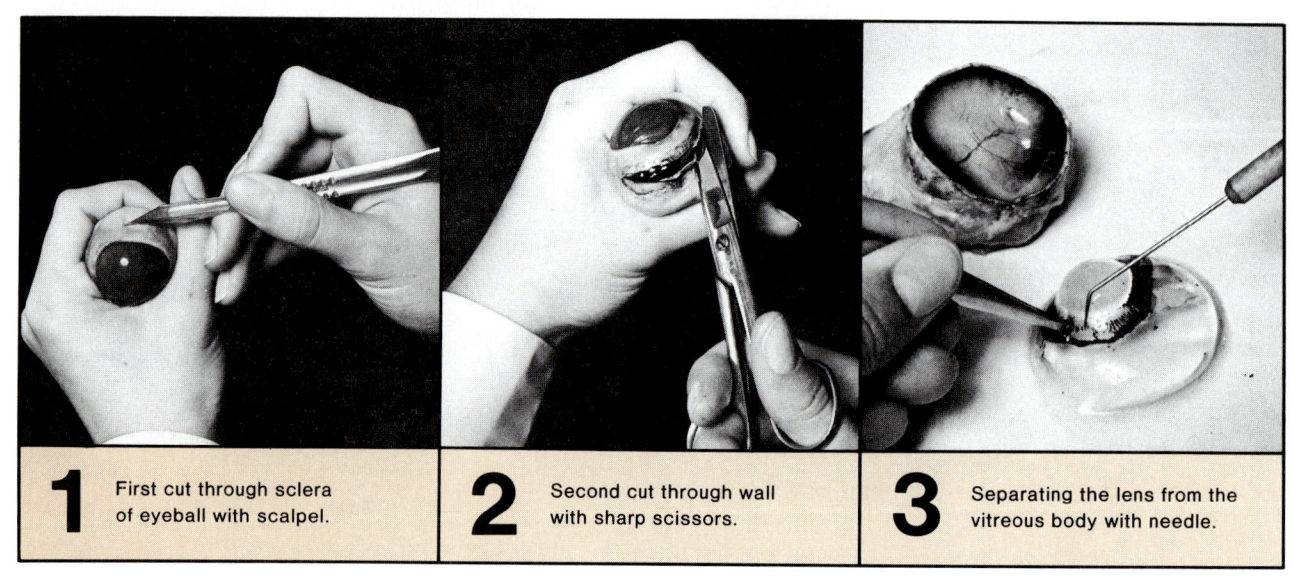

| 1 | First cut through sclera of eyeball with scalpel. | 2 | Second cut through wall with sharp scissors. | 3 | Separating the lens from the vitreous body with needle. |

Figure 28.4 Three steps in beef eye dissection.

ular, fewer in number, and often show small hemorrhages. In *papilledema,* or choked disk, the optic disk is blurred, enlarged, and often hemorrhagic; the veins are also considerably enlarged. These are only a few examples of pathology showing up in the fundus.

The instrument that one uses for examining the fundus is called an **ophthalmoscope.** In this exercise you will have an opportunity to examine the interior of the eyes of your laboratory partner. Your partner, in turn, will examine your eyes. It will be necessary to make this examination in a darkened room. Before this examination can be made, however, it is essential that you understand the operation of the ophthalmoscope.

The Ophthalmoscope

Figure 28.6 reveals the construction of a Welch Allyn ophthalmoscope. Within its handle are two C-size batteries that power an illuminating bulb that is located in the viewing head. Note that at the top of the handle there is a rheostat control for regulating the intensity of the light source. Only after depressing the lock button can this control be rotated.

The head of the instrument has two rotatable notched disks: a large lens selection disk and a smaller aperture selection disk. A viewing aperture is located at the upper end of the head.

While looking through the viewing aperture, the examiner is able to select one of twenty-three small lenses by rotating the **lens selection disk** with the index finger held as shown in figure 28.7. Twelve of the lenses on this disk are positive (convex) and eleven of them are negative (concave). Numbers that appear in the **diopter window** indicate which lens is in place. The positive lenses are represented as black numbers; negative lens numbers are red. A black "0" in the window indicates that no lens is in place.

If the eyes of both subject and examiner are normal (*emmetropic*), no lens is needed. If the eye of the subject or examiner is far-sighted (*hypermetropic*), the positive lenses will be selected. Near-sighted (*myopic*) eyes require the use of negative lenses. The degree of myopia or hypermetropia is indicated by the magnitude of the number. Since the eyes of both the examiner and subject affect the lens selection, the selection becomes entirely empirical.

The **aperture selection disk** enables the examiner to change the character of the light beam that

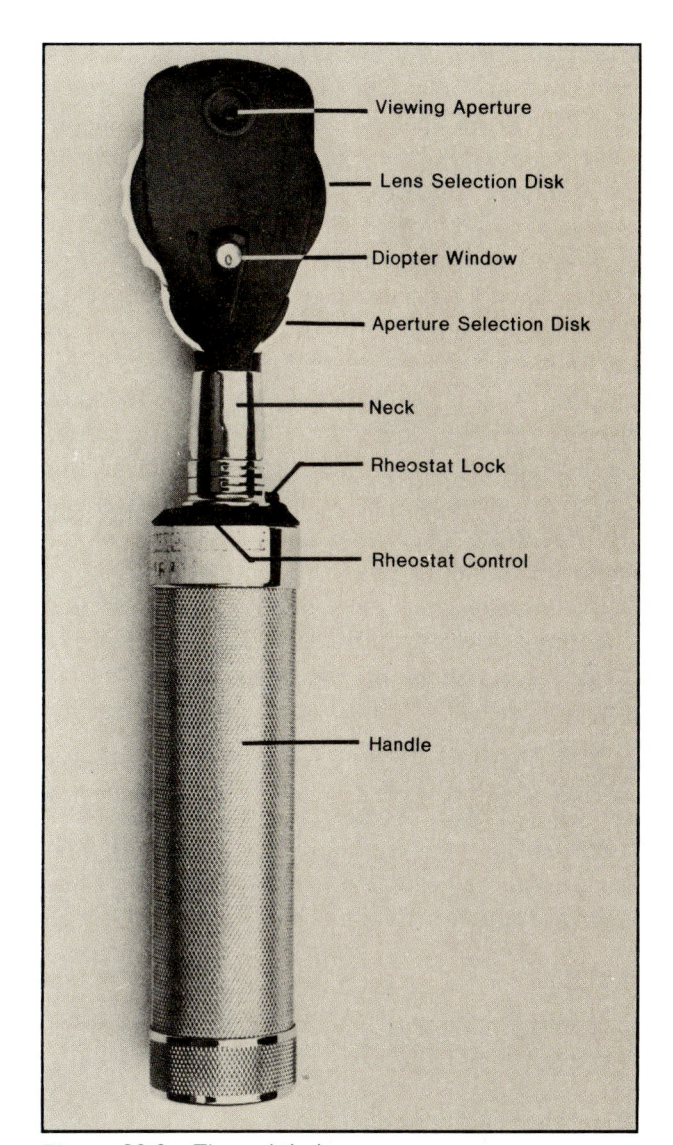

Figure 28.6 The ophthalmoscope.

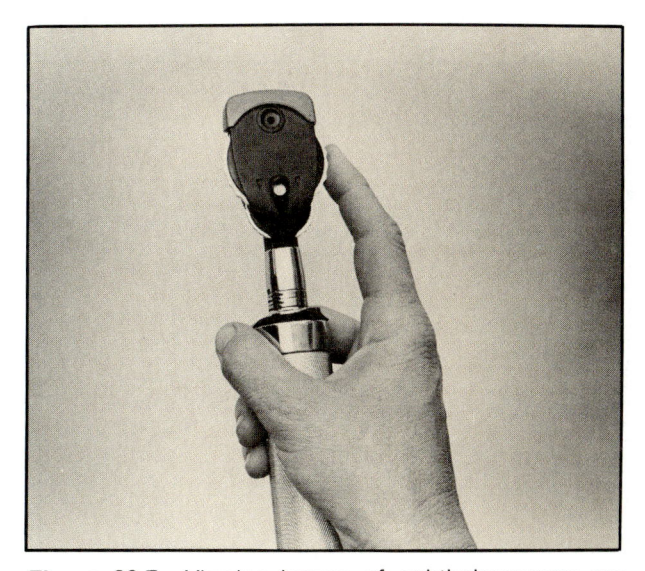

Figure 28.7 Viewing lenses of ophthalmoscope are rotated into position by moving the lens selection disk with index finger.

is projected into the eye. The light may be projected as a grid, straight line, white spot, or green spot. **The green spot is most frequently used** because it is less irritating to the eye of the subject, and it causes the blood vessels to show up more clearly.

Using an ophthalmoscope for the first time seems difficult for some users and relatively easy for others. The examiner with emmetropic eyes has a definite advantage over one with myopia, astigmatism, or hypermetropia. Even for individuals with normal eyes, there is the troublesome reflection of light from the retina back into the examiner's eye. The best way to minimize this problem is to **direct the light beam toward the edge of the pupil** rather than through the center.

A precautionary statement *must* be heeded concerning light exposure: **Avoid subjecting an eye to more than one minute light exposure.** After one minute exposure, allow several minutes of rest for recovery of the retina.

Procedure

Prior to using the ophthalmoscope in the darkened room, it will be necessary for you to become completely familiar with its mechanics.

Materials:

> ophthalmoscope
> metric tape or ruler

Desk Study of Ophthalmoscope

Turn on the light source by depressing the lock button and rotating the rheostat control. Observe how the light intensity can be varied from dim to very bright. Rotate the aperture selection disk as you hold the ophthalmoscope about two inches away from your desk top. Keep the instrument parallel to the desk surface. How many different light patterns are there? Select the large white spot for the next phase of this study.

Rotate the lens selection disk until a black 5 appears in the diopter window. While peering through the viewing window at the print on this page, bring the letters into sharp focus. Have your lab partner measure with a metric tape the distance in millimeters between the ophthalmoscope and the printed page when the lettering is in sharp focus. Record this distance on the Laboratory Report. Do the same thing for the 10D, 20D, and 40D lenses, recording all measurements.

Now, set the lens selection disk on "0" and the light source on the green spot. The instrument is properly set now for the beginning of an eye examination. Read over the following procedure *in its entirety* before entering the darkened room.

The Examination

Figures 28.8 and 28.9 illustrate how the ophthalmoscope is held in different viewing situations. Note that the examiner uses the right hand when examining the right eye and the left when examining the left eye. Proceed as follows:

1. With the "0" in the diopter window and the light turned on, grasp the ophthalmoscope, as shown in figure 28.8. Note that the index finger rests on the lens selection disk.

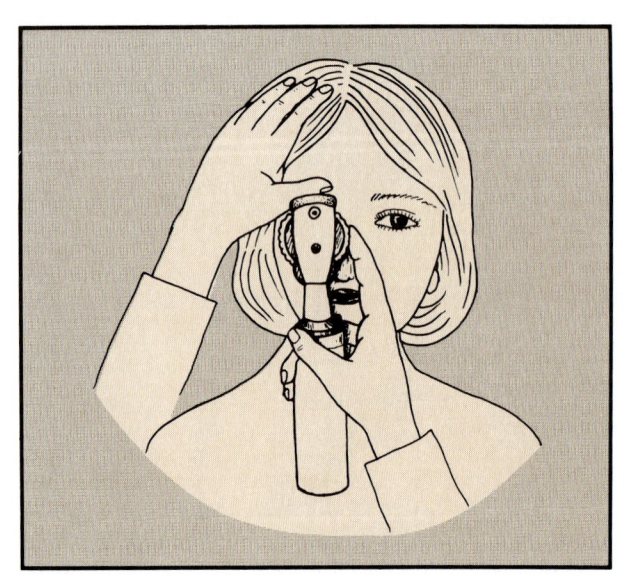

Figure 28.8 When examining the right eye, the ophthalmoscope is held with the right hand.

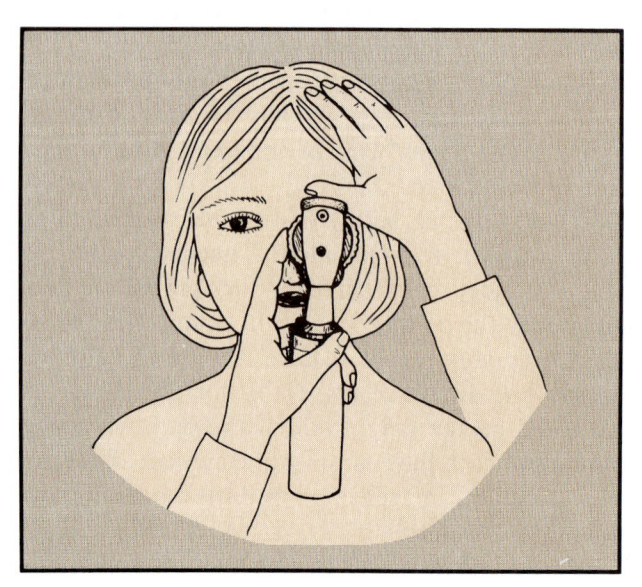

Figure 28.9 When examining the left eye, the ophthalmoscope is held with the left hand.

2. Place the viewing aperture in front of your right eye and steady the ophthalmoscope by resting the top of it against your eyebrow. See figure 28.10.

Start viewing the subject's right eye at a distance of about 12 inches. Keep your subject on your right and instruct your subject to **look straight ahead at a fixed object** at eye level.

3. Direct the beam of light into the pupil and examine the lens and vitreous body. As you look through the pupil, a red *reflex* will be seen. If the image is not sharp, adjust the focus with the lens selection disk.

4. While keeping the pupil in focus, move in to within two inches of the subject, as illustrated in figure 28.11. The red reflex should become more pronounced. **Try to direct the light beam toward the edge of the pupil** rather than in the center to minimize reflection from the retina.

5. Search out the **optic disk** and adjust the focus, as necessary, to produce a sharp image. Observe how blood vessels radiate out from the optic disk. Follow one or more of them to the periphery.

Locate the **macula.** It is situated about two disk diameters *laterally* from the optic disk. Note that it lacks blood vessels. It is easiest to observe when the subject is asked to look directly into the light, a position that **must be limited to one second only.**

6. Examine the entire retinal surface. Look for any irregularities, depressions, or protrusions from its surface. It is not unusual to see a roundish elevation, not unlike a pimple, on its surface.

To examine the periphery, instruct the subject to: (1) **look up** for examination of the superior retina, (2) **look down** for examination of the inferior retina, and (3) **look laterally and medially** for those respective areas.

7. **Caution:** Remember to limit the examinations to **one minute!** After this time limit is reached, examine the left eye, using the left hand to hold the ophthalmoscope and reversing the entire procedure.

8. Switch roles with your laboratory partner. When you have examined each other's eyes, examine the eyes of other students. Report any unusual conditions to your instructor.

Histological Studies

Most prepared slides available for laboratory study are made from either the rabbit or the monkey. Both animals are suitable. Proceed as follows to identify structures depicted in the photomicrographs of figures HA-15 and HA-16 of the Histology Atlas.

Materials:

prepared slides:

monkey eye, x.s. (H10.635, H10.64, or H10.76)
rabbit eye, sagittal section (H10.61 or 10.62)

The Cornea With the lowest powered objective on your microscope scan a cross section of the eye of a rabbit or monkey until you find the cornea. Refer to illustrations A and B, figure HA-15. Note that the cornea consists of three layers: the epithelium, stroma, and endothelium. For fine detail, as in illustration B, use high-dry.

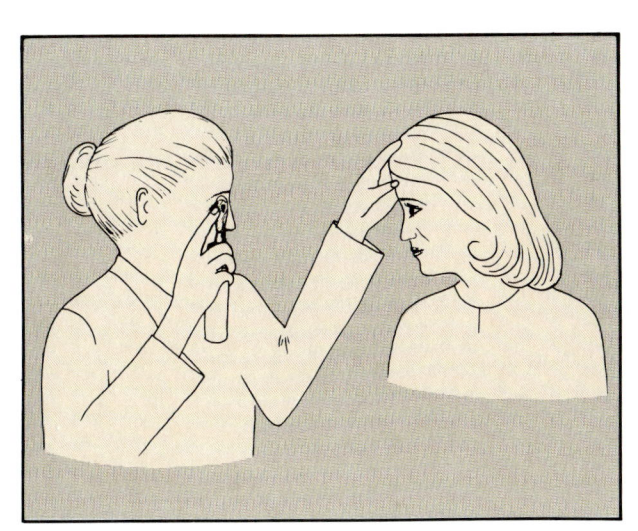

Figure 28.10 When viewing the lens and vitreous body, use this position, relative to subject.

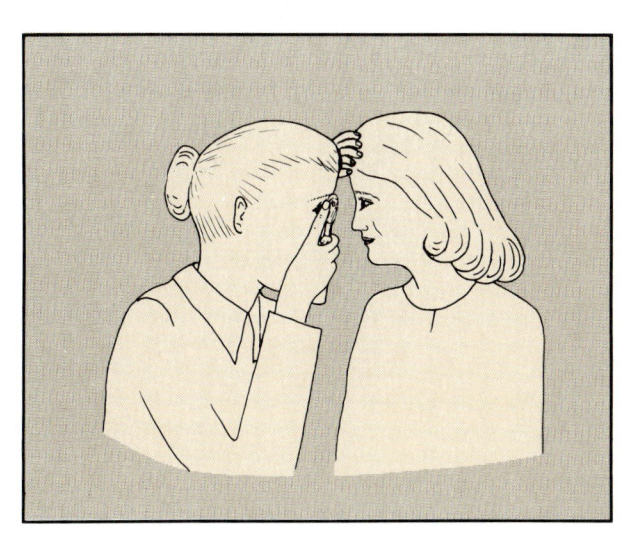

Figure 28.11 When examining the retinal surfaces, move in close as illustrated here.

The **corneal epithelium** is the outer portion that consists of stratified squamous. While the outermost cells of this layer are flattened squamous cells, the basal cells are columnar.

The **corneal endothelium** is the innermost layer of cells, which is adjacent to the aqueous humor. This thin layer consists of low cuboidal cells.

The **corneal stroma** (*substantia propria*) comprises nine-tenths of the thickness of the cornea. It consists of collagenous fibrils, fibroblasts, and cementing substance. The fibrils are arranged in lamellae that run parallel to the corneal surface. The components of this stroma are held together by a mucopolysaccharide cement. The chemical structure and fibril arrangement contribute to the transparency of the cornea.

The Lens Note that the lens is enclosed in a homogenous elastic **capsule** to which the **suspensory ligament** is attached. The lens is formed from epithelial cells that become elongated to a fibrous shape (lens fibers), losing most of their organelles and nuclei. All that remains in a mature lens fiber are a few microtubules and clumps of free ribosomes. These cells are not entirely inert, and they persist throughout life.

The Ciliary Muscle This ring of smooth muscle tissue is a part of the body wall of the eye. Identify the **ciliary processes,** which form ridges on the ciliary muscle. The latter provide an anchor for the suspensory ligaments.

Body Wall of Eye Examine a section through the body wall at the back of the eye. Identify the sclera, choroid coat, and retina. Note that the **sclera** consists of closely packed collagenous fibers, elastic fibers, and fibroblasts.

Note, also, the large amount of pigment in the **choroid coat** that is produced by **melanocytes.** This is the layer that supplies nourishment to the retina and scleroid coat. Look for blood vessels.

The **retina** is the inner photosensitive layer of the body wall.

Retinal Layers The retina is composed of five main classes of neurons: the photoreceptors (rods and cones), bipolar cells, ganglion cells, horizontal cells, and amacrine cells. The first three form a direct pathway from the retina to the brain. The horizontal and amacrine cells form laterally directed pathways that modify and control the message being passed along the direct pathway.

Study a section of the retina and identify the various layers. Refer to figure HA-16 for reference. Any Turtox slide of monkey eye section is suitable for retinal study.

At the base of the retina, where it meets the choroid layer, are the **rods** and **cones.** The nuclei for these photoreceptors are located in the **outer nuclear layer.** To stimulate these receptors light must pass through all the other cell layers.

Nuclei of the amacrine and bipolar neurons are located in the **inner nuclear layer.** Dendrites of these association neurons make synaptic connections with axons of the rods and cones in the **outer synaptic layer.**

The nuclei of ganglion cells are located closest to the exposed surface of the retina: in a layer designated as the **ganglion cell layer.** The dendrites of ganglion cells make synaptic connections with amacrine and bipolar cells in the **inner synaptic layer.** Nonmyelinated axons of the ganglion cells fill up the **nerve fiber layer;** they converge at the optic disk to form the optic nerve. Some neuroglial cell nuclei can be seen in the nerve fiber layer.

The Fovea Centralis Study a slide that reveals the structure of the fovea (H10.635). Compare your slide with the photomicrographs in illustrations B and C in figure HA-16.

Laboratory Report

Complete the Laboratory Report for this exercise.

The human ear serves a dual function in that it is (1) a receptor for sound, and (2) one of the mechanisms for maintaining equilibrium. Separate components in each ear function in these two respects.

In the first portion of this exercise those anatomical structures that pertain to hearing will be studied. Some of the mechanics of hearing will also be explored. Those parts of the ear that function in maintaining equilibrium will be studied last.

Characteristics of Sound

Sound waves moving through the air are propagated in wave forms that possess characteristics relative to the vibratory motion that generates them. The ear is able to distinguish tones that differ in pitch, loudness, and quality. *Pitch* is determined by the frequency of vibration; *loudness* pertains to the intensity of the vibration; and *quality* relates to the nature of the vibrations as revealed by the wave shape.

Figure 29.1 illustrates several curves depicting both the shapes of sound waves and the characteristics of the vibrations that produce them. The sine curves A and B in illustration I differ in frequency, with B producing the tone of higher pitch. Curves A and C in the middle group are of the same fre-

quency; they differ only in amplitude, or loudness. Although the amplitude of A is twice that of C, the loudness of A will be four times that of C. This is because the intensity (I) of sound is directly proportional to the square of the amplitude (a):

$$I = 2\pi^2 \, V f^2 \, a^2 \, d$$

V = velocity of wave propagation
f = frequency
d = density of medium

Waves A and D in illustration III differ in shape, D having some components of higher frequency that are not present in A. These curves represent sounds of different quality.

The ability of the ear to distinguish differences in pitch, amplitude, and quality depend on: (1) the conduction and pressure amplification of sound waves through the ossicles of the middle ear; (2) the stimulation of receptor cells in the cochlea; and (3) the conveyance of action potentials in the cochlear nerve to the auditory centers in the brain for interpretation. The interference of any component of this system results in hearing loss. The types of hearing loss will be studied as hearing tests are performed. Let us now explore the anatomy of the ear as it functions in normal anatomy.

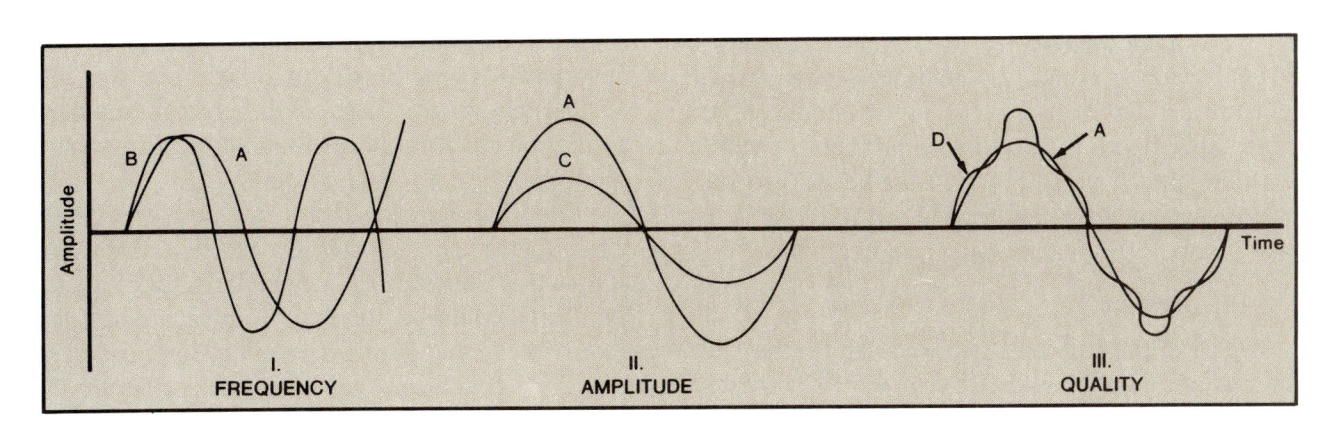

Figure 29.1 Differences in sound waves.

Components of the Ear

Anatomically, the human ear consists of three distinct divisions: the external ear, the middle ear, and the internal ear. Figure 29.2 is a diagrammatic representation of its various components.

The External Ear

The outer or external ear consists of two parts: the auricle and external auditory meatus. The **auricle,** or **pinna,** is the outer shell of skin and elastic cartilage that is attached to the side of the head. The **external auditory meatus** is a canal about one inch in length that extends from the auricle into the head through the temporal bone. The skin lining the canal contains some small hairs and modified apocrine sweat glands that produce a waxy secretion called *cerumen.* The inner end of this meatus terminates at the **tympanic membrane,** or eardrum. The auricle serves to collect and direct sound waves into the tympanic membrane through the meatus.

The Middle Ear

This division of the ear consists of a small cavity in the temporal bone between the tympanic membrane and the inner ear. It contains three small bones (*ossicles*) that are united to form a lever system. The outermost ossicle, which is attached to the tympanic membrane, is the **malleus,** a hammer or club-shaped bone. The middle bone, an anvil-shaped structure, is the **incus.** The innermost bone, which fits into the **oval window** of the inner ear, is stirrup-shaped and is called the **stapes.**

It is the role of these ossicles to transfer the forces from the eardrum to the cochlear fluids of the inner ear through the oval window. Although most sound waves reach the inner ear via the ossicles (*ossicular conduction*), some sounds, specifically very loud ones, reach the cochlea through the bones of the skull (*bone conduction*).

Leading downward from the middle ear to the nasopharynx is a duct, the **auditory** (Eustachian) **tube,** which allows air pressure in the middle ear to be equalized with the outside atmosphere. A valve at the nasopharynx end of the tube keeps the tube closed. Acts of yawning or swallowing cause it to open temporarily for pressure equalization.

The Internal Ear

This part of the ear consists of two labyrinths: the osseous and membranous labyrinths. The **osseous labyrinth** is shown in illustration B. It is the hol-lowed out portion of the temporal bone that contains an inner tubular structure of membranous tissue, the **membranous labyrinth.** The entire membranous labyrinth is shown in figure 29.4. Some portions of the membranous labyrinth are shown in cutaway portions of the osseous labyrinth in illustration B, figure 29.2.

Within the membranous labyrinth is a fluid, the *endolymph.* Between the membranous and osseous labyrinths is a different fluid, the *perilymph.* These fluids act as conduction media for the forces involved in hearing and maintaining equilibrium.

The osseous labyrinth consists of three semicircular canals, the vestibule, and the cochlea. The **vestibule** is that portion that has the oval window on its side into which the stapes fits. The three **semicircular canals** branch off the vestibule to one side, and the **cochlea,** which is shaped like a snail's shell, emerges from the other side.

On the osseous labyrinth are two nerves, which are branches of the eighth cranial, or vestibulocochlear, nerve. The **vestibular nerve** is the upper nerve branch, which passes from the sensory areas of the semicircular ducts, saccule, and utricle. The other branch is the **cochlear nerve,** which emerges from the cochlea.

The cochlea consists of a coiled, bony tube with three chambers extending along its full length. Illustration C in figure 29.2 reveals a cross section of the cochlear tube. The upper chamber, or **scala vestibuli** (label 16), is so-named because it is continuous with the vestibule. The lower larger chamber is the **scala tympani.** The **round window** (label 1) is a membrane-covered opening that is on the osseous wall of the scala tympani. Between these two chambers is a triangular cross section that represents the **cochlear duct.** This duct is bounded on its upper surface by the **vestibular membrane** and on its lower surface by the **basilar membrane.** On the upper surface of the basilar membrane lies the **organ of Corti,** which contains the receptor cells of hearing. All of these chambers contain fluid: perilymph in the scala vestibuli and scala tympani; endolymph in the cochlear duct.

Illustration D reveals the detailed structure of the organ of Corti. Note how the hair tips of the **hair cells** are embedded in a gelatinouslike flap, the **tectorial membrane.** Leading from each hair cell is a nerve fiber that passes through the basilar membrane and becomes part of the cochlear nerve. The upper margins of the hair cells are held in place by

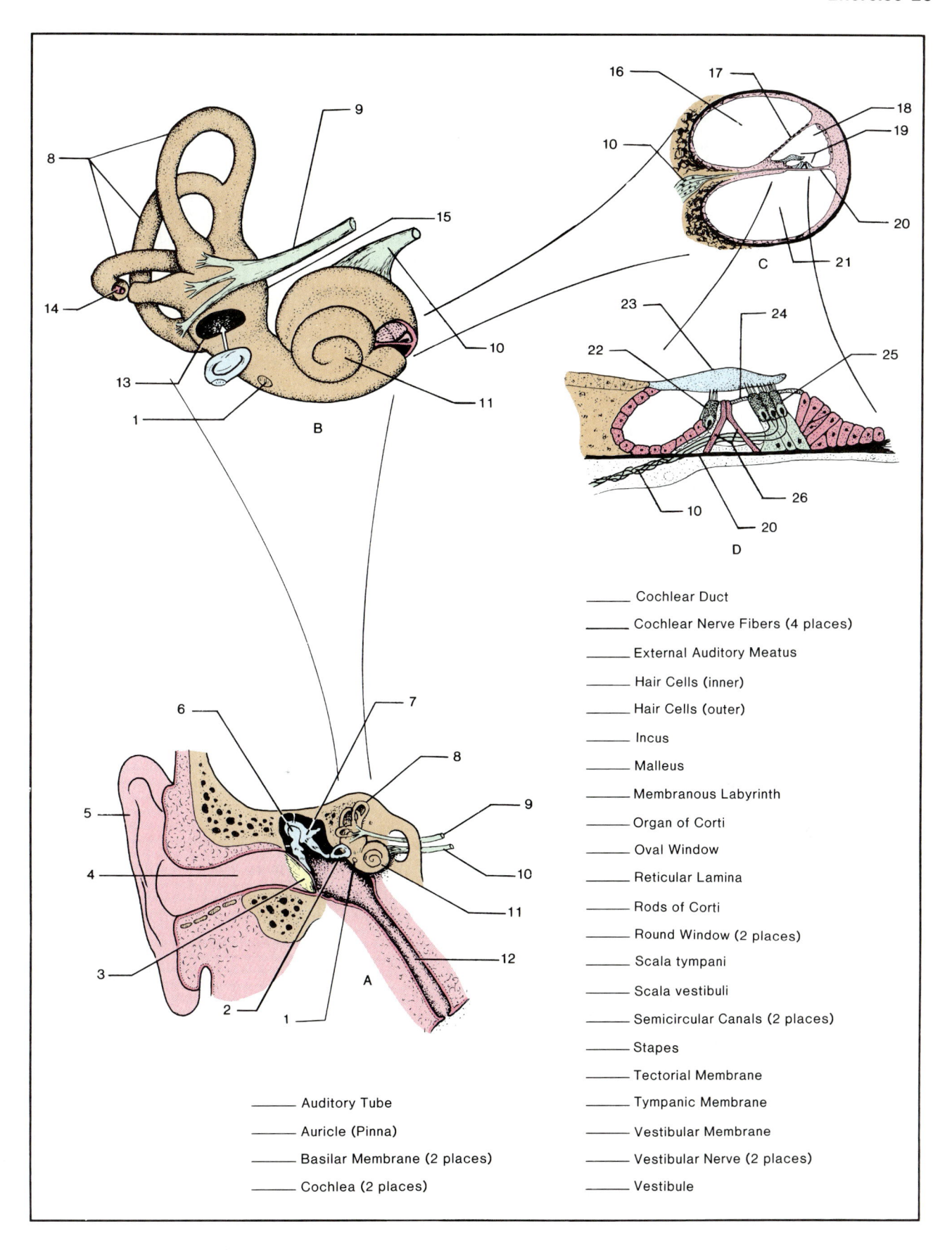

Figure 29.2 Anatomy of the ear.

_____ Cochlear Duct
_____ Cochlear Nerve Fibers (4 places)
_____ External Auditory Meatus
_____ Hair Cells (inner)
_____ Hair Cells (outer)
_____ Incus
_____ Malleus
_____ Membranous Labyrinth
_____ Organ of Corti
_____ Oval Window
_____ Reticular Lamina
_____ Rods of Corti
_____ Round Window (2 places)
_____ Scala tympani
_____ Scala vestibuli
_____ Semicircular Canals (2 places)
_____ Stapes
_____ Tectorial Membrane
_____ Tympanic Membrane
_____ Vestibular Membrane
_____ Vestibular Nerve (2 places)
_____ Vestibule

_____ Auditory Tube
_____ Auricle (Pinna)
_____ Basilar Membrane (2 places)
_____ Cochlea (2 places)

the **reticular lamina.** Between the reticular lamina and the basilar membrane are reinforcing structures called the **rods of Corti.** The significance of all these structures must be taken into account in any plausible theory of hearing.

Assignment:

Label figure 29.2.

The Physiology of Hearing

As stated previously, hearing occurs when action potentials are received by the auditory centers of the brain. These action potentials, which pass along the cochlear nerve fibers of the eighth cranial nerve, are initiated by the hair cells in the organ of Corti. Activation of the hair cells depends on forces within the cochlear fluids, basilar membrane structure, secondary energy transfer, and endocochlear potential. A discussion of roles of each of these follows.

Role of Cochlear Fluids In figure 29.3 the cochlea has been uncoiled to reveal the relationships of its various chambers. When the stapes moves in and out of the oval window, sound wave energy moves through the scala vestibuli and into the scala tympani. Since the perilymph is incompressible, the elasticity of the round window membrane accommodates the pressure changes by moving in and out in synchrony with the movements of the stapes.

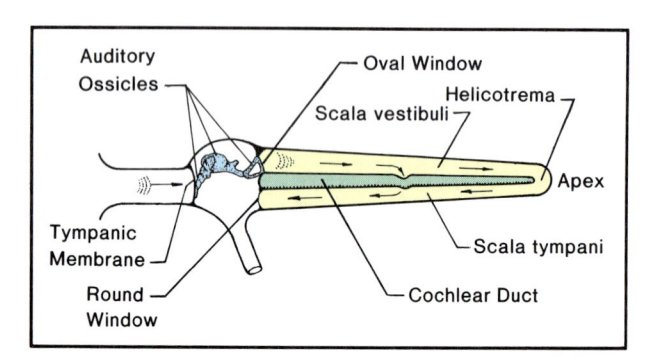

Figure 29.3 Pathway of sound wave transmission in the ear.

The energy of sound waves moving through the cochlea reaches the round window in two ways: (1) directly into the scala tympani through the helicotrema at the apex of the cochlea, and (2) through the flexible cochlear duct to the scala tympani. Arrows in figure 29.3 illustrate both routes of energy propagation.

Basilar Membrane Structure The first structure of the organ of Corti that reacts to vibrations of different sound frequencies is the basilar membrane. Within this membrane are approximately 20,000 fibers that project from the bony center of the cochlea toward the outer wall. The fibers closest to the stapes are short (.04 mm) and stiff; they vibrate when stimulated by vibrations caused by high frequency sounds. The fibers at the end of the cochlea near the helicotrema are long (.5 mm), more limber, and vibrate in harmony with low frequency sounds. These fibers are elastic reedlike structures that are not fixed at their distal ends. Because they are free at one end, they are able to vibrate like reeds of a harmonica to specific frequencies.

Secondary Energy Transfer Once fibers at a particular point on the basilar membrane are set into motion by a specific sound frequency, the rods of Corti transfer the energy from the basilar membrane to the reticular lamina, which supports the upper portion of the hair cells (see illustration D, figure 29.2). This secondary transfer of energy causes all these components to move as a unit, with the end result that the hairs of the hair cells are bent and stressed. The back and forth bending of the hairs, in turn, causes alternate changes in the electrical potential across the hair cell membrane. This alternating potential, known as the *receptor potential* of the hair cell, stimulates the nerve endings that are at the base of each hair cell, and an action potential in the cochlear nerve fibers is initiated.

Endocochlear Potential The sensitivity of the hair cells to depolarization is greatly enhanced by the chemical differences between the perilymph and endolymph. Perilymph has a high sodium-to-potassium ratio; endolymph has a high potassium-to-sodium ratio. These ionic differences result in an *endocochlear potential* of 80 millivolts. It is significant that the tops of the hair cells project through the reticular lamina into the endolymph of the scala media, but the lower portions of these cells lie bathed in perilymph. It is believed that this potential difference of 80 mv between the top and bottom of each hair cell greatly sensitizes the cell to slight movement of the hairs.

Frequency Range The variability in length and stiffness of the fibers within the basilar membrane enables the ear to differentiate sound waves as low as 30 cycles per second near the apex of the cochlea, and as high as 20,000 cps near the base of the cochlea. In between these two extremes, at various spots on the basilar membrane, the membrane responds to the in-between frequencies. This method of pitch localization by the basilar membrane is called the *place principle*.

Loudness Determination As noted in figure 29.1, the loudness of a sound is reflected in the sound wave. Increased loudness of sounds causes an increase in the amplitude of vibration of the basilar membrane. With an increase in basilar membrane vibration, more and more hair cells become stimulated, causing *spatial summation* of impulses; that is, more nerve fibers are carrying more impulses, and this is interpreted by the brain as increased loudness.

Assignment:

Answer the questions on the Laboratory Report that pertain to the physiology of hearing.

The Vestibular Apparatus

The part of the ear that functions in equilibrium is known as the *vestibular apparatus*. It incorporates the semicircular ducts, saccule and utricle of the membranous labyrinth (figure 29.4).

Although the vestibular apparatus plays the most important role in the maintenance of equilibrium, it should be kept in mind that three other mechanisms are also involved. These other mechanisms are: (1) visual evaluation of horizon position, (2) proprioceptor sensation in joint capsules, and (3) cutaneous sensations through certain exteroceptors.

Note in figure 29.4 that the **semicircular ducts** lie at right angles to each other in three different planes: horizontal, frontal and sagittal. Each duct has an enlarged portion, the **ampulla,** near one end that opens into a sac, the utricle. Within each ampulla is a cluster of hair cells called the **crista ampullaris.** Agitation of the endolymph occasioned by movements of the head stimulates the hair cells,

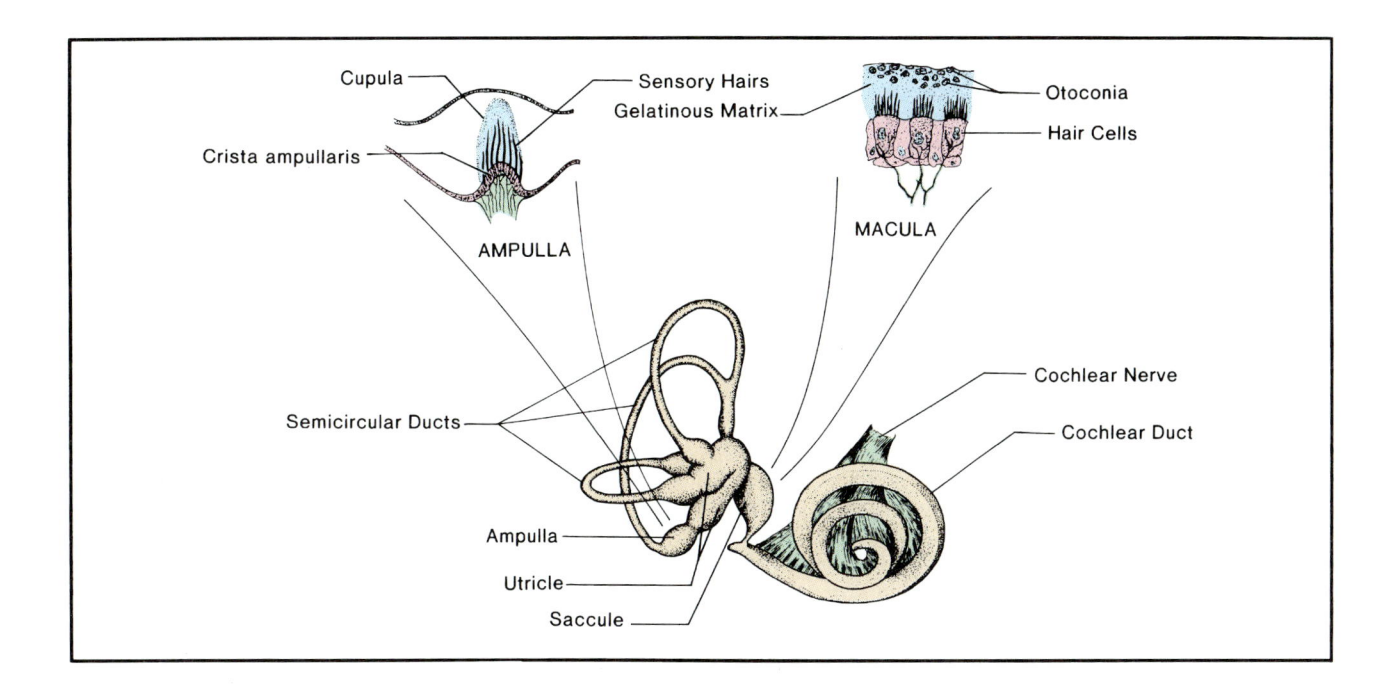

Figure 29.4 The membranous labyrinth.

and impulses are initiated in the vestibular nerve endings. These semicircular ducts function in the maintentance of *dynamic* (moving) *equilibrium.*

The utricle and saccule lie within the vestibule of the osseous labyrinth. They contain sensory hair cells which function in the maintenance of *static equilibrium.* As stated above, the **utricle** is that part of the vestibular apparatus to which the semicircular ducts are attached. The **saccule** is the portion that connects directly to the coiled up **cochlear duct.**

In the inner walls of the saccule and utricle are hair cells that are covered by a gelatinous suspension of **otoconia** (ear dust). When the head is in some position other than vertical the force of gravity acting on the calcaneous otoconia bends the hairs, triggering impulses along the vestibular nerve. The entire sensory mass of hair cells, gelatinous matrix and otoconia is called a **macula.**

Assignment:

Label figure 29.4

Histological Study

Examine slides H10.53 amd H10.54 to study the parts of the cochlea and crista ampullaris shown in figure HA-17 of the Histology Atlas. Both of these slides were made from guinea pig tissue. In particular, attempt to identify all the structures of the organ of Corti that are shown in illustration C. Note in illustration B that the cupula is obscured by the collapsed wall of the ampulla.

Laboratory Report

Complete the Laboratory Report for this exercise.

HISTOLOGY ATLAS

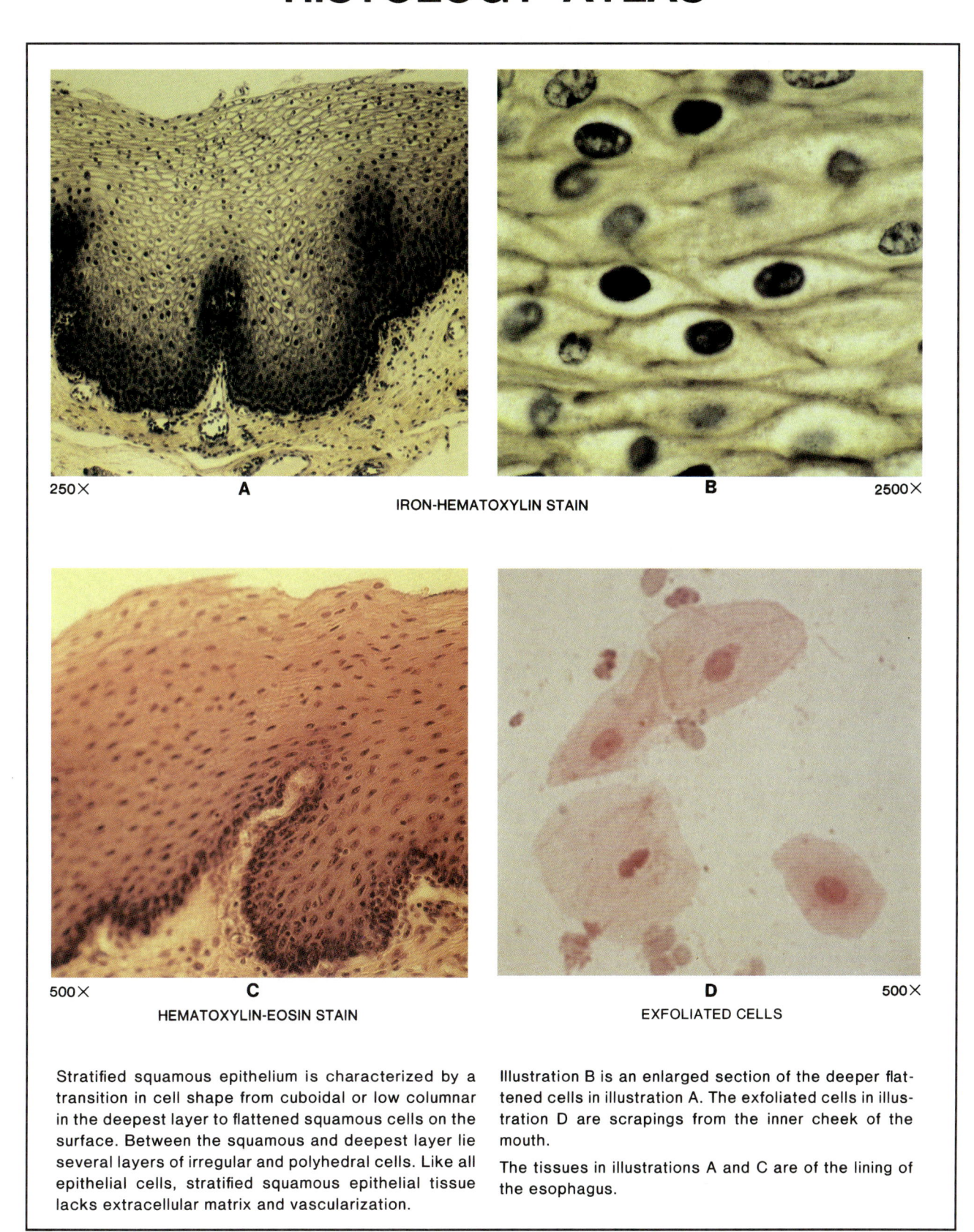

250×   **A**   **B**   2500×

IRON-HEMATOXYLIN STAIN

500×   **C**   **D**   500×

HEMATOXYLIN-EOSIN STAIN   EXFOLIATED CELLS

Stratified squamous epithelium is characterized by a transition in cell shape from cuboidal or low columnar in the deepest layer to flattened squamous cells on the surface. Between the squamous and deepest layer lie several layers of irregular and polyhedral cells. Like all epithelial cells, stratified squamous epithelial tissue lacks extracellular matrix and vascularization.

Illustration B is an enlarged section of the deeper flattened cells in illustration A. The exfoliated cells in illustration D are scrapings from the inner cheek of the mouth.

The tissues in illustrations A and C are of the lining of the esophagus.

Figure HA–1   Stratified squamous epithelium.

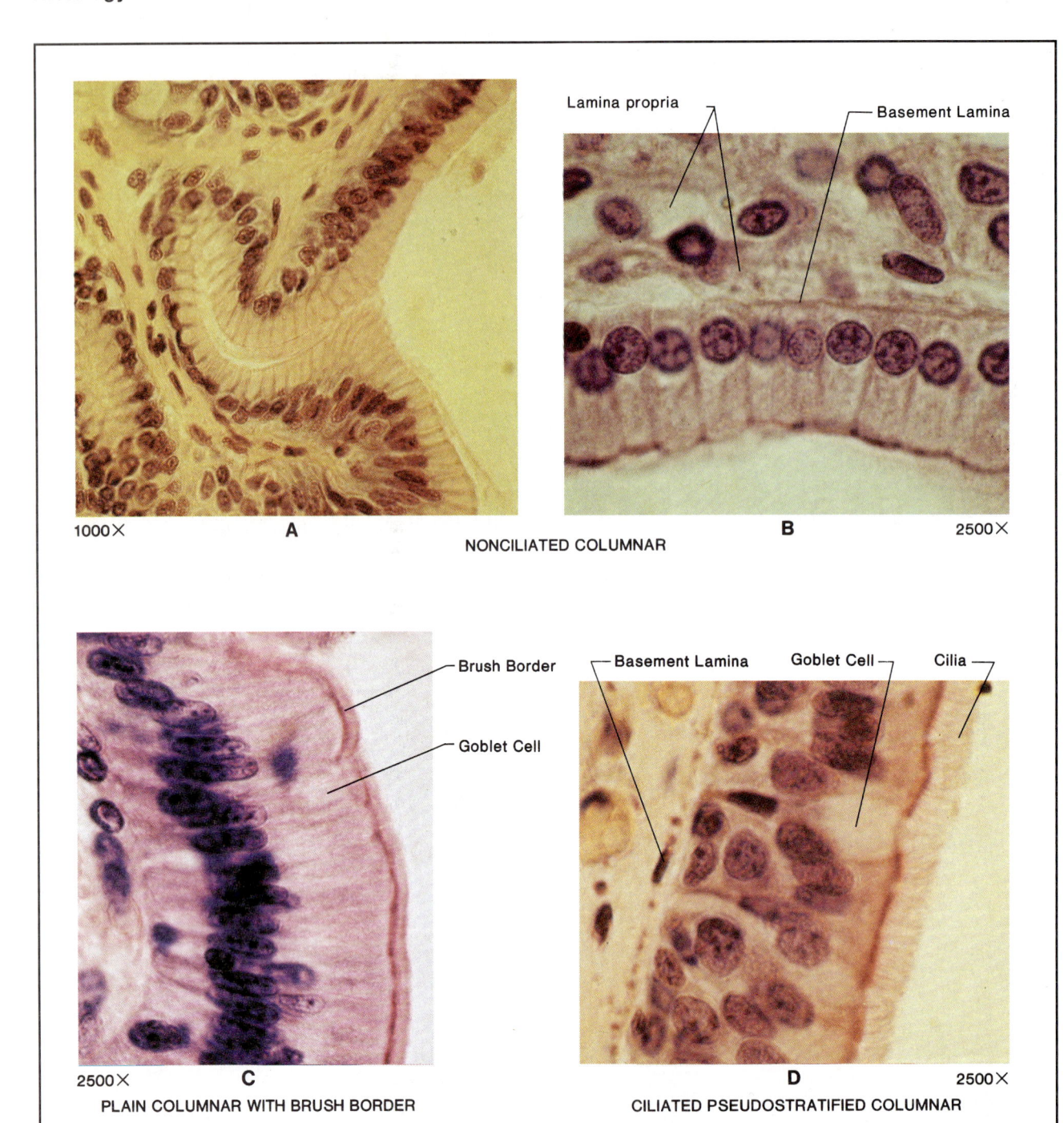

1000×   **A**

NONCILIATED COLUMNAR

B   2500×

Lamina propria — Basement Lamina

2500×   **C**

PLAIN COLUMNAR WITH BRUSH BORDER

Brush Border

Goblet Cell

D   2500×

CILIATED PSEUDOSTRATIFIED COLUMNAR

Basement Lamina — Goblet Cell — Cilia

Columnar epithelia of the digestive and respiratory tracts exhibit large numbers of goblet cells that produce mucus. Although only illustrations C and D have them labeled, they can also be seen in illustration A.

The distinct differences between cilia and a brush border are seen in illustrations C and D. While cilia form from centrioles, brush borders are modified microvilli. Another modification of microvilli are cilialike structures called stereocilia. These nonmotile organelles are seen on columnar cells that line the vas deferens (see figure HA-34).

Note the distinct line of demarcation that constitutes the basement lamina in illustrations B and D. This thin layer between the epithelial cells and the lamina propria consists of a colloidal complex of protein, polysaccharide, and reticular fibers.

The lamina propria, to which all epithelial tissues are connected, consists of connective tissue, vascular and lymphatic channels, lymphocytes, plasma cells, eosinophils, and mast cells.

Figure HA–2   Columnar epithelium.

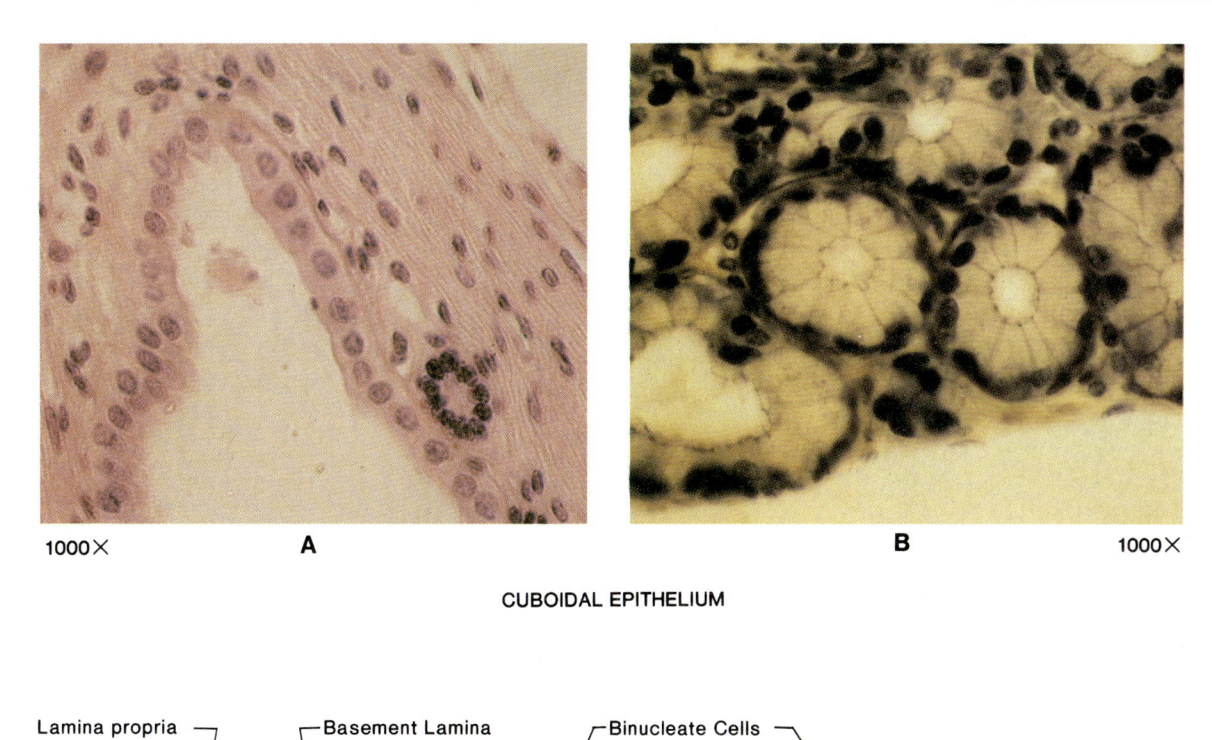

1000×   **A**   **B**   1000×

CUBOIDAL EPITHELIUM

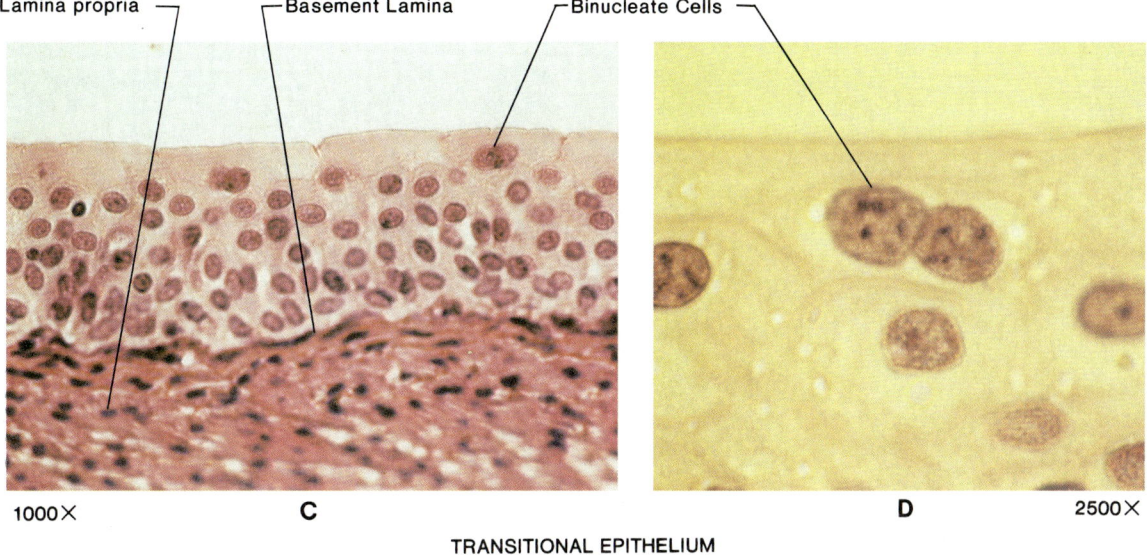

Lamina propria   Basement Lamina   Binucleate Cells

1000×   **C**   **D**   2500×

TRANSITIONAL EPITHELIUM

While cuboidal cells are usually thought of as having a squarish appearance, as in illustration A, they often take on a pyramidal structure when observed surrounding the lumen of a duct or a small gland as in illustration B. Cuboidal epithelia may serve both absorptive and secretory functions, as in the case of tubules in the kidney.

Transitional epithelium is a stratified epithelium whose surface cells do not fall into squamous, cuboidal, or columnar categories. Note that the surface cells are dome-shaped and often binucleate, while the basal cells are more like stratified columnar cells. Between the surface cells and basal cells can be seen layers of pear-shaped cells in a loose configuration. This type of tissue is seen in the wall of the urinary bladder, the urethra, and certain places in the kidneys. The loose nature of the cells makes it desirable in places where organ distention demands elasticity of tissue.

Figure HA–3   Cuboidal and transitional epithelium.

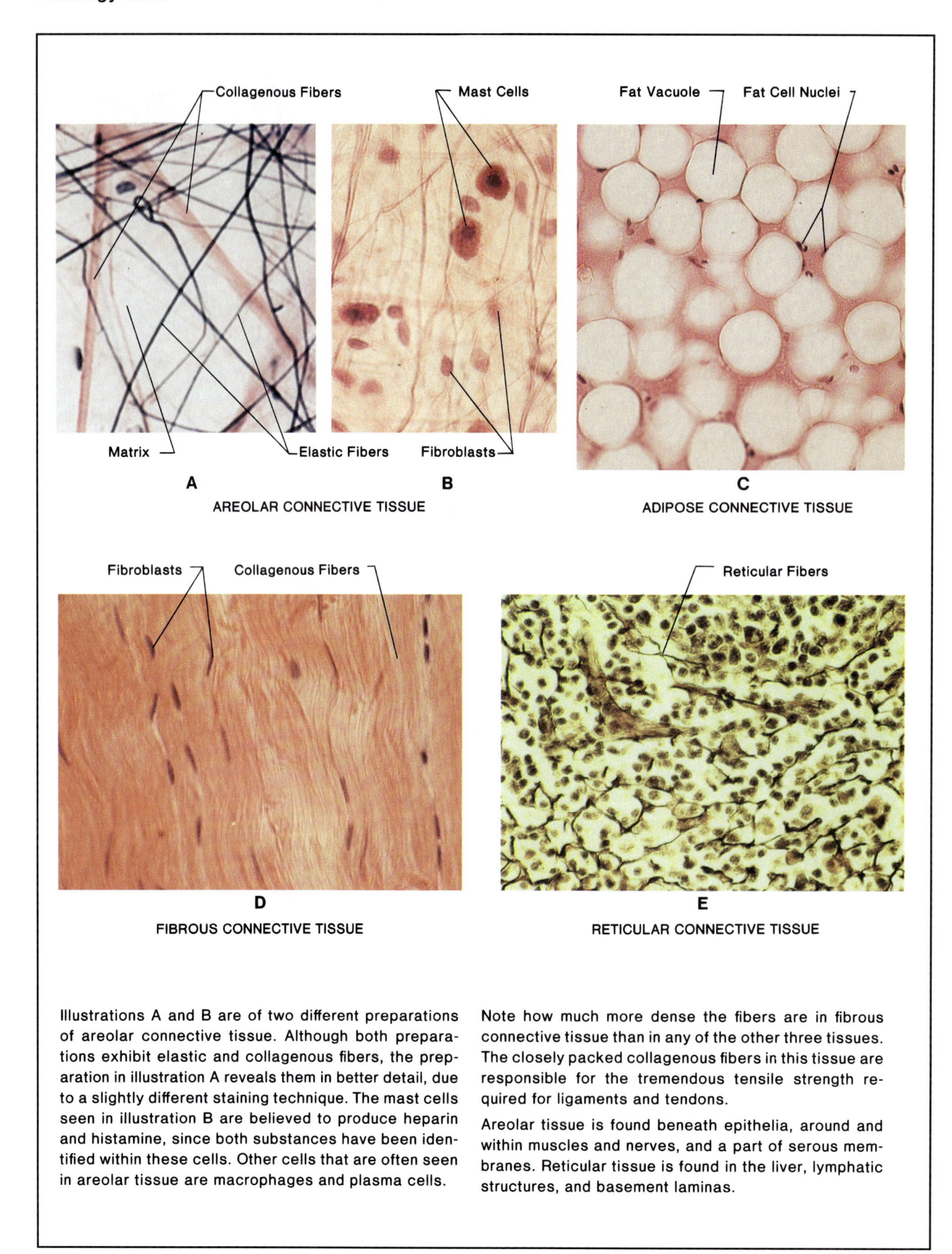

Collagenous Fibers — Mast Cells — Fat Vacuole — Fat Cell Nuclei

Matrix — Elastic Fibers — Fibroblasts

A — **B**
AREOLAR CONNECTIVE TISSUE

C
ADIPOSE CONNECTIVE TISSUE

Fibroblasts — Collagenous Fibers — Reticular Fibers

D
FIBROUS CONNECTIVE TISSUE

E
RETICULAR CONNECTIVE TISSUE

Illustrations A and B are of two different preparations of areolar connective tissue. Although both preparations exhibit elastic and collagenous fibers, the preparation in illustration A reveals them in better detail, due to a slightly different staining technique. The mast cells seen in illustration B are believed to produce heparin and histamine, since both substances have been identified within these cells. Other cells that are often seen in areolar tissue are macrophages and plasma cells.

Note how much more dense the fibers are in fibrous connective tissue than in any of the other three tissues. The closely packed collagenous fibers in this tissue are responsible for the tremendous tensile strength required for ligaments and tendons.

Areolar tissue is found beneath epithelia, around and within muscles and nerves, and a part of serous membranes. Reticular tissue is found in the liver, lymphatic structures, and basement laminas.

Figure HA–4 Connective tissues (1000×).

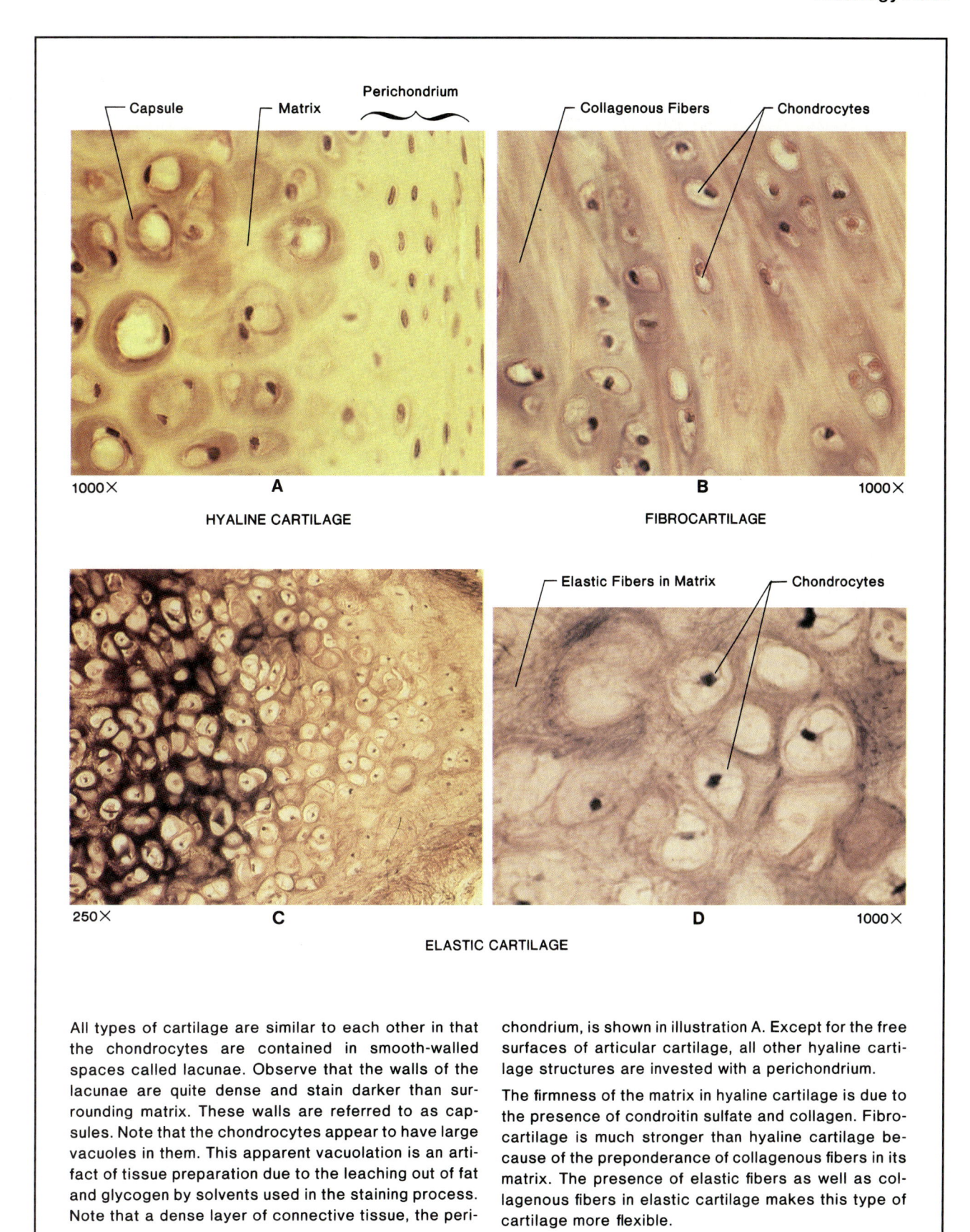

Figure HA-5 Types of cartilage.

All types of cartilage are similar to each other in that the chondrocytes are contained in smooth-walled spaces called lacunae. Observe that the walls of the lacunae are quite dense and stain darker than surrounding matrix. These walls are referred to as capsules. Note that the chondrocytes appear to have large vacuoles in them. This apparent vacuolation is an artifact of tissue preparation due to the leaching out of fat and glycogen by solvents used in the staining process. Note that a dense layer of connective tissue, the perichondrium, is shown in illustration A. Except for the free surfaces of articular cartilage, all other hyaline cartilage structures are invested with a perichondrium.

The firmness of the matrix in hyaline cartilage is due to the presence of condroitin sulfate and collagen. Fibrocartilage is much stronger than hyaline cartilage because of the preponderance of collagenous fibers in its matrix. The presence of elastic fibers as well as collagenous fibers in elastic cartilage makes this type of cartilage more flexible.

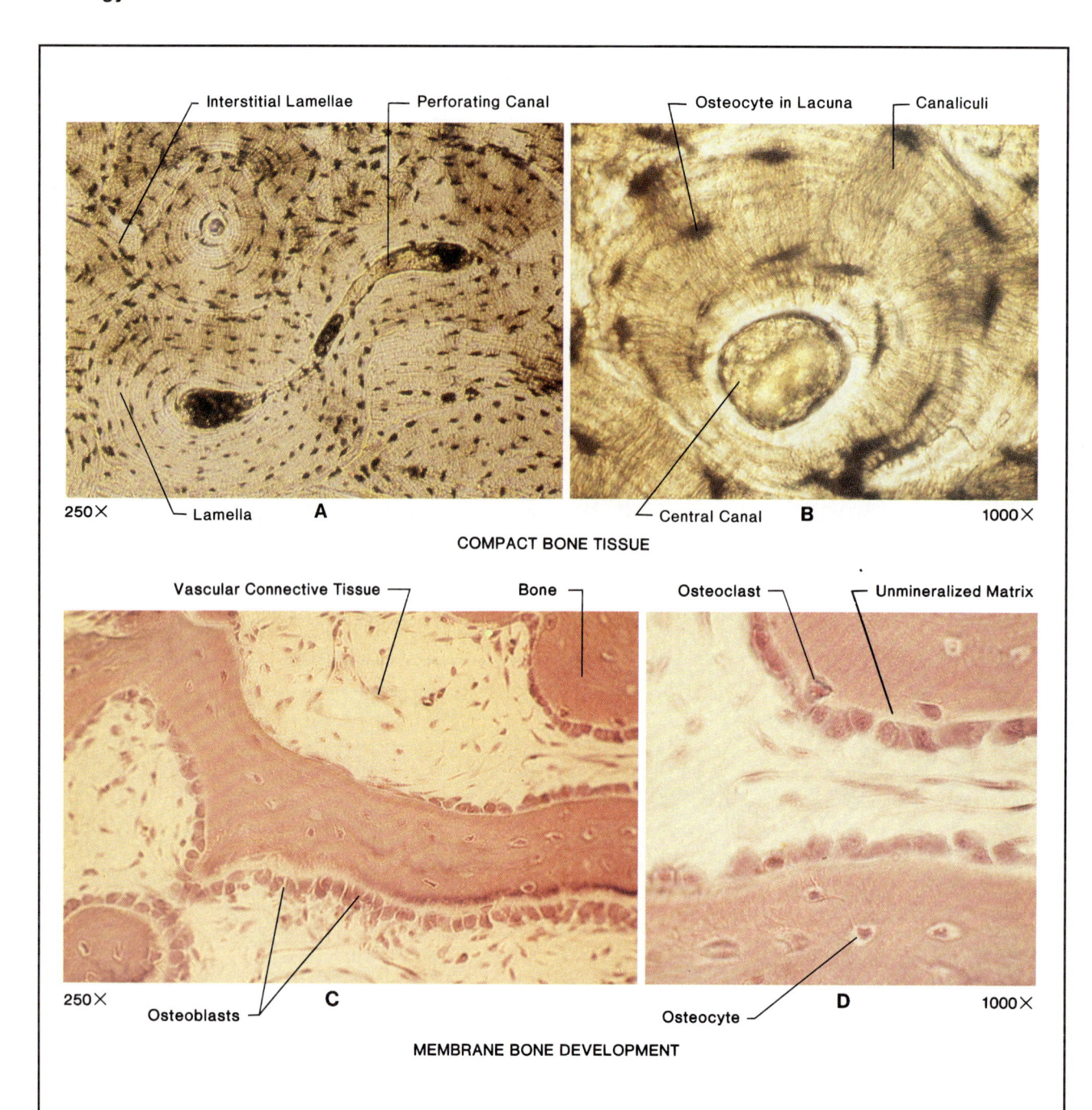

250× · Interstitial Lamellae · Perforating Canal · Lamella · **A** · Osteocyte in Lacuna · Canaliculi · Central Canal · **B** · 1000×

COMPACT BONE TISSUE

Vascular Connective Tissue · Bone · Osteoclast · Unmineralized Matrix · 250× · Osteoblasts · **C** · Osteocyte · **D** · 1000×

MEMBRANE BONE DEVELOPMENT

Bone formation has two origins: (1) from cartilage and (2) from osteogenic mesenchymal connective tissue. Compact bone of the long bones forms from cartilage; bones of the skull, on the other hand, develop as shown in illustrations C and D. The latter are often referred to as "membrane bones."

Note the loci of the different types of bone cells in the above illustrations. Illustrations C and D reveal that osteoblasts in membranous bone formation are seen on the leading edge of the forming bone. The first stage is the secretion of matrix by the osteoblasts. Reticular fibers are then added to the matrix by surrounding mesenchymal cells. Finally, mineralization occurs due to osteoblastic activity.

Osteoclasts are larger multinucleated cells that are involved in shaping bone structure by bone resorption. These cells are surrounded by a clear area (Howship's lacuna), evidence of mineral resorption. The osteoclast seen in illustration D is in an early stage of development; thus, Howship's lacuna is not very large. Once a bone cell becomes completely surrounded by bone, it is referred to as an osteocyte. Nourishment in mature compact bone reaches osteocytes through canaliculi.

Figure HA–6   Bone histology.

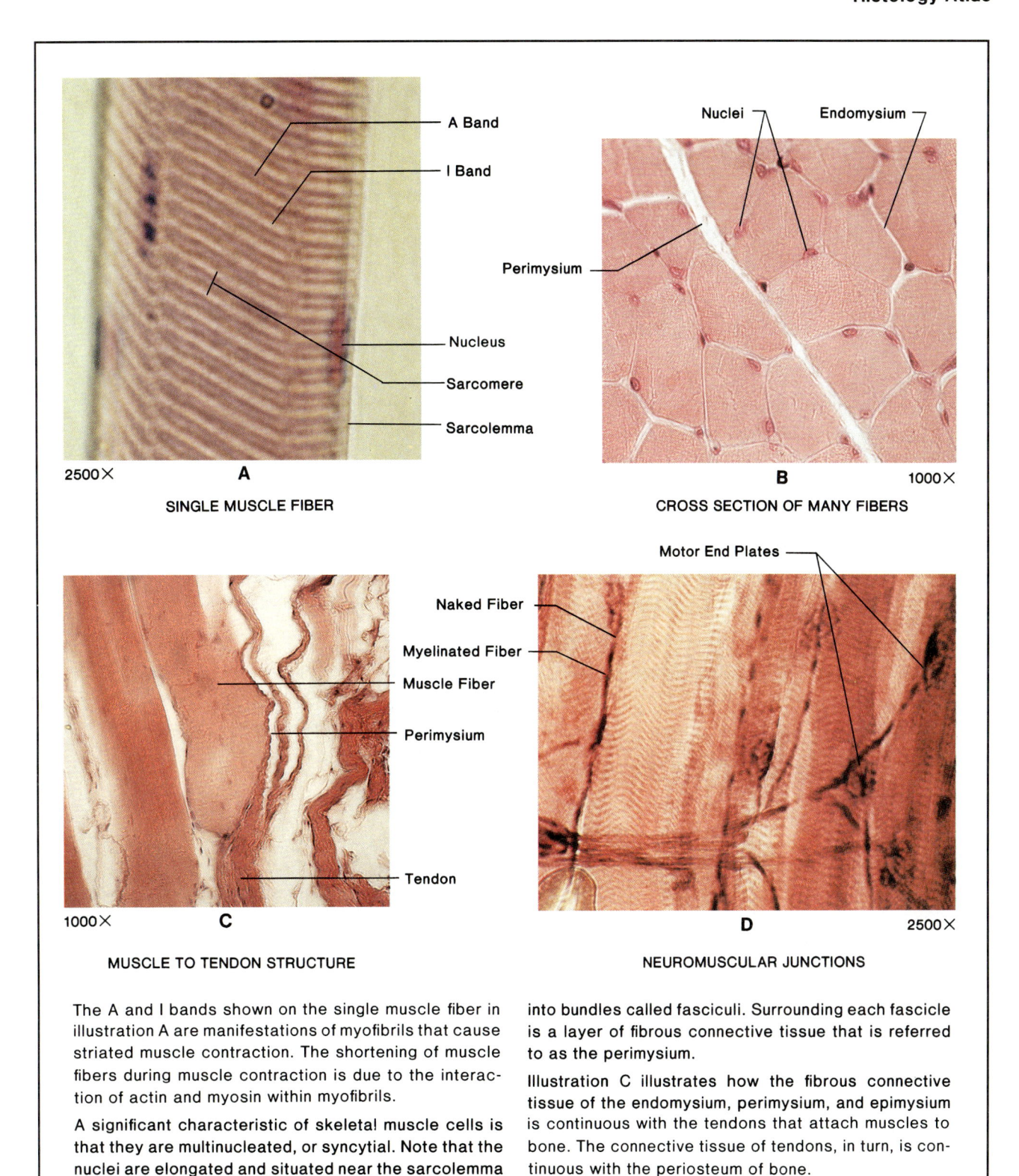

A 2500×

A Band
I Band
Nucleus
Sarcomere
Sarcolemma

SINGLE MUSCLE FIBER

B 1000×

Nuclei Endomysium
Perimysium

CROSS SECTION OF MANY FIBERS

C 1000×

Naked Fiber
Myelinated Fiber
Muscle Fiber
Perimysium
Tendon

MUSCLE TO TENDON STRUCTURE

D 2500×

Motor End Plates

NEUROMUSCULAR JUNCTIONS

The A and I bands shown on the single muscle fiber in illustration A are manifestations of myofibrils that cause striated muscle contraction. The shortening of muscle fibers during muscle contraction is due to the interaction of actin and myosin within myofibrils.

A significant characteristic of skeletal muscle cells is that they are multinucleated, or syncytial. Note that the nuclei are elongated and situated near the sarcolemma of the cell. The peripheral location of the nuclei shows up well in illustration B.

Illustration B reveals that muscle fibers are separated from each other by endomysium, and grouped together into bundles called fasciculi. Surrounding each fascicle is a layer of fibrous connective tissue that is referred to as the perimysium.

Illustration C illustrates how the fibrous connective tissue of the endomysium, perimysium, and epimysium is continuous with the tendons that attach muscles to bone. The connective tissue of tendons, in turn, is continuous with the periosteum of bone.

Note in illustration D how the myelinated motor nerve fibers lose their myelin sheaths and become "naked" where they join the motor end plates.

Figure HA–7 Skeletal muscle microstructure.

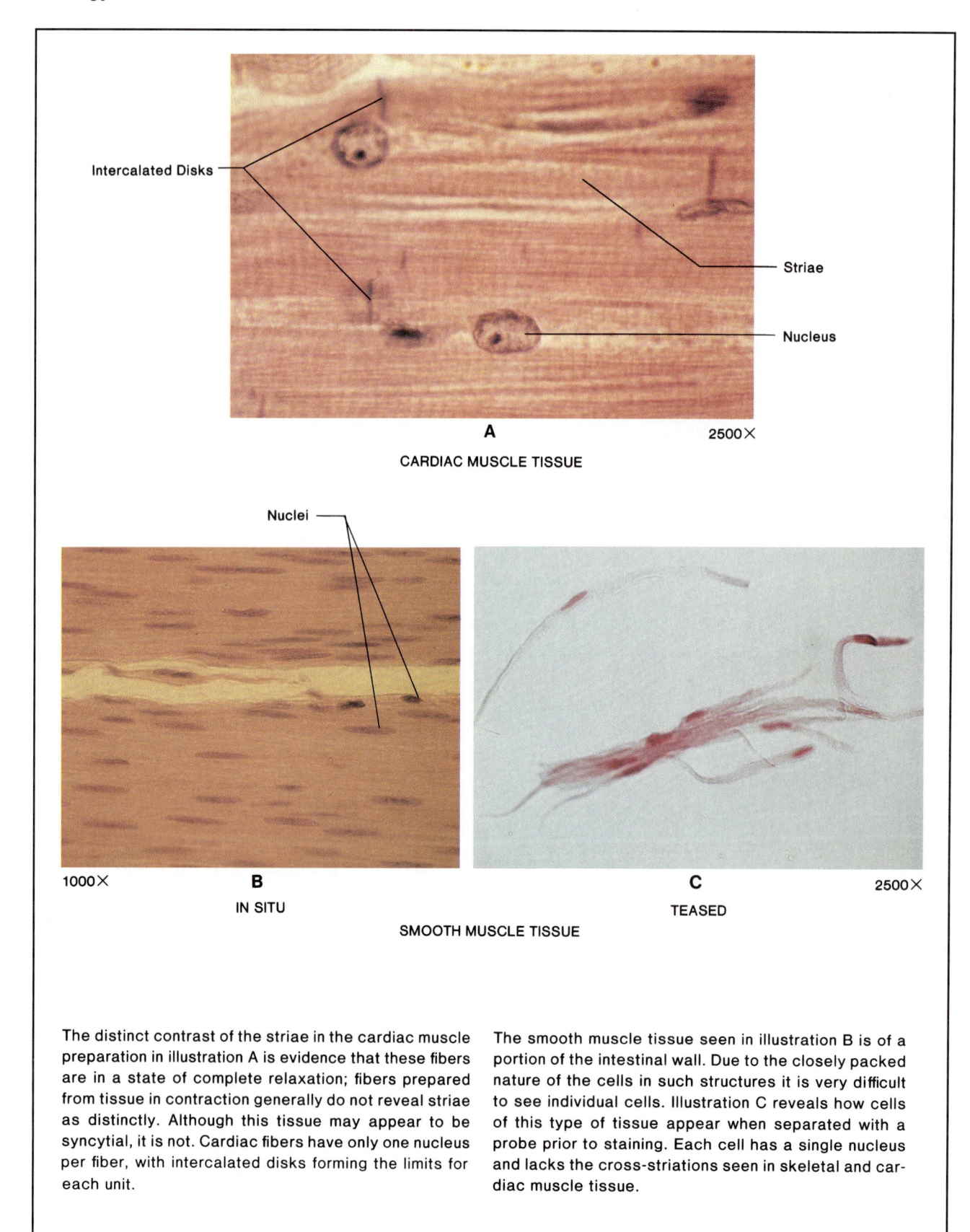

Intercalated Disks

Striae

Nucleus

A 2500×
CARDIAC MUSCLE TISSUE

Nuclei

1000× **B** **C** 2500×
IN SITU TEASED
SMOOTH MUSCLE TISSUE

The distinct contrast of the striae in the cardiac muscle preparation in illustration A is evidence that these fibers are in a state of complete relaxation; fibers prepared from tissue in contraction generally do not reveal striae as distinctly. Although this tissue may appear to be syncytial, it is not. Cardiac fibers have only one nucleus per fiber, with intercalated disks forming the limits for each unit.

The smooth muscle tissue seen in illustration B is of a portion of the intestinal wall. Due to the closely packed nature of the cells in such structures it is very difficult to see individual cells. Illustration C reveals how cells of this type of tissue appear when separated with a probe prior to staining. Each cell has a single nucleus and lacks the cross-striations seen in skeletal and cardiac muscle tissue.

Figure HA–8 Cardiac and smooth muscle tissue.

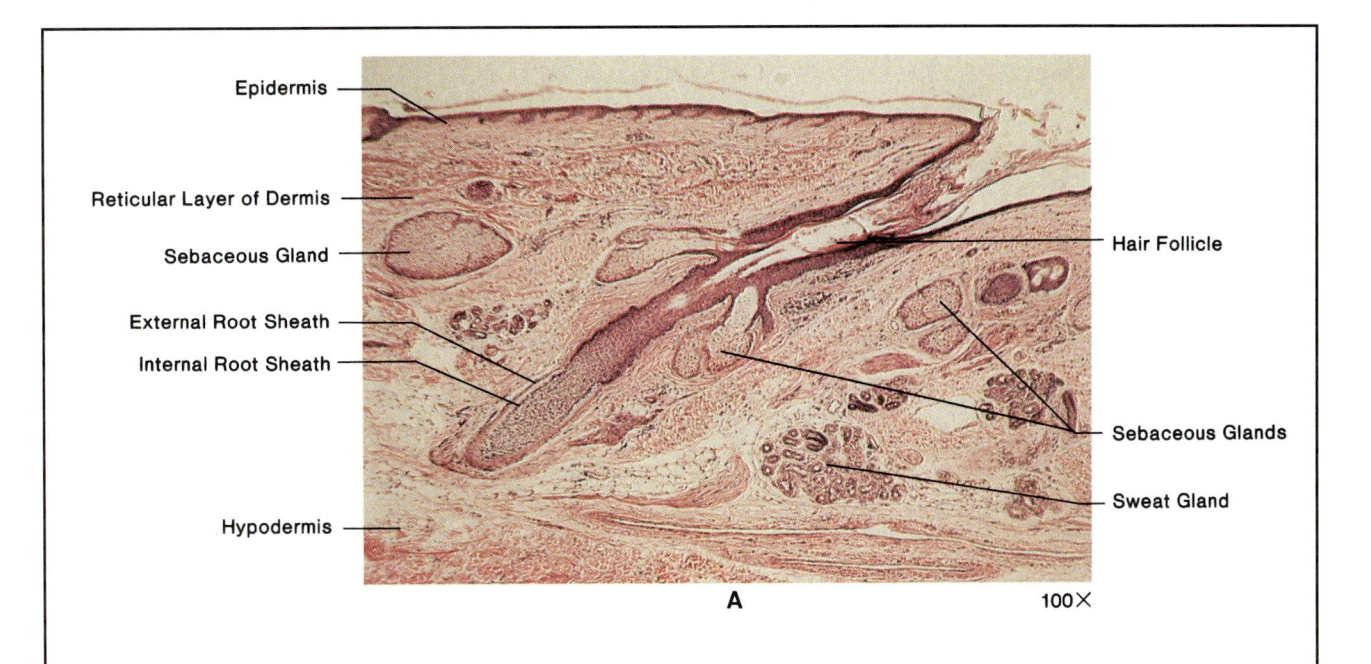

Epidermis

Reticular Layer of Dermis

Sebaceous Gland

External Root Sheath

Internal Root Sheath

Hypodermis

Hair Follicle

Sebaceous Glands

Sweat Gland

A   100×

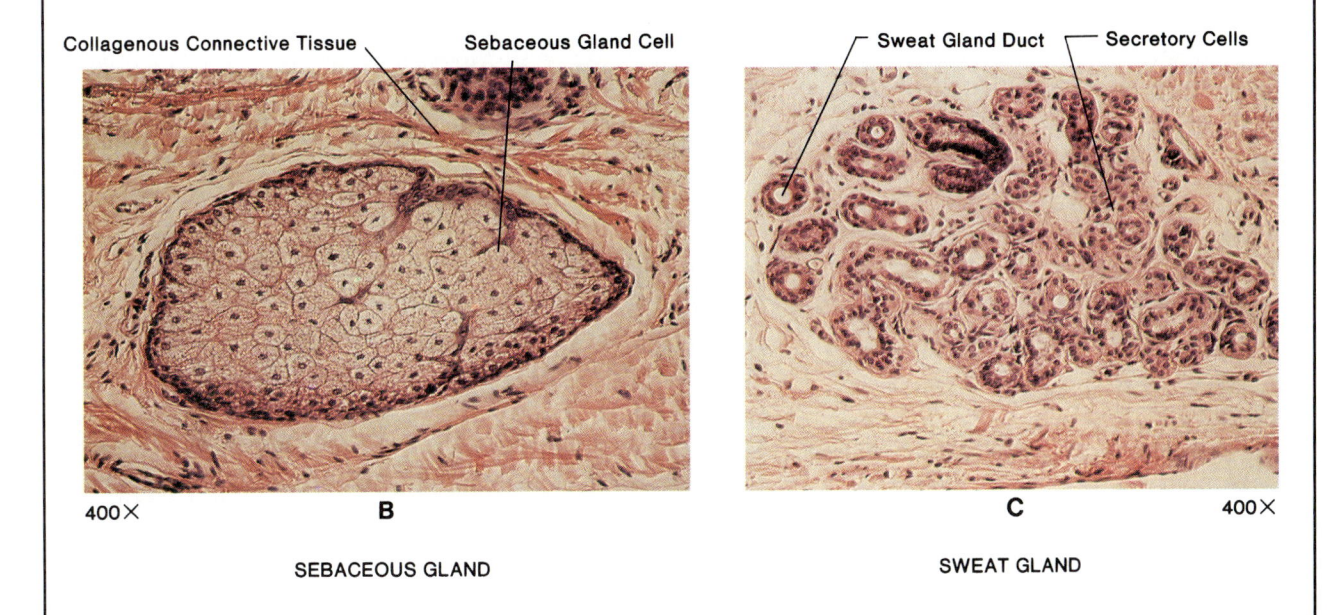

Collagenous Connective Tissue   Sebaceous Gland Cell

Sweat Gland Duct   Secretory Cells

400×   **B**

C   400×

SEBACEOUS GLAND

SWEAT GLAND

The relationship of the sebaceous and sweat glands to other structures of the skin is illustrated on this page. The low magnification of illustration A reveals that the epidermis is a very thin layer as compared to the dermis. Except for the palms and soles of the feet, the epidermis is usually only 0.1 mm thick. The dermis or corium, which underlies the epidermis, varies from 0.3 to 4.0 mm thick in different parts of the body. Note that both the sebaceous and sweat glands are located in the reticular layer of the dermis.

Note that the sweat glands are tubulo-alveolar structures lined with cuboidal or columnar epithelium. The sebaceous glands, on the other hand, consist of rounded masses of cells, cuboidal at the periphery, and polygonal in the center. The secretion of sebaceous glands is formed by the breaking down of the central cells into an oily complex which is forced out into the space between the follicle and hair shaft. Although not shown in illustration A, the sweat glands open out directly onto the surface of the skin.

Figure HA–9   Scalp histology.

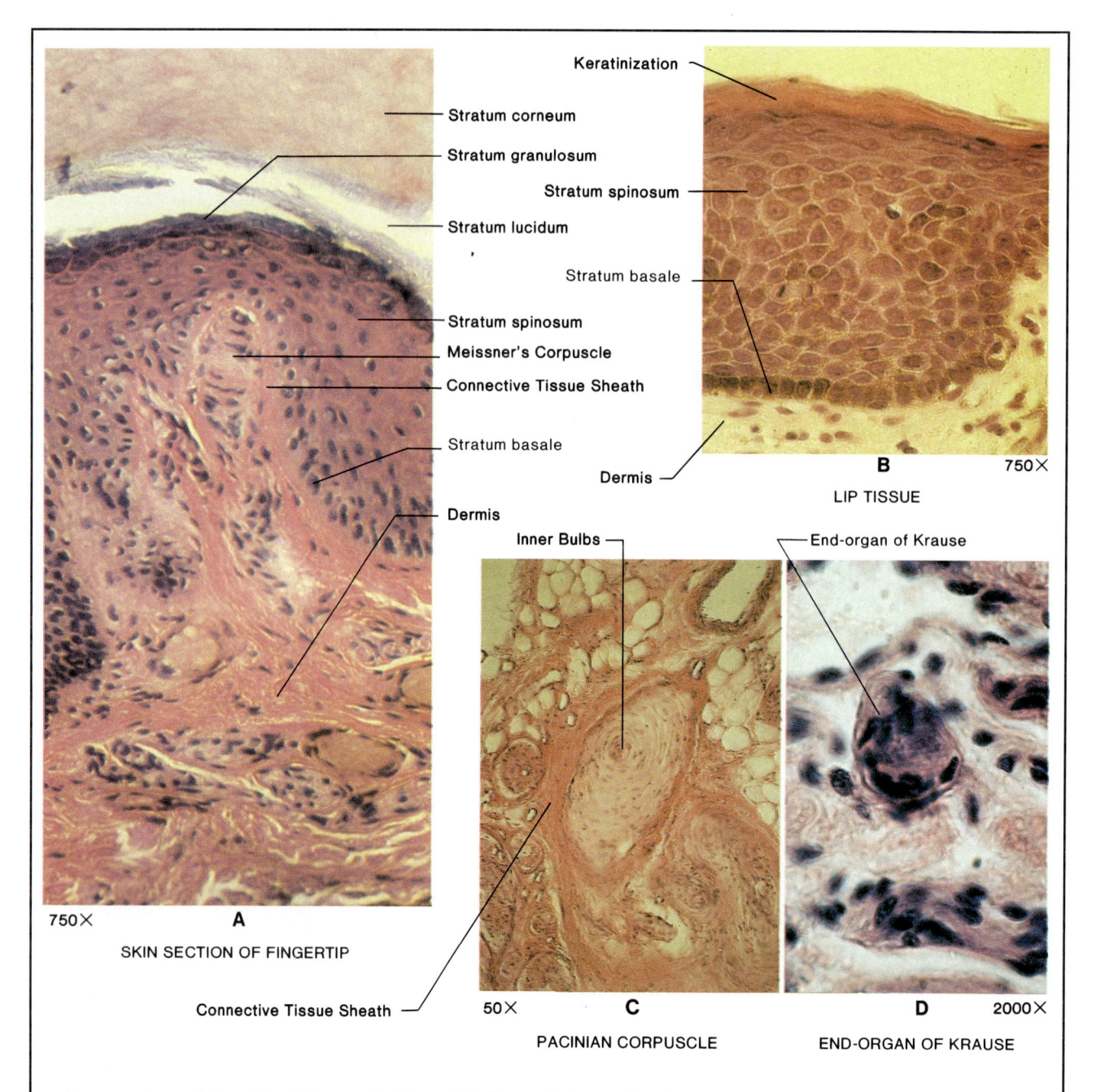

Keratinization

Stratum corneum

Stratum granulosum

Stratum lucidum

Stratum spinosum

Stratum spinosum

Meissner's Corpuscle

Connective Tissue Sheath

Stratum basale

Stratum basale

Dermis

Dermis

Inner Bulbs

End-organ of Krause

B 750×

LIP TISSUE

750× **A**

SKIN SECTION OF FINGERTIP

Connective Tissue Sheath

50× **C**

PACINIAN CORPUSCLE

D 2000×

END-ORGAN OF KRAUSE

A comparison of the skin of the scalp (figure HA-9), a fingertip (illustration A), and the lip (illustration B) reveals that the integument differs in construction in different regions of the body. These differences are due to the presence or absence of hair and the degree of keratinization. The fingertips, palms, and soles of the feet have epidermal layers with a thick stratum corneum and no hair follicles. Skin on the lips has some keratinization, but to a much lesser degree than the fingertips.

Three receptors of the skin are illustrated here: Meissner's, Pacinian, and Krause corpuscles. Meissner's corpuscle, which is seen in illustration A,

is located in the papillary layer of the dermis. Note that it is encased in a sheath of connective tissue. These receptors are sensors of discriminative touch.

Pacinian corpuscles (illustration C) consist of laminated collagenous material and several inner bulbs. Pressure on the lamina triggers impulses in nerve endings in the bulbs. They are so large that they can be seen without magnification.

End-organs of Krause are small corpuscles that are sensitive to cold temperatures. They, too, are quite numerous in the skin.

Figure HA–10   Skin structure.

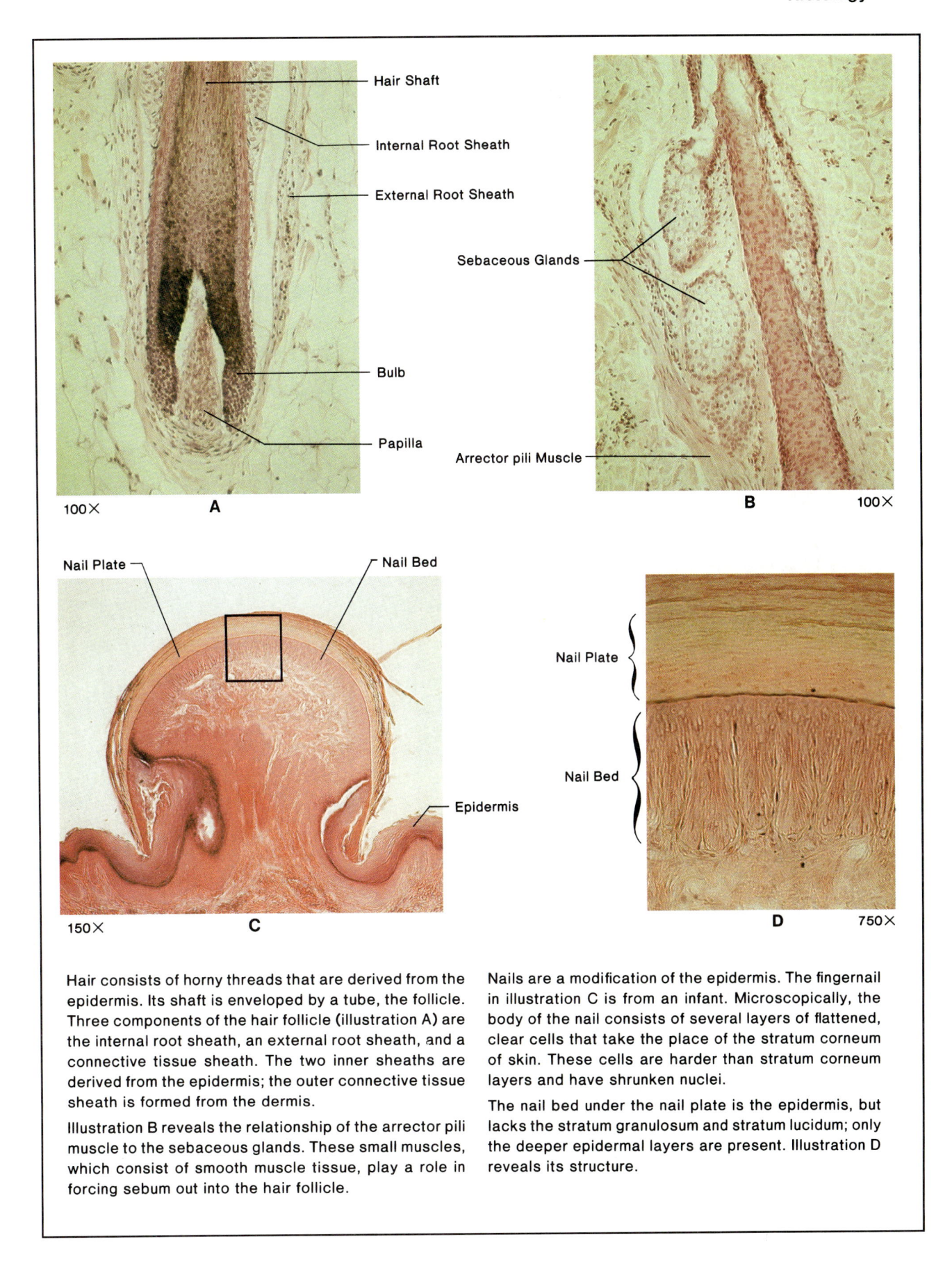

Hair Shaft

Internal Root Sheath

External Root Sheath

Bulb

Papilla

100× **A**

Sebaceous Glands

Arrector pili Muscle

B 100×

Nail Plate — Nail Bed

Epidermis

150× **C**

Nail Plate

Nail Bed

D 750×

Hair consists of horny threads that are derived from the epidermis. Its shaft is enveloped by a tube, the follicle. Three components of the hair follicle (illustration A) are the internal root sheath, an external root sheath, and a connective tissue sheath. The two inner sheaths are derived from the epidermis; the outer connective tissue sheath is formed from the dermis.

Illustration B reveals the relationship of the arrector pili muscle to the sebaceous glands. These small muscles, which consist of smooth muscle tissue, play a role in forcing sebum out into the hair follicle.

Nails are a modification of the epidermis. The fingernail in illustration C is from an infant. Microscopically, the body of the nail consists of several layers of flattened, clear cells that take the place of the stratum corneum of skin. These cells are harder than stratum corneum layers and have shrunken nuclei.

The nail bed under the nail plate is the epidermis, but lacks the stratum granulosum and stratum lucidum; only the deeper epidermal layers are present. Illustration D reveals its structure.

Figure HA–11   Hair and nail structure of the integument.

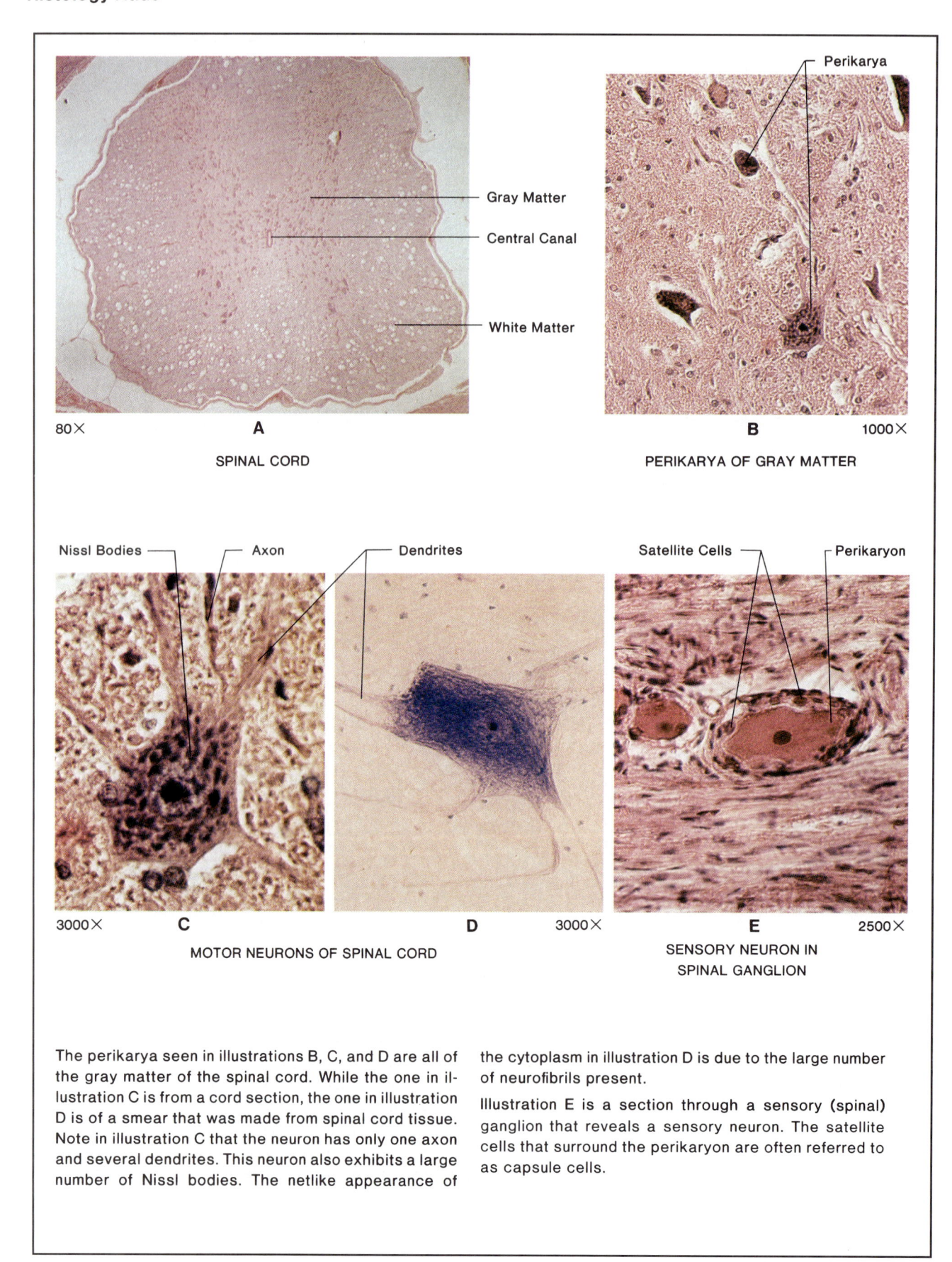

A 80×

SPINAL CORD

Gray Matter

Central Canal

White Matter

B 1000×

PERIKARYA OF GRAY MATTER

Perikarya

Nissl Bodies — Axon — Dendrites — Satellite Cells — Perikaryon

C 3000×

D 3000×

E 2500×

MOTOR NEURONS OF SPINAL CORD

SENSORY NEURON IN
SPINAL GANGLION

The perikarya seen in illustrations B, C, and D are all of the gray matter of the spinal cord. While the one in illustration C is from a cord section, the one in illustration D is of a smear that was made from spinal cord tissue. Note in illustration C that the neuron has only one axon and several dendrites. This neuron also exhibits a large number of Nissl bodies. The netlike appearance of the cytoplasm in illustration D is due to the large number of neurofibrils present.

Illustration E is a section through a sensory (spinal) ganglion that reveals a sensory neuron. The satellite cells that surround the perikaryon are often referred to as capsule cells.

Figure HA–12 Neurons of the spinal cord and spinal ganglia.

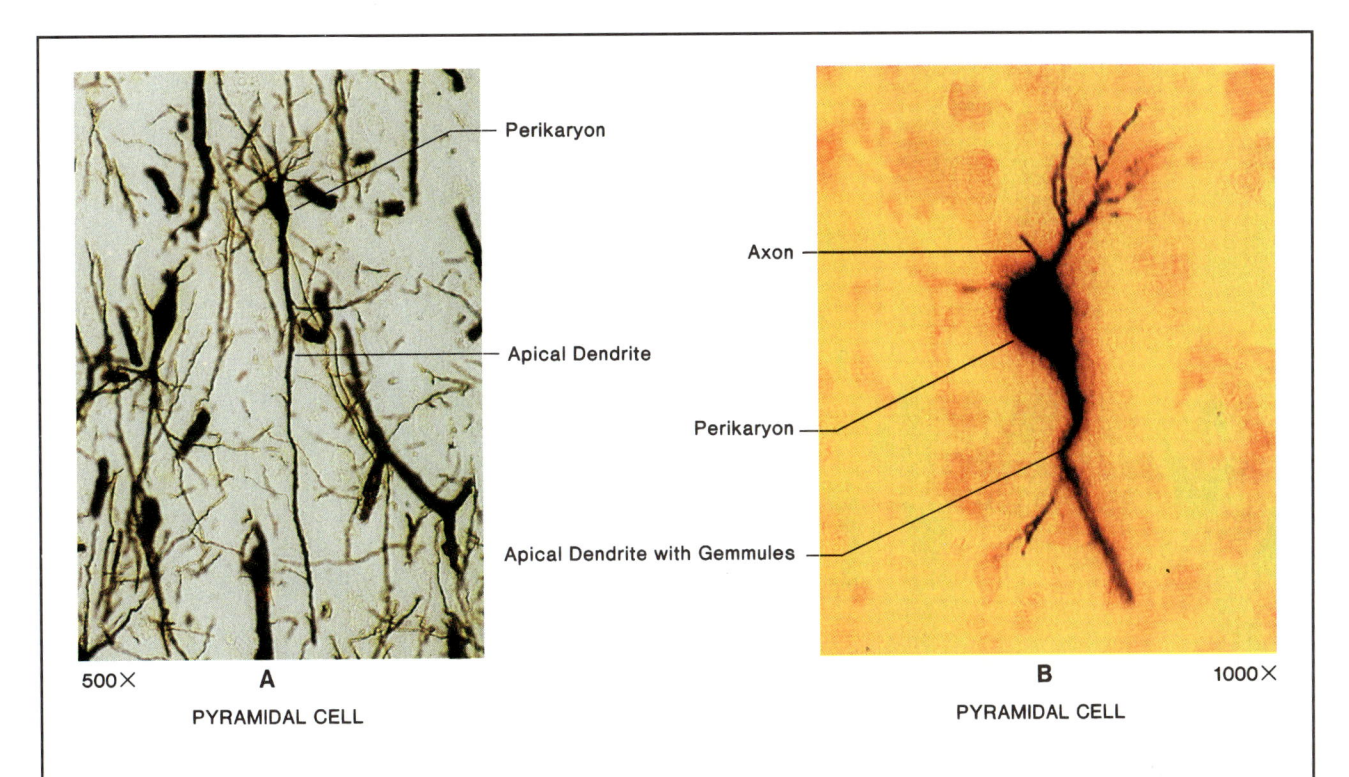

500×   **A**
PYRAMIDAL CELL

Perikaryon

Apical Dendrite

Apical Dendrite with Gemmules

Axon

Perikaryon

B   1000×
PYRAMIDAL CELL

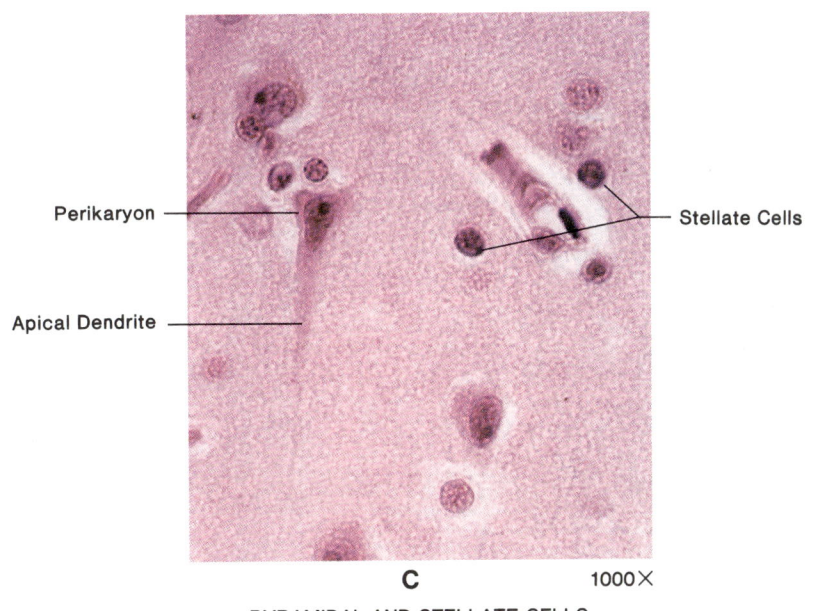

Perikaryon

Apical Dendrite

Stellate Cells

C   1000×
PYRAMIDAL AND STELLATE CELLS

The principal nerve cells of the cerebrum are pyramidal cells. Note in each of the above photomicrographs that a long apical dendrite extends from the perikaryon. The apical dendrite is always oriented toward the surface of the cerebrum. In illustration B there is evidence of "gemmules" on the surface of the dendrite. Gemmules are small processes that greatly increase the surface area of dendrites, allowing large neurons to receive as many as 100,000 separate axon terminals or synapses.

Note the difference in size between the axon and dendrites in illustration B. The axon is much smaller in diameter and has a smoother surface due to the absence of gemmules.

The stellate cells shown in illustration C are association neurons that provide connections between pyramidal cells of the cerebrum. These interneurons are also present in the cerebellum, where they provide linkage between the Purkinje cells.

Figure HA–13   Neurons of the cerebrum.

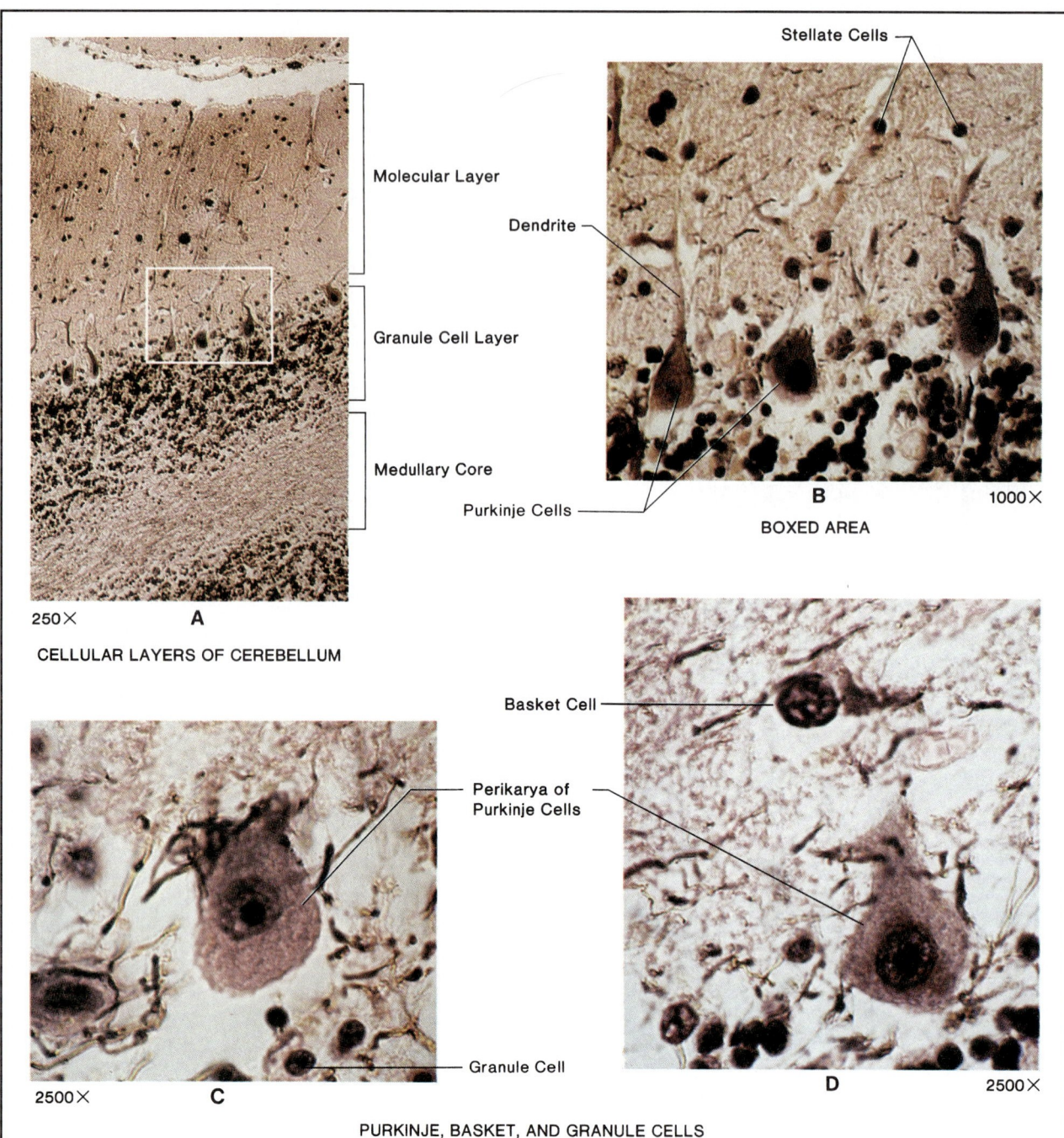

Molecular Layer

Granule Cell Layer

Medullary Core

250× **A**

CELLULAR LAYERS OF CEREBELLUM

Stellate Cells

Dendrite

Purkinje Cells

B 1000×

BOXED AREA

Basket Cell

Perikarya of
Purkinje Cells

Granule Cell

2500× **C**

D 2500×

PURKINJE, BASKET, AND GRANULE CELLS

Illustration A is a section through the cerebellum that depicts an outermost molecular layer, a middle granule cell layer, and an inner medullary core.

The most distinctive neurons of the cerebellum are the Purkinje cells. Note in illustration A that these neurons form a layer deep within the molecular layer near the edge of the granule cell layer. Each flask-shaped cell has a thick dendrite that is directed toward the cerebellar cortex. A short distance out from the perikaryon

the dendrite branches out into two thick branches, which, in turn, divide many times to arborize out into the molecular layer. The axon of each Purkinje cell extends from the perikaryon through the granular and medullary layers, and finally, through collaterals, reenters the molecular layer to contact other Purkinje cells.

Stellate, basket, and granule cells are all multipolar association neurons. Note the proximity of the perikarya of the basket cells to the Purkinje cells.

Figure HA–14 Neurons of the cerebellum.

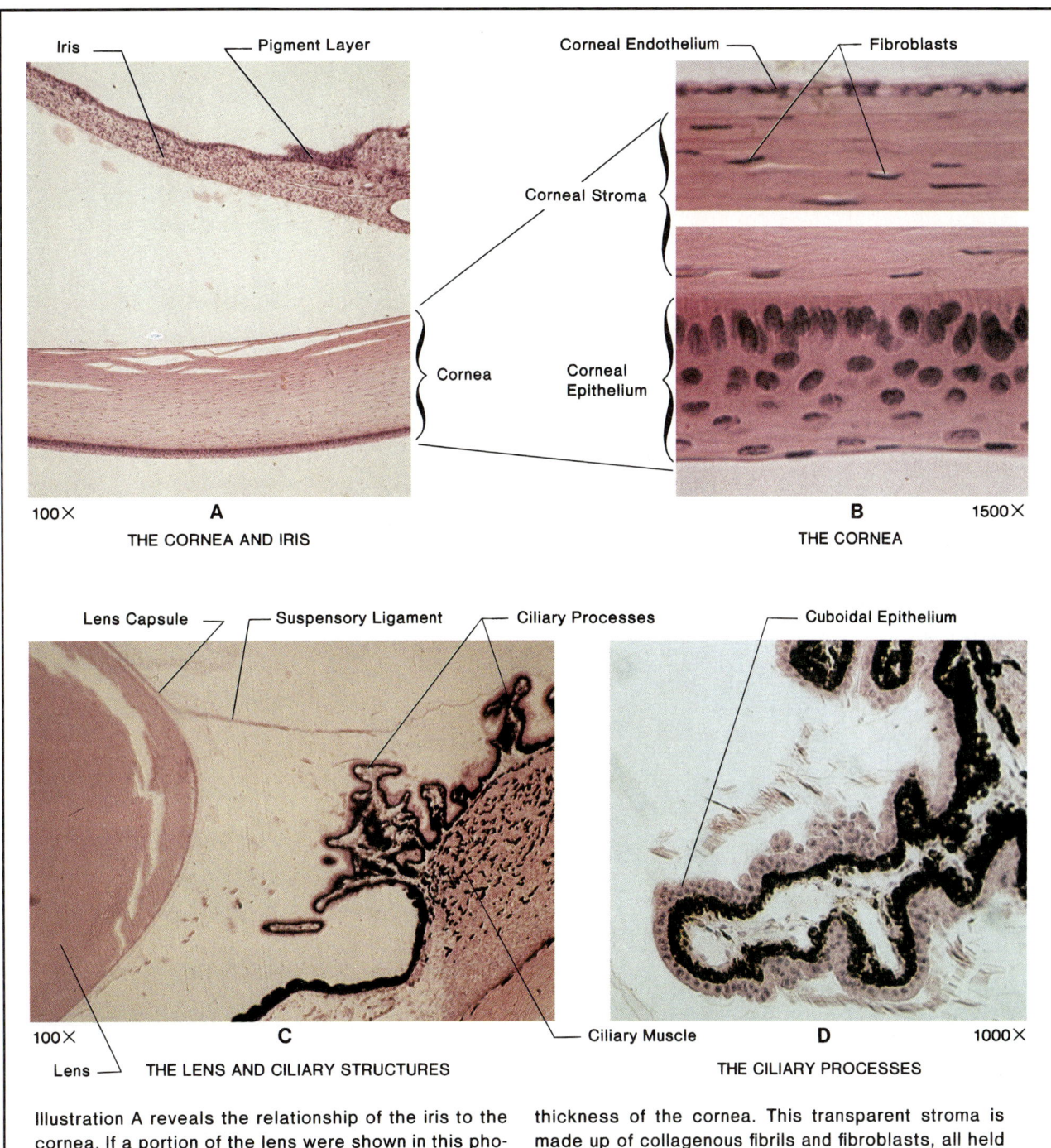

100× **A**
THE CORNEA AND IRIS

B 1500×
THE CORNEA

100× **C**
THE LENS AND CILIARY STRUCTURES

D 1000×
THE CILIARY PROCESSES

Illustration A reveals the relationship of the iris to the cornea. If a portion of the lens were shown in this photomicrograph, it would be above the iris, since the iris lies between the lens and the cornea.

Illustration B is a compacted enlargement of the cornea, in which many of the middle layers have been removed so that all significant layers can be seen. Note that the outer corneal epithelium consists of stratified squamous epithelium, and that the inner corneal endothelium consists of a single layer of low cuboidal cells. Between these two layers is the corneal stroma (*substantia propria*), which makes up nine-tenths of the

thickness of the cornea. This transparent stroma is made up of collagenous fibrils and fibroblasts, all held together with a mucopolysaccharide cement.

Note in illustration C that the lens is encased in an elastic capsule to which the suspensory ligament is attached. The lens is formed from epithelial cells that become elongated and lose their nuclei. Note, also, that the ciliary processes shown in illustration D are covered with cuboidal epithelial cells. It is these cells that produce the aqueous humor that fills the space between the lens and the cornea.

Figure HA–15   The cornea, lens, iris, and ciliary structures.

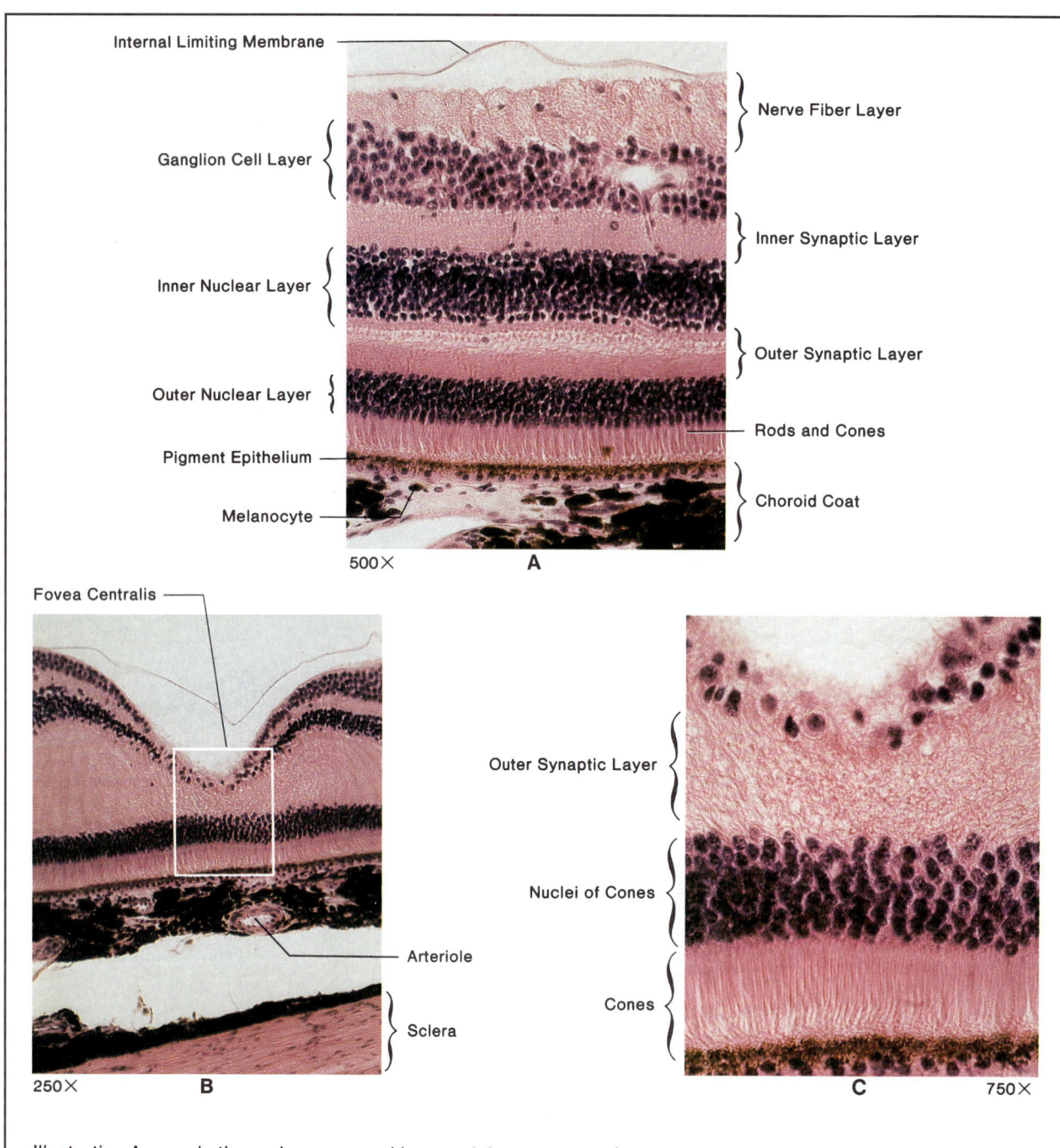

Illustration A reveals the various neuronal layers of the retina. Note that the photoreceptors (rods and cones) are in the deepest layer next to the choroid coat. Light striking the retina must pass through all these layers to reach the receptors.

The nuclei seen in the outer nuclear layer are of the rods and cones. The outer synaptic (*plexiform*) layer is where the synapses are made between axons of the rods and cones and the dendrites of bipolar cells and the processes of horizontal cells. The inner nuclear layer contains nuclei of bipolar neurons and association neurons (horizontal and amacrine cells). The inner synaptic (*plexiform*) layer is the place where synaptic connections are made between the cells of the inner nuclear layer and the ganglion cells. The nerve fiber layer consists of nonmyelinated axons of the ganglion cells. These fibers converge on the optic disk to form the optic nerve. Illustrations B and C reveal the nature of the fovea centralis. Note that the receptors in the fovea consist only of cones and that the inner synaptic and nerve fiber layers are lacking.

Figure HA–16   The retina of the eye.

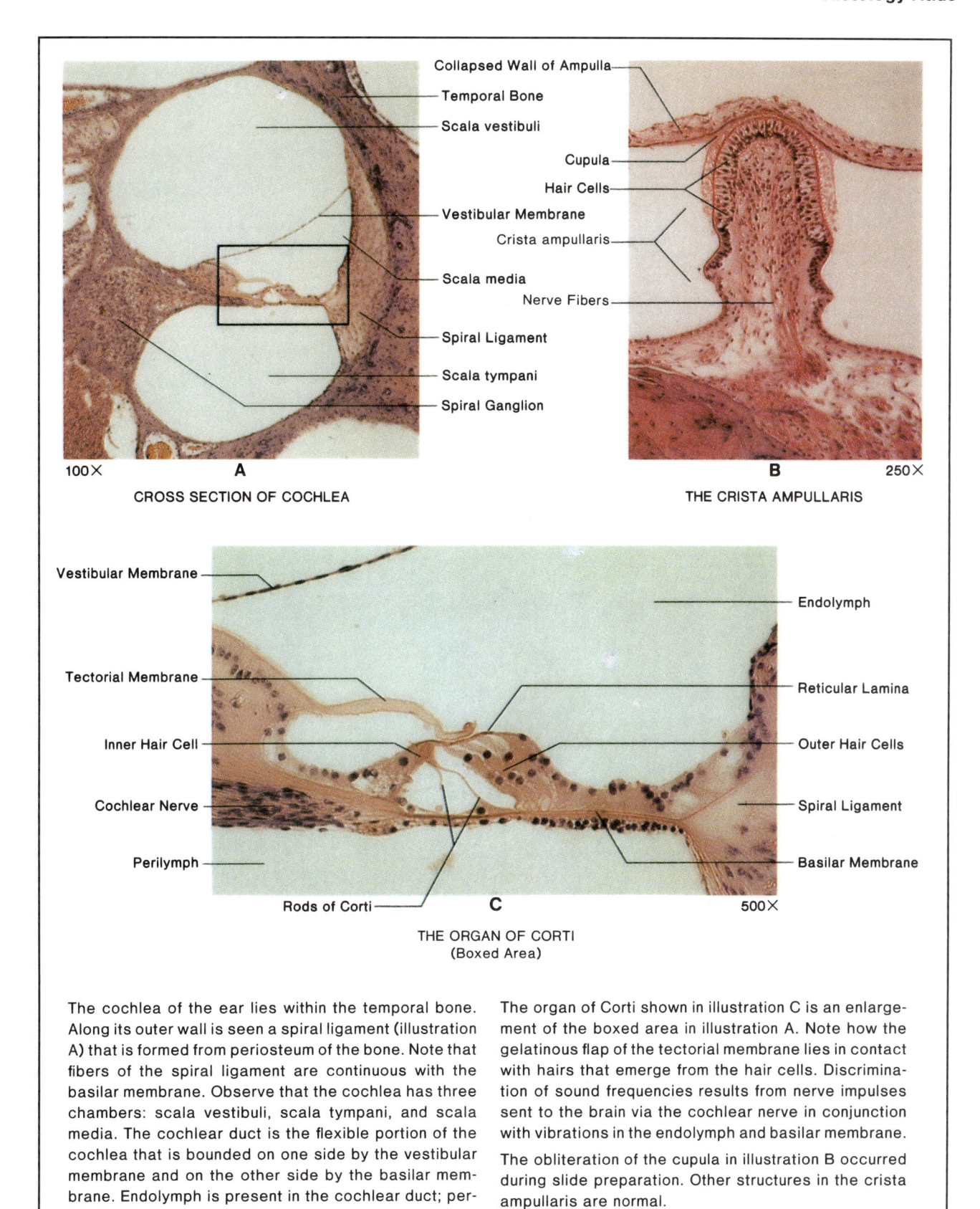

Figure HA–17 The cochlea and crista ampullaris.

The cochlea of the ear lies within the temporal bone. Along its outer wall is seen a spiral ligament (illustration A) that is formed from periosteum of the bone. Note that fibers of the spiral ligament are continuous with the basilar membrane. Observe that the cochlea has three chambers: scala vestibuli, scala tympani, and scala media. The cochlear duct is the flexible portion of the cochlea that is bounded on one side by the vestibular membrane and on the other side by the basilar membrane. Endolymph is present in the cochlear duct; perilymph fills the scala vestibuli and scala tympani.

The organ of Corti shown in illustration C is an enlargement of the boxed area in illustration A. Note how the gelatinous flap of the tectorial membrane lies in contact with hairs that emerge from the hair cells. Discrimination of sound frequencies results from nerve impulses sent to the brain via the cochlear nerve in conjunction with vibrations in the endolymph and basilar membrane.

The obliteration of the cupula in illustration B occurred during slide preparation. Other structures in the crista ampullaris are normal.

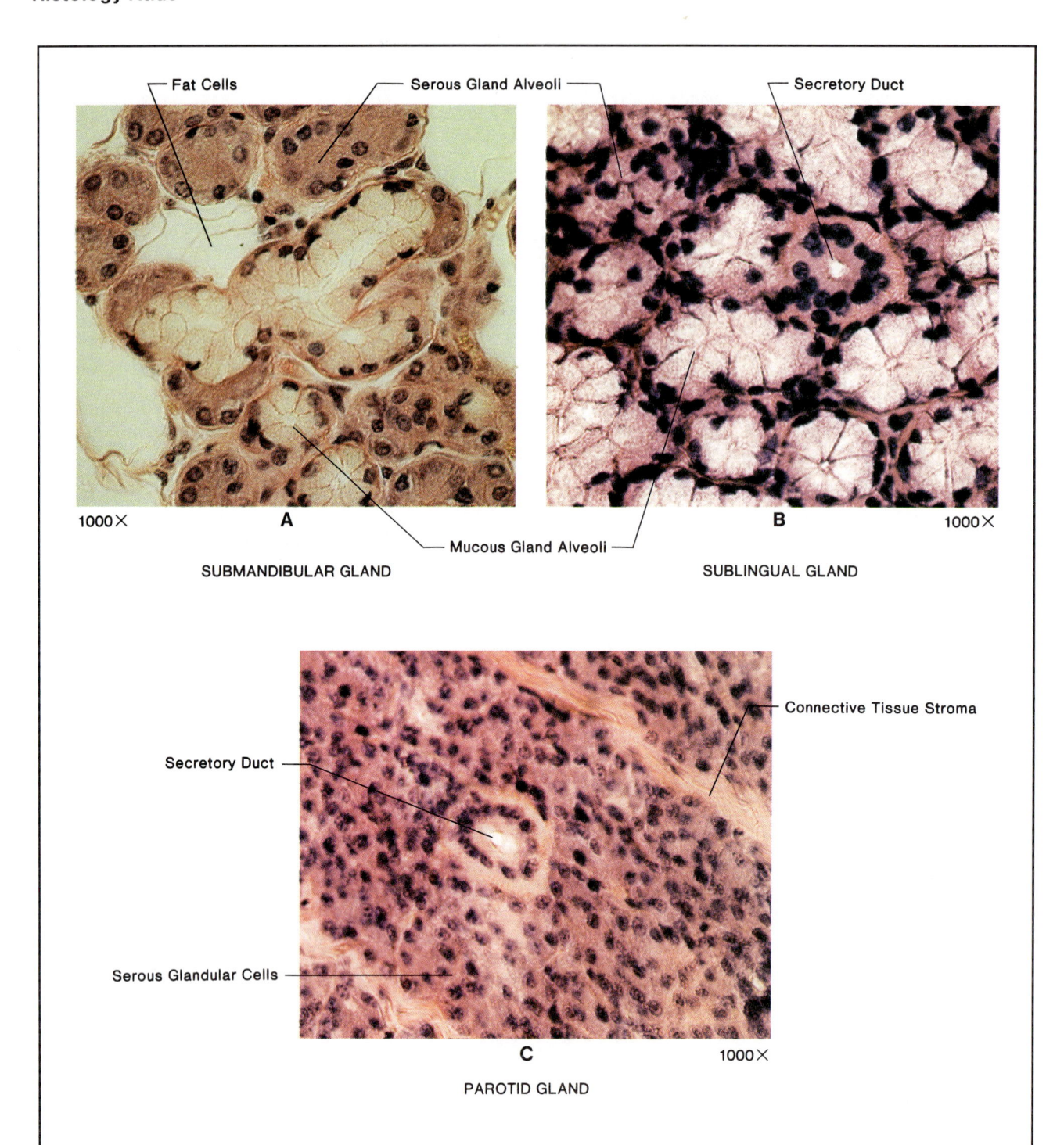

Fat Cells — Serous Gland Alveoli — Secretory Duct

1000× **A**

Mucous Gland Alveoli

SUBMANDIBULAR GLAND

B 1000×

SUBLINGUAL GLAND

Connective Tissue Stroma

Secretory Duct

Serous Glandular Cells

C 1000×

PAROTID GLAND

Whether a salivary gland produces mucus or the less viscous serous fluid is easily determined by microscopic examination of its tissue. Note in illustrations A and B that mucus-producing cells are much paler and larger than cells that produce serous fluid. The presence of both types of secretory cells in the submandibular and sublingual glands indicates that these glands secrete a mixture of mucus and serous fluid into the oral cavity. Although the submandibular gland is primarily serous, the sublingual produces mostly mucus. The absence of mucous acini in the parotid glands indicates that only serous fluid is produced by these glands.

Figure HA–18 Histology of major salivary glands.

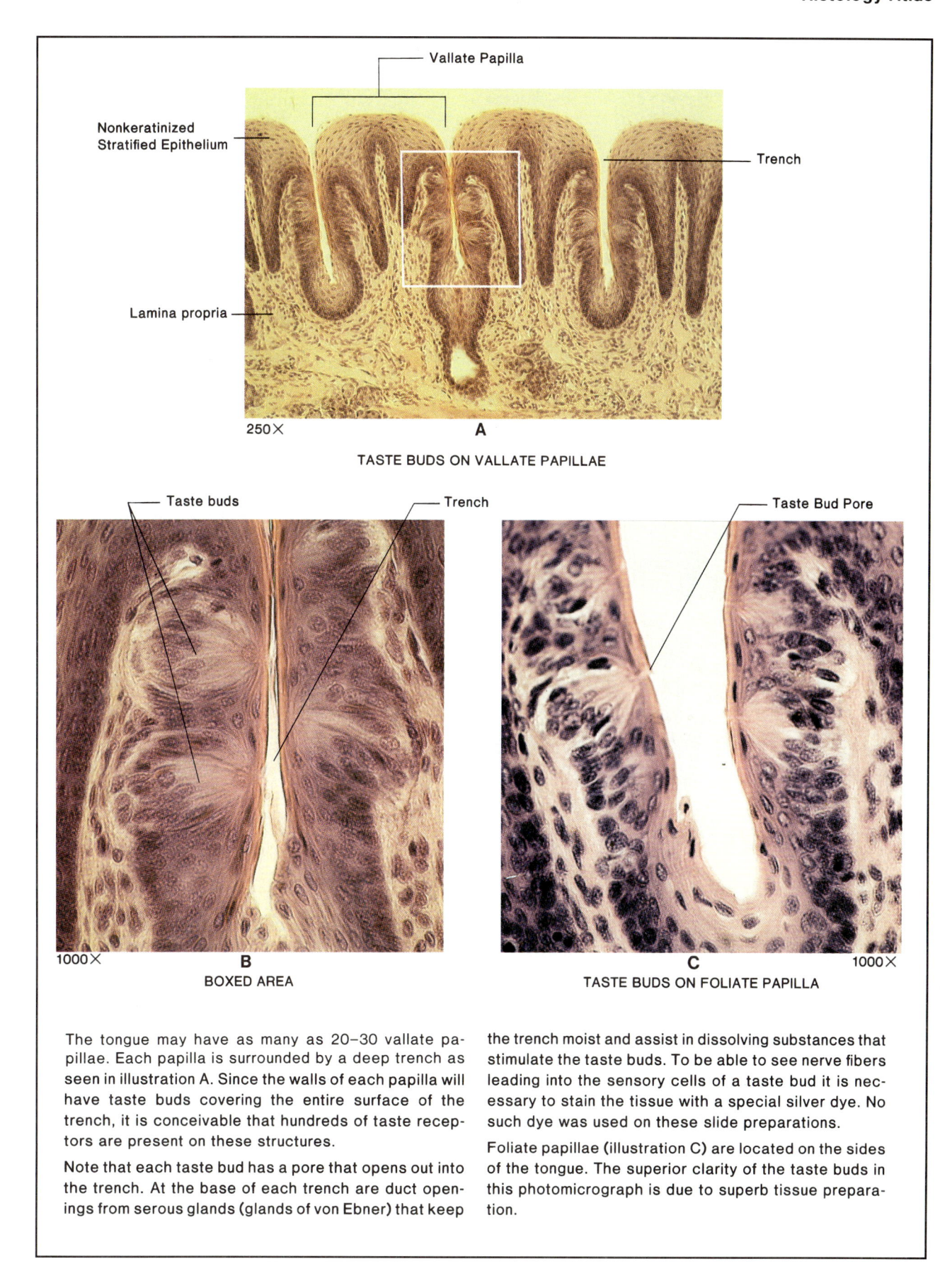

Vallate Papilla

Nonkeratinized
Stratified Epithelium

Trench

Lamina propria

250×   **A**

TASTE BUDS ON VALLATE PAPILLAE

Taste buds   Trench   Taste Bud Pore

1000×   **B**   1000×

BOXED AREA

C

TASTE BUDS ON FOLIATE PAPILLA

The tongue may have as many as 20–30 vallate papillae. Each papilla is surrounded by a deep trench as seen in illustration A. Since the walls of each papilla will have taste buds covering the entire surface of the trench, it is conceivable that hundreds of taste receptors are present on these structures.

Note that each taste bud has a pore that opens out into the trench. At the base of each trench are duct openings from serous glands (glands of von Ebner) that keep the trench moist and assist in dissolving substances that stimulate the taste buds. To be able to see nerve fibers leading into the sensory cells of a taste bud it is necessary to stain the tissue with a special silver dye. No such dye was used on these slide preparations.

Foliate papillae (illustration C) are located on the sides of the tongue. The superior clarity of the taste buds in this photomicrograph is due to superb tissue preparation.

Figure HA–19   Taste buds.

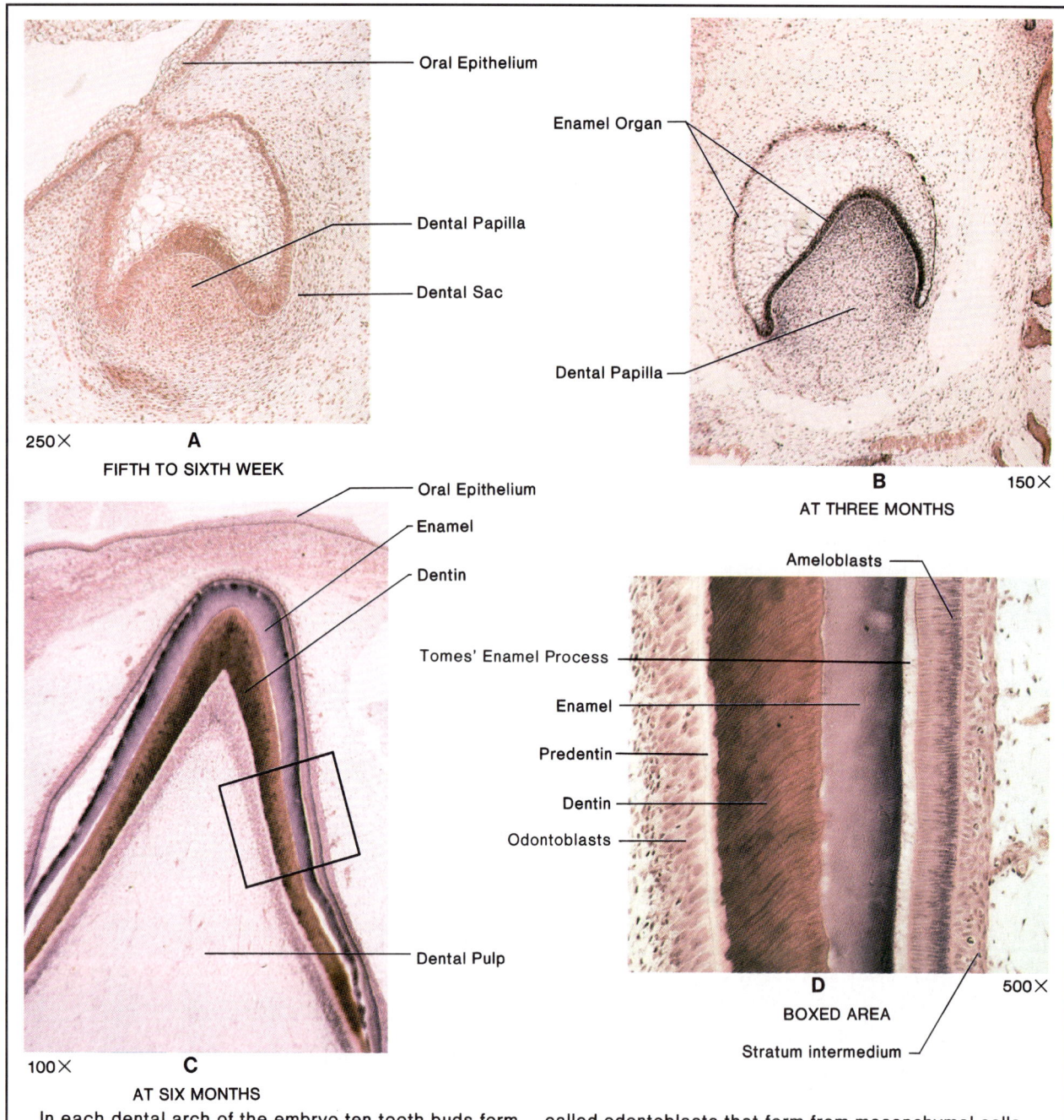

In each illustration:

- Oral Epithelium
- Dental Papilla
- Dental Sac

250× **A**
FIFTH TO SIXTH WEEK

- Enamel Organ
- Dental Papilla

B 150×
AT THREE MONTHS

- Oral Epithelium
- Enamel
- Dentin
- Dental Pulp

100× **C**
AT SIX MONTHS

- Ameloblasts
- Tomes' Enamel Process
- Enamel
- Predentin
- Dentin
- Odontoblasts

D 500×
BOXED AREA
- Stratum intermedium

In each dental arch of the embryo ten tooth buds form by proliferation of cells in the oral epithelium. At first the buds are solid and rounded, but as the cells multiply they push inward (invaginate) as shown in illustration A. The oral epithelium (ectoderm) forms a two-layered structure called the enamel organ. Mesenchymal cells (mesoderm) in the distal portion of the bud push in to form the dental papilla. Illustration C reveals that by the fifth or sixth month the enamel organ produces the enamel of the tooth, and the cells of the dental papilla differentiate to form dentin.

Dentin is laid down just before the appearance of enamel. It is produced by a layer of elongated cells called odontoblasts that form from mesenchymal cells of the dental papilla. Note in illustration D that uncalcified dentin, or predentin, is formed first. Predentin is quickly converted to mature dentin, which consists of collagenous fibers and a calcified component called apatite.

Enamel is produced by cells called ameloblasts. Note in illustration D that these cells produce a clear layer called Tomes' enamel process, which becomes converted to mature enamel by calcification with mineral salts. As new enamel forms, the ameloblasts move outward away from the dentin and odontoblasts. When the tooth erupts, the ameloblasts are sloughed off.

Figure HA-20   Embryological stages in tooth development.

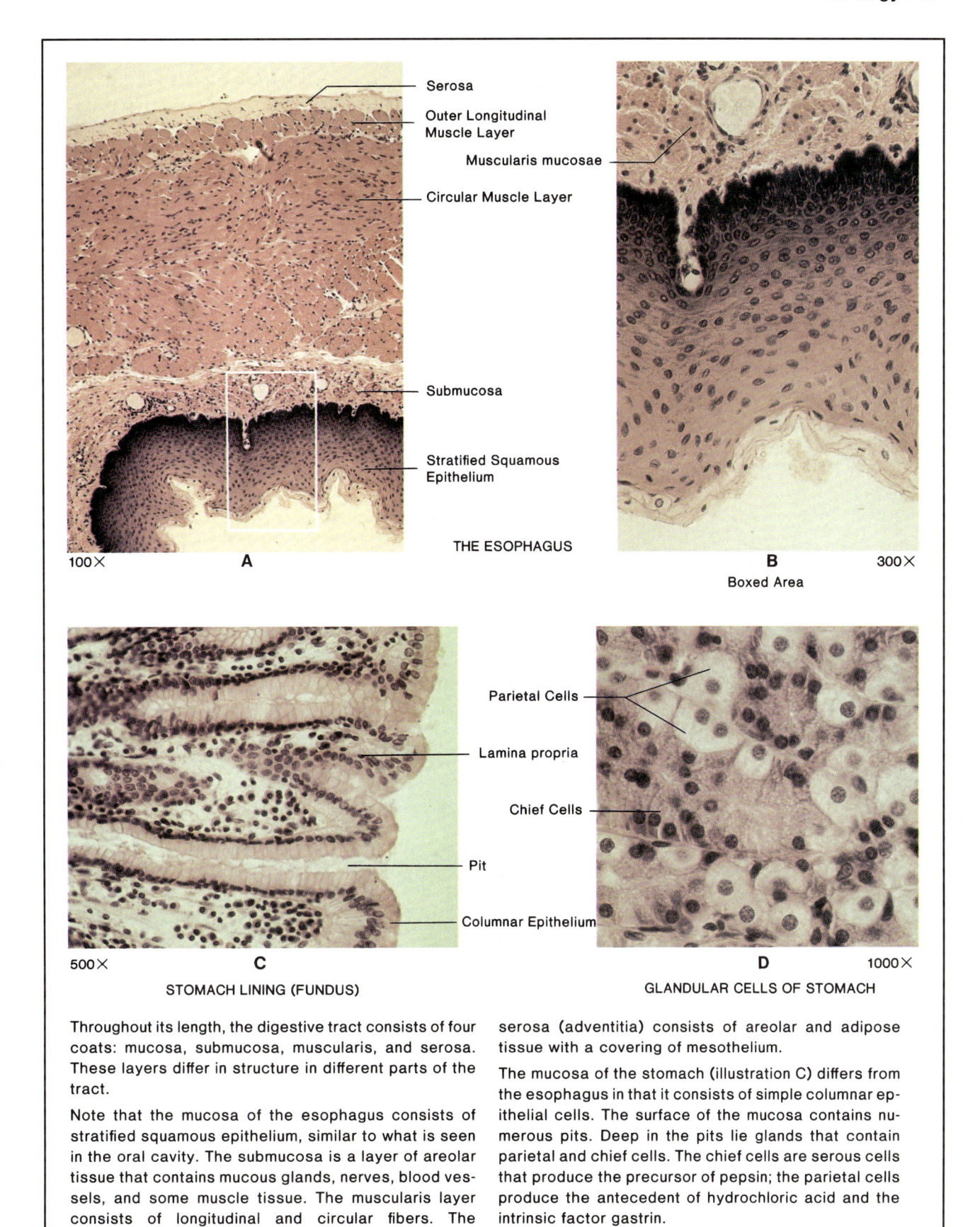

Serosa

Outer Longitudinal Muscle Layer

Muscularis mucosae

Circular Muscle Layer

Submucosa

Stratified Squamous Epithelium

THE ESOPHAGUS

100×   **A**

B   300×

Boxed Area

Parietal Cells

Lamina propria

Chief Cells

Pit

Columnar Epithelium

500×   **C**

D   1000×

STOMACH LINING (FUNDUS)

GLANDULAR CELLS OF STOMACH

Throughout its length, the digestive tract consists of four coats: mucosa, submucosa, muscularis, and serosa. These layers differ in structure in different parts of the tract.

Note that the mucosa of the esophagus consists of stratified squamous epithelium, similar to what is seen in the oral cavity. The submucosa is a layer of areolar tissue that contains mucous glands, nerves, blood vessels, and some muscle tissue. The muscularis layer consists of longitudinal and circular fibers. The serosa (adventitia) consists of areolar and adipose tissue with a covering of mesothelium.

The mucosa of the stomach (illustration C) differs from the esophagus in that it consists of simple columnar epithelial cells. The surface of the mucosa contains numerous pits. Deep in the pits lie glands that contain parietal and chief cells. The chief cells are serous cells that produce the precursor of pepsin; the parietal cells produce the antecedent of hydrochloric acid and the intrinsic factor gastrin.

Figure HA–21   The esophagus and stomach.

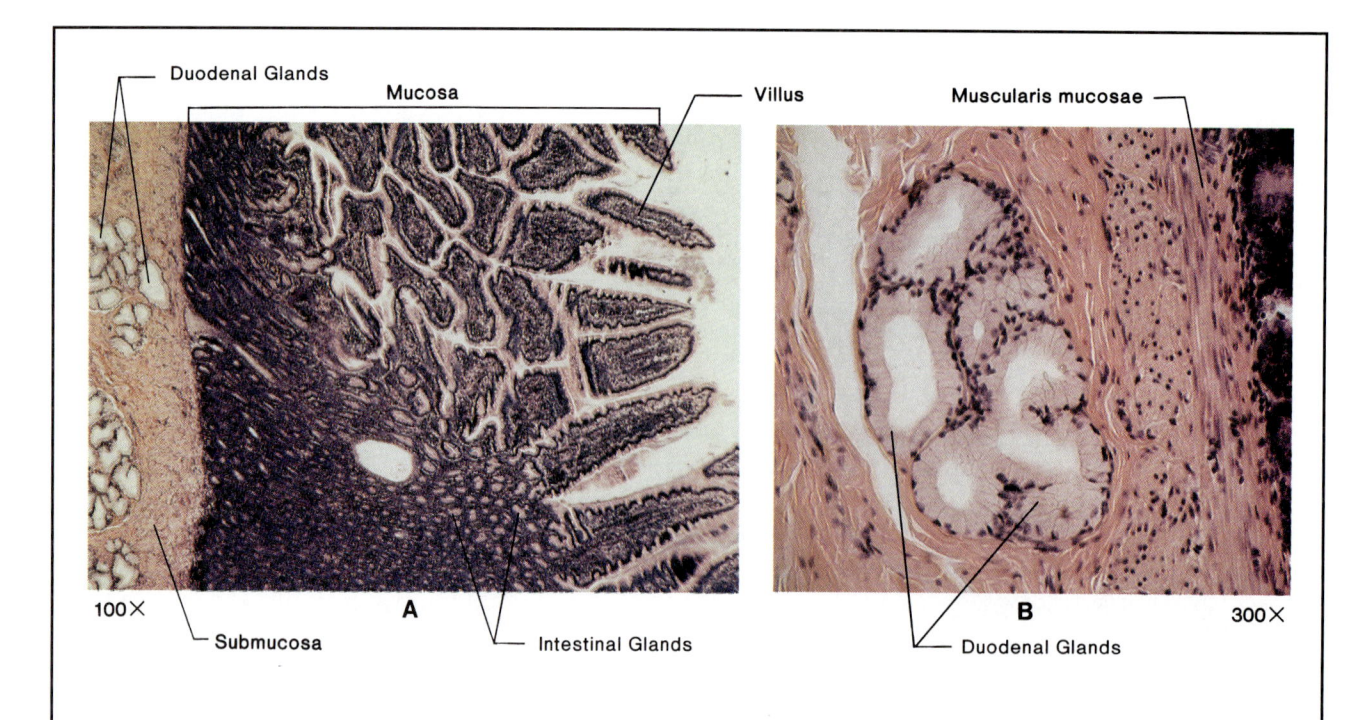

Duodenal Glands

Mucosa

Villus

Muscularis mucosae

100×

A

Submucosa

Intestinal Glands

B

300×

Duodenal Glands

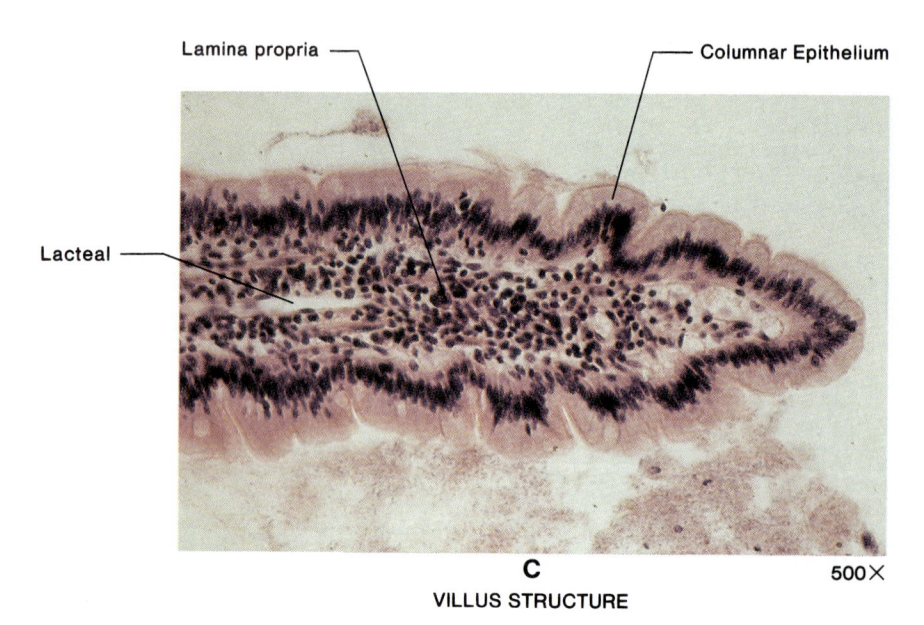

Lamina propria

Columnar Epithelium

Lacteal

C

500×

VILLUS STRUCTURE

The mucosa of the duodenum consists of the epithelium and the lamina propria. Within the lamina propria are numerous intestinal glands (crypts of Lieberkühn). The entire mucosal surface is covered with millions of small fingerlike projections called villi.

Where the lamina propria meets the muscularis mucosae, the mucosa ends. Note the large number of mucus-secreting duodenal (Brunner's) glands (illustration B) that are located in the submucosa.

Illustration C reveals the structure of a single villus. The entire epithelium consists of simple columnar cells interspersed with goblet cells. The core of the villus is the lamina propria, which contains loose connective tissue, smooth muscle fibers, blood vessels, and a lymphatic vessel, the lacteal. The muscularis layer (not shown in illustration C) contains an inner circular layer of smooth muscle tissue, and an outer longitudinal layer of smooth fibers. The outer surface of the duodenum is covered by the serosa.

Figure HA–22 The duodenum.

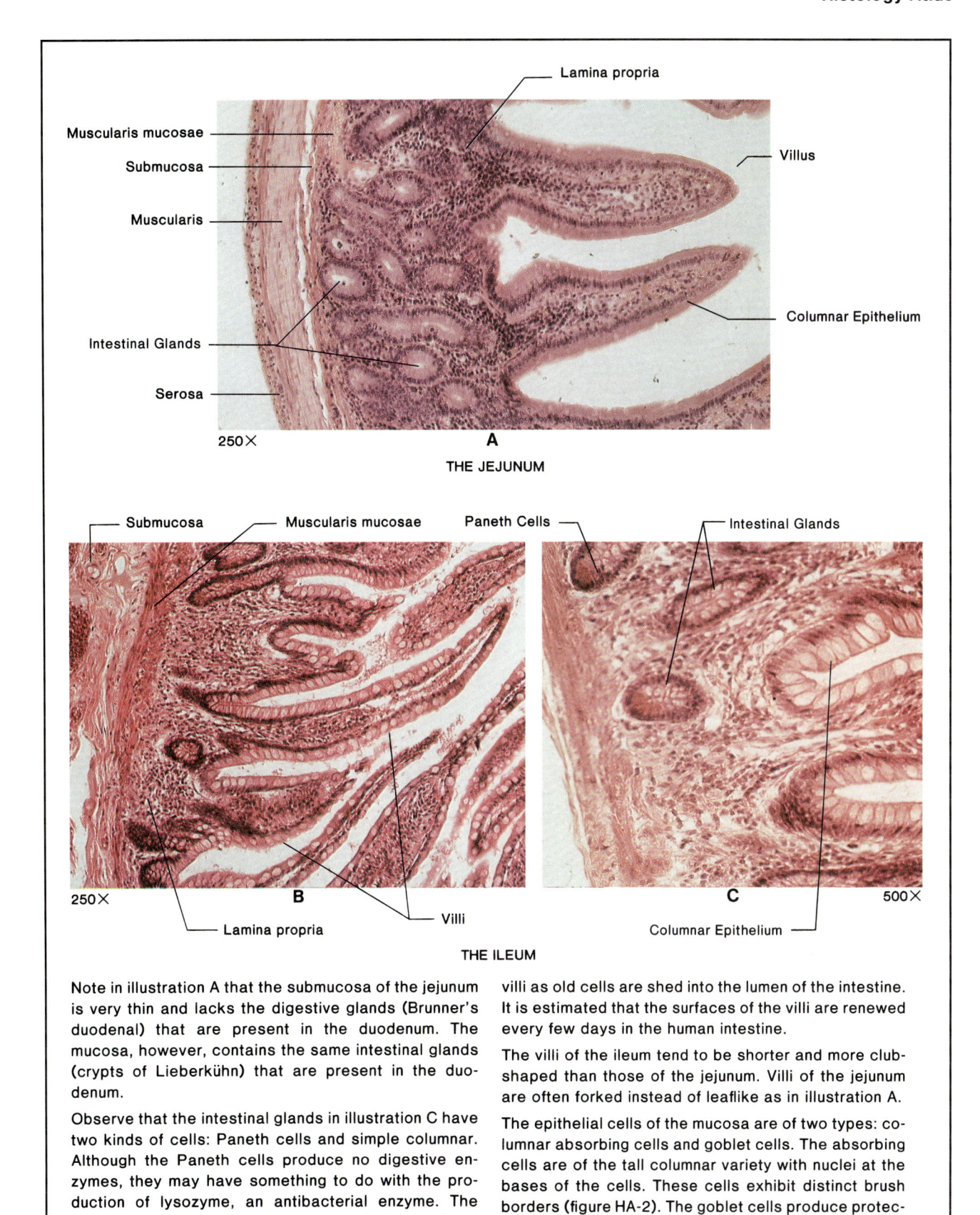

Lamina propria

Muscularis mucosae

Submucosa

Muscularis

Intestinal Glands

Serosa

Villus

Columnar Epithelium

250×

A

THE JEJUNUM

Submucosa   Muscularis mucosae   Paneth Cells   Intestinal Glands

250×   **B**

Lamina propria   Villi

C   500×

Columnar Epithelium

THE ILEUM

Note in illustration A that the submucosa of the jejunum is very thin and lacks the digestive glands (Brunner's duodenal) that are present in the duodenum. The mucosa, however, contains the same intestinal glands (crypts of Lieberkühn) that are present in the duodenum.

Observe that the intestinal glands in illustration C have two kinds of cells: Paneth cells and simple columnar. Although the Paneth cells produce no digestive enzymes, they may have something to do with the production of lysozyme, an antibacterial enzyme. The columnar cells, which resemble the columnar cells of the epithelium, provide new cells for the surfaces of the villi as old cells are shed into the lumen of the intestine. It is estimated that the surfaces of the villi are renewed every few days in the human intestine.

The villi of the ileum tend to be shorter and more club-shaped than those of the jejunum. Villi of the jejunum are often forked instead of leaflike as in illustration A.

The epithelial cells of the mucosa are of two types: columnar absorbing cells and goblet cells. The absorbing cells are of the tall columnar variety with nuclei at the bases of the cells. These cells exhibit distinct brush borders (figure HA-2). The goblet cells produce protective mucus.

Figure HA–23   The jejunum and ileum.

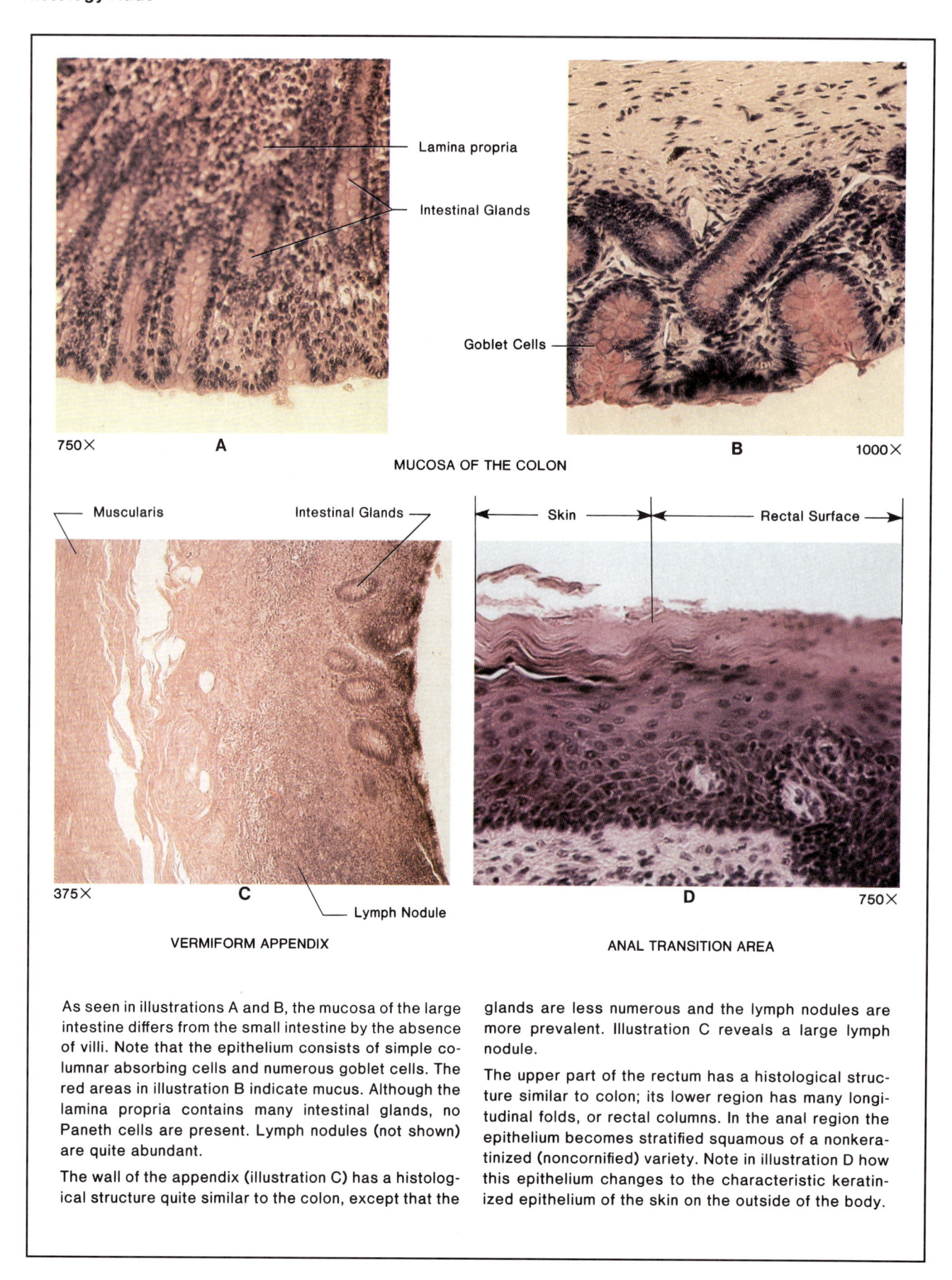

MUCOSA OF THE COLON

A — Lamina propria, Intestinal Glands — 750×

B — Goblet Cells — 1000×

VERMIFORM APPENDIX

C — Muscularis, Intestinal Glands, Lymph Nodule — 375×

ANAL TRANSITION AREA

D — Skin, Rectal Surface — 750×

As seen in illustrations A and B, the mucosa of the large intestine differs from the small intestine by the absence of villi. Note that the epithelium consists of simple columnar absorbing cells and numerous goblet cells. The red areas in illustration B indicate mucus. Although the lamina propria contains many intestinal glands, no Paneth cells are present. Lymph nodules (not shown) are quite abundant.

The wall of the appendix (illustration C) has a histological structure quite similar to the colon, except that the glands are less numerous and the lymph nodules are more prevalent. Illustration C reveals a large lymph nodule.

The upper part of the rectum has a histological structure similar to colon; its lower region has many longitudinal folds, or rectal columns. In the anal region the epithelium becomes stratified squamous of a nonkeratinized (noncornified) variety. Note in illustration D how this epithelium changes to the characteristic keratinized epithelium of the skin on the outside of the body.

Figure HA–24   The lower digestive tract.

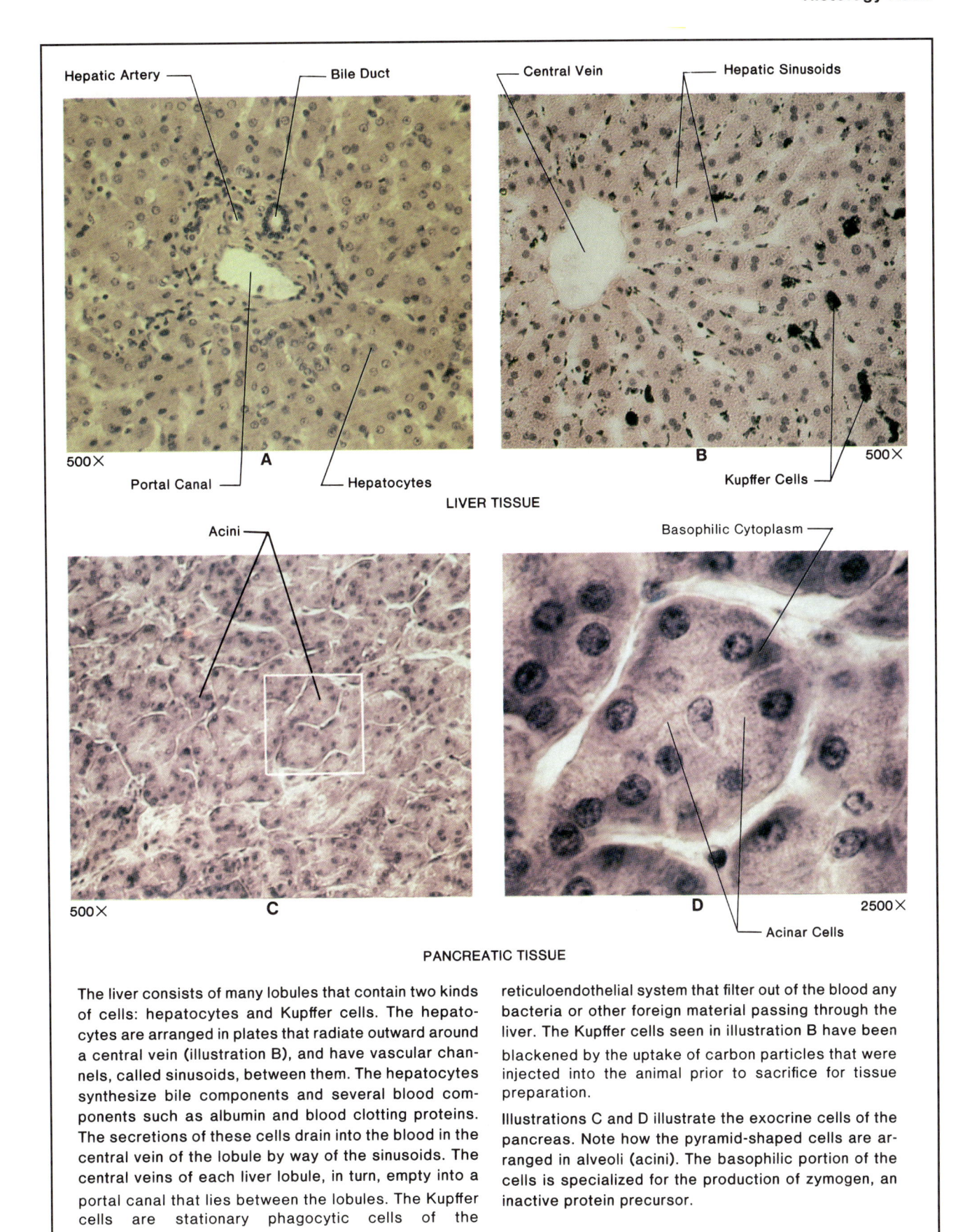

LIVER TISSUE

PANCREATIC TISSUE

The liver consists of many lobules that contain two kinds of cells: hepatocytes and Kupffer cells. The hepatocytes are arranged in plates that radiate outward around a central vein (illustration B), and have vascular channels, called sinusoids, between them. The hepatocytes synthesize bile components and several blood components such as albumin and blood clotting proteins. The secretions of these cells drain into the blood in the central vein of the lobule by way of the sinusoids. The central veins of each liver lobule, in turn, empty into a portal canal that lies between the lobules. The Kupffer cells are stationary phagocytic cells of the reticuloendothelial system that filter out of the blood any bacteria or other foreign material passing through the liver. The Kupffer cells seen in illustration B have been blackened by the uptake of carbon particles that were injected into the animal prior to sacrifice for tissue preparation.

Illustrations C and D illustrate the exocrine cells of the pancreas. Note how the pyramid-shaped cells are arranged in alveoli (acini). The basophilic portion of the cells is specialized for the production of zymogen, an inactive protein precursor.

Figure HA–25   Liver and pancreas histology.

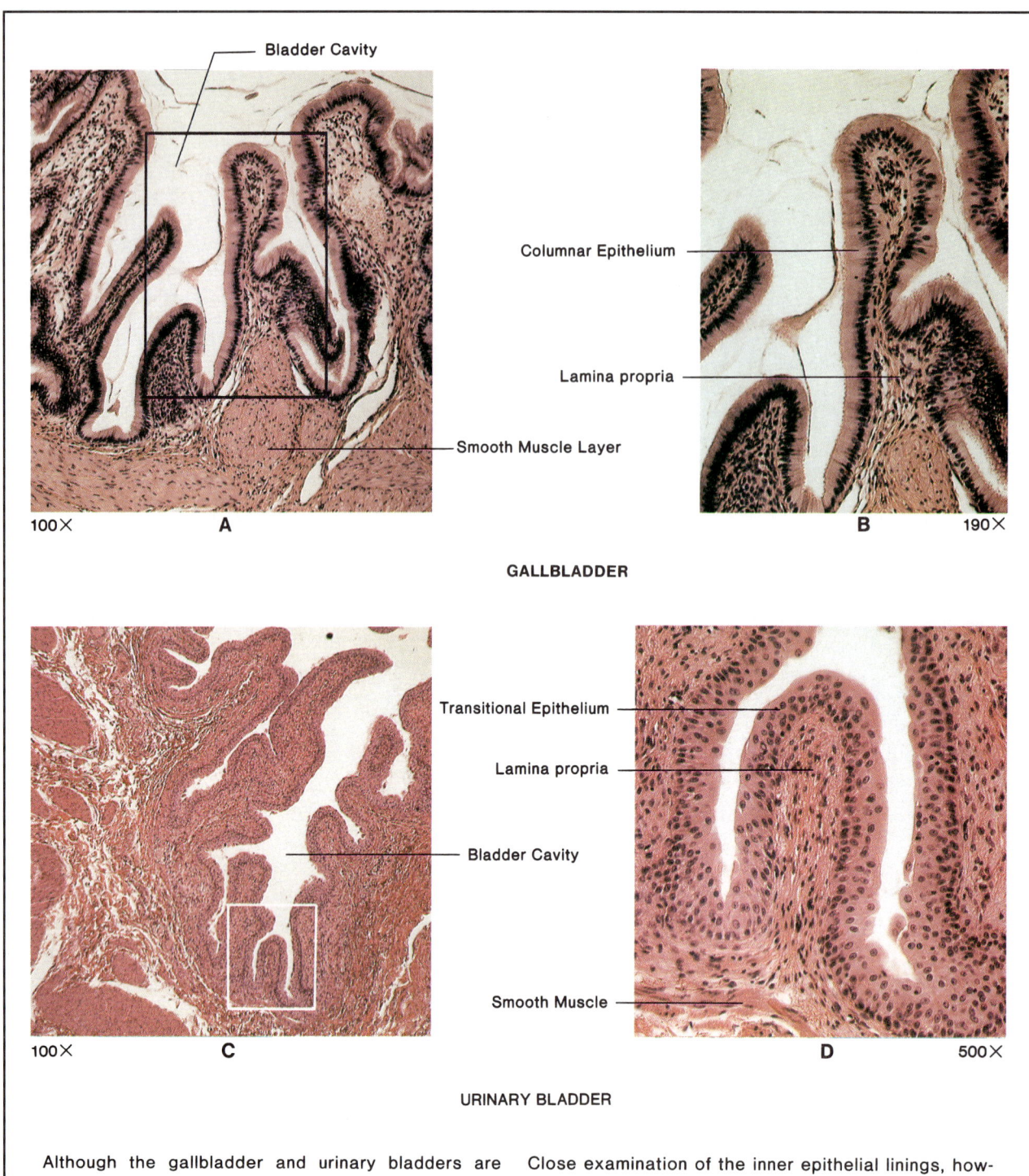

GALLBLADDER

URINARY BLADDER

Although the gallbladder and urinary bladders are organs of two different systems, they have similarities as well as distinct differences when compared side by side.

At first glance the considerable infolding of the mucosa of both bladders is evident. As both bladders fill up with their contents (bile or urine), the extensive infolding allows for expansion to contain the fluids that pour into them.

Close examination of the inner epithelial linings, however, reveals distinct differences. Note that the epithelium of the gallbladder consists of a single layer of columnar cells, and the urinary bladder mucosa is much thicker, being made up of transitional epithelium. These differences are as one would expect: columnar cells in most of the digestive tract and transitional epithelium in the urinary system.

Figure HA–26 The gall and urinary bladders.

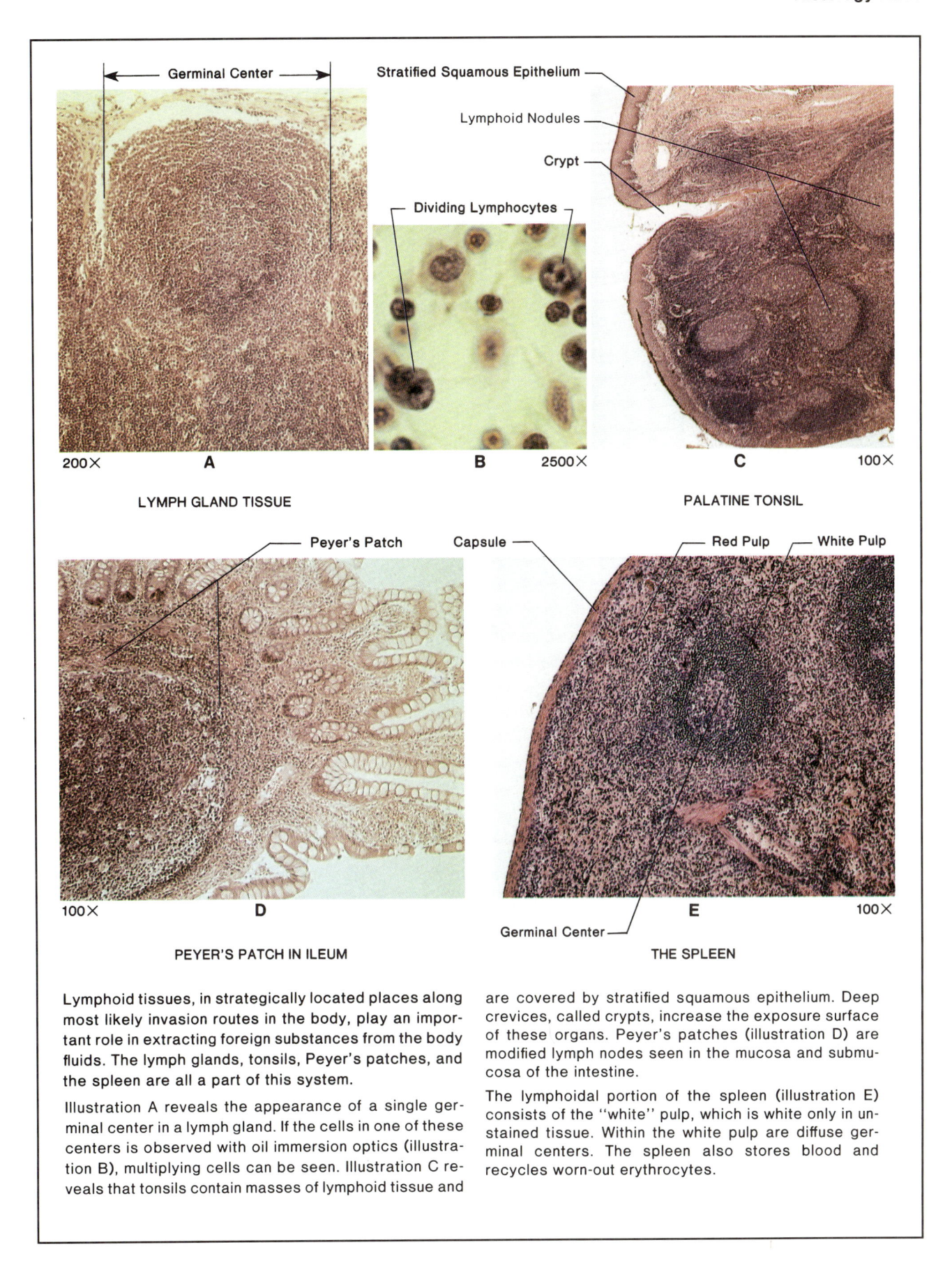

Germinal Center

Stratified Squamous Epithelium

Lymphoid Nodules

Crypt

Dividing Lymphocytes

200× **A**

B 2500×

C 100×

LYMPH GLAND TISSUE

PALATINE TONSIL

Peyer's Patch

Capsule

Red Pulp

White Pulp

100× **D**

E 100×

Germinal Center

PEYER'S PATCH IN ILEUM

THE SPLEEN

Lymphoid tissues, in strategically located places along most likely invasion routes in the body, play an important role in extracting foreign substances from the body fluids. The lymph glands, tonsils, Peyer's patches, and the spleen are all a part of this system.

Illustration A reveals the appearance of a single germinal center in a lymph gland. If the cells in one of these centers is observed with oil immersion optics (illustration B), multiplying cells can be seen. Illustration C reveals that tonsils contain masses of lymphoid tissue and

are covered by stratified squamous epithelium. Deep crevices, called crypts, increase the exposure surface of these organs. Peyer's patches (illustration D) are modified lymph nodes seen in the mucosa and submucosa of the intestine.

The lymphoidal portion of the spleen (illustration E) consists of the "white" pulp, which is white only in unstained tissue. Within the white pulp are diffuse germinal centers. The spleen also stores blood and recycles worn-out erythrocytes.

Figure HA–27 Lymphoid tissues in lymph gland, palatine tonsil, ileum, and spleen.

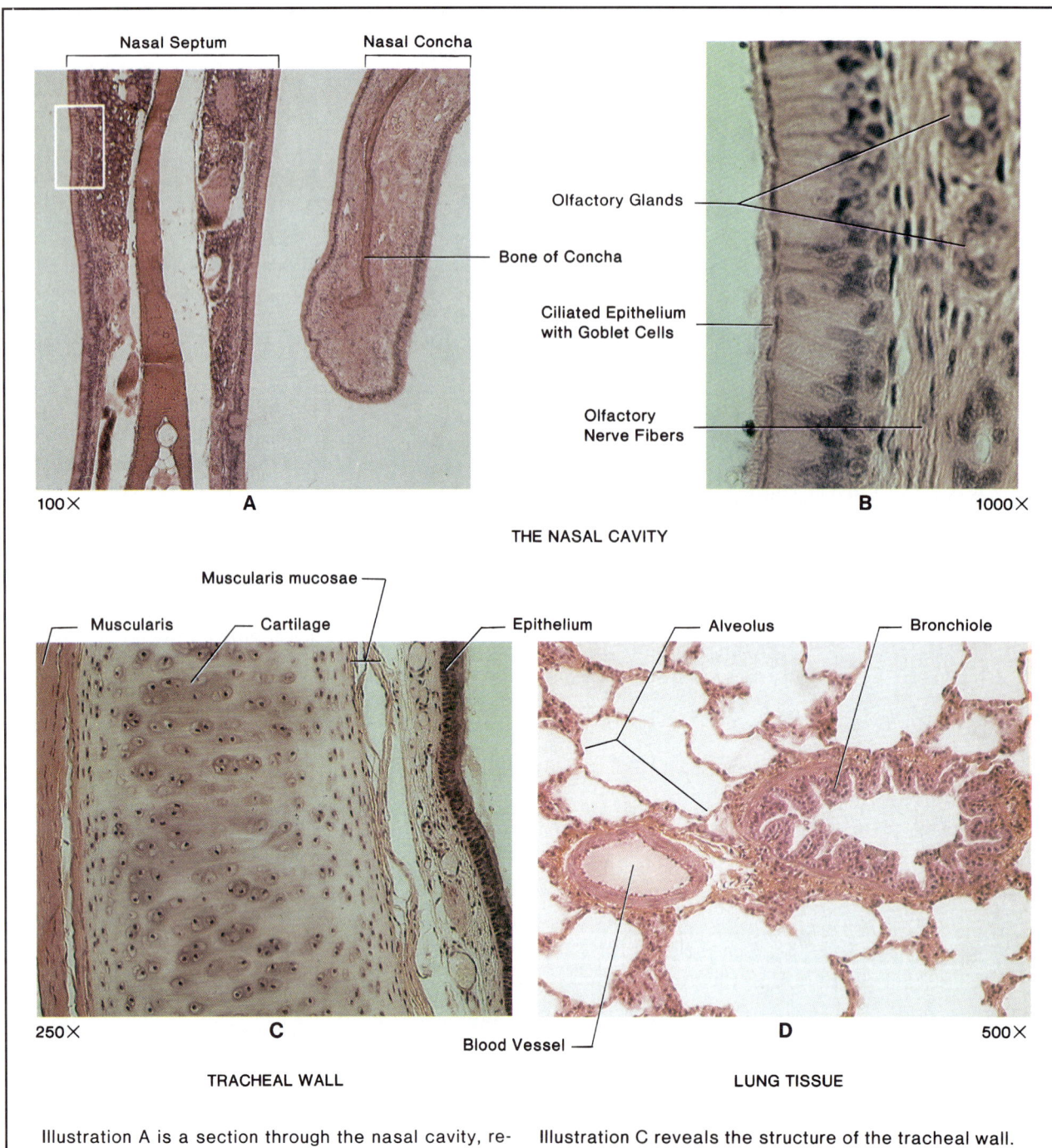

Nasal Septum · Nasal Concha

Bone of Concha

100× A

Olfactory Glands

Ciliated Epithelium
with Goblet Cells

Olfactory
Nerve Fibers

B 1000×

THE NASAL CAVITY

Muscularis mucosae

Muscularis · Cartilage · Epithelium · Alveolus · Bronchiole

250× C

Blood Vessel

TRACHEAL WALL

D 500×

LUNG TISSUE

Illustration A is a section through the nasal cavity, revealing the structure of the nasal septum and a portion of a nasal concha. Note in illustration B (enlargement of the boxed area in illustration A) that the nasal epithelium consists of ciliated columnar cells. Interspersed between these columnar cells are olfactory receptors that are not readily visible here due to the absence of silver dye staining. The olfactory (Bowman's) glands in the lamina propria produce a secretion made up of mucus and serous fluid. This secretion helps to keep the epithelium moist and dissolves molecules that stimulate the olfactory receptors.

Illustration C reveals the structure of the tracheal wall. Tracheal rigidity is provided by hyaline cartilaginous rings. The epithelium consists of pseudostratified ciliated epithelium (see illustration D, figure HA-2). The section of lung tissue in illustration D depicts a cluster of alveoli, a bronchiole, and a small artery. Note that several alveoli open into a larger atrium, which empties ultimately into a bronchiole. Observe that the inner wall of a bronchiole consists of cuboidal or low columnar epithelium. Cilia are present in the proximal portion of bronchioles and absent distally.

Figure HA–28 Histology of respiratory structures.

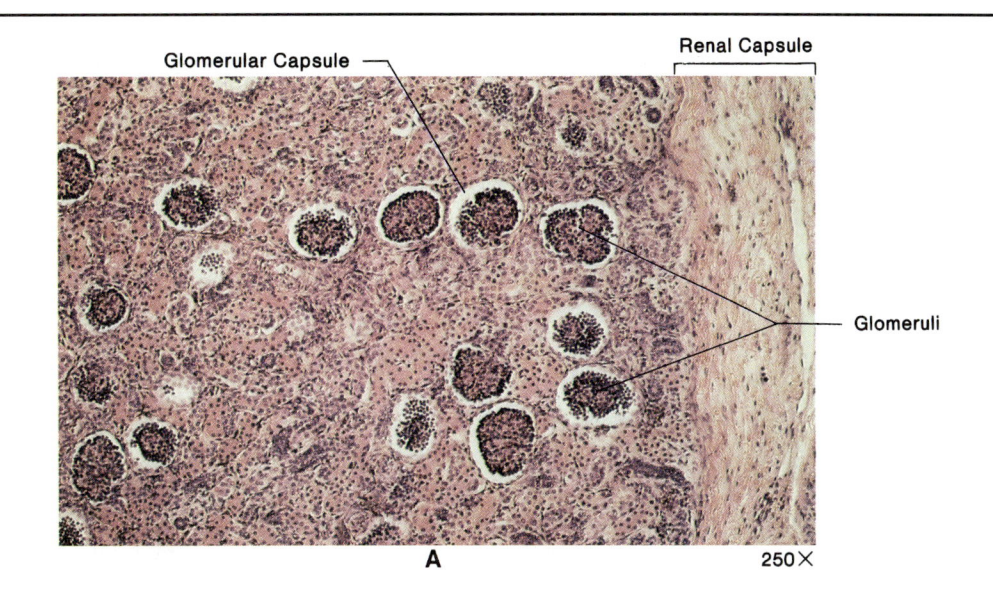

Glomerular Capsule

Renal Capsule

Glomeruli

A   250×

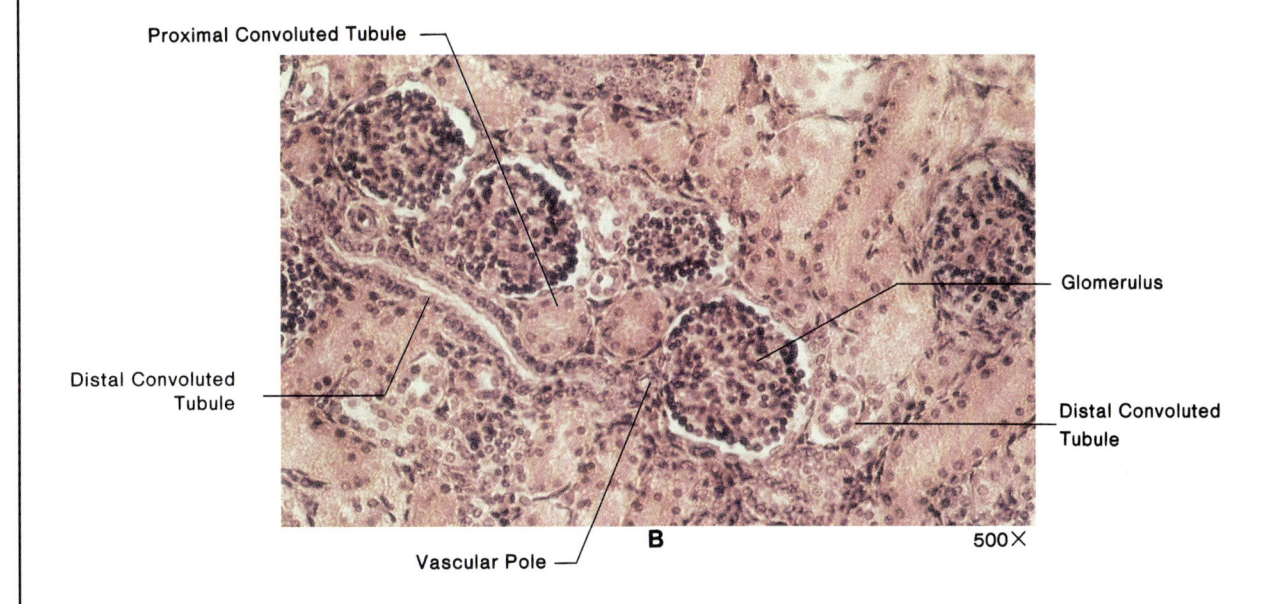

Proximal Convoluted Tubule

Distal Convoluted Tubule

Glomerulus

Distal Convoluted Tubule

Vascular Pole

B   500×

Illustration A reveals the structure of the outermost portion of the cortex of the kidney. The entire organ is enclosed by a thick fibrous capsule.

Blood enters each glomerulus through its vascular pole (shown in illustration B). High vascular pressure in the glomeruli results in the production of a glomerular filtrate consisting of water, glucose, amino acids, and other substances. This glomerular filtrate is collected by the glomerular capsule and passes down the length of the nephron collecting tubule, being altered in composition as it approaches the calyx of the kidney. Note that the proximal convoluted tubules can be differentiated from the distal convoluted tubules by the size of the cuboidal cells that comprise their walls: large in the proximal tubule and small in the distal tubule. Eighty percent of water absorption occurs in the proximal convoluted tubules.

Figure HA-29   Histology of the cortex of the kidney.

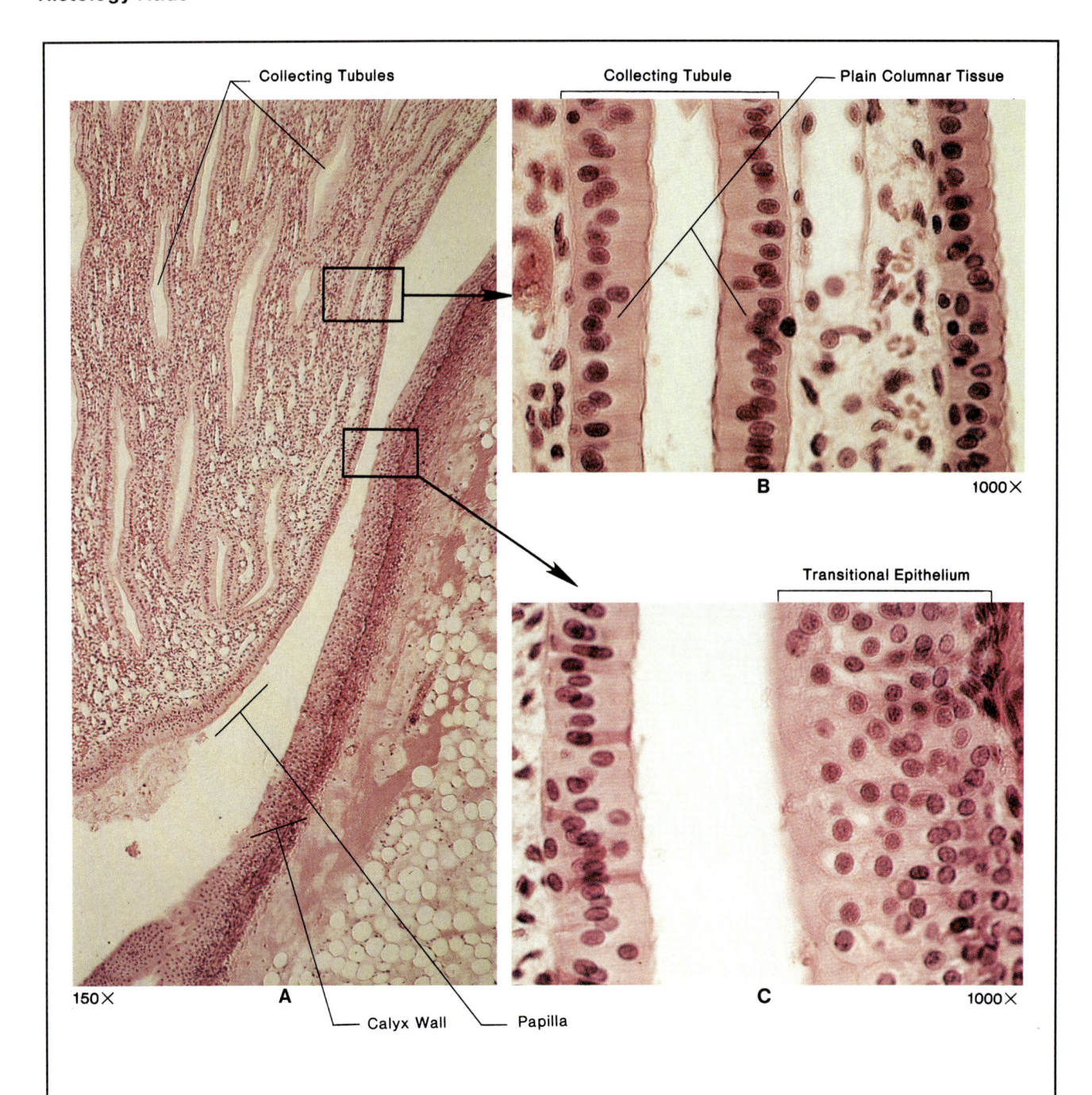

Figure HA-30 Histology of the papilla and calyx of the kidney.

Illustration A portrays a portion of the tip of a pyramid and the wall of the calyx. Illustrations B and C reveal the histological nature of these two structures. The collecting tubules, which collect urine from several nephrons, are lined with distinct low columnar epithelium. Examination of these cells with oil immersion optics will reveal the existence of a distinct brush border. Both absorption and secretion takes place through these columnar cells.

Note in illustration C that the wall of the calyx is lined with transitional epithelium. This same type of tissue is seen lining the ureters and the urinary bladder (see illustrations C and D, figure HA-26).

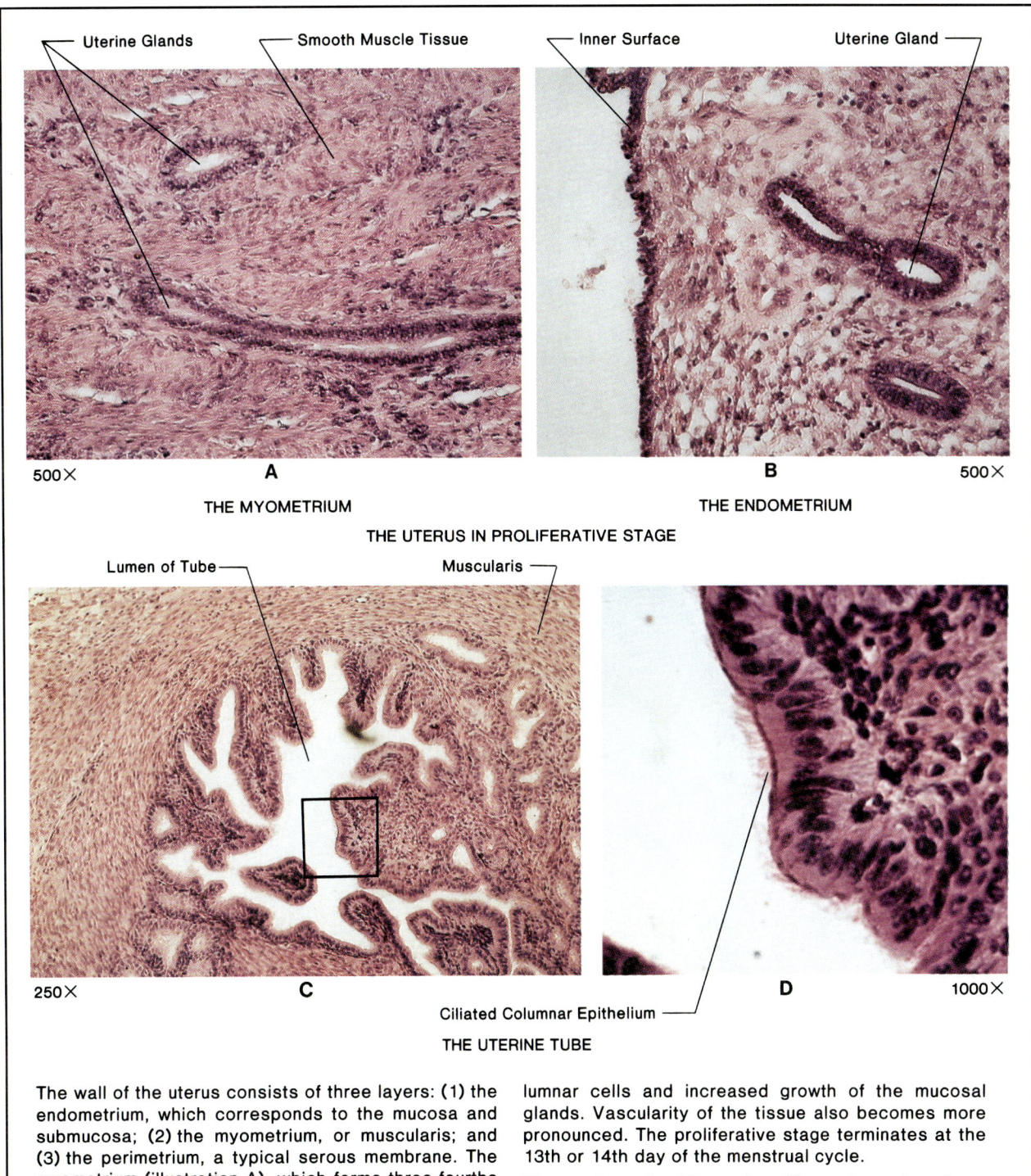

Uterine Glands — Smooth Muscle Tissue

500× **A**

THE MYOMETRIUM

Inner Surface — Uterine Gland

B 500×

THE ENDOMETRIUM

THE UTERUS IN PROLIFERATIVE STAGE

Lumen of Tube — Muscularis

250× **C**

Ciliated Columnar Epithelium

D 1000×

THE UTERINE TUBE

The wall of the uterus consists of three layers: (1) the endometrium, which corresponds to the mucosa and submucosa; (2) the myometrium, or muscularis; and (3) the perimetrium, a typical serous membrane. The myometrium (illustration A), which forms three-fourths of the uterine wall, consists of three layers of smooth muscle fibers: an inner longitudinal layer, a middle circular layer, and an outer oblique layer. Some glands extend into it from the endometrium. The endometrial surface cells are columnar and partially ciliated. During the proliferative stage (immediately after menstruation) the endometrium undergoes regeneration of the co-

lumnar cells and increased growth of the mucosal glands. Vascularity of the tissue also becomes more pronounced. The proliferative stage terminates at the 13th or 14th day of the menstrual cycle.

The uterine tube (illustration C) consists of an inner mucosa, a middle muscularis, and an outer serosa. The mucosa epithelium consists of a mixture of ciliated and nonciliated columnar cells (see illustration D). The muscularis consists of inner circular and outer longitudinal layers of smooth muscle fibers. There is no muscularis mucosae as seen in the digestive tract.

Figure HA–31   The uterus and Fallopian tube.

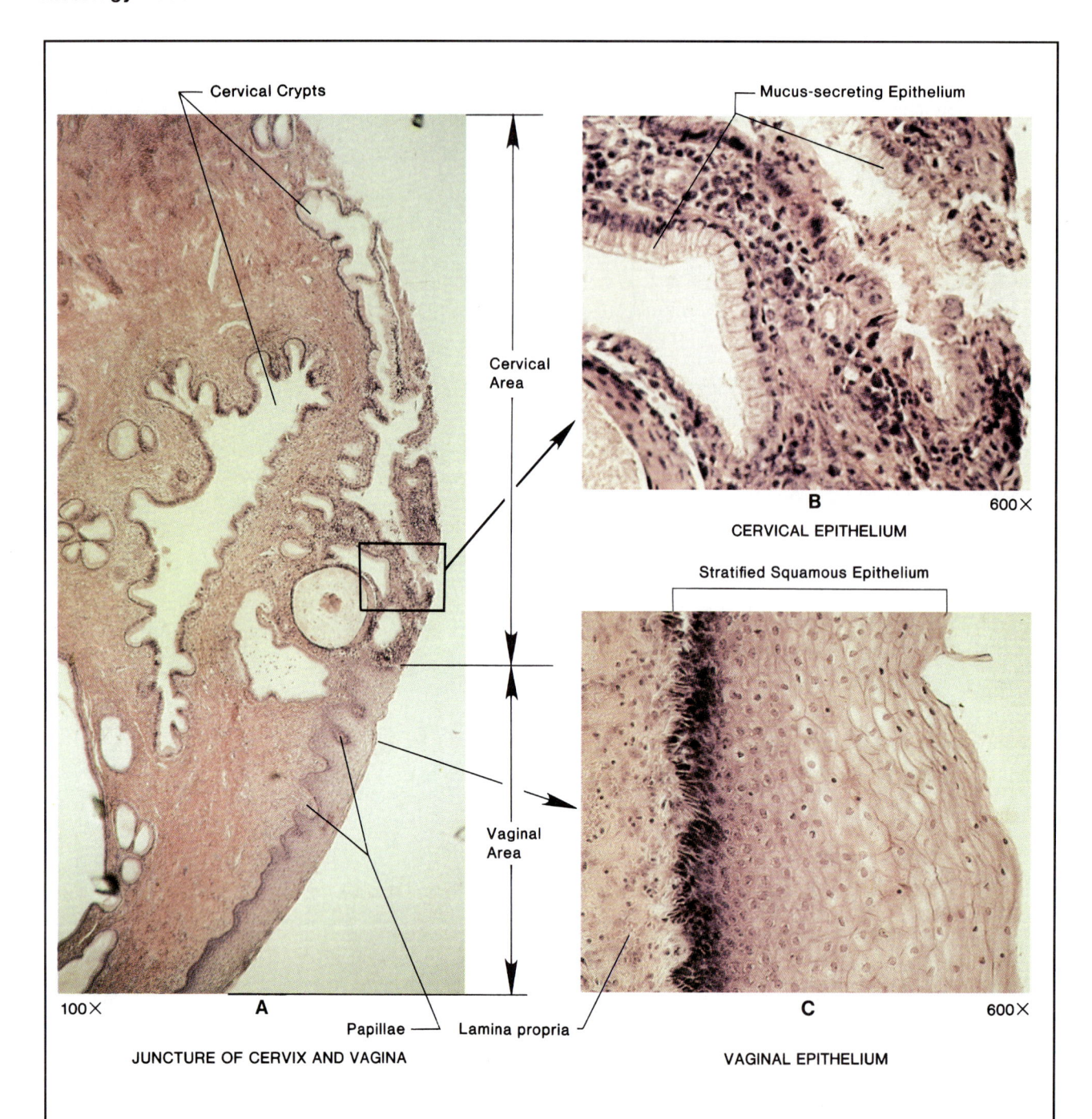

Cervical Crypts

Cervical Area

100× **A**

JUNCTURE OF CERVIX AND VAGINA

Papillae — Lamina propria

Mucus-secreting Epithelium

B 600×

CERVICAL EPITHELIUM

Stratified Squamous Epithelium

C 600×

VAGINAL EPITHELIUM

Vaginal Area

Illustration A shows the contrasting histological differences that exist between the epithelia of the vagina and cervix. Note in illustration C that the vaginal epithelium consists of nonkeratinized stratified squamous epithelium. Examination of the lamina propria of the vaginal mucosa with high-dry or oil immersion optics will reveal the presence of large numbers of lymphocytes. Note in illustration A that the epithelium has a large number of papillae.

The most distinguishing characteristic of the cervical portion of the uterus is the presence of approximately one hundred mucus-secreting cervical crypts. As indicated in illustration B, the epithelium of these crypts consists, primarily, of plain columnar cells; some ciliated cells are also present, however. Approximately 20 to 60 mg of mucus are produced daily. During ovulation mucus production increases to over 700 mg daily. Mucus plays an important role in fertility since it is the first secretion met by the sperm entering the female tract. Occasionally the exit of a crypt will become occluded, causing a cyst to form. The large round structure near the box in illustration A is such a structure.

Figure HA–32   The cervix and vagina.

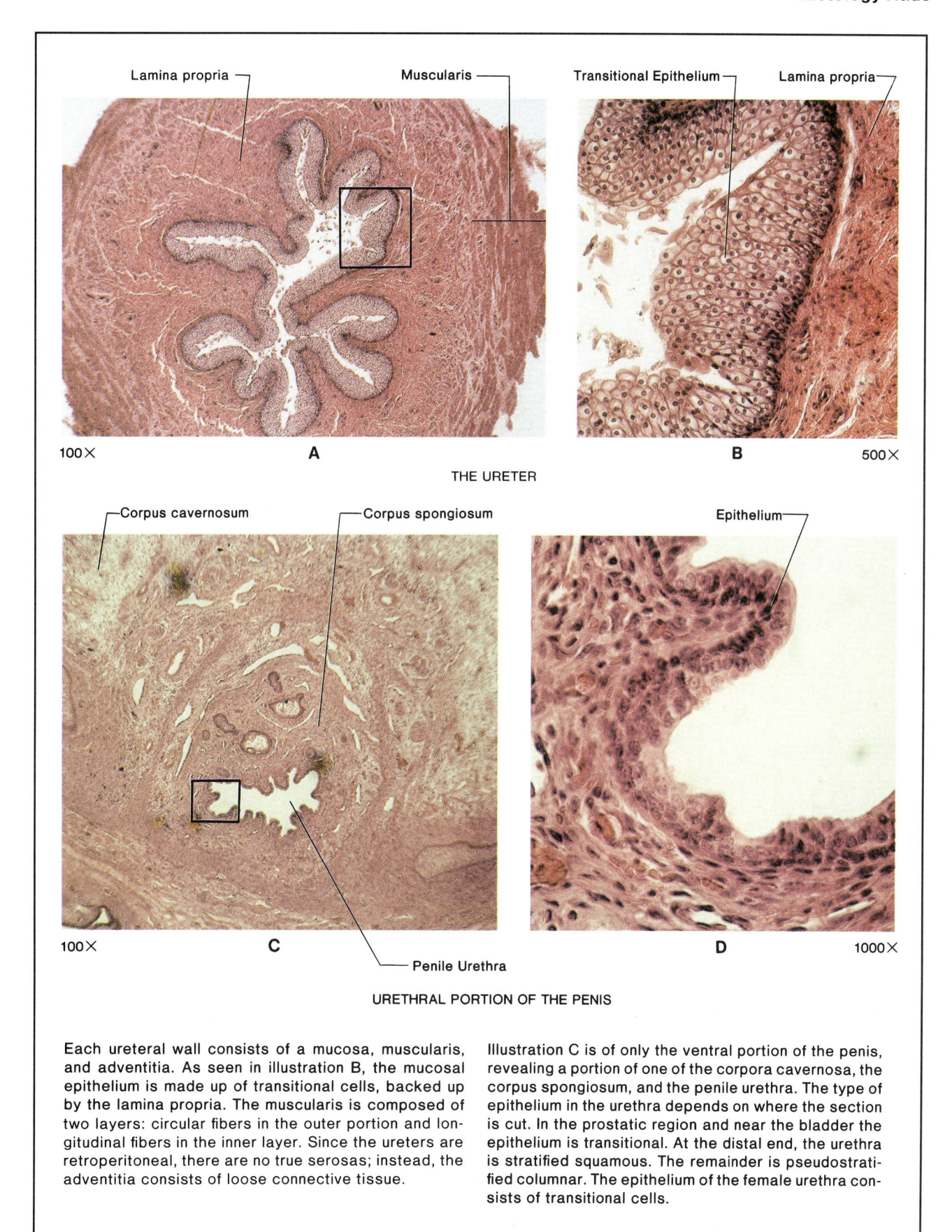

Lamina propria — Muscularis

Transitional Epithelium — Lamina propria

100× **A**

THE URETER

B 500×

Corpus cavernosum — Corpus spongiosum

Epithelium —

100× **C**

— Penile Urethra

D 1000×

URETHRAL PORTION OF THE PENIS

Each ureteral wall consists of a mucosa, muscularis, and adventitia. As seen in illustration B, the mucosal epithelium is made up of transitional cells, backed up by the lamina propria. The muscularis is composed of two layers: circular fibers in the outer portion and longitudinal fibers in the inner layer. Since the ureters are retroperitoneal, there are no true serosas; instead, the adventitia consists of loose connective tissue.

Illustration C is of only the ventral portion of the penis, revealing a portion of one of the corpora cavernosa, the corpus spongiosum, and the penile urethra. The type of epithelium in the urethra depends on where the section is cut. In the prostatic region and near the bladder the epithelium is transitional. At the distal end, the urethra is stratified squamous. The remainder is pseudostratified columnar. The epithelium of the female urethra consists of transitional cells.

Figure HA–33   The ureter and penile urethra.

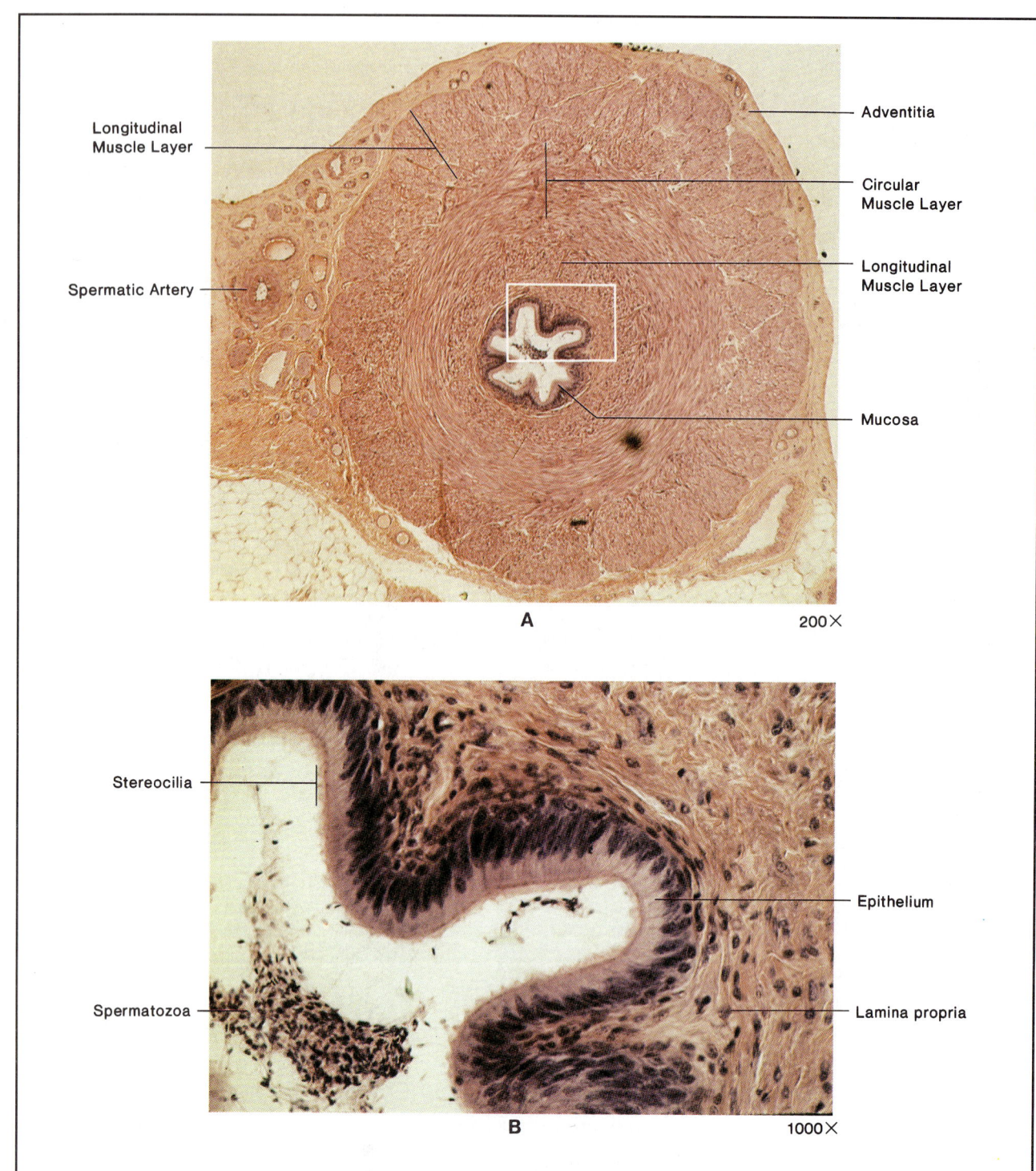

Longitudinal Muscle Layer

Spermatic Artery

Adventitia

Circular Muscle Layer

Longitudinal Muscle Layer

Mucosa

A 200×

Stereocilia

Spermatozoa

Epithelium

Lamina propria

B 1000×

The vas deferens (spermatic duct) is a thick-walled muscular tube that transports spermatozoa from the epididymis to the ejaculatory duct where fluid from the seminal vesicles joins the spermatozoa. The wall has three distinct areas: an outer adventitia, a middle muscularis (three-layered), and an inner mucosa. Note that the muscularis is very thick with two layers of longitudinal fibers and a middle layer of circular fibers. Peri-

staltic waves produced by these muscles help to propel the spermatozoa during ejaculation.

The mucosa, consisting of the lamina propria and epithelium, is unique in that the columnar cells that make up the epithelium have stereocilia. These structures are nonmotile enlarged microvilli that cover the exposed surfaces of the cells.

Figure HA–34   The vas deferens.

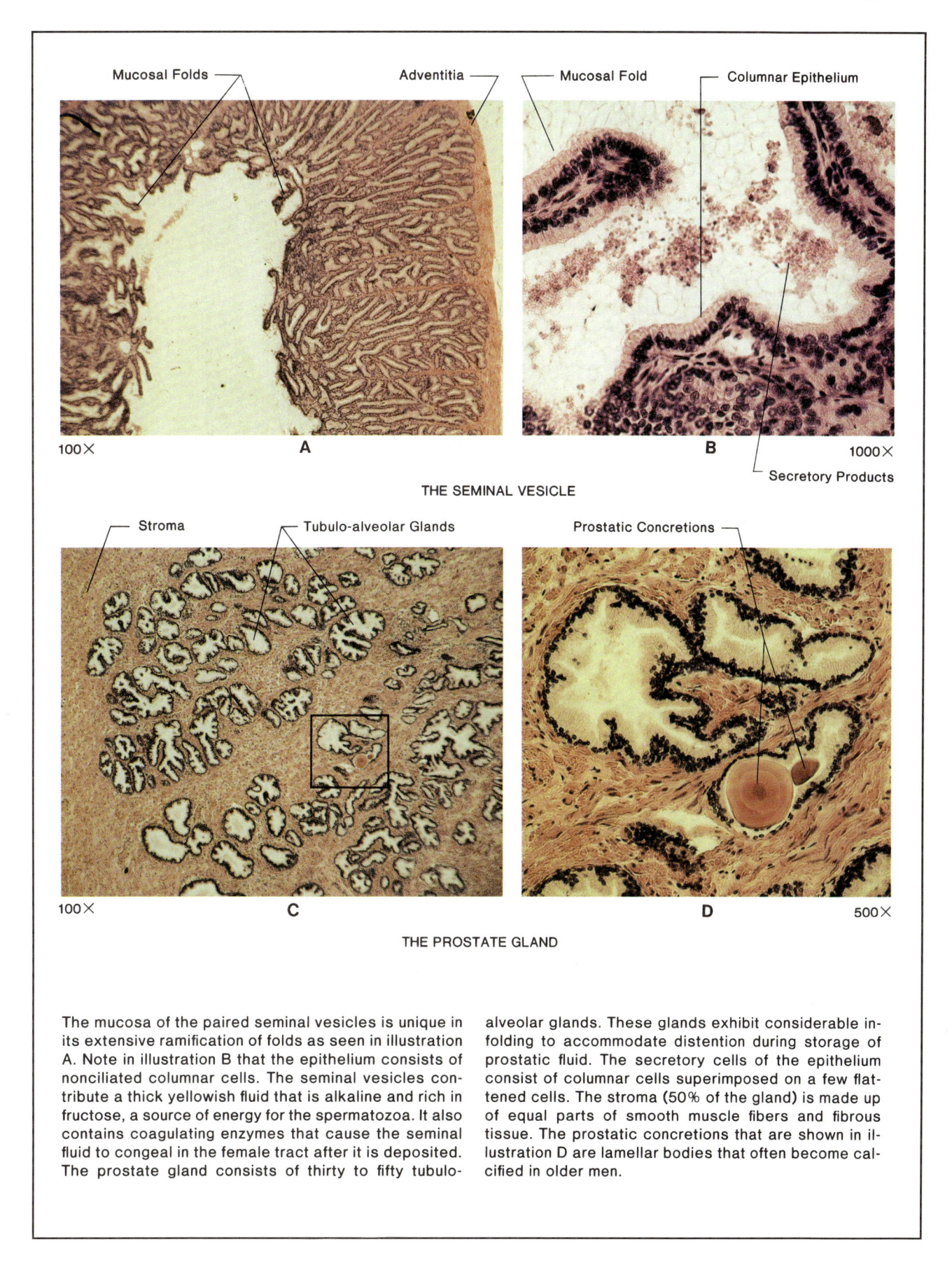

THE SEMINAL VESICLE

THE PROSTATE GLAND

The mucosa of the paired seminal vesicles is unique in its extensive ramification of folds as seen in illustration A. Note in illustration B that the epithelium consists of nonciliated columnar cells. The seminal vesicles contribute a thick yellowish fluid that is alkaline and rich in fructose, a source of energy for the spermatozoa. It also contains coagulating enzymes that cause the seminal fluid to congeal in the female tract after it is deposited. The prostate gland consists of thirty to fifty tubulo-alveolar glands. These glands exhibit considerable infolding to accommodate distention during storage of prostatic fluid. The secretory cells of the epithelium consist of columnar cells superimposed on a few flattened cells. The stroma (50% of the gland) is made up of equal parts of smooth muscle fibers and fibrous tissue. The prostatic concretions that are shown in illustration D are lamellar bodies that often become calcified in older men.

Figure HA-35 Seminal vesicle and prostate gland.

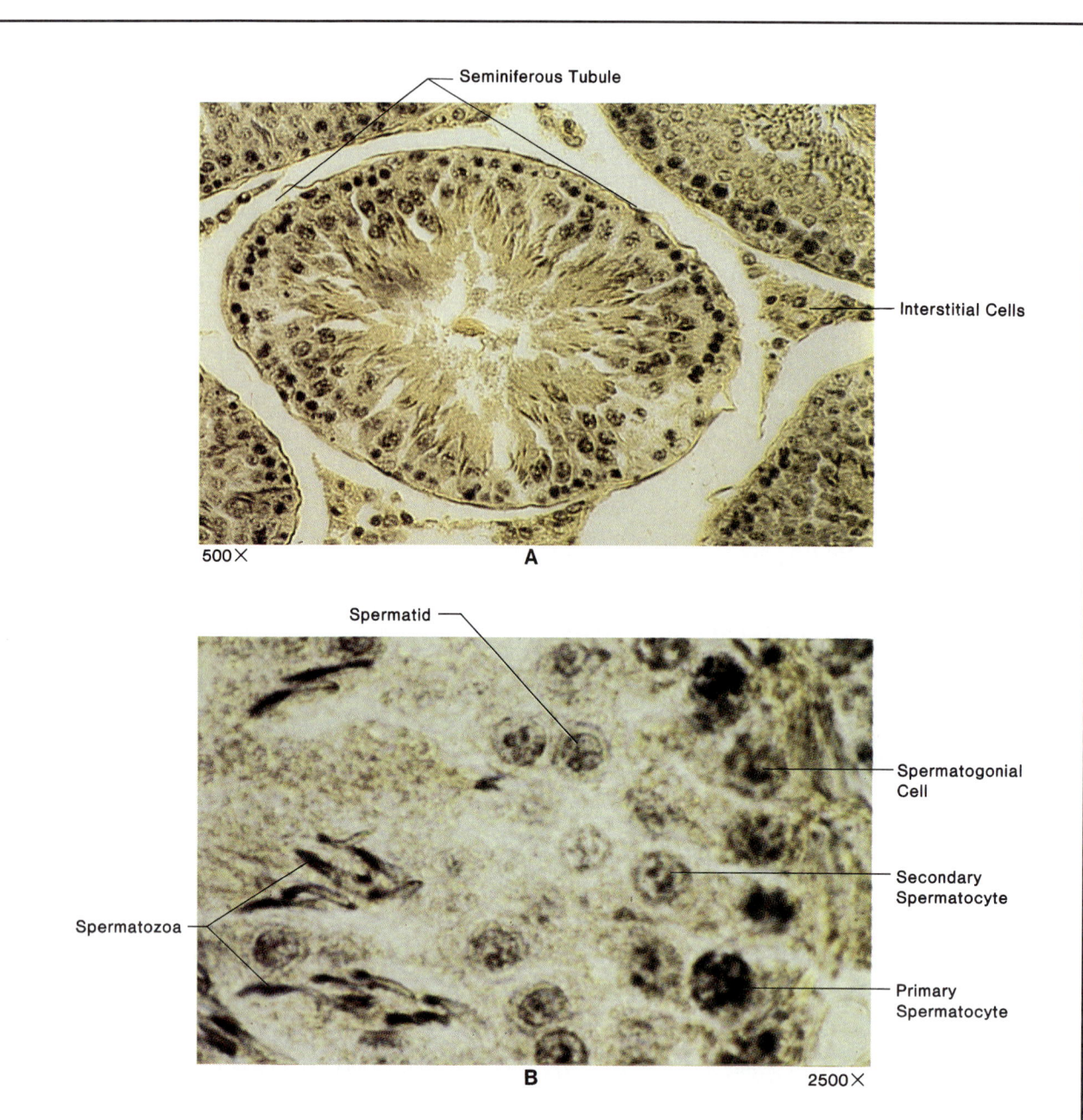

Seminiferous Tubule

Interstitial Cells

500× — A

Spermatid

Spermatogonial Cell

Secondary Spermatocyte

Primary Spermatocyte

Spermatozoa

B — 2500×

The production of spermatozoa, known as spermatogenesis, occurs in the seminiferous tubules of the testes. Illustration A reveals the structure of a single tubule. Between the tubules can be seen the interstitial cells that secrete testosterone into the circulatory system.

All spermatozoa originate from the primordial germ cells, or spermatogonia, that are located at the periphery of the seminiferous tubule. These cells have a diploid complement of 46 chromosomes. The first step in this process is the synapsis (union) of the homologous chromosomes to form tetrads in the primary spermatocyte. Note the proximity of the primary spermatocyte to the spermatogonial cells in illustration B.

The next step is for the primary spermatocyte to divide, meiotically, to produce two secondary spermatocytes. This meiotic division produces two cells (secondary spermatocytes) that have a haploid number (23) of chromosomes. Note in illustration B that the secondary spermatocytes are closer to the lumen of the seminiferous tubule. Finally, the two secondary spermatocytes divide meiotically, again, to produce a total of four spermatids which contain 23 chromosomes each. The spermatids continue to develop into mature spermatozoa.

Figure HA–36   Spermatogenesis.

Part 6 Metabolic Support

Anabolic and catabolic activities of all cells of the body require the support of the circulatory, respiratory, digestive, and urinary systems. Sources of energy (food) must be made available by the digestive system. Food molecules and oxygen must be transported by the circulatory system from their points of origin (intestines and lungs) to all cells. As metabolic wastes are produced by the multitude of cells, they must be carried by the blood to the kidneys to be excreted. It is about these various systems of metabolic support that this unit is concerned.

Precautions for Exercise 30

In Exercise 30 you will have an opportunity to prepare a microscope slide of your own blood. Since it will be necessary to make a small puncture in the skin of your finger it is important that certain sanitary precautions be observed. If these measures are not observed one or both of the following conditions could result: (1) self-infection from environmental contaminants, and (2) transmission of infections (i.e., hepatitis, AIDS, etc.) from one person to another. If the following routine is observed, no self-infection or cross-transmission should occur.

• Sponge down your table top at the beginning of the period with an appropriate disinfectant.

• Wash your hands with soap and water before and after doing any blood tests.

• If you are perforating another person's finger for a blood sample, avoid contact with the blood or use rubber gloves.

• Use disposable lancets only one time. Dispose of the lancet into a receptacle that contains disinfectant. Do not toss used lancets into the waste basket!

• Before perforating the finger for a blood sample, disinfect the skin with alcohol.

• At the end of the period wash up all equipment with soap and water.

• Scrub down the table top at the end of the period and wash your hands again with soap and water. A final rinse of the hands with disinfectant will provide additional protection.

30 The Blood

The blood is an opaque, rather viscous fluid that is bright red when oxygenated and dark red when depleted of oxygen. Its specific gravity is normally around 1.06 and its pH is slightly alkaline. When centrifuged, blood becomes separated into a dark red portion made up of **formed elements** and a clear straw-colored portion called **plasma.** The formed element content of blood is around 47 percent in men and 42 percent in women.

In this exercise we will study the formed elements in human blood. This study may be made from a prepared stained microscope slide or from a slide made from your own blood. Figures 30.1 and 30.3 will be used to identify the various types of blood cells. If you are going to prepare a slide from your own blood, *be sure to review the sanitary precautions that are provided on the previous page.*

The formed elements of blood consist of ***erythrocytes*** (red blood cells), ***leukocytes*** (white blood cells), and ***blood platelets.*** As illustrated in figure 30.1, the erythrocytes are non-nucleated cells with depressed centers that contain hemoglobin. They are the most numerous elements in blood: around 4.5 to 5.5 million cells per cubic millimeter.

The leukocytes are of two types: granulocytes and agranulocytes. The *granulocytes* are so-named because they have conspicuous granules in their cytoplasm. Neutrophils, eosinophils, and basophils fall into this category. The *agranulocytes* lack pronounced granules in the cytoplasm; the monocytes and lymphocytes are of this type.

The blood platelets are noncellular elements in the blood that assist in the blood clotting process.

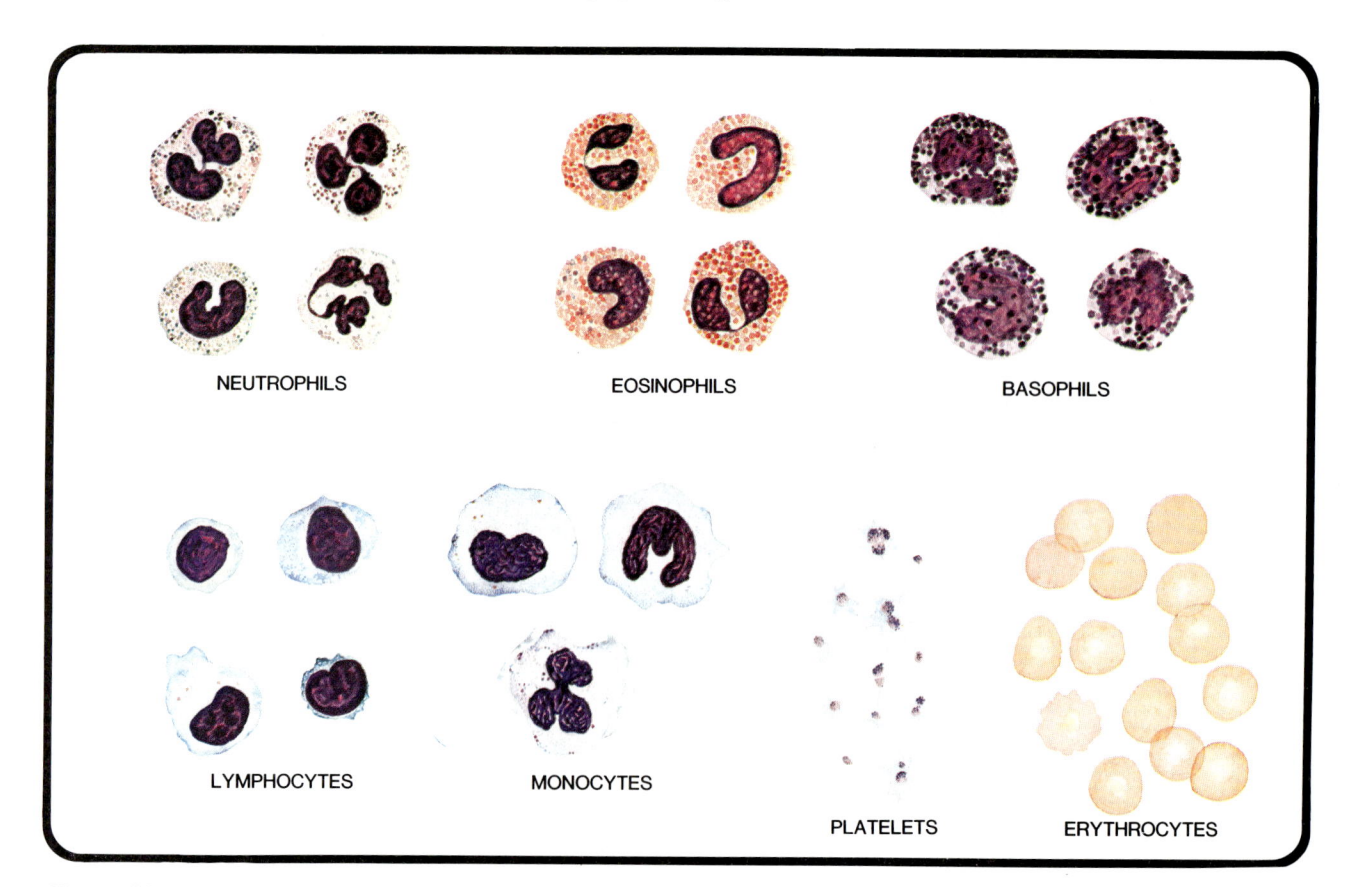

NEUTROPHILS   EOSINOPHILS   BASOPHILS

LYMPHOCYTES   MONOCYTES   PLATELETS   ERYTHROCYTES

Figure 30.1   Formed elements of blood.

K. P. Talaro

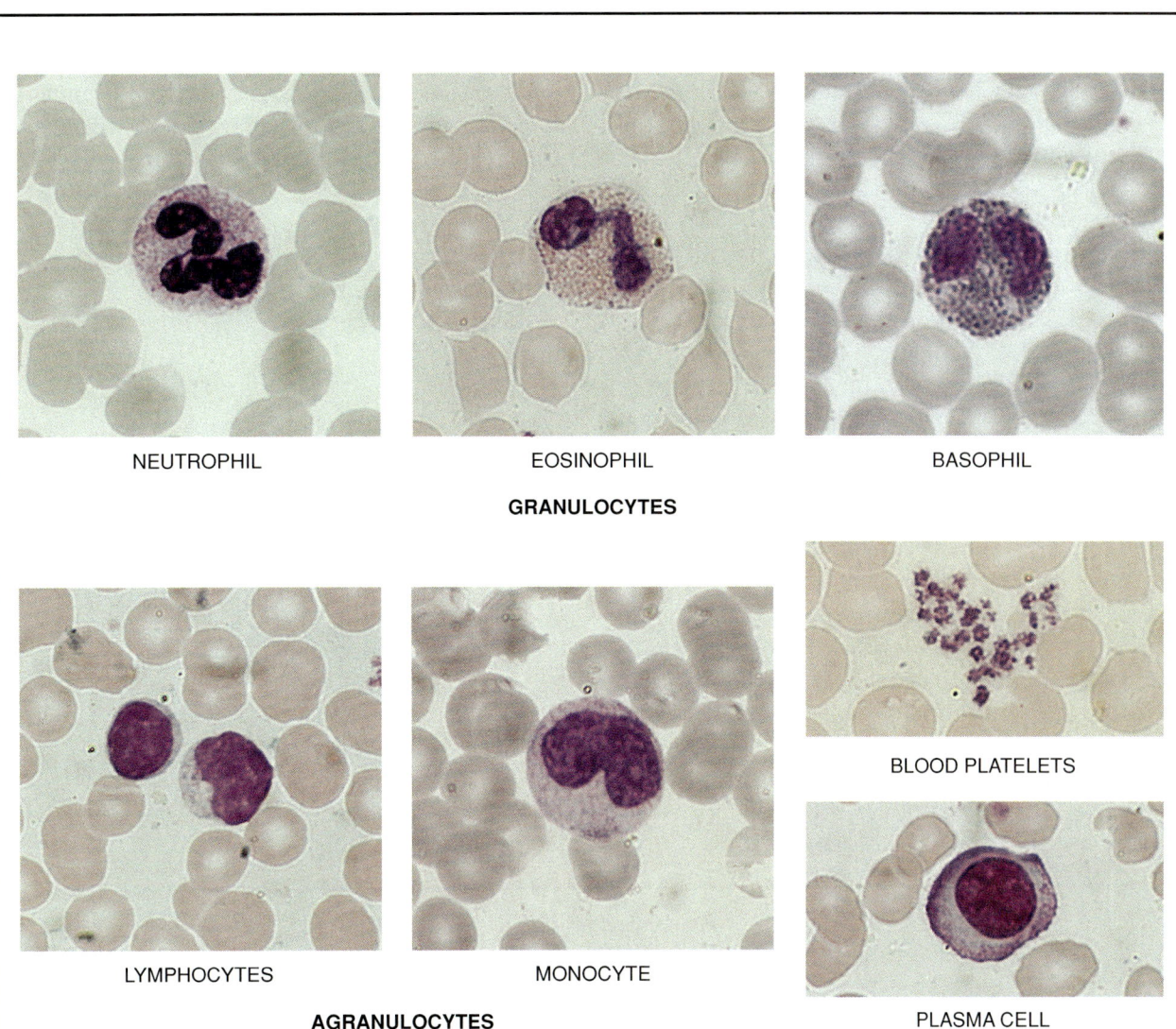

NEUTROPHIL	EOSINOPHIL	BASOPHIL

GRANULOCYTES

LYMPHOCYTES	MONOCYTE	BLOOD PLATELETS

AGRANULOCYTES

PLASMA CELL
(abnormal)

Neutrophils differ from the other two granulocytes in having smaller and paler granules in the cytoplasm. Nuclei of these leukocytes are characteristically lobulated with thin bridges between the lobules (see figure 30.1). During infections, when many of these are being produced in the bone marrow, the nuclei are horseshoe-shaped; these juvenile cells are often called "stab cells."

Eosinophils, generally, have bilobed nuclei as above; however, juveniles have nuclei that are horseshoe-shaped (figure 30.1). Note that the eosinophilic granules in the cytoplasm are large and pronounced.

Basophils, which are few in number, are distinguished from the other granulocytes by the presence of dark basophilic granules in the cytoplasm. The nuclei of these cells are large and varied in shape. The fact that heparin has been identified in these cells indicates that they probably secrete this substance into the blood.

Two sizes of lymphocytes—large and small— are shown above and in figure 30.1. The small ones, which are more abundant than the large ones, have large, dense nuclei surrounded by a thin layer of basophilic cytoplasm. The large lymphocytes have indented nuclei and more cytoplasm than small lymphocytes.

Blood platelets, which form from megakaryocytes in the bone marrow, function in the formation of blood clots.

Plasma cells are only rarely seen in the blood. The photomicrograph above was made from the blood of a patient with plasma cell leukemia. Although they resemble lymphocytes, the plasma cells have more cytoplasm that is very basophilic.

Figure 30.2 Photomicrographs of formed elements in the blood (5,000×).

In this study of the formed elements we will attempt to determine the percentage of each type of leukocyte on a slide. By scanning an entire slide and counting the various types, you will have an opportunity to encounter most, if not all, types. The erythrocytes and blood platelets will be ignored.

The normal percentage ranges for the various leukocytes are as follows: neutrophils 50–70%, lymphocytes 20–30%, monocytes 2–6%, eosinophils 1–5%, and basophils 0.5–1%. Because of the extremely low percentage of eosinophils and basophils, it is necessary to examine at least 100 leukocytes to increase the possiblity of encountering one or two of them on a slide.

Deviations from the above percentages may indicate serious pathological conditions. High neutrophil counts, or *neutrophilia,* often signal localized infections such as appendicitis or abcesses in some part of the body. *Neutropenia,* a condition in which there is a marked decrease in the number of neutrophils, occurs in typhoid fever, undulant fever, and influenza. *Eosinophilia* (high eosinophil count) may indicate allergic conditions or invasions by parasitic roundworms such as *Trichinella spiralis,* the pork worm. Counts of eosinophils may rise to as much as 50% of total leukocytes in cases of tri-

chinosis. High lymphocyte counts, or *lymphocytosis,* are present in whooping cough and some viral infections. A white cell count which determines the relative percentages of each type of leukocyte is called a **differential white blood cell count.** It is this type of a count that will be performed here in this laboratory period.

If a prepared slide is to be used, ignore the instructions below under the heading of "Preparation of Slide" and proceed to the heading "Performing the Cell Count."

Materials:

prepared blood slide stained with Wright's or Giemsa's stains (H2.851 or H2.852)
for staining a blood smear:
2 or 3 clean microscope slides (polished edges)
sterile disposable lancets
sterile absorbent cotton
Wrights stain
distilled water in dropping bottle
70% alcohol
wax pencil
bibulous paper.

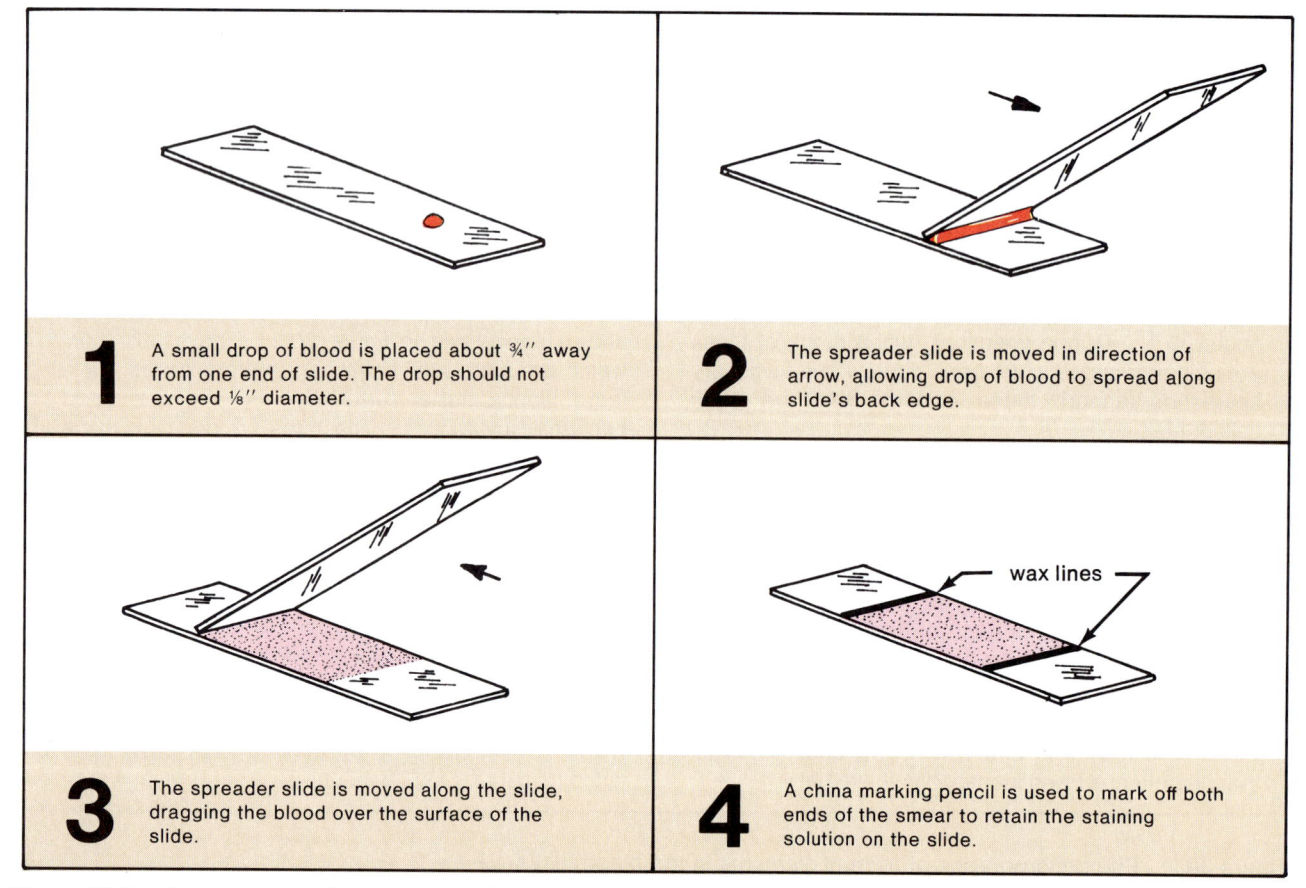

1 A small drop of blood is placed about ¾″ away from one end of slide. The drop should not exceed ⅛″ diameter.

2 The spreader slide is moved in direction of arrow, allowing drop of blood to spread along slide's back edge.

3 The spreader slide is moved along the slide, dragging the blood over the surface of the slide.

4 A china marking pencil is used to mark off both ends of the smear to retain the staining solution on the slide.

wax lines

Figure 30.3 Smear preparation technique for stained blood slide.

Preparation of a Slide

Figure 30.3 illustrates the procedure that will be used to make a stained slide of a blood smear. The most difficult step in making such a slide is getting a good spread of the blood, which is thick at one end and thin at the other end. If done properly, the smear will have a gradient of cellular density that will make it possible to choose an area that is ideal for study. The angle at which the spreading slide is held in making the smear will determine the thickness of the smear. It may be necessary for you to make more than one slide to get an ideal one.

1. Clean three or four slides with soap and water. Handle them with care to avoid getting their flat surfaces dirty with the fingers. Although only two slides may be used, it is often necessary to repeat the spreading process, thus the extra slides.
2. Scrub the middle finger with 70% alcohol and stick it with a lancet. Put a drop of blood on the slide ¾'' from one end and spread with another slide in the manner illustrated in figure 30.4. *Note that the blood is dragged over the slide, not pushed.* Do not pull the slide over the smear a second time. If you don't get an even smear the first time, repeat the process on a fresh clean slide. To get a smear that will be the proper thickness, hold the spreading slide at an angle somewhat greater than 45°.
3. Draw a line on each side of the smear with a wax pencil to confine the stain that is to be added.
4. Cover the film with Wright's stain, *counting the drops* as you add them. Stain for **4 minutes** and then add the same number of drops of distilled water to the stain and let stand for another **10 minutes.** Blow gently on the mixture every few minutes to keep the solutions mixed.

5. Gently wash off the slide under running water for 30 seconds and shake off the excess. Blot dry with bibulous paper.

Performing the Cell Count

Whether you are using a prepared slide or one that you have just stained, the procedure is essentially the same. Ideally, one should use an oil immersion lens for this procedure; high-dry optics can be used, but are not as reliable for best results. Proceed as follows:

1. Scan the slide with the low power objective to find an area where cell distribution is best. A good area is one in which the cells are not jammed together or scattered too far apart.
2. Once an ideal area has been located, place a drop of immersion oil on the slide near one edge and lower the oil immersion objective into the oil. If the high-dry objective is to be used, omit placing oil on the slide.
3. Systematically scan the slide, following the pathway indicated in figure 30.4. As each leukocyte is encountered identify it, using figures 30.1 and 30.2 for reference.

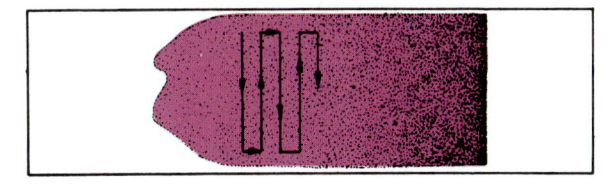

Figure 30.4   The path of the cell count.

4. Tabulate your count on the Laboratory Report sheet according to the instructions there. It is best to remove your Lab Report sheet from the back of the manual for identification and tabulation.

Laboratory Report

Complete the Laboratory Report for this exercise.

31 The Heart

In this study of the anatomy of the human heart we will use a sheep heart for dissection and comparison. Before beginning the dissection, however, study figures 31.1 and 31.2.

Internal Anatomy

Figure 31.1 reveals the internal anatomy of the human heart. Red colored vessels carry oxygenated blood and blue ones carry deoxygenated blood.

Chambers of the Heart

Note that the heart has four chambers: two small upper atria and two larger ventricles. The atria receive all the blood that enters the heart and the ventricles pump it out. Note that the **right atrium** in the frontal section is on the left side of the illustration and the **left atrium** is on the right. Observe, also, that although the **right ventricle** is somewhat larger than the **left ventricle,** the left ventricle has a thicker wall. Separating the two ventricles is a partition, the **ventricular septum.**

Wall of the Heart

The wall of the heart consists of three layers: the myocardium, the endocardium, and the epicardium. The **myocardium** is the muscular portion of the wall that is composed of cardiac muscle tissue. Note in the enlarged section of the wall that the myocardium makes up the bulk of the wall thickness.

Lining the inner surface of the heart is the **endocardium.** It is a thin serous membrane that is continuous with the endothelial lining of the arteries and veins. An infection of this membrane is called *endocarditis.*

Attached to the outer surface of the heart is another serous membrane, the **epicardium,** or **visceral pericardium.** The production of serous fluid by this membrane on the outer surface of the heart enables the heart to move freely within the pericardial sac. Note that the **pericardial sac,** or **parietal pericardium,** consists of two layers: an inner

serous layer and another fibrous layer. Between the heart and the parietal pericardium is the **pericardial cavity** (label 19). Its dimension has been exaggerated here.

Vessels of the Heart

The major vessels of the heart are the two venae cavae, the pulmonary artery, the four pulmonary veins, and the aorta. The **superior vena cava** is the upper blue vessel on the right atrium; it conveys deoxygenated blood to the right atrium from the head and arms. The **inferior vena cava** is the lower blue vessel that empties deoxygenated blood from the trunk and legs into the right atrium. From the right atrium blood passes to the right ventricle, where it leaves the heart through the **pulmonary trunk.** This artery branches into the **right** and **left pulmonary arteries,** which carry blood to the lungs.

Blood is drained from the lungs by means of the four **pulmonary veins** (four small red vessels), which carry it to the left atrium. This blood passes into the left ventricle and finally out through the **aorta.** The initial emergence of the aorta is obscured, but it can be seen as the large red vessel at the top of the heart. The aorta carries oxygenated blood to the systemic circulation.

Note what appears to be a short vessel between the pulmonary trunk and the aorta. It is called the **ligamentum arteriosum.** During prenatal life this ligament is a functional blood vessel, the *ductus arteriosus,* that allows blood to pass from the pulmonary trunk to the aorta.

Valves of the Heart

The heart has two atrioventricular and two semilunar valves. Between the right atrium and the right ventricle is the **tricuspid valve.** Between the left atrium and the left ventricle is the **bicuspid,** or **mitral valve.** The differences between these two valves are seen in the superior sectional view of figure 31.1. Note that the tricuspid valve has three

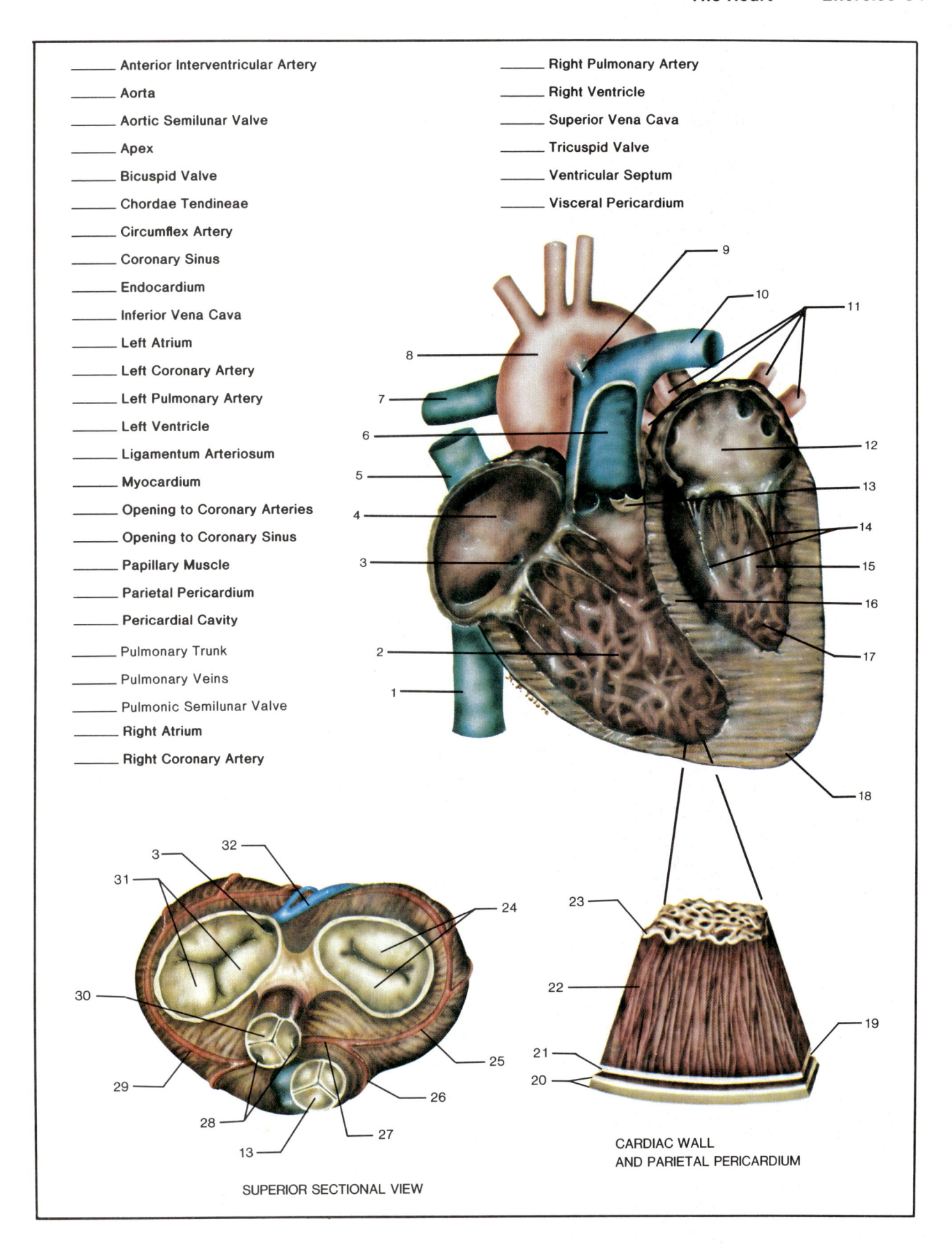

_____ Anterior Interventricular Artery

_____ Aorta

_____ Aortic Semilunar Valve

_____ Apex

_____ Bicuspid Valve

_____ Chordae Tendineae

_____ Circumflex Artery

_____ Coronary Sinus

_____ Endocardium

_____ Inferior Vena Cava

_____ Left Atrium

_____ Left Coronary Artery

_____ Left Pulmonary Artery

_____ Left Ventricle

_____ Ligamentum Arteriosum

_____ Myocardium

_____ Opening to Coronary Arteries

_____ Opening to Coronary Sinus

_____ Papillary Muscle

_____ Parietal Pericardium

_____ Pericardial Cavity

_____ Pulmonary Trunk

_____ Pulmonary Veins

_____ Pulmonic Semilunar Valve

_____ Right Atrium

_____ Right Coronary Artery

_____ Right Pulmonary Artery

_____ Right Ventricle

_____ Superior Vena Cava

_____ Tricuspid Valve

_____ Ventricular Septum

_____ Visceral Pericardium

SUPERIOR SECTIONAL VIEW

CARDIAC WALL AND PARIETAL PERICARDIUM

Figure 31.1 Internal anatomy of the heart.

flaps or cusps, and the bicuspid valve has only two cusps. Observe, also, that the edges of the cusps have fine cords, the **chordae tendineae,** which are anchored to **papillary muscles** on the wall of the heart (see frontal section). These cords and muscles prevent the cusps from being forced up into the atria during systole (ventricular contraction).

The other two valves are the **pulmonic semilunar** and **aortic semilunar valves.** They are located at the bases of the pulmonary trunk and the aorta. They prevent blood in those vessels from flowing back into the heart during diastole (relaxation phase). Note in the superior sectional view that each of these valves has three small cusps.

The Coronary Circulation

The vessels that supply the heart muscle with blood comprise the *coronary circulatory system.* Oxygenated blood in the aorta passes into right and left coronary arteries through two small openings at a point just superior to the aortic semilunar valve. The **openings to the coronary arteries** are seen in the wall of the aorta in the superior sectional view in figure 31.1. The **left coronary artery** has two principal branches: a **circumflex artery** that passes around the heart in the left atrioventricular sulcus and the **anterior interventricular artery,** which lies in the interventricular sulcus on the anterior surface of the heart. The **right coronary artery** lies in the right atrioventricular sulcus and has branches that supply the posterior and anterior surfaces of the ventricular muscle.

Once the coronary blood has been relieved of its oxygen and nutrients, it is picked up by the various veins that parallel the arteries and empty into the **coronary sinus** (label 2, posterior aspect, figure 31.2). Blood in the coronary sinus is emptied into the right atrium. Its point of entry can be seen in the superior and frontal sectional views of figure 31.1.

Assignment:

Label figure 31.1.

External Anatomy

The study of the external anatomy of the heart is relatively simple once the internal anatomy is understood. Figure 31.2 reveals two external views of the heart.

Anterior Aspect

Note that the heart lies within the **mediastinum** at a slight tilt to the left so that the **apex,** or tip of the heart, is somewhat on the left side. The obscured appearance of the coronary vessels in this view is due to the fact that the **parietal pericardium** lies intact over the organ. The clarity of the structures on the posterior view is due to the fact that the parietal pericardium has been removed.

Differentiating the right ventricle from the left ventricle is best determined by locating the *interventricular sulcus* first. This sulcus is the slight depression over the ventricular septum that contains the **anterior interventricular artery** and the **great cardiac vein.** The yellow material seen in the sulcus consists of fatty deposits. The left ventricle is on the left side of the interventricular sulcus, and the right ventricle is to the right of it.

Observe that the aorta forms an **aortic arch** over the heart and descends behind the heart. That part that is near the heart is called the **ascending aorta.** The part that passes down behind the heart is called the **descending aorta.** Only a short portion of the descending aorta is seen at the bottom of the illustration.

Locate the right and left pulmonary arteries that emerge from under the aortic arch. Also, identify the ligamentum arteriosum between the pulmonary trunk and the aorta. The superior vena cava shows up well near the top of the right atrium. Only a short portion of the inferior vena cava is seen at the bottom of this view. The **right coronary artery** and the **small cardiac vein** are visible in the atrioventricular sulcus.

Posterior Aspect

The posterior view of the heart in figure 31.2 reveals more clearly the position of the four pulmonary veins. The two right pulmonary veins are located near the venae cavae. Note how close together the venae cavae are located. The appearance of a single blue vessel lying below the aorta is actually the site of division of the pulmonary trunk into right and left pulmonary arteries.

The following coronary arteries are seen on this side of the heart: (1) the **right coronary artery,** which lies in the right atrioventricular sulcus; (2) the **posterior descending right coronary artery,** which is the downward extension of the right coronary artery; (3) the **posterior interventricular artery** (label 1); and (4) the **circumflex artery.**

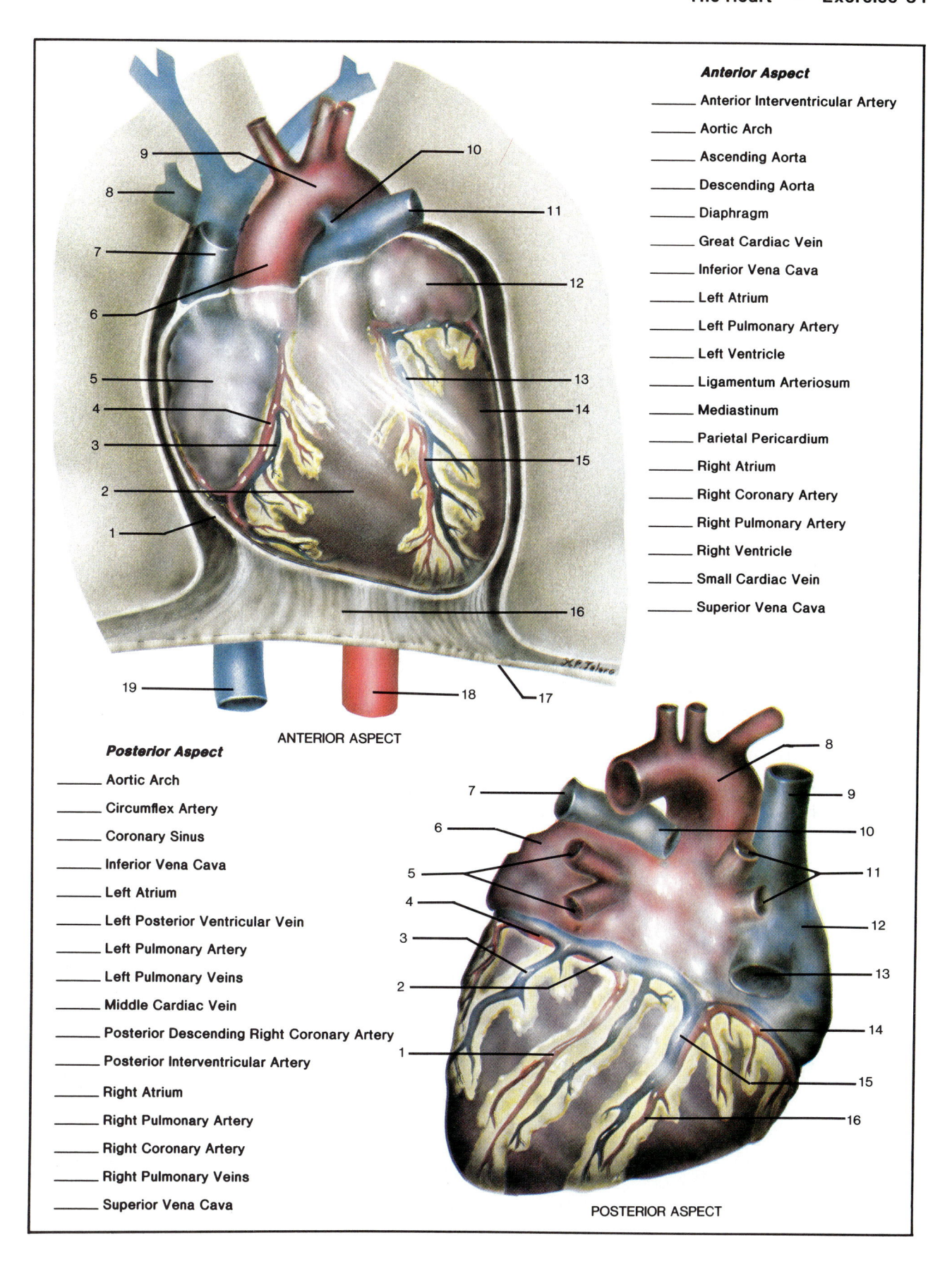

Figure 31.2 External anatomy of the heart.

Anterior Aspect

_____ Anterior Interventricular Artery
_____ Aortic Arch
_____ Ascending Aorta
_____ Descending Aorta
_____ Diaphragm
_____ Great Cardiac Vein
_____ Inferior Vena Cava
_____ Left Atrium
_____ Left Pulmonary Artery
_____ Left Ventricle
_____ Ligamentum Arteriosum
_____ Mediastinum
_____ Parietal Pericardium
_____ Right Atrium
_____ Right Coronary Artery
_____ Right Pulmonary Artery
_____ Right Ventricle
_____ Small Cardiac Vein
_____ Superior Vena Cava

ANTERIOR ASPECT

Posterior Aspect

_____ Aortic Arch
_____ Circumflex Artery
_____ Coronary Sinus
_____ Inferior Vena Cava
_____ Left Atrium
_____ Left Posterior Ventricular Vein
_____ Left Pulmonary Artery
_____ Left Pulmonary Veins
_____ Middle Cardiac Vein
_____ Posterior Descending Right Coronary Artery
_____ Posterior Interventricular Artery
_____ Right Atrium
_____ Right Pulmonary Artery
_____ Right Coronary Artery
_____ Right Pulmonary Veins
_____ Superior Vena Cava

POSTERIOR ASPECT

The major coronary veins on this side are (1) the **middle cardiac vein,** which parallels the posterior descending right coronary artery; (2) the **left posterior ventricular vein** (label 3); and (3) the **posterior interventricular vein.** All these coronary veins empty into the **coronary sinus** (label 2).

Assignment:

Label figure 31.2.

Sheep Heart Dissection

While dissecting the sheep heart, attempt to identify as many structures as possible that are shown in figures 31.1 and 31.2.

Materials:

sheep heart, fresh or preserved
dissecting instruments and tray

1. Rinse the heart with cold water to remove excess preservative or blood. Allow water to flow through the large vessels to irrigate any blood clots out of its chambers.
2. Look for evidence of the **parietal pericardium.** This fibroserous membrane is usually absent from laboratory specimens, but there may be remnants of it attached to the large blood vessels of the heart.
3. Attempt to isolate the **visceral pericardium** (*epicardium*) from the outer surface of the heart. Since it consists of only one layer of squamous cells, it is very thin. With a sharp

scalpel try to peel a small portion of it away from the myocardium.

4. Identify the **right** and **left ventricles** by squeezing the walls of the heart as shown in illustration 1, figure 31.3. The right ventricle will have the thinner wall.
5. Identify the **anterior interventricular sulcus** (between the two ventricles), which is usually covered with fatty tissue. Carefully trim away the fat in this sulcus to expose the **anterior interventricular artery** and the **great cardiac vein.**
6. Locate the **right** and **left atria** of the heart. The right atrium is seen on the left side of illustration 1, figure 31.3.
7. Identify the **aorta,** which is the large vessel just to the right of the right atrium as seen in illustration 1, figure 31.3. Carefully peel away some of the fat around the aorta to expose the **ligamentum arteriosum.**
8. Locate the **pulmonary trunk** which is the large vessel between the aorta and the left atrium as seen when looking at the anterior side of the heart. If the vessel is of sufficient length, trace it to where it divides into the **right** and **left pulmonary arteries.**
9. Examine the posterior surface of the heart. It should appear as in illustration 2, figure 31.3. Note that only the right atrium and two ventricles can be seen on this side. The left atrium is obscured by fat from this aspect. Look for the four thin-walled **pulmonary veins** that are embedded in the fat. Probe into these vessels and you will see that they lead into the left atrium.

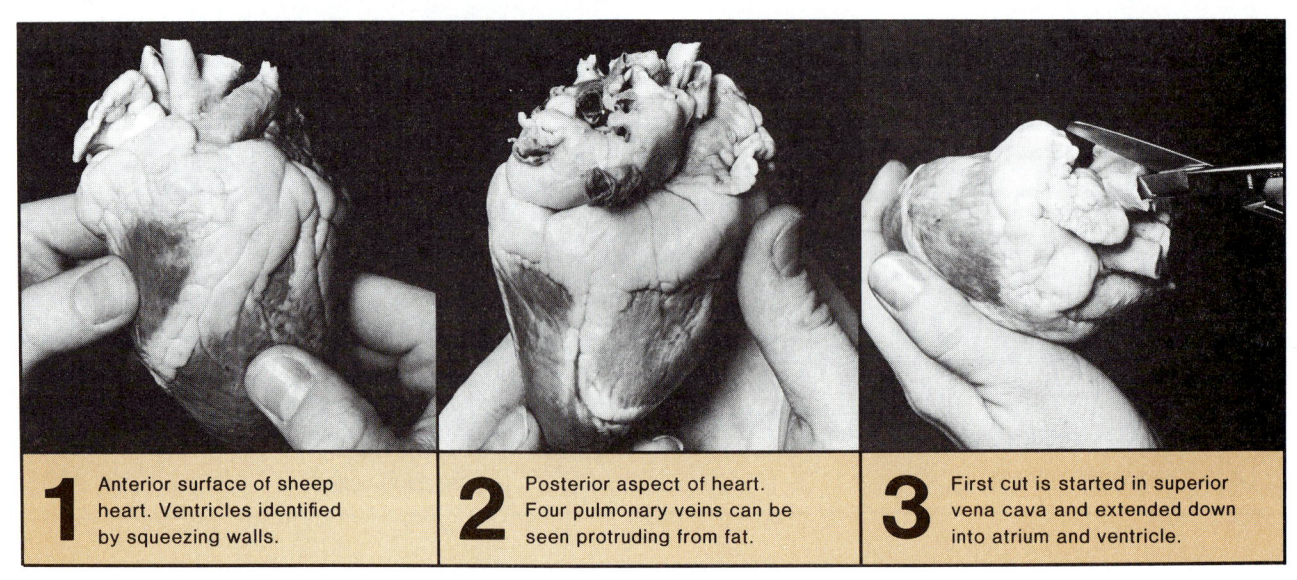

1 Anterior surface of sheep heart. Ventricles identified by squeezing walls.

2 Posterior aspect of heart. Four pulmonary veins can be seen protruding from fat.

3 First cut is started in superior vena cava and extended down into atrium and ventricle.

Figure 31.3 Sheep heart dissection.

10. Locate the **superior vena cava,** which is attached to the upper part of the right atrium. Insert one blade of your dissecting scissors into this vessel (illustration 3, figure 31.3), and cut through it into the atrium to expose the **tricuspid valve** between the right atrium and right ventricle. Don't cut into the ventricle at this time.

11. Fill the right ventricle with water, pouring it in through the tricuspid valve. Gently squeeze the walls of the ventricle to note the closing action of the valve's cusps.

12. Drain the water from the heart and continue the cut with scissors from the right atrium through the tricuspid valve down to the apex of the heart.

13. Open the heart and flush it again with cold water. Examine the interior. The open heart should look like illustration 1, figure 31.4.

14. Examine the interior wall of the right atrium. This inner surface has ridges, giving it a comb-like appearance; thus, it is called **pectinate muscle** (*pecten,* comb). Between the inferior vena cava and the tricuspid valve you should see the **opening to the coronary sinus.** It is through this opening that blood of the coronary circulation is returned to the venous circulation. This opening can be seen in illustration 1, figure 31.4.

15. Insert a probe under the cusps of the mitral valve. Are you able to see three flaps?

16. Locate the **papillary muscles** and **chordae tendineae.** How many papillary muscles do you

see in the right ventricle? Identify the **moderator band,** which is a reinforcement cord between the ventricular septum and the ventricular wall. Its presence prevents excessive stress from occurring in the myocardium of the right ventricle.

17. With scissors, cut the right ventricular wall up along its lower margin parallel to the anterior interventricular sulcus to the pulmonary trunk. Continue the cut through the exit of the right ventricle into the pulmonary artery. Spread the cut surfaces of this new incision to expose the **pulmonic semilunar valve.** Wash the area with cold water to dispel blood clots.

18. Insert one blade of your scissors into the left atrium, as shown in illustration 2, figure 31.4. Cut through the atrium into the left ventricle. Also, cut from the left ventricle into the aorta, slitting this vessel longitudinally.

19. Examine the **bicuspid** (mitral) **valve,** which lies between the left atrium and left ventricle. With a probe, identify the two cusps.

20. Examine the pouches of the **aortic semilunar valve.** Compare the number of pouches of this valve with the pulmonic valve.

21. Look for the two **openings to the coronary arteries,** which are in the walls of the aorta just above the aortic semilunar valve. Force a blunt probe into each hole. Note how they lead into the two coronary arteries.

Laboratory Report

Complete the Laboratory Report for this exercise.

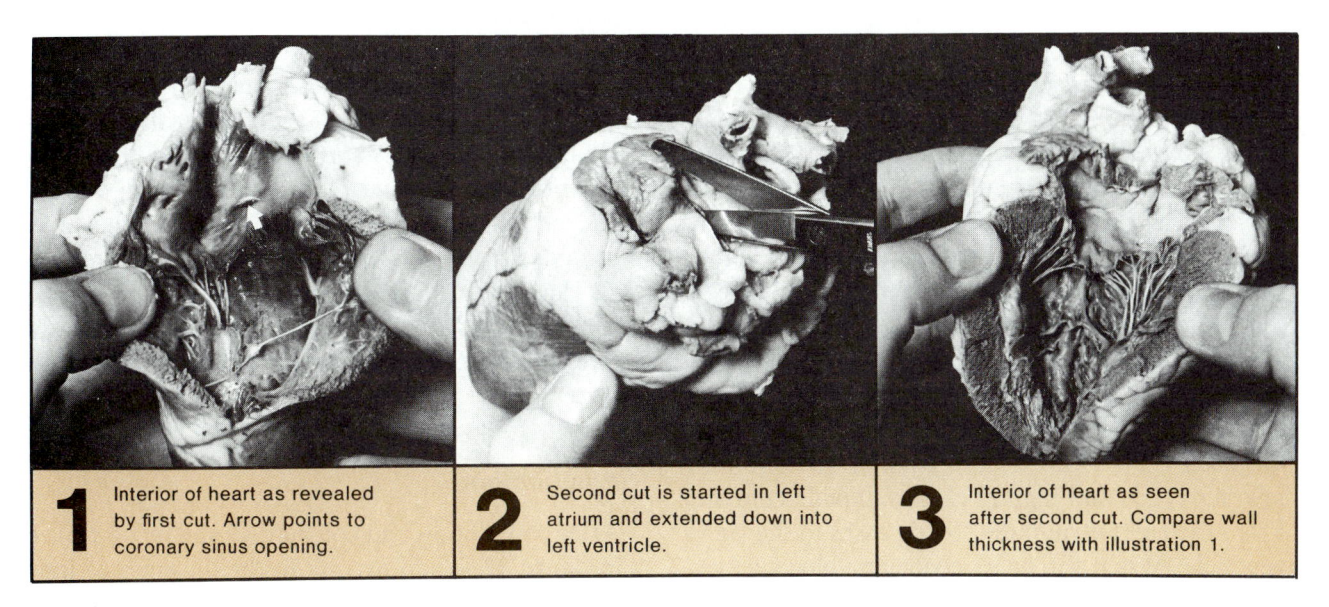

1. Interior of heart as revealed by first cut. Arrow points to coronary sinus opening.

2. Second cut is started in left atrium and extended down into left ventricle.

3. Interior of heart as seen after second cut. Compare wall thickness with illustration 1.

Figure 31.4 Sheep heart dissection.

32 The Arteries and Veins

In this exercise, we will study the general plan of circulation of the blood. First, by completing the diagram in figure 32.1, the general direction of blood flow will be determined. This will be followed by a more detailed study of the specific arteries and veins in all parts of the body. Once the arteries and veins of figures 32.2 and 32.3 have been identified, the circulatory system of the cat will be studied. In most respects its circulatory system is much like the human. It is essential that figures 32.1, 32.2, and 32.3 be completely labeled prior to beginning the cat study.

The Circulatory Plan

Figure 32.1 is an incomplete flow diagram of the heart and major regions of the body. The problem of this assignment is to connect the blood vessels of the heart with the various organs and regions so that all parts are properly supplied and drained of blood. After all the blood vessels have been drawn in, those that contain oxygenated blood should be **colored with red** and those with deoxygenated blood should be **colored blue.** The following description explains the circulatory plan.

The circulatory system consists of three separate circuits, or "systems": the pulmonary, systemic, and coronary. The *pulmonary system* carries blood from the heart through the lungs and back to the heart. The *systemic system* supplied blood to all parts of the body except the lungs and heart muscle. The *coronary system* is the shortest circuit which supplies only the myocardium of the heart. Figure 32.1 shows only the pulmonary and systemic circuits.

Blood enters the right atrium (left side of illustration) from the **superior** and **inferior venae cavae,** which have collected blood from all parts of the body. This blood is dark colored because it is low in oxygen and high in carbon dioxide content. From the right atrium the blood passes to the right ventricle. When the heart contracts, blood leaves the right ventricle through the **pulmonary trunk** to the lungs, where it picks up oxygen and gives off

carbon dioxide. The blood leaves the lungs by way of the **pulmonary veins** and passes back to the left atrium of the heart. Blood in the pulmonary veins is brightly colored due to its high oxygen content. The pulmonary arteries, veins, and capillaries constitute the *pulmonary system.* The systemic circulatory system includes the remainder of the circulatory system discussed in the next two paragraphs.

From the left atrium the blood passes to the left ventricle. When the heart contracts, blood leaves the left ventricle through the **aortic arch.** This blood, which is rich in oxygen, passes to all parts of the body. The aortic arch has branches that go to the head and arms. (For simplicity, only one blood vessel is shown passing to these regions.) Passing downward on the right side of the illustration, the aortic arch becomes the **aorta,** which has branches going to the liver, digestive organs, kidneys, pelvis, and legs. The branch that enters the liver is the **hepatic artery.** The intestines are supplied by the **superior mesenteric artery,** and the kidneys receive blood through the **renal arteries.** The pelvis and legs are supplied by several arteries, but only one is shown for simplicity.

The blood leaving most of the organs of the trunk empties directly into a large collecting vein, the inferior vena cava. The **renal veins** from the kidneys and **hepatic vein** from the liver empty into the inferior vena cava. Several veins drain the legs and pelvic region. Blood from the intestines does not go directly to the inferior vena cava; instead, all blood from this region passes to the liver by way of the **portal vein.** This route of the blood from the intestines to the liver is called the *portal circulation.*

Assignment:

After completing and coloring all the blood vessels in figure 32.1, add arrows to the diagram to indicate the direction of blood flow. Label all blood vessels, also.

The Arterial Division

The principal arteries of the body are shown in the left hand illustration of figure 32.2. Blood leaving the left ventricle of the heart is carried in a large curved artery, the **aortic arch.** From the upper surface of this vessel emerge three arteries: the left subclavian, the left common carotid, and the brachiocephalic artery.

The **left subclavian** artery is the artery that passes from the aortic arch into the left shoulder behind the clavicle. In the armpit (*axilla*) the subclavian becomes the **axillary** artery. The axillary, in turn, becomes the **brachial** artery in the upper arm. This latter artery divides into the radial and ulnar arteries in the forearm. The **radial** artery follows the radial bone and the **ulnar** artery follows the ulnar bone.

The **brachiocephalic** (innominate) artery is the short vessel coming off the aortic arch on the right side of the body. It gives rise to two arteries. The branch that extends upward to the head is the **right**

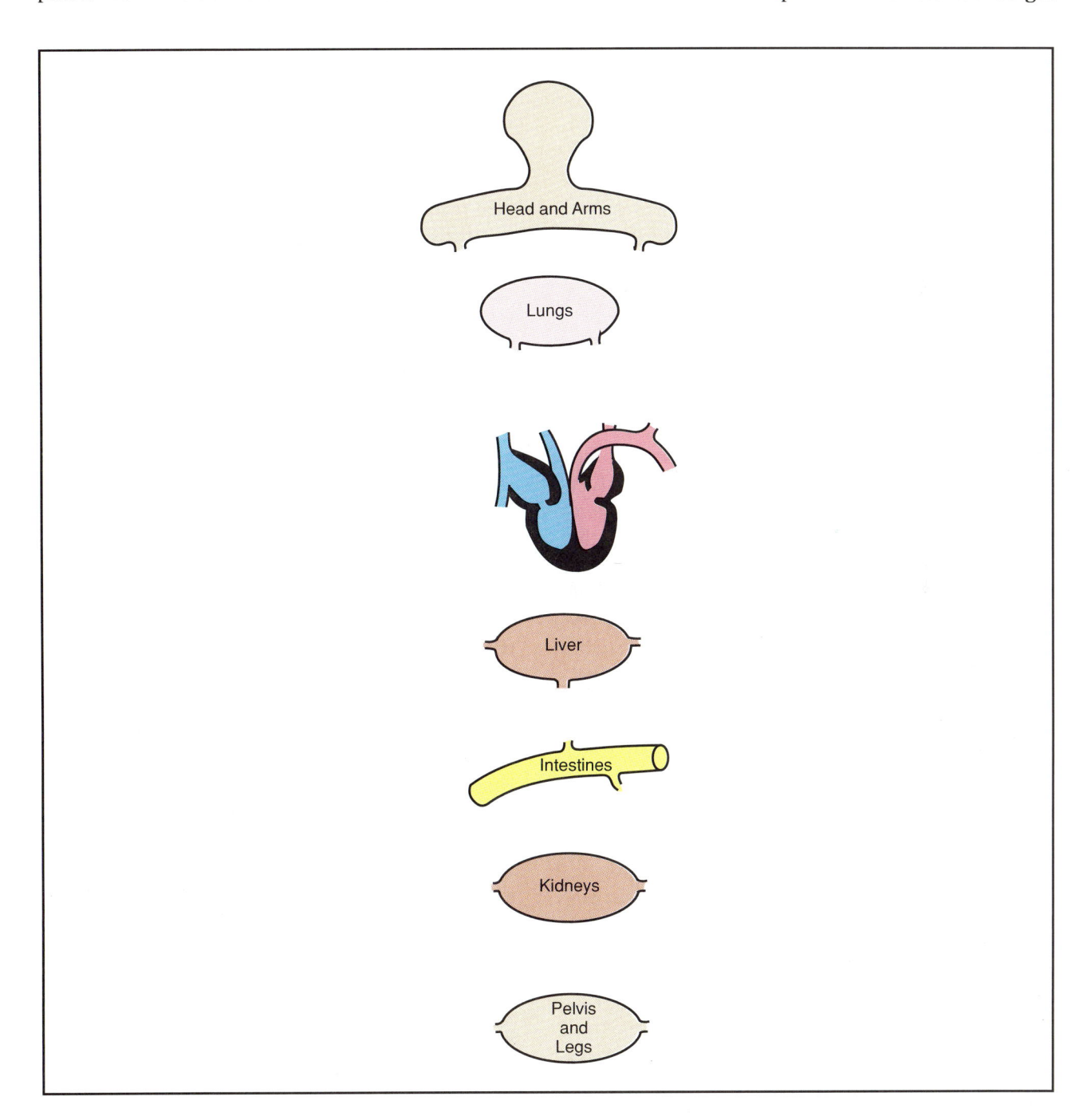

Figure 32.1 The circulatory plan.

common carotid artery. It furnishes the right side of the head with blood. The **right subclavian** artery is an outward extension of the brachiocephalic artery from the base of the right common carotid. It passes behind the right clavicle.

The third branch of the aortic arch is the **left common carotid.** It supplies the left side of the head with oxygenated blood.

As it passes down through the thorax, the aortic arch becomes the **descending aorta.** Although the aorta has many branches leading to various organs, only the larger ones are shown in figure 32.2. The first branch, emerging just below the heart, is the **celiac** artery. It supplies the stomach, liver, and spleen. Just below the celiac is the **superior mesenteric** artery, which supplies most of the small intestine and part of the large intestine. Inferior to the superior mesenteric are a pair of **renal** arteries that supply the kidneys. The single branch of the aorta just below the renals is the **inferior mesenteric** artery, which supplies part of the large intestine and rectum with blood.

In the lumbar region the aorta divides into the right and left **common iliac** arteries. Each common iliac passes downward a short distance and then divides into a smaller inner branch, the **internal iliac** (hypogastric) artery, and a larger branch, the **external iliac** artery, which continues on down into the leg. The external iliac becomes the **femoral** artery in the upper three-fourths of the thigh. In the general region of the origin of the femoral artery, the **deep femoral** branches off of it. This artery courses backward and downward along the medial surface of the femur. In the knee region the femoral becomes the **popliteal** artery. Just below the knee the popliteal divides into the **posterior tibial** and **anterior tibial** arteries.

Assignment:

Label the arterial portion of figure 32.2.

The Venous Division

Starting at the heart in figure 32.2, we see the **superior vena cava** emptying into the upper part of the right atrium and the **inferior vena cava** leading into the lower part of the right atrium.

In the neck region are seen four veins: two medial **internal jugular** veins and two smaller lateral **external jugulars.** The internal jugulars empty into the brachiocephalic veins and the externals

empty into the subclavian veins. The **brachiocephalic** veins are the short veins that empty into the superior vena cava.

Three veins, the cephalic, basilic, and brachial, collect blood in the upper arm. The **cephalic** vein courses along the lateral aspect of the arm and empties into the **axillary** vein. The **basilic** lies on the medial side of the arm, and the **brachial** lies along the posterior surface of the humerus. Both the basilic and brachial empty into a short **axillary** vein that becomes the **subclavian** in the shoulder region. Between the basilic and cephalic veins in the elbow region is seen the **median cubital** vein. An **accessory cephalic** vein lies on the lateral portion of the forearm and empties into the cephalic in the elbow region.

Blood in the legs is returned to the heart by superficial and deep sets of veins. The superficial veins are just beneath the skin. The deep veins accompany the arteries. Both sets are provided with valves which are more numerous in the deep ones. The **posterior tibial** vein (label 24) is one of the deep veins that lies behind the tibia. It collects blood from the calf and foot. In the knee region the posterior tibial vein becomes the **popliteal** vein. Above the knee this vessel becomes the **femoral** vein, which, in turn, empties into the **external iliac** vein in the upper leg region. The external and **internal iliac** (label 11) empty into the **common iliac** vein. The inferior vena cava, thus, receives blood from the two common iliacs, renal veins, and many others not shown in this diagram.

A large superficial vein of the leg, the **great saphenous,** originates from the **dorsal venous arch** on the superior surface of the foot, and enters the femoral vein at the top of the thigh.

Although many short veins empty into the inferior vena cava, only the hepatic, renals, and spermatics are shown in figure 32.2. The **hepatic** is the short one just under the heart that contains blood from the liver. The two **renals** are inferior to the hepatic. Note that the left renal has a branch, the **left spermatic** (or **left ovarian**) that carries blood away from the left testis or ovary. The **right spermatic** (or **right ovarian**) empties into the inferior vena cava at a point just inferior to where the right renal vein joins the inferior vena cava.

The presence of valves in veins can be vividly demonstrated on the back of your own hand. If you apply pressure to a prominent vein on the back of your left hand near the knuckles with the middle

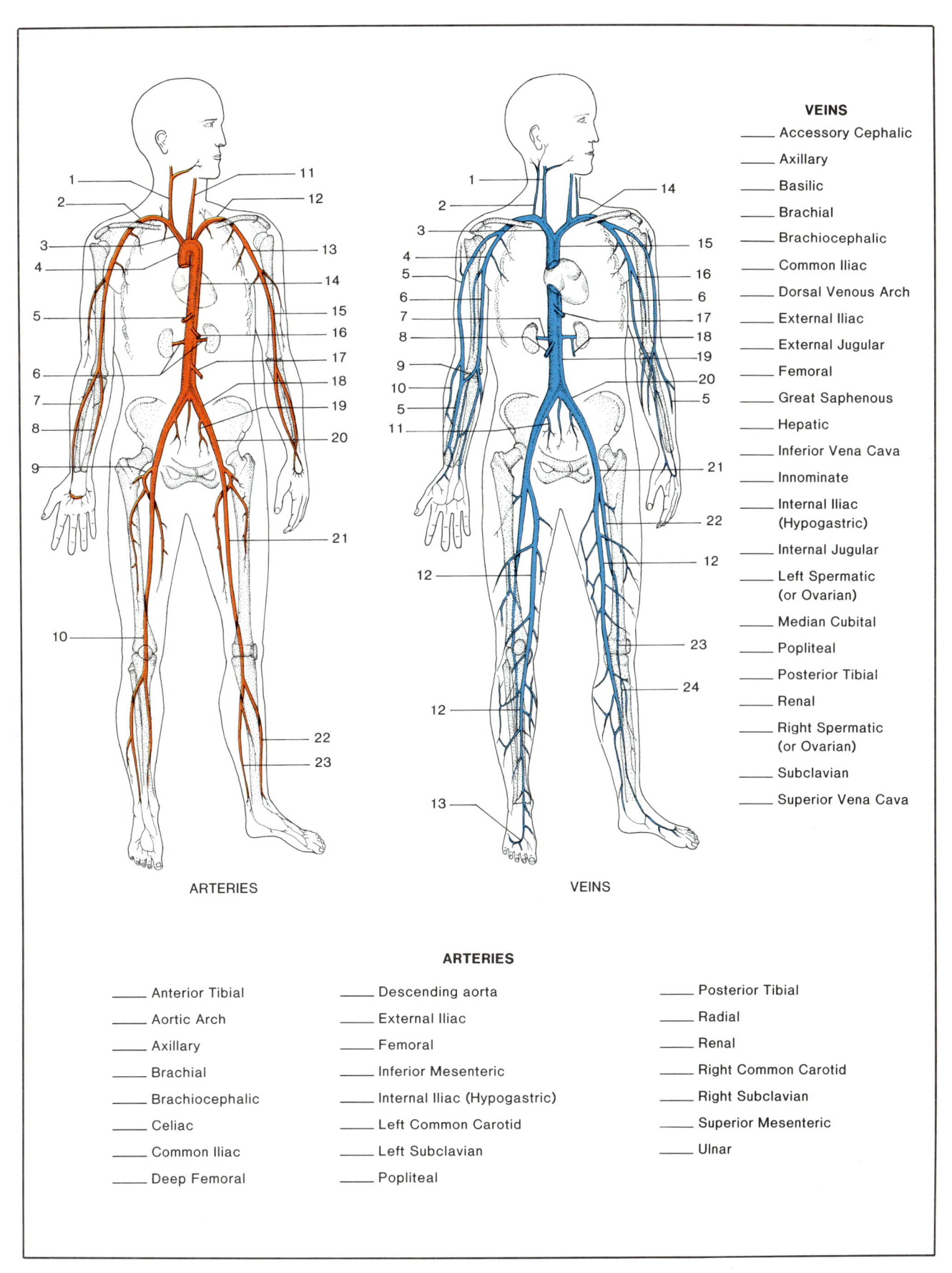

Figure 32.2 Arteries and veins.

VEINS

_____ Accessory Cephalic
_____ Axillary
_____ Basilic
_____ Brachial
_____ Brachiocephalic
_____ Common Iliac
_____ Dorsal Venous Arch
_____ External Iliac
_____ External Jugular
_____ Femoral
_____ Great Saphenous
_____ Hepatic
_____ Inferior Vena Cava
_____ Innominate
_____ Internal Iliac (Hypogastric)
_____ Internal Jugular
_____ Left Spermatic (or Ovarian)
_____ Median Cubital
_____ Popliteal
_____ Posterior Tibial
_____ Renal
_____ Right Spermatic (or Ovarian)
_____ Subclavian
_____ Superior Vena Cava

ARTERIES

VEINS

ARTERIES

_____ Anterior Tibial
_____ Aortic Arch
_____ Axillary
_____ Brachial
_____ Brachiocephalic
_____ Celiac
_____ Common Iliac
_____ Deep Femoral

_____ Descending aorta
_____ External Iliac
_____ Femoral
_____ Inferior Mesenteric
_____ Internal Iliac (Hypogastric)
_____ Left Common Carotid
_____ Left Subclavian
_____ Popliteal

_____ Posterior Tibial
_____ Radial
_____ Renal
_____ Right Common Carotid
_____ Right Subclavian
_____ Superior Mesenteric
_____ Ulnar

finger of your right hand and then strip the blood in the vein away from the point of pressure with your index finger, you will note that blood does not flow back toward the point of pressure. This indicates that valves prevent backward flow.

Assignment:

Label the veins in figure 32.2.

Portal Circulation

Figure 32.3 reveals the venous system that comprises the human portal circulation. All the veins shown here from the stomach, spleen, pancreas, and intestine drain into the **portal** vein (label 2) which empties into the liver. Figure 32.4 is of the same system in the cat.

The large vessel that collects blood from the ascending colon (label 4) and the ileum (label 5) is the **superior mesenteric** vein. It empties directly into the portal vein. Blood from the descending colon (label 7) and rectum is collected by the **inferior mesenteric,** which empties into the **splenic,** or *lienal,* vein. The latter blood vessel parallels the length of the pancreas, receiving blood from the pancreas via several short **pancreatic** veins. Near the spleen, the

splenic vein also receives blood from the stomach through the **short gastric** vein.

From the stomach a venous loop empties blood from the medial surface of the stomach into the portal vein. The upper portion of the loop is the **coronary** vein; the lower portion is the **pyloric vein.**

Assignment:

Label figure 32.3.

Cat Dissection

To facilitate differentiation of arteries and veins in the cat, the animal has been injected with red and blue latex: red for arteries and blue for veins. When tracing blood vessels it is necessary that each vessel be freed from adjacent tissue so that it is clearly visible. A sharp dissecting needle is indispensable for this purpose. It is essential, however, that considerable care be taken to avoid accidental severance of the blood vessels. Once they are cut they become difficult to follow.

In this study of the arteries and veins it will be necessary to refer to illustrations in other portions of this manual that pertain to other organ systems. By the time you have completed this circulatory study you should be familiar with the respiratory,

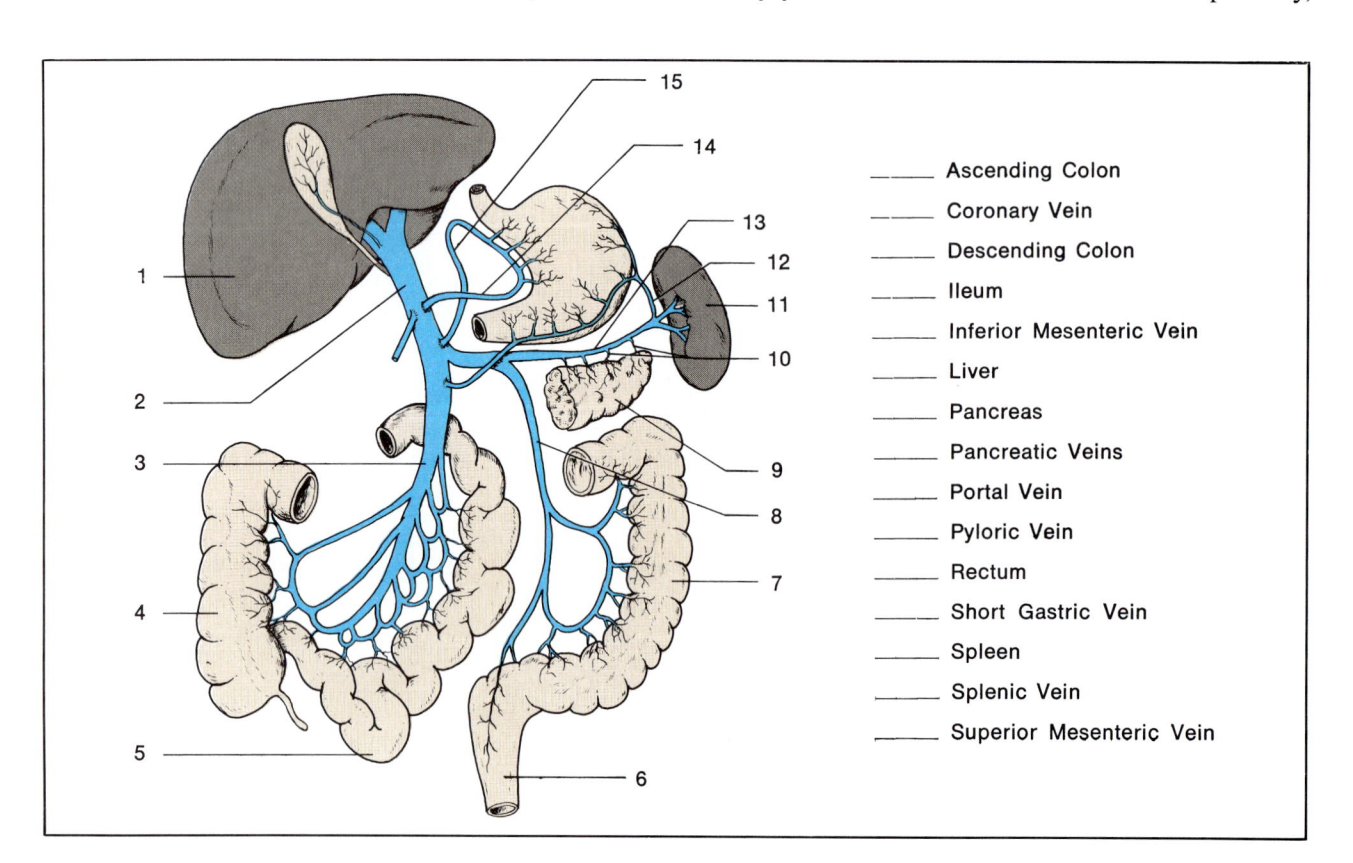

_____ Ascending Colon
_____ Coronary Vein
_____ Descending Colon
_____ Ileum
_____ Inferior Mesenteric Vein
_____ Liver
_____ Pancreas
_____ Pancreatic Veins
_____ Portal Vein
_____ Pyloric Vein
_____ Rectum
_____ Short Gastric Vein
_____ Spleen
_____ Splenic Vein
_____ Superior Mesenteric Vein

Figure 32.3 Portal circulation, human.

digestive, excretory, and reproductive organs of the cat. Great care should be taken, however, to avoid damaging the organs of the various systems at this time since they will be required for later study.

Exposing the Organs

Open up the ventral surface of the animal by starting a longitudinal incision in the thoracic wall that is about one centimeter to the right or left of midline. This cut should pass through the rib cartilages and is easily performed with a sharp scalpel or scissors. Extend the incision, cranially, to the apex of the thorax and, posteriorly, to the pubic region. In addition, make two lateral cuts caudal to the diaphragm.

Spread apart the walls of the thorax to expose its viscera. Greater exposure can be achieved by cutting away part of the chest wall on each side, using heavy-duty scissors to break through the ribs. In addition, trim away portions of the abdominal wall on each side of the original longitudinal incision to expose the abdominal organs.

Organ Identification

By comparing your dissection with figure 35.4 identify the **lungs, thymus gland, thyroid gland, dia-**

phragm, trachea, and larynx. In addition, squeeze the surface of the **heart** with your thumb and fore-finger, noting the thickness and texture of the **pericardium** that envelops it. Remove the pericardium to expose the vessels on the heart. Now, refer to figure 36.9 to identify the **liver, stomach, spleen, pancreas,** and the various portions of the **small** and **large intestines.**

Veins of the Thorax

Since the veins of the thoracic region lie over most of the arteries, it is best to study them first. By referring to figures 32.5 and 32.6 identify the veins in the following sequence.

Veins Entering the Heart

The **superior vena cava, inferior vena cava,** and three groups of **pulmonary veins** empty blood into the heart. Only the superior vena cava is shown in figure 32.6. Probe around the heart to find all these vessels. Each group of pulmonary veins, which empty into the left atrium, is composed of two or three veins.

Veins Emptying into the Superior Vena Cava

Locate the **azygous** vein. It is a large vein that empties into the dorsal surface of the superior vena

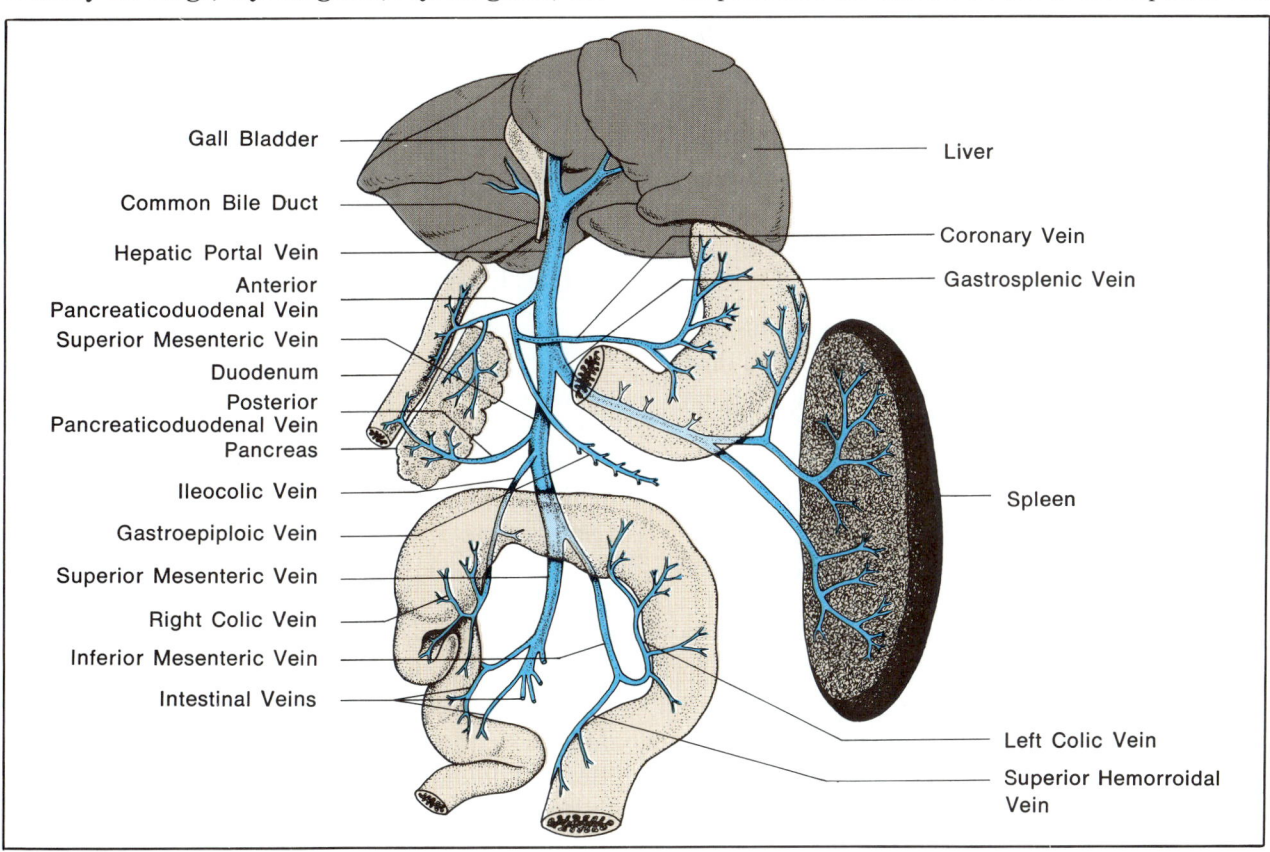

Figure 32.4   Portal circulation, cat.

cava (s.v.c.) close to where the s.v.c. enters the right atrium of the heart. Since it is obscured by the heart and lungs, it will be necessary to force these organs to the left to locate it. Note that this vein lies along the right side of the vertebral column, collecting blood from the **intercostal, esophageal,** and **bronchial** veins. Trace the azygous vein to these branches.

Identify the **internal mammary** (*sternal*) vein which enters the s.v.c. opposite the third rib.

Examine the dorsal surface of the s.v.c. to identify the spot where the **right vertebral** and **right costocervical** veins enter it. These two veins unite to form a short vessel before entering the s.v.c. A stub of this vessel, labeled VE, is shown in figure 32.6. Note that the **left costocervical** vein is shown entering the left innominate vein in figure 32.6. A short stub of the left vertebral is also shown joining the left costocervical.

Identify the **right** and **left brachiocephalic** veins (BC) that empty into the s.v.c. These veins receive blood from the head and arms.

Veins that Drain into the Brachiocephalic Veins

Note that the right brachiocephalic receives blood from two vessels, and the left brachiocephalic from four veins. The **external jugular** and **subclavian** veins empty into both brachiocephalics. The left brachiocephalic receives blood also from the **left vertebral** and **left costocervical.** Identify all of these vessels on your specimen.

Vessels that Drain into the External Jugulars

The principal veins that empty into the external jugulars are the **transverse scapular** and **internal jugulars.** Locate them first in figure 31.6, and then on your specimen. Note that the internal jugulars parallel the common carotid arteries.

Refer to figure 32.5 to locate the **transverse jugular** vein that connects the two external jugular veins in the chin region; then, identify it on your specimen. Locate also, the **posterior** and **anterior facial** veins in figure 32.5.

The **thoracic duct,** a part of the lymphatic system, also empties into the external jugular vein. Its point of entrance is very close to where the left external jugular enters the left subclavian. This vessel is difficult to find. It will be necessary to push the left lung to the right and look at the back of the left thoracic cavity near the vertebral column

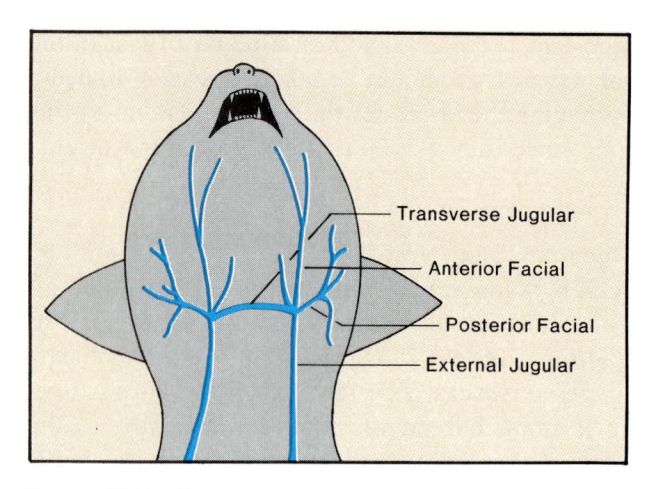

Figure 32.5 External jugular vein branches.

to find it. It has a beaded structure due to the presence of valves.

Veins Emptying into the Subclavian Vein

The principal veins that empty into the subclavian are the **subscapular** and **axillary.** Locate them on your specimen. Note that the axillary receives blood from the **thoracodorsal** and **brachial** veins. Locate them, also.

Arteries of the Thorax

Once you have identified the veins of the thorax you can study the arteries by gingerly manipulating the veins to one side. Do not cut away the veins, however. By referring to figures 32.7 and 32.8 identify the arteries as follows:

Arteries Emerging from the Heart

Locate the **aortic arch** and **pulmonary trunk** by referring to figure 32.7. Trace the pulmonary trunk to where it divides into the right and left pulmonary arteries.

Dissect away the connective tissue at the base of the aorta to locate the coronary arteries. Note their pathways on the surface of the heart.

Branches of the Aortic Arch

Note that in the cat there are only two branches emerging from the upper surface of the aortic arch: the **brachiocephalic** and the **left subclavian.** How does this compare with humans? Note, also, that the **right common carotid, right subclavian,** and **left common carotid** arteries branch off the brachiocephalic.

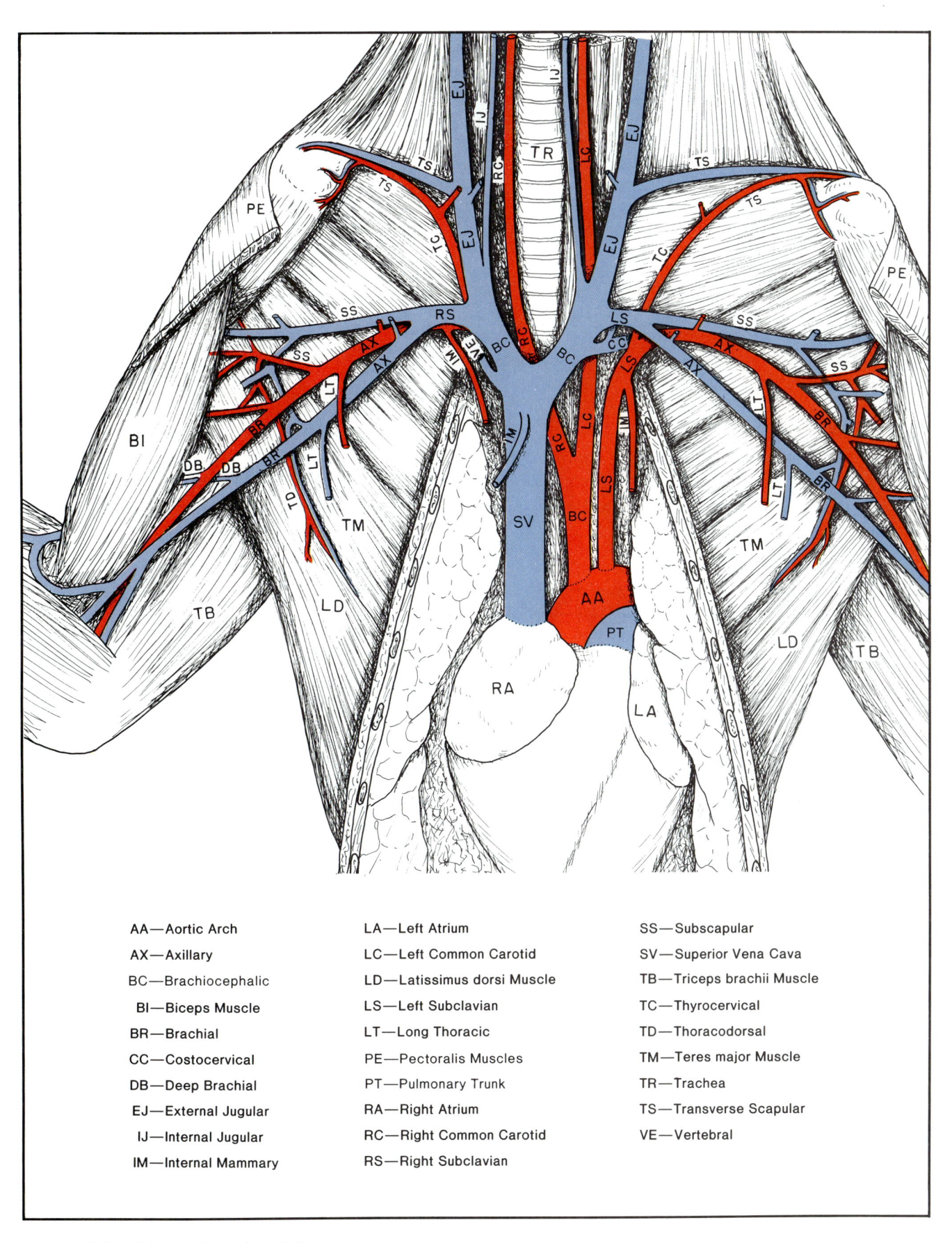

Figure 32.6 Veins and arteries of thorax.

AA—Aortic Arch

AX—Axillary

BC—Brachiocephalic

BI—Biceps Muscle

BR—Brachial

CC—Costocervical

DB—Deep Brachial

EJ—External Jugular

IJ—Internal Jugular

IM—Internal Mammary

LA—Left Atrium

LC—Left Common Carotid

LD—Latissimus dorsi Muscle

LS—Left Subclavian

LT—Long Thoracic

PE—Pectoralis Muscles

PT—Pulmonary Trunk

RA—Right Atrium

RC—Right Common Carotid

RS—Right Subclavian

SS—Subscapular

SV—Superior Vena Cava

TB—Triceps brachii Muscle

TC—Thyrocervical

TD—Thoracodorsal

TM—Teres major Muscle

TR—Trachea

TS—Transverse Scapular

VE—Vertebral

Branches of the Subclavian Arteries

Locate the vertebral, costocervical, internal mammary, and the thyrocervical arteries that branch off the subclavian arteries. The **vertebral** carries blood to the brain, passing through the transverse foramina of the cervical vertebrae.

The **costocervical** supplies blood to deep muscles of the back and neck. The **internal mammary** arteries supply the ventral body wall, and the **thyrocervical** arteries supply blood to the neck and shoulder.

Note that the thyrocervical becomes the **transverse scapular** and that the subclavian becomes the **axillary.** The axillary eventually becomes the **brachial** artery in the arm.

Branches of the Axillary Artery

Identify the **ventral thoracic, long thoracic,** and **subscapular** arteries that branch off the axillary artery. These branches supply blood to the latissimus dorsi and pectoral muscles.

Note that the subscapular becomes the **thoracodorsal** artery, and the axillary becomes the **brachial.** If the brachial is followed down past the elbow it becomes the **radial** artery.

Branches of Each Common Carotid

Each common carotid has an inferior and a superior thyroid artery. The **inferior thyroid** is a small vessel that originates near the base of the common carotid. Probe around this area to locate it. The **superior thyroid** is shown in figure 32.9. Locate this one also.

If your specimen is properly injected you should be able to locate the **occipital, external carotid,** and **internal carotid** that branch off the common carotid.

Branches of the Thoracic Aorta

Pull the viscera of the thorax to the right to expose the aorta in the thoracic cavity. Since the aorta lies

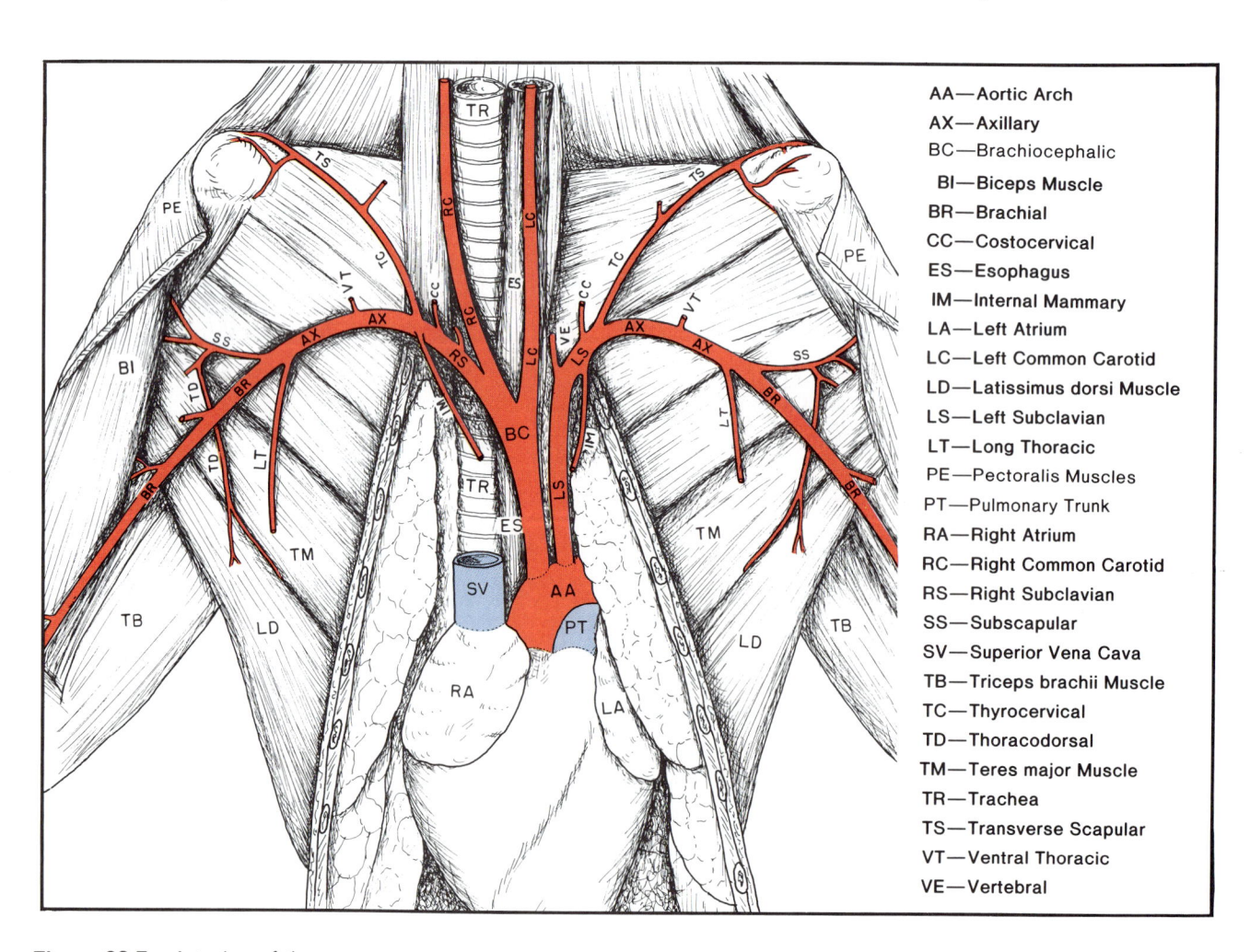

AA—Aortic Arch
AX—Axillary
BC—Brachiocephalic
BI—Biceps Muscle
BR—Brachial
CC—Costocervical
ES—Esophagus
IM—Internal Mammary
LA—Left Atrium
LC—Left Common Carotid
LD—Latissimus dorsi Muscle
LS—Left Subclavian
LT—Long Thoracic
PE—Pectoralis Muscles
PT—Pulmonary Trunk
RA—Right Atrium
RC—Right Common Carotid
RS—Right Subclavian
SS—Subscapular
SV—Superior Vena Cava
TB—Triceps brachii Muscle
TC—Thyrocervical
TD—Thoracodorsal
TM—Teres major Muscle
TR—Trachea
TS—Transverse Scapular
VT—Ventral Thoracic
VE—Vertebral

Figure 32.7 Arteries of thorax.

dorsal to the parietal pleura, peel away this membrane to expose it.

Locate the ten pairs of **intercostal** arteries that emerge from the thoracic portion of the aorta to supply the intercostal muscles. Also, locate the **bronchial** arteries that emerge from the aorta opposite the fourth intercostal space or from the fourth intercostal artery. They accompany the bronchi to the lungs. Next, identify the **esophageal** arteries that supply blood to the esophagus.

Branches of the Abdominal Aorta

Remove the peritoneum from the dorsal abdominal wall just below the diaphragm to expose the **celiac artery.** Note in figure 32.8 that this is the first branch of the abdominal portion of the aorta. Follow it out to its three branches: **hepatic, left gastric,** and **splenic** arteries.

Identify the **superior mesenteric, renal, internal spermatic** or **ovarian, inferior mesenteric,** and **iliolumbar** arteries, in that order, noting the organs that they supply. Note that a pair of **adrenolumbar** arteries emerge caudad to the superior mesenteric. These arteries supply the adrenal glands, diaphragm, and muscles of the body wall.

There are also seven pairs of small **lumbar** arteries that assist the iliolumbar arteries in providing the abdominal body wall with blood. Can you locate them?

Note that in the cat there are no common iliac arteries; instead, two large branches, the **external iliac** arteries pass into the hind legs. Each external iliac eventually becomes the **femoral** in the thigh region.

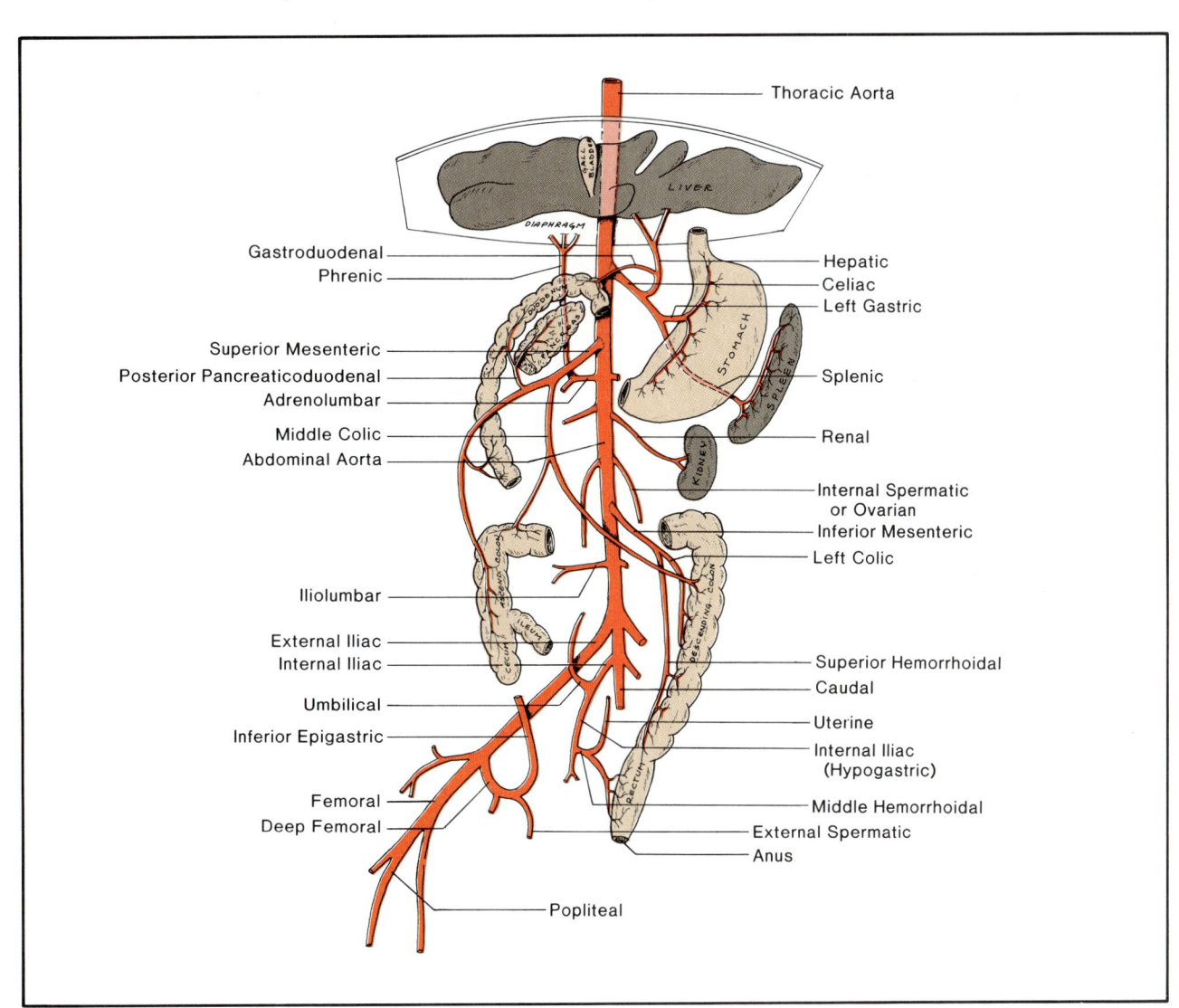

Figure 32.8 Arteries of abdomen and leg.

Caudad to the external iliacs are a pair of **internal iliac** arteries branching off the aorta. The aorta terminates as the **caudal** artery.

Drainage into the Inferior Vena Cava

Figure 32.10 reveals the ramifications of the venous system that drains into the **inferior vena cava** (i.v.c.). Note that the i.v.c. passes through the diaphragm and lies to the right of the abdominal aorta. The tributaries of this vein usually parallel similarly named arteries.

Scrape away some of the liver tissue on its anterior surface to locate the **hepatic** veins that empty into the i.v.c.

Study the **adrenolumbar** and **renal** veins. Note that the right adrenolumbar empties into the i.v.c., while the left one empties into the left renal vein. Note, also, that the **spermatic (ovarian)** veins differ in their drainage, with only the right one emptying directly into the i.v.c.

Locate the **iliolumbar** veins that convey blood from the body wall in the lumber region to the i.v.c.

Identify the right and left **common iliac** veins that convey blood from the legs to the inferior vena cava.

Tributaries of the Common Iliac Veins

Note in illustration 32.10 that the **caudal** vein empties into the left common iliac instead of being a direct extension of the i.v.c. This is not always the case, however.

Trace the common iliac in one leg down to where it branches to form the **external iliac** and **internal iliac.** Note that, as in humans, the external iliac becomes the **femoral** in the thigh region. Follow

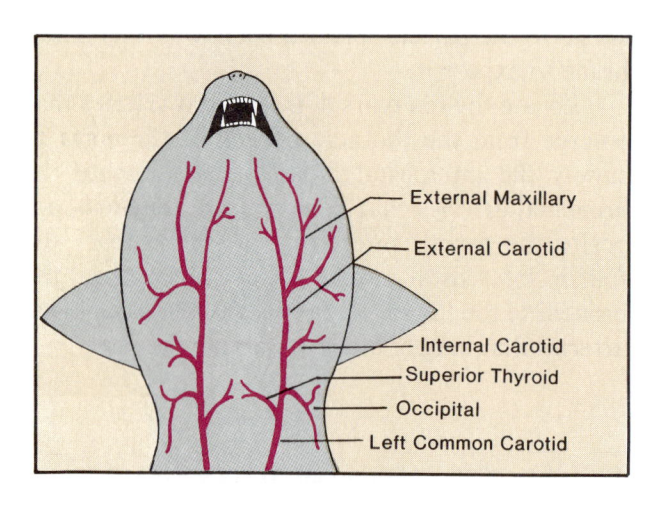

Figure 32.9 Carotid artery branches.

the femoral further into the leg to locate the **greater saphenous** and **popliteal** veins.

The Hepatic Portal System

The veins of this drainage system are seen in figures 32.4 and 32.10. Using either illustration, proceed as follows:

Note that, as in humans, blood from the stomach, spleen, pancreas, small intestine (duodenum), and large intestine (colon), empties into the **hepatic portal,** or simply, **portal** vein.

Locate the following tributaries that empty into this large vessel: **gastrosplenic, superior mesenteric, inferior mesenteric,** and **pancreaticoduodenal** veins. Pay particular attention to the organs that supply them with blood.

Laboratory Report

Complete the Laboratory Report for this exercise.

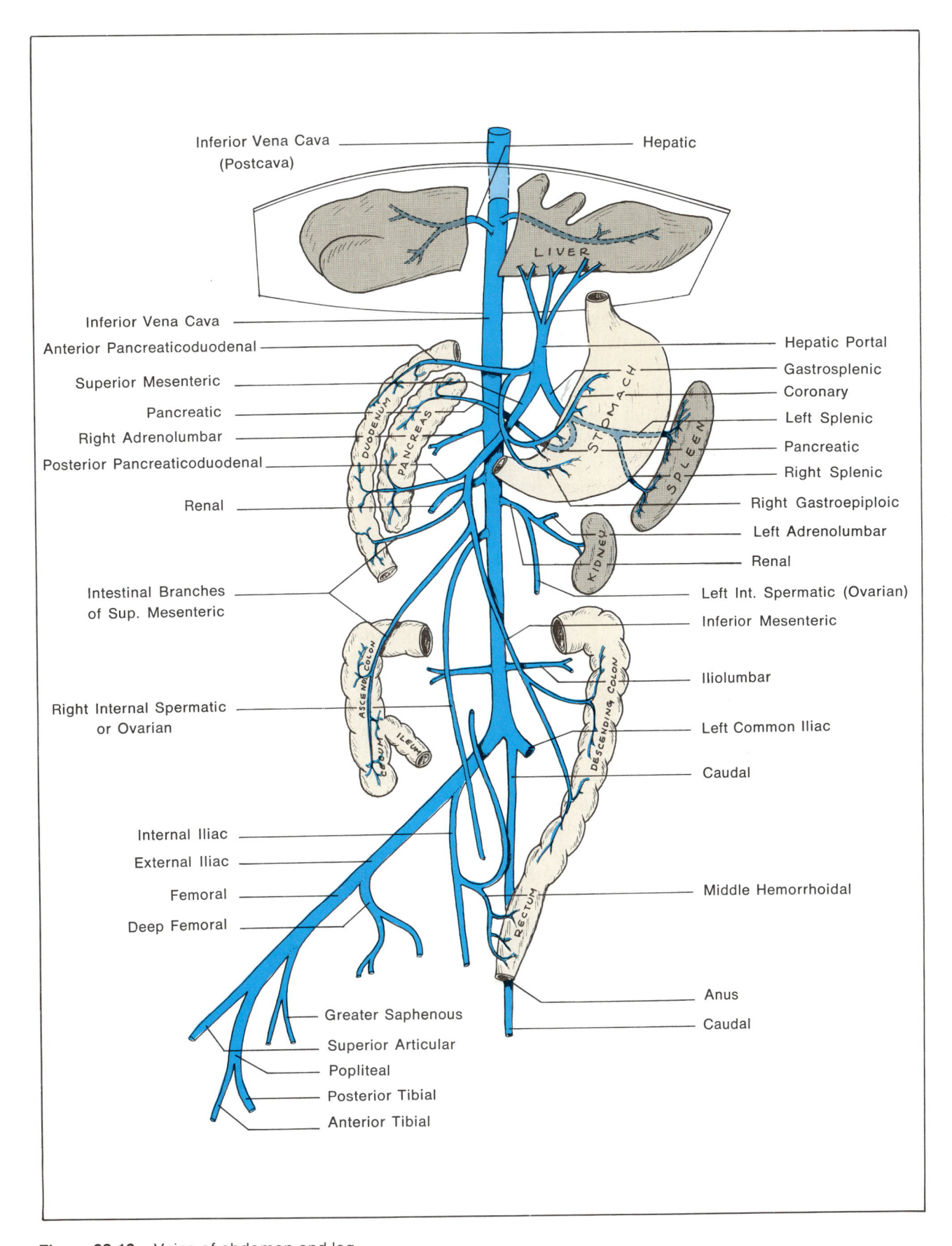

Figure 32.10 Veins of abdomen and leg.

33 Fetal Circulation

During human embryological development the circulatory system is necessarily somewhat different from that after birth. The fact that the lungs are nonfunctional before birth dictates that less blood should go to the lungs. Also, because the food and oxygen supply must come from the mother by way of the placenta, blood vessels to and from the placenta through the umbilical cord must be present and functional.

Figure 33.1 illustrates, in a diagrammatic way, the circulatory pathway through the fetal heart. It is the purpose of this short exercise to trace the blood through the veins and arteries of figure 33.1 so that you understand the pathway of the blood prior to birth and comprehend the changes that must occur after birth.

In the lower left-hand corner of the illustration is seen a large vessel with two smaller vessels wrapped around it. The large vessel is the **umbilical vein,** which carries blood from the placenta of the mother. It contains all the nutrients and oxygen required by the developing fetus. The two small vessels wrapped around the umbilical vein are the **umbilical arteries.** These arteries return blood laden with carbon dioxide and wastes to the placenta. Near the liver of the fetus the umbilical vein narrows to become a short narrow vessel, the **ductus venosus.** At the entrance to the ductus venosus is a **sphincter muscle** that closes off that vessel when the umbilical cord is severed at birth. This helps prevent excessive loss of blood from the infant. The ductus venosus empties into the **inferior vena cava,** where rich oxygenated blood from the placenta is mixed with unoxygenated blood. Most of this mixed blood in the inferior vena cava flows through the right atrium directly into the left atrium through an opening, the **foramen ovale.** Observe that this opening has a flaplike valve over it. Some blood in the right atrium, however, does flow into the right ventricle.

When the heart contracts, blood leaves the right ventricle through the pulmonary trunk, which, in turn, divides to form the **right and left pulmonary arteries.** At the same time, oxygenated blood leaves the left ventricle through the ascending aorta to supply blood to the head, arms, trunk, and legs.

Note that between the pulmonary arteries and the aortic arch is a short vessel called the **ductus arteriosus.** This vessel transfers a considerable amount of blood directly into the aorta instead of allowing it to go to the lungs; enough blood passes to the lungs through the pulmonary arteries, however, to supply the needs of growing lung tissue.

The remainder of the circulatory system resembles the adult plan in that the aorta passes down through the body and divides into two common iliac arteries; each common iliac, in turn, divides to form an external iliac and a hypogastric (internal iliac) artery. Unlike the adult circulatory system, the hypogastric arteries in the fetus are much larger than the external iliacs.

Note that fetal blood is returned to the placenta via the **hypogastric arteries** that pass along each side of the bladder. From the bladder these arteries pass upward along the anterior abdominal body wall to entwine around the umbilical vein to become the **umbilical arteries.**

Once the fetus is separated from the placenta at birth, changes occur in the heart, veins, and arteries to provide a new route for the blood. As stated, one of the first things that happens is the closure of the umbilical vein by the sphincter muscle to help in the prevention of blood loss. Coagulation of blood in this vessel, as well as ligature by the physician, also assists in this respect. Within five days after birth the umbilical vein becomes the *round ligament* (ligamentum teres), which extends from the umbilicus to the liver in the adult.

As soon as the infant begins to breathe, more blood is drawn to the lungs via the pulmonary arteries. The abandonment of the path through the ductus arteriosus causes this vessel to collapse and begin its gradual transformation to connective tissue of the *ligamentum arteriosum.*

With the increase in blood volume and blood pressure in the left atrium, due to a greater blood flow from the lungs, the flap on the foramen ovale closes this opening. Eventually, connective tissue permanently seals off this valve.

The ductus venosus becomes a fibrous band, the *ligamentum venosum* of the liver. Those parts of

the hypogastric arteries that lie along the bladder form into fibrous cords *(lateral umbilical ligaments)* and vesical arteries. The lateral umbilical ligaments extend anteriorly and upward from the bladder to the inner abdominal wall. The superior, middle, and inferior vesical arteries supply blood to the urinary bladder.

Laboratory Report

Label figure 33.1 and answer the questions on Laboratory Report 33,34 that pertain to this exercise.

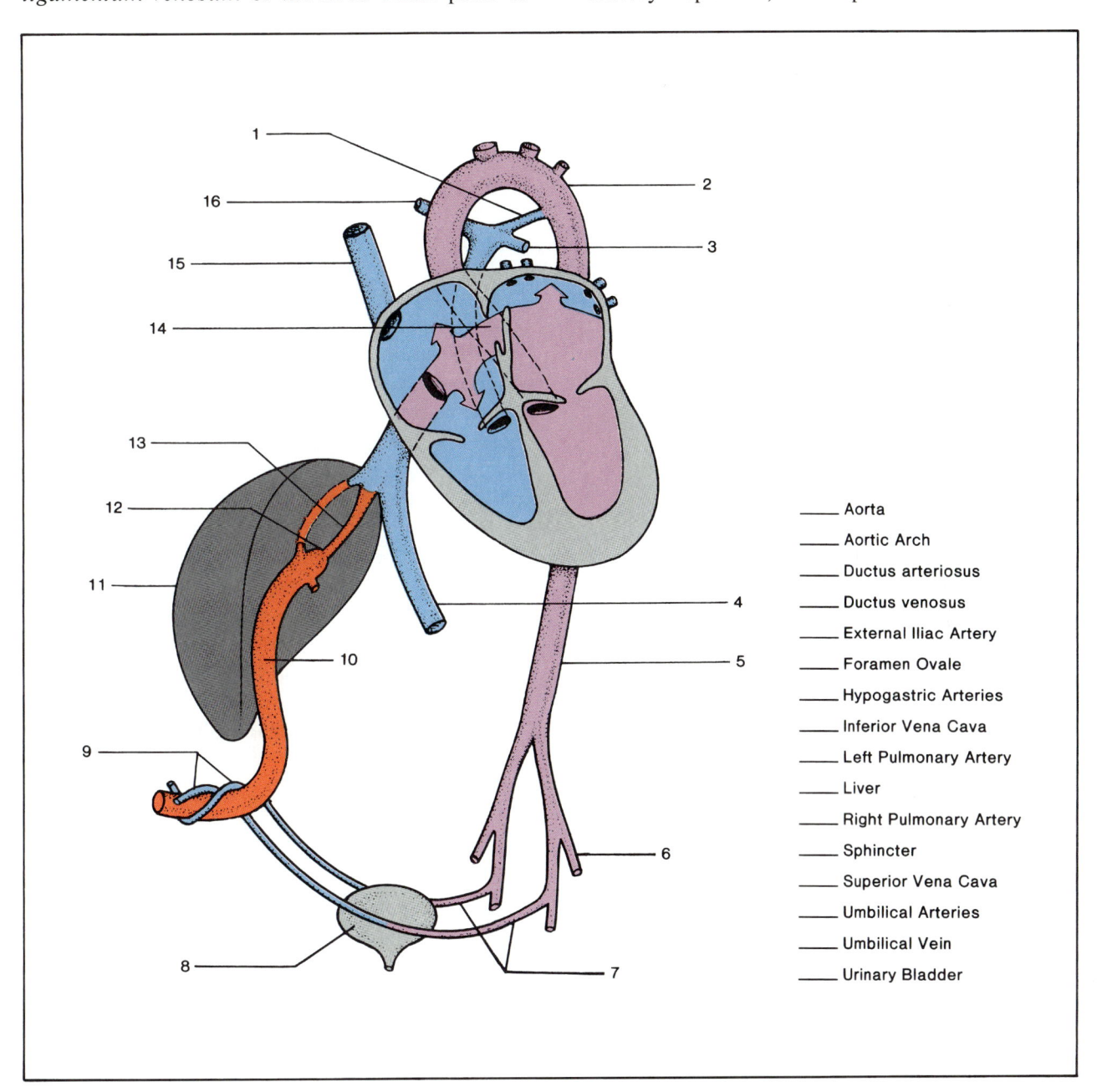

_____ Aorta

_____ Aortic Arch

_____ Ductus arteriosus

_____ Ductus venosus

_____ External Iliac Artery

_____ Foramen Ovale

_____ Hypogastric Arteries

_____ Inferior Vena Cava

_____ Left Pulmonary Artery

_____ Liver

_____ Right Pulmonary Artery

_____ Sphincter

_____ Superior Vena Cava

_____ Umbilical Arteries

_____ Umbilical Vein

_____ Urinary Bladder

Figure 33.1 Fetal circulation.

34 The Lymphatic System and the Immune Response

The lymphatic system consists of a drainage system of lymphatic vessels that returns tissue fluid from the interstitial cell spaces to the blood. On its journey back to the blood, the lymph in these vessels is cleansed of bacteria and other foreign material by macrophages (reticuloendothelial system) in the lymph nodes. In addition to macrophages, the lymph nodes are packed with lymphocytes that play a leading role in cellular and humoral immunity. In this exercise we will explore the genesis and physiology of lymphocytes as well as the overall anatomy of the lymphatic system.

Lymph Pathway

The smallest vessels of the lymphatic system are the *lymph capillaries*. These tiny vessels have closed ends, are microscopic, and are situated among the cells of the various tissues of the body. The lymph capillaries unite to form the **lymphatic vessels** (*lymphatics*) that are the visible vessels shown in the arms and legs in figure 34.1. The irregular appearance of the walls of these vessels is due to the fact that they contain many valves to restrict the backward flow of lymph.

As lymph moves toward the center of the body through the lymphatics, it eventually passes through one or more of the small oval **lymph nodes.** Note that these nodes are clustered in the neck, groin, axillae, and abdominal cavity; they are also found in smaller clusters in other parts of the body. They vary in size from that of a pinhead to an almond.

Two collecting vessels, the thoracic and right lymphatic ducts, collect the lymph from different regions of the body. The largest one is the **thoracic duct,** which collects all the lymph from the legs, abdomen, left half of the thorax, left side of the head, and left arm. Its lower extremity consists of a saclike enlargement, the **cisterna chyli.** Lymph from the intestines passes through lymphatics in the mesentery to the cisterna chyli. The lymph from this region contains a great deal of fat and is usually referred to as *chyle*. The thoracic duct empties into the left subclavian vein near the left internal jugular vein. The **right lymphatic duct** is a short vessel that drains lymph from the right arm and right side of the head into the right subclavian vein near the right internal jugular.

Lymph Node Structure

Each lymph node has a slight depression on one side, the **hilum,** through which blood vessels and the **efferent lymphatic vessel** emerge. **Afferent lymphatic vessels** may enter the lymph node at various points. Although each lymph node has only one efferent vessel, it may have several afferent lymphatic vessels. Surrounding the entire node is a **capsule** of fibrous connective tissue. Just inside the capsule lies the **cortex,** which consists of (1) sinuses reinforced with reticular tissue and (2) **germinal centers** *(nodules).* The germinal centers represent structural units of the node. They arise from small nests of lymphocytes or lymphoblasts and reach about one millimeter in diameter. The central portion of a lymph node is the **medulla.**

Assignment:

Label figure 34.1.

Genesis of Lymphocytes

The term *lymphocyte* usually refers to a family of cells characterized by the absence of specific granules and the presence of a centrally located nucleus. Lymphocytes in the blood are small to medium in size (4–10 μm); those in lymph are usually larger (up to 15 μm). Although all lymphocytes are morphologically similar, there are considerable physiological differences between individual cells. In addition to being present in blood, lymph, and lymph nodes, they are also seen in the bone marrow, thymus, spleen, and lymphoid masses associated with the digestive, respiratory, and urinary passages.

Two different kinds of lymphocytes account for what are known as humoral and cellular immunity. *Humoral immunity* is that type of immunity which is achieved through circulating **antibody.** *Cellular immunity* is immunity in which *sensitized lymphocytes* (**lymphoblasts**) act against foreign cells;

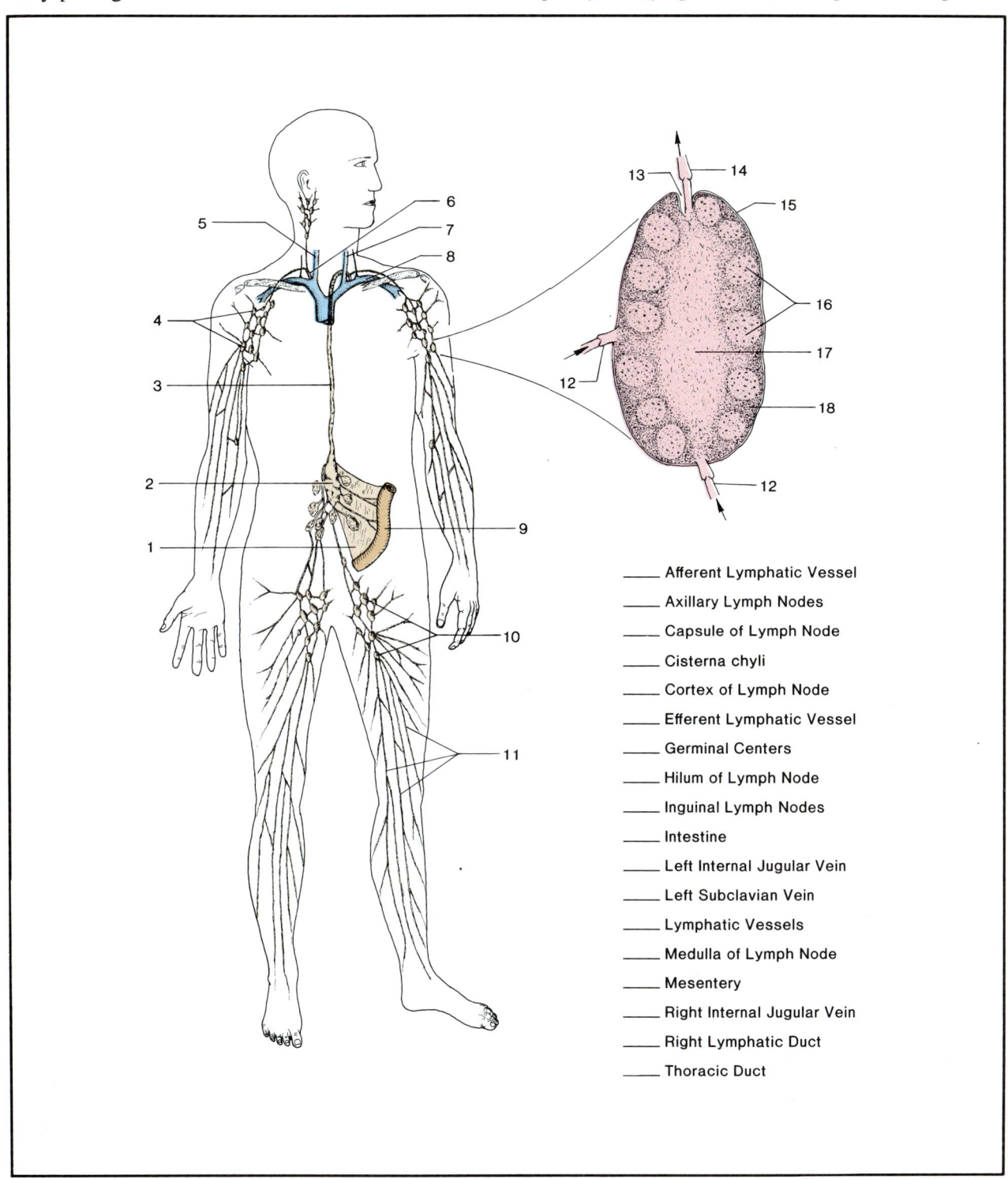

_____ Afferent Lymphatic Vessel
_____ Axillary Lymph Nodes
_____ Capsule of Lymph Node
_____ Cisterna chyli
_____ Cortex of Lymph Node
_____ Efferent Lymphatic Vessel
_____ Germinal Centers
_____ Hilum of Lymph Node
_____ Inguinal Lymph Nodes
_____ Intestine
_____ Left Internal Jugular Vein
_____ Left Subclavian Vein
_____ Lymphatic Vessels
_____ Medulla of Lymph Node
_____ Mesentery
_____ Right Internal Jugular Vein
_____ Right Lymphatic Duct
_____ Thoracic Duct

Figure 34.1 The lymphatic system.

these sensitized cells are responsible for tissue rejection in organ transplants and grafts. Both types of immunity are *acquired,* since they are not present at birth and since they develop in the presence of foreign biological agents.

The lymphocytes that are responsible for antibody formation are called **B-lymphocytes,** or B-cells (*B* for bursa). The lymphocytes that are responsible for cellular immunity are **T-lymphocytes,** or T-cells (*T* for thymus).

Both types of lymphocytes originate from **lymphocytic stem cells** in the bone marrow before birth and shortly after birth. The stem cells are released into the blood and follow one of two pathways for "processing," as illustrated in figure 34.2. The cells that settle in the thymus for modification become T-cells; the remaining cells are processed in some other unknown area to become B-cells. Birds possess a *bursa of Fabricius* on the hindgut, where B-cells are formed; in man an equivalent of this organ is being sought. At present, it is speculated that lymphoid tissue in the fetal liver or even in the bone marrow may be responsible for B-cell processing.

Once the T-lymphocytes have matured in the thymus, they leave the thymus via the blood and colonize in specific loci of the lymph nodes and spleen. T-cells have a long life. In the presence of antigens they are transformed to **lymphoblasts,** which are responsible for cellular immunity.

The stem cells that mature in the B-cell processing tissues leave these tissues through the blood as B-lymphocytes and colonize in specific regions of the lymph nodes and spleen also. When these B-cells come in contact with the appropriate antigens they are transformed into **plasma cells** that produce the antibodies of humoral immunity.

Laboratory Assignment

Materials:

    prepared slide of lymph node (H13.11)
       microscope

1. Examine a prepared slide of a lymph node and compare it with the photomicrographs in figure HA-27 of the Histology Atlas. Locate a **germinal center.**
2. Examine the **lymphocytes** under high-dry or oil immersion to see if you can identify cells that are dividing.
3. Make drawings, if required.
4. Answer all questions on Laboratory Report 33,34 that pertain to this exercise.

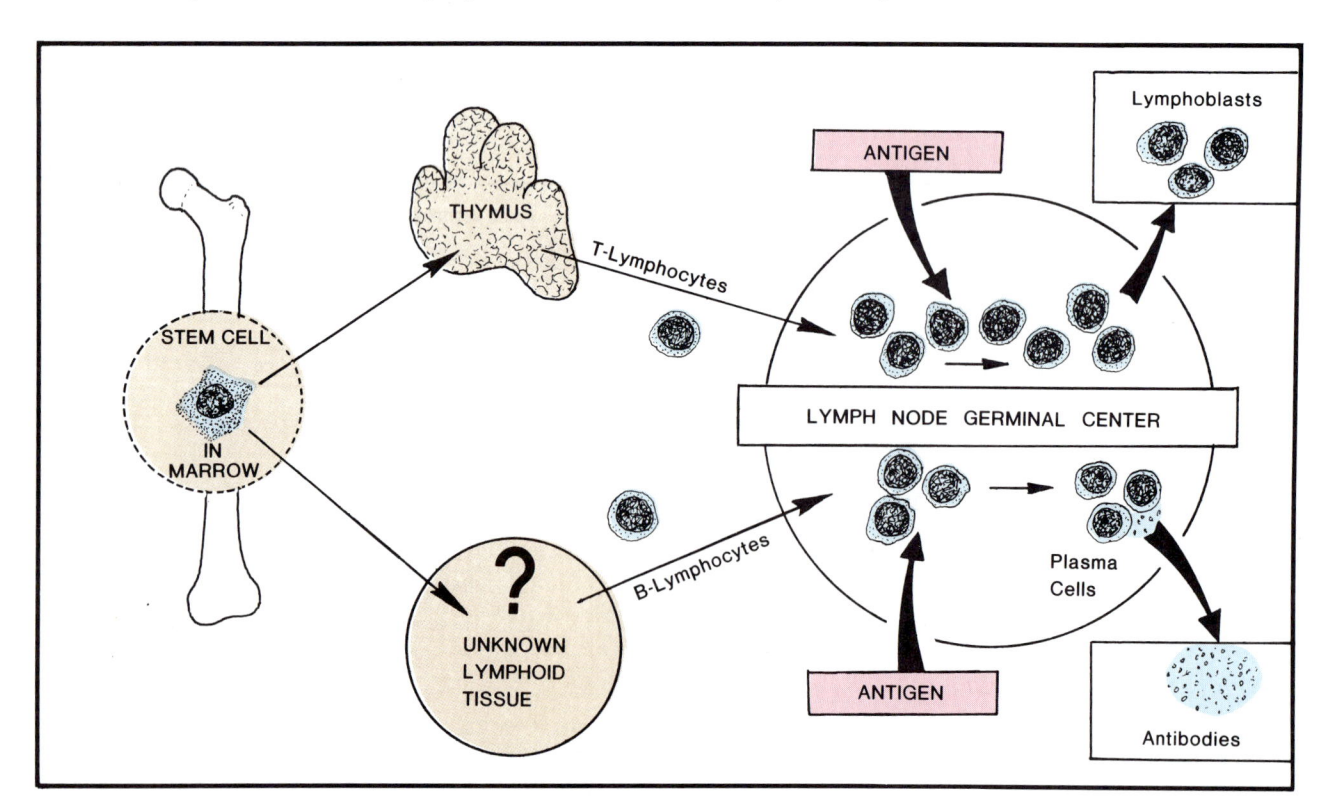

Figure 34.2 The genesis of lymphoblasts and plasma cells.

35 The Respiratory System

Both gross and microscopic anatomy of the respiratory system will be studied in this exercise. Although the cat will be the primary dissection specimen here, sheep and frog materials are also available for certain observations. Before any laboratory dissections are performed, however, it is desirable that figures 35.1, 35.2, and 35.3 be labeled.

Materials:

> models of median section of head and larynx
> frog, pithed
> sheep pluck
> dissecting instruments and trays
> prepared slides of rat trachea and lung tissue
> Ringer's solution
> bone or autopsy saw

The Lungs, Trachea, and Larynx

Figure 35.1 illustrates the respiratory passages from the larynx to the lungs. Note that the larynx (voice box) consists of three cartilages: an upper **epiglottis,** a large middle **thyroid cartilage,** and a smaller **cricoid cartilage.** Figure 35.2 reveals these cartilages in greater detail.

Below the larynx extends the **trachea** to a point in the center of the thorax where it divides to form two short **bronchi.** Note that both the trachea and bronchi are reinforced with rings of cartilage of the hyaline type. Each bronchus divides further into many smaller tubes called **bronchioles.** At the terminus of each bronchiole is a cluster of tiny sacs, the **alveoli,** where gas exchange with the blood takes place. Each lung is made up of approximately 150 million of these sacs.

Free movement of the lungs in the thoracic cavity is facilitated by the pleural membranes. Covering each lung is a **pulmonary** (*visceral*) **pleura** and attached to the thoracic wall is a **parietal pleura.** Between these two pleurae is a potential cavity, the **pleural** (*intrapleural*) **cavity.** Normally, the lungs are firmly pressed against the body wall with little

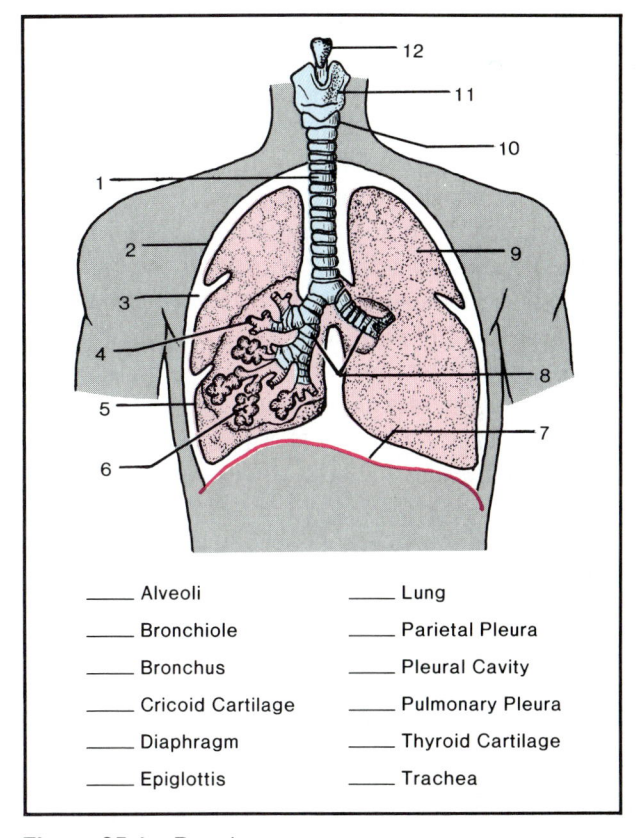

____ Alveoli	____ Lung
____ Bronchiole	____ Parietal Pleura
____ Bronchus	____ Pleural Cavity
____ Cricoid Cartilage	____ Pulmonary Pleura
____ Diaphragm	____ Thyroid Cartilage
____ Epiglottis	____ Trachea

Figure 35.1 Respiratory tract.

or no space between the two pleurae. The bottom of the lungs rests against the muscular **diaphragm,** the principal muscle of respiration. The parietal pleura is attached to the diaphragm also.

Assignment:

Label figure 35.1

The Upper Respiratory Tract

In addition to breathing, the upper respiratory tract also functions in eating and speech; thus, a study of the respiratory organs in this region necessarily includes organs concerned with these other activities. Figure 35.3 is of this area.

The two principal cavities of the head are the nasal and oral cavities. The upper **nasal cavity,** which serves as the passageway for air, is separated from the lower **oral cavity** by the **palate.** The anterior portion of the palate is reinforced with bone and is called the **hard palate.** The posterior part, which terminates in a fingerlike projection, the **uvula,** is the **soft palate.**

The oral cavity consists of two parts: the **oral cavity proper,** the larger cavity that contains the tongue; and the **oral vestibule,** which is between the lips and teeth.

During breathing, air enters the nasal cavity through the nostrils, or **nares.** The lateral walls of this cavity have three pairs of fleshy lobes, the superior, middle, and inferior **nasal conchae.** These lobes serve to warm the air as it enters the body.

Above and behind the soft palate is the **pharynx.** That part of the pharynx posterior to the tongue, where swallowing is initiated, is the **oropharynx.** Above it is the **nasopharynx.** Two openings to the **auditory** (*Eustachian*) **tubes** are seen on the walls of the nasopharynx.

After air passes through the nasal cavity, nasopharynx, and oropharynx, it passes through the larynx and trachea to the lungs. The cartilages (labels 8, 10, and 11) of the larynx vary considerably in size and histology. The upper **epiglottis** consists of elastic cartilage; it helps to prevent food from entering the respiratory passages during swallowing. The **thyroid cartilage,** which consists of hyaline cartilage, forms the side walls of the larynx and the protuberance known as the "Adam's apple." Inferior to the thyroid cartilage is the **cricoid cartilage,** which consists of hyaline cartilage. Note that on the inner wall of the larynx is depicted a **vocal fold** that is, essentially, the true vocal cord of the larynx. The paired vocal cords are actuated by muscles through the **arytenoid cartilages** (label 5, figure 35.2) to produce sounds. One of these vocal cords exists on each side of the larynx. The vocal folds should not be confused with the **ventricular folds** (label 9, figure 35.3) that lie superior to the vocal folds. The ventricular folds are also known as "false vocal cords." Posterior to the larynx and trachea lies the **esophagus,** which carries food from the pharynx to the stomach.

In several areas of the oral cavity and nasopharynx are seen islands of lymphoidal tissue called *tonsils.* The **pharyngeal tonsils,** or *adenoids,* are situated on the roof of the nasopharynx; the **lingual tonsils** are on the posterior inferior portion of the tongue; and the **palatine tonsils** are on each side of the tongue on the lateral walls of the oropharynx.

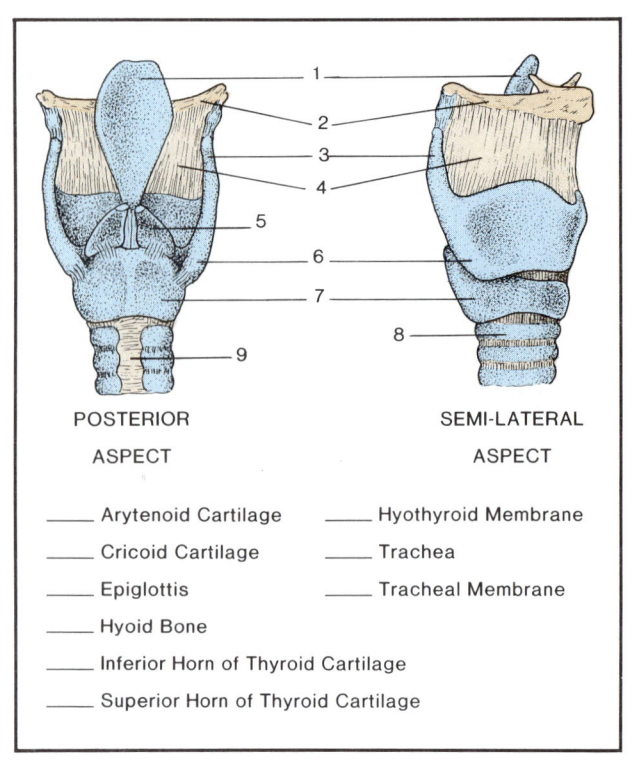

Figure 35.2 Human larynx.

These masses of tissue are as important as the lymph nodes of the body in protection against infection. The palatine tonsils are ones most frequently removed by surgical methods.

Assignment:

Label figures 35.2 and 35.3.

Study models of the head and larynx. Be able to identify all structures.

Cat Dissection

Examination of the upper and lower respiratory passages of the cat will require some dissection. The amount of dissection to be performed will depend on what systems have been previously studied on your specimen. Figures 34.3, 34.4, and 34.5 will be used for reference.

Materials:

autopsy saw
embalmed cat
dissecting tray

Upper Respiratory Tract

To identify all the cavities and structures of the cat's head that are shown in figure 34.3, it is necessary

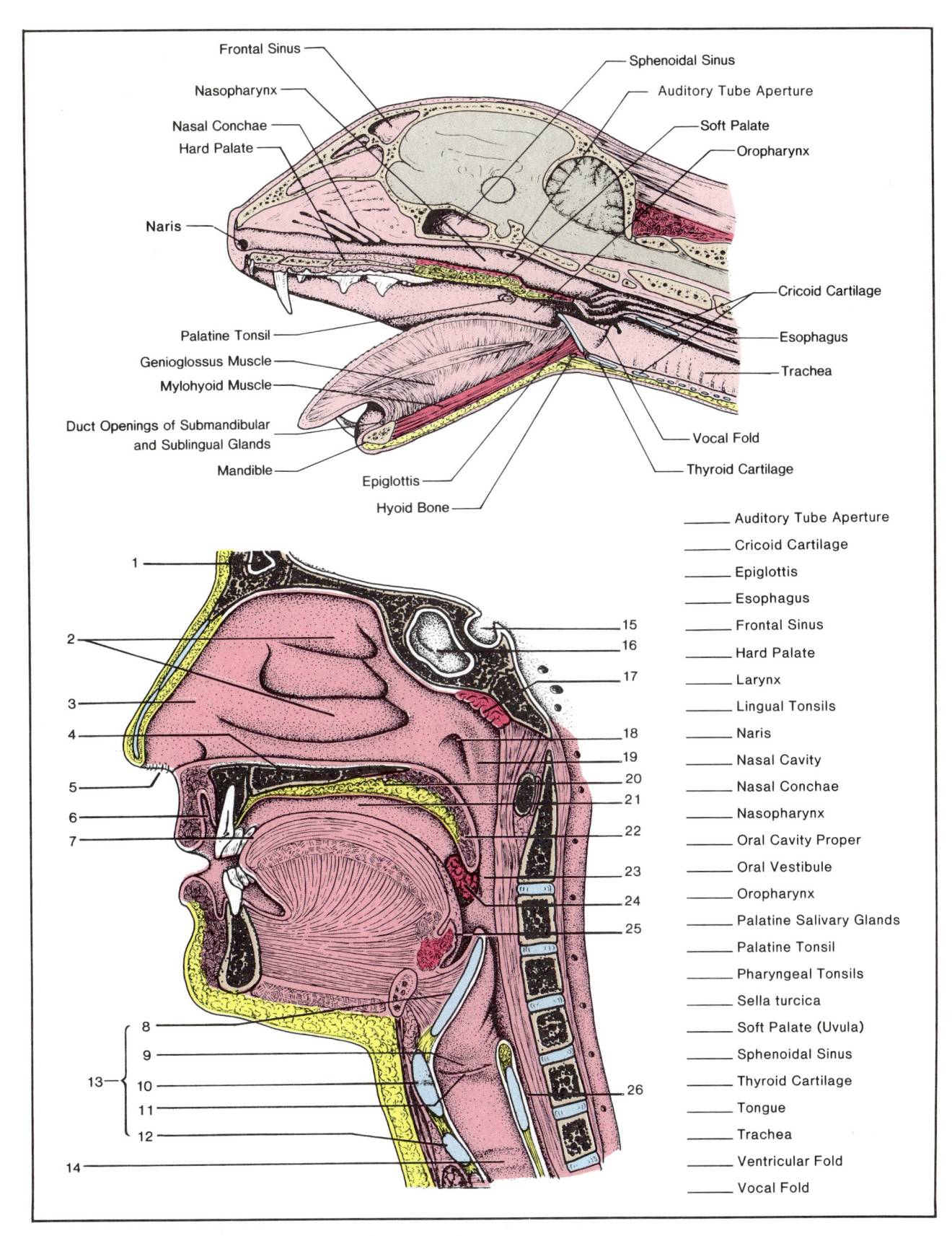

Frontal Sinus

Sphenoidal Sinus

Nasopharynx

Auditory Tube Aperture

Nasal Conchae

Soft Palate

Hard Palate

Oropharynx

Naris

Cricoid Cartilage

Esophagus

Trachea

Palatine Tonsil

Genioglossus Muscle

Mylohyoid Muscle

Duct Openings of Submandibular and Sublingual Glands

Vocal Fold

Mandible

Thyroid Cartilage

Epiglottis

Hyoid Bone

_____ Auditory Tube Aperture

_____ Cricoid Cartilage

_____ Epiglottis

_____ Esophagus

_____ Frontal Sinus

_____ Hard Palate

_____ Larynx

_____ Lingual Tonsils

_____ Naris

_____ Nasal Cavity

_____ Nasal Conchae

_____ Nasopharynx

_____ Oral Cavity Proper

_____ Oral Vestibule

_____ Oropharynx

_____ Palatine Salivary Glands

_____ Palatine Tonsil

_____ Pharyngeal Tonsils

_____ Sella turcica

_____ Soft Palate (Uvula)

_____ Sphenoidal Sinus

_____ Thyroid Cartilage

_____ Tongue

_____ Trachea

_____ Ventricular Fold

_____ Vocal Fold

Figure 35.3 Upper respiratory passages, human and cat.

to use a mechanical bone saw or an electric autopsy saw to cut the head down the median line. The instructor will designate certain students to make sagittal sections that can be studied by all members of the class. Most specimens will be left intact to facilitate the study of other systems.

If an autopsy saw is used, it is essential that the head of the specimen be held by one student while another student does the cutting. The instructor will demonstrate the procedure. Although an electric autopsy saw is relatively safe because of its reciprocating action, there are certain precautions that must be observed.

The principal rules of safety are (1) Cut only **away from** the assistant's hands. (2) While cutting, brace the hands against the table for steadiness; don't try to "free-hand" it. (3) The cutter's hands should never be allowed to tire; frequent rests are essential.

Use the large cutting edge for straight cuts and the small cutting edge for sharp curves. Cut only deep enough to get through the bone; use the scalpel for soft tissues. Once the head has been cut through, it should be washed free of all loose debris.

First identify the **nares** and **nasal cavity.** As in humans, the nasal cavity lies superior to the palate. Also, identify the **nasal conchae,** which are shaped somewhat differently in cats than in humans. Identify that region designated as the **nasopharynx.** Observe that it has a small **auditory tube aperture** in approximately the same position as the human. Insert a probe into it.

Press against the palate with a blunt probe to note where the **hard palate** ends and the **soft palate** begins. Locate the **oropharynx,** which is at the back of the mouth near the base of the tongue. Observe that the cat has a very small **palatine tonsil** on each side of the oropharynx. Does it appear to lie in a recess, as is true of the same tonsil in humans?

Lower Respiratory Passages

After identifying the above structures on the sagittal section, open the thoracic cavity if it has not

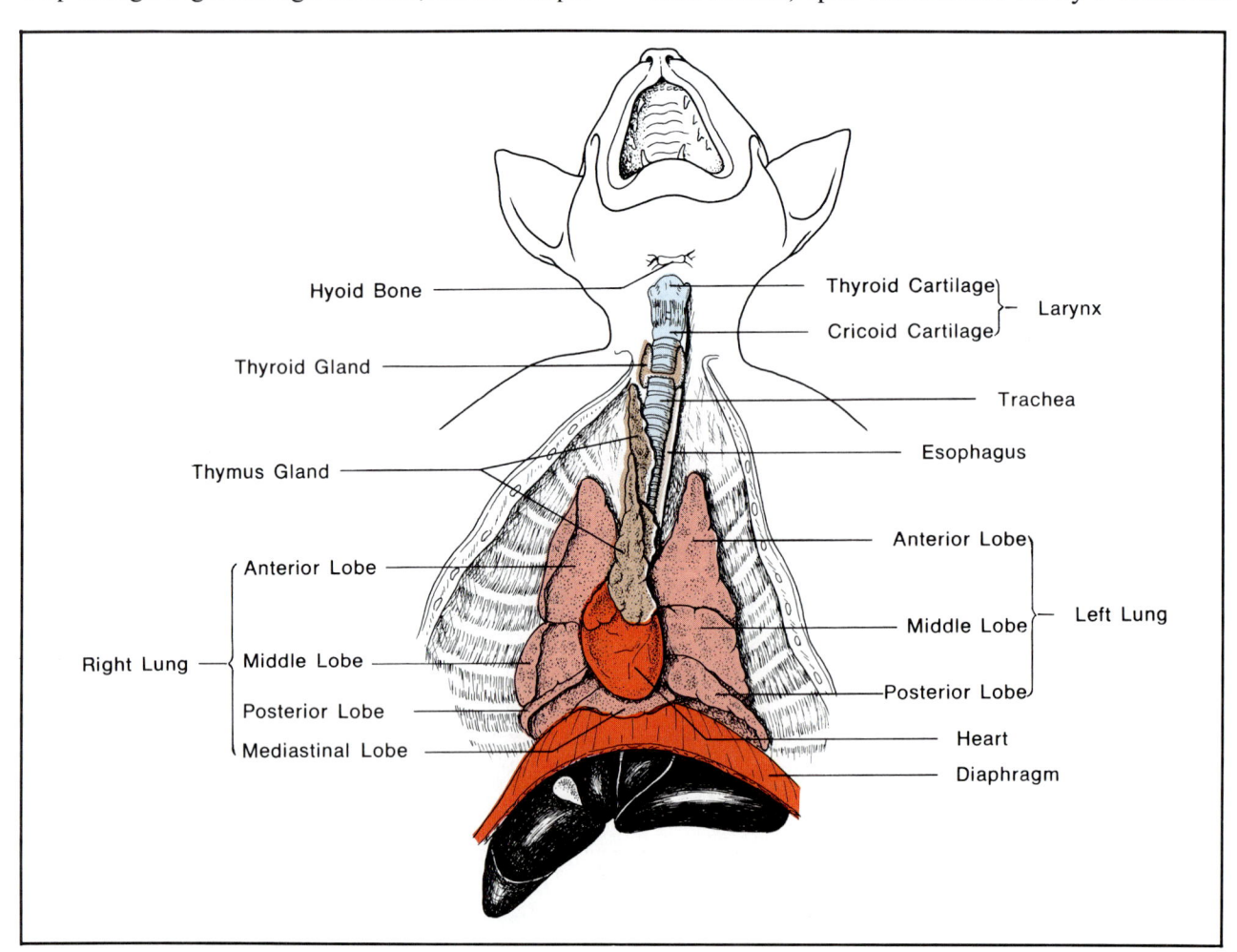

Figure 35.4 Thoracic organs of cat.

already been done. If the circulatory system has been studied, it will already be open.

To open the chest cavity, make a longitudinal incision about one centimeter to the right or left of midline. Such a cut will be primarily through muscle and cartilage rather than bone. The incision may be cut partially through with a scalpel and completed with scissors. Avoid damaging the internal organs. Extend the cut up the throat to the mandible.

Continue the incision down the abdominal wall past the liver. Make two cuts laterally from the midline in the region of the liver. Spread apart the thoracic walls and sever the diaphragm from the wall with scissors. To enable the thoracic walls to remain open, make a shallow longitudinal cut with a scalpel along the inside surface of each side that is sufficiently deep to weaken the ribs. When the walls are folded back, the thoracic wall on each side should break at the cut. Your specimen should look like figure 35.4.

Examine the larynx to identify the large flap-like **epiglottis,** the **thyroid cartilage,** and the **cricoid cartilage.** Refer to figure 35.5 to note the details of the larynx. Locate the **arytenoid cartilages** and the paired vocal folds that lie within the cavity of the larynx.

Trace the **trachea** down into the lungs. In humans the right lung has three lobes and the left lung has only two. How does this compare with the cat? Cut out a short section of the trachea and examine a cross section through the **cartilaginous rings.** Are they continuous all the way around the trachea? Can you see where the trachea branches to form the **bronchi?** Make a frontal section through one lung and look for further branching of the bronchus.

Sheep Pluck Dissection

A "sheep pluck" consists of the trachea, lungs, larynx, and heart of a sheep as removed during routine slaughter. Since it is fresh material rather than formalin-preserved, it is more lifelike than the organs of an embalmed cat. If plucks are available, proceed as follows to dissect one.

Materials:

    sheep plucks, less the liver
    dissecting instruments
    drinking straws or serological pipettes

1. Lay out a fresh sheep pluck on a tray. Identify the major organs, such as the **lungs, larynx, trachea, diaphragm** remnants, and **heart.**
2. Examine the larynx more closely. Can you identify the **epiglottis, thyroid,** and **cricoid cartilages?** Look into the larynx. Can you see the **vocal folds?**
3. Cut a cross section through the upper portion of the trachea and examine a sectioned cartilaginous ring. Is it similar to the cat?
4. Force your index finger down into the trachea, noting the smooth and slimy nature of the inner lining. What kind of tissue lines the trachea that makes it so smooth and slippery?
5. Note that each lung is divided into lobes. How many lobes make up the right lung? The left

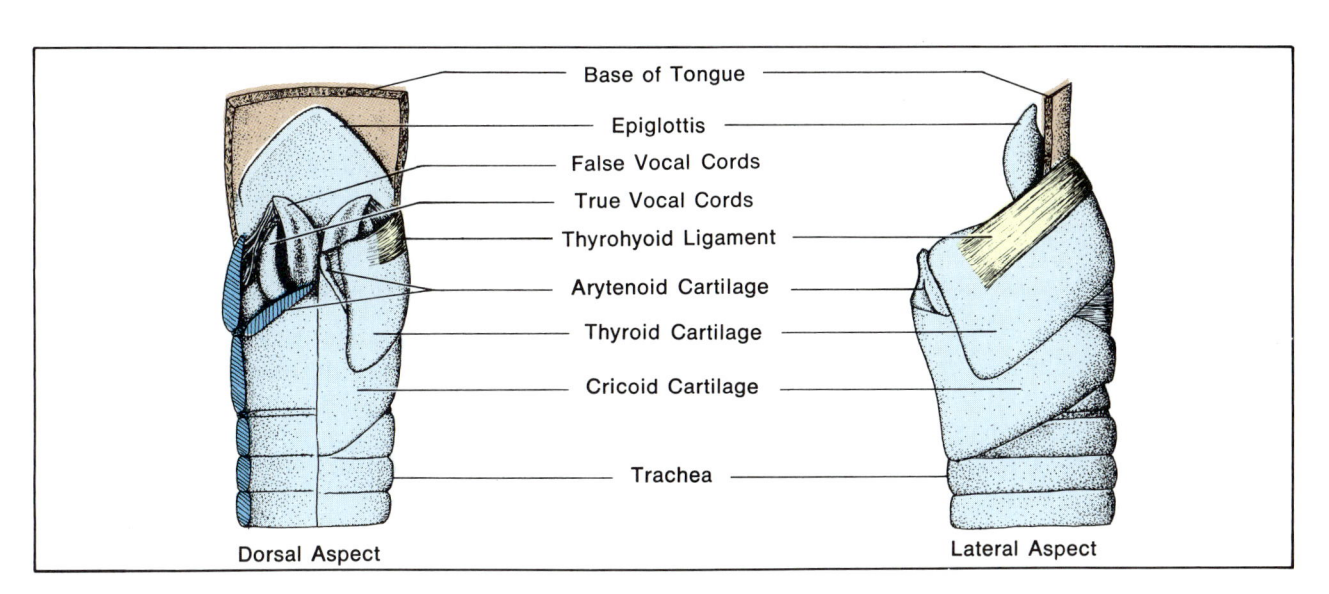

Dorsal Aspect

Base of Tongue
Epiglottis
False Vocal Cords
True Vocal Cords
Thyrohyoid Ligament
Arytenoid Cartilage
Thyroid Cartilage
Cricoid Cartilage
Trachea

Lateral Aspect

Figure 35.5 Larynx of cat.

lung? Compare with the human lung (figure 35.1).

6. Rub your fingers over the surface of the lung. What membrane on the surface of the lung makes it so smooth?

7. Free the connective tissue around the **pulmonary artery** and expose its branches leading into the lung. Also, locate the **pulmonary veins** that empty into the left atrium. Can you find the **ligamentum arteriosum,** which is between the pulmonary trunk and aorta?

8. With a sharp scalpel, free the trachea from the lung tissue and trace it down to where it divides into the **bronchi.**

9. With a pair of scissors, cut off the trachea at the level of the top of the heart.

10. Now, cut the trachea down its posterior surface on the median line with a pair of scissors. The posterior surface of the trachea is opposite the heart. Extend this cut down to where it branches into the two primary bronchi. (Observe that the upper right lobe has a separate bronchus leading into it. This bronchus branches off some distance above where the primary bronchi divide from the trachea.)

11. Continue opening up the respiratory tree until you get down deep into the center of the lung. Note the extensive branching.

12. Insert a plastic straw or a serological pipette into one of the bronchioles and blow into the lung. If a pipette is used, **put the mouthpiece of the pipette into the bronchiole and blow on the small end.** Note the great expansive capability of the lung.

13. Cut off a lobe of the lung and examine the cut surface. Note the sponginess of the tissue.

14. Record all your observations on the Laboratory Report.

Important: Wash your hands with soap and water at the end of the period.

Frog Lung Observation

To study the nature of living lung tissue in an animal, we will do a microscopic study of the lung of a frog shortly after pithing and dissection. A frog lung is less complex than the human lung, but it is made of essentially the same kind of tissue. Proceed as follows:

Materials:

> frog, recently double pithed
> dissecting instruments and dissecting trays
> dissecting microscope
> Ringer's solution in wash bottle

1. Pin the frog, ventral side up, in a wax-bottomed dissecting pan.

2. With your scissors, make an incision through the skin along the midline of the abdomen.

3. Make transverse cuts in both directions at each end of the incision and lay back the flaps of skin.

   Now, carefully make an incision through the right or left side of the abdomen over the lung and parallel to the midline. Take care not to cut too deeply. The inflated lung should now be visible.

4. With a probe, gently lift the lung out through the incision. Do not perforate the lung! From this point keep the lung moist with Ringer's solution.

5. If the lungs of your frog are not inflated, insert a medicine dropper into the slitlike glottis on the floor of the oral cavity and blow air into them by squeezing the bulb. Deflated lungs may be the result of excessive squeezing during pithing.

6. Observe the shape and general appearance of the frog lung. Note that it is basically saclike.

7. Place the frog under a dissecting microscope and examine the lungs. Locate the network of ridges on the inner walls. The thin-walled regions between the ridges represent the alveoli. Look carefully to see if you can detect blood cells moving slowly across the alveolar surface. Careful examination of the lungs may reveal the presence of parasitic worms. They are quite common in frogs.

8. When you have completed this study, dispose of the frog, as directed, and clean the pan and instruments.

Histological Study

Prepared slides of the nasal cavity, trachea, and lung tissue will be available for study. If Turtox slides are used, the tissues will probably be from monkey or human organs. Tissues from other mammals, such as the mouse or rabbit, may also be available.

Use figure HA-28 in the Histology Atlas for reference, and follow these suggestions in making your study.

Materials:

prepared slides of nasal septum (H6.1), trachea (H6.41), and lung tissue (H6.51)

Nasal Septum Scan this slide first with low power to locate the nasal septum and nasal concha. Refer to illustration A, figure HA-28, for reference. Identify the bony tissue and nasal epithelium.

Study the ciliated epithelium and the tissues beneath it with high-dry magnification. Look for the **olfactory** (*Bowman's*) **glands** (illustration B) which are located in the lamina propria. The secretion of these glands helps to keep the epithelial surface moist and facilitates the solution of substances that stimulate the olfactory receptors. Observe that a large number of unmyelinated **olfactory fibers** lie between the glands and the ciliated epithelium. These fibers carry nerve impulses from olfactory receptors that are dispersed among the cells of the epithelium.

Trachea Identify the hyaline cartilage, ciliated epithelium, lamina propria, and muscularis mucosae. Look for goblet cells on the epithelial layer. Refer to illustration C, figure HA-28.

Lung Tissue Examine with the high-dry objective. Look for the thin-walled **alveoli,** a **bronchiole,** and blood vessels. Consult illustration D for reference.

Laboratory Report

Complete the Laboratory Report for this exercise.

36 The Digestive System

The study of the alimentary tract, liver, and pancreas will be pursued in this exercise. Cat dissection will provide an in-depth study of the various components.

The Alimentary Canal

Figure 36.1 is a simplified illustration of the digestive system. The alimentary canal, which is about thirty feet in length, has been foreshortened in the intestines for clarity. The following text, which pertains to this illustration, is related to the passage of food through its full length.

Materials:

manikin

When food is taken into the oral cavity, it is chewed and mixed with saliva that is secreted by many glands of the mouth. The most prominent of these glands are the parotid, submandibular, and sublingual glands. The **parotid glands** are located in the cheeks in front of the ears, one on each side of the head. The **sublingual glands** are located under the tongue and are the most anterior ones of the three pairs. The **submandibular** glands are situated posterior to the sublinguals, just inside of the body of the mandible. (Figure 36.4 shows the position of these glands more precisely.)

After the food has been completely mixed with saliva it passes to the **stomach** by way of a long tube, the **esophagus.** The food is moved along the esophagus by wavelike constrictions called *peristaltic waves.* These constrictions originate in the **oropharynx,** which is the cavity at the top of the esophagus, posterior to the tongue. The upper opening of the stomach through which the food enters is the **cardiac valve.** The upper rounded portion, or **fundus,** of the stomach holds the bulk of the food to be digested. The lower portion, or **pyloric region,** is smaller in diameter, more active, and accomplishes most of the digestion that occurs in the stomach. That region between the fundus and the pyloric portion is the **body.** After the food has been

acted on by the various enzymes of the gastric fluid, it is forced into the small intestine through the **pyloric valve** of the stomach.

The *small intestine* is approximately 23 feet long and consists of three parts: the duodenum, jejunum, and ileum. The first 10 to 12 inches make up the **duodenum.** The **jejunum** comprises the next 7 or 8 feet, and the last coiled portion is the **ileum.** Complete digestion and absorption of food takes place in the small intestine.

Indigestible food and water pass from the ileum into the large intestine, or **colon,** through the **ileocecal valve.** This valve is shown in a cutaway section. The large intestine has four sections: the ascending, transverse, descending, and sigmoid colons. The **ascending colon** is the portion of the large intestine that the ileum empties into. At its lower end is an enlarged compartment or pouch, the **cecum,** which has a narrow tube extending down from it which is the **appendix.** The ascending colon ascends on the right side of the abdomen until it reaches the under surface of the liver where it bends abruptly to the left, becoming the **transverse colon.** The **descending colon** passes down the left side of the abdomen where it changes direction again, becoming the **sigmoid colon.** The last portion of the alimentary canal is the **rectum,** which is about five inches long and terminates with an opening, the **anus.**

Leading downward from the inferior surface of the **liver** is the **hepatic duct.** This duct joins the **cystic duct,** which connects with the round saclike **gallbladder.** Bile, which is produced in the liver, passes down the hepatic duct and up the cystic duct to the gallbladder where it is stored until needed. When the gallbladder contracts, bile is forced down the cystic duct into the **common bile duct,** which extends from the juncture of the cystic and hepatic ducts to the intestine.

Between the duodenum and the stomach lies another gland, the **pancreas.** Its duct, the **pancreatic duct,** joins the common bile duct and empties into the duodenum.

Assignment:

Label figure 36.1. Disassemble the manikin and identify all of these structures.

Answer the questions on the Laboratory Report pertaining to this part of the exercise.

Oral Anatomy

A typical normal mouth is illustrated in figure 36.2. To provide maximum exposure of the oral structures, the lips (*labia*) have been retracted away from the teeth, and the cheeks (*buccae*) have been cut. The lips are flexible folds that meet laterally at the *angle* of the mouth, where they are continuous with the cheeks. The lining of the lips, cheeks, and other oral surfaces consists of mucous membrane, the *mucosa.* Near the median line of the mouth on the inner surface of the lips, the mucosa is thickened to form folds, the **labial frenula,** or *frena.* Of the two frenula, the upper one is usually stronger. The delicate mucosa that covers the neck of each tooth is the **gingiva.**

The hard and soft palates are distinguishable as differently shaded areas on the roof of the mouth.

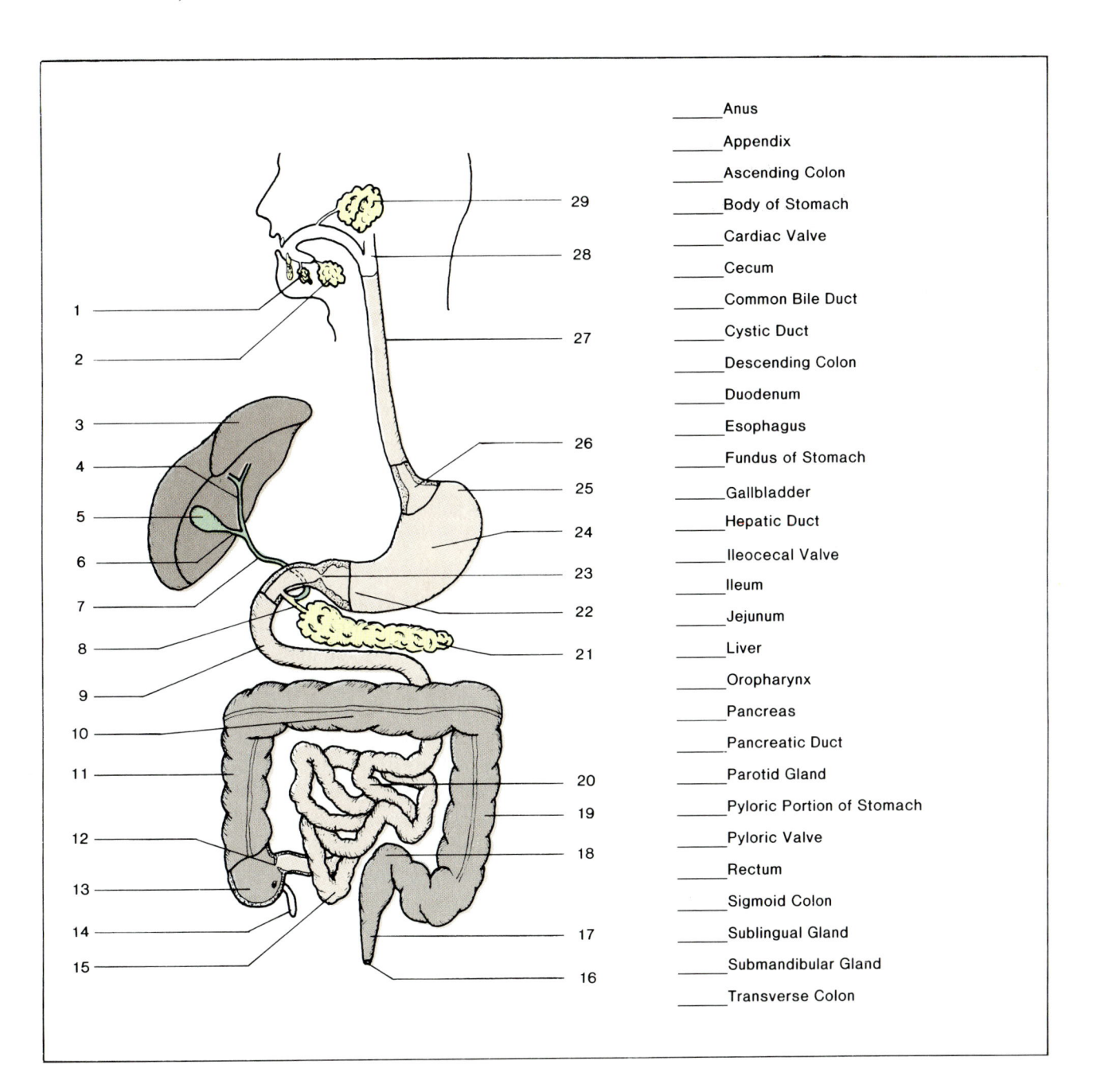

_____ Anus	
_____ Appendix	
_____ Ascending Colon	
_____ Body of Stomach	
_____ Cardiac Valve	
_____ Cecum	
_____ Common Bile Duct	
_____ Cystic Duct	
_____ Descending Colon	
_____ Duodenum	
_____ Esophagus	
_____ Fundus of Stomach	
_____ Gallbladder	
_____ Hepatic Duct	
_____ Ileocecal Valve	
_____ Ileum	
_____ Jejunum	
_____ Liver	
_____ Oropharynx	
_____ Pancreas	
_____ Pancreatic Duct	
_____ Parotid Gland	
_____ Pyloric Portion of Stomach	
_____ Pyloric Valve	
_____ Rectum	
_____ Sigmoid Colon	
_____ Sublingual Gland	
_____ Submandibular Gland	
_____ Transverse Colon	

Figure 36.1 The alimentary canal.

The lighter shaded area is the **hard palate.** Posterior to it is a darker area, the **soft palate.** The **uvula** is a part of the soft palate. It is the fingerlike projection that extends downward over the back of the tongue. It varies considerably in size and shape in different individuals.

On each side of the tongue at the back of the mouth are the **palatine tonsils.** Each tonsil lies in a recess bounded anteriorly by a membrane, the **glossopalatine arch,** and posteriorly by a membrane, the **pharyngopalatine arch.** The tonsils consist of lymphoid tissue covered by epithelium. The epithelial covering of these structures dips inward into the lymphoid tissue forming glandlike pits called **tonsillar crypts** (label 11, figure 36.3). These crypts connect with channels that course through the lymphoid tissue of the tonsil. If they are infected, however, their protective function is impaired and they may actually serve as foci of infection. Inflammation of the palatine tonsils is called *tonsillitis.* Enlargement of the tonsils tends to obstruct the throat cavity and interfere with the passage of air to the lungs.

Assignment:

Label figure 36.2.

The Tongue

Figure 36.3 shows the tongue and adjacent structures. It is a mobile mass of striated muscle completely covered with mucous membrane. The tongue is subdivided into three parts: the apex, body, and root. The **apex** of the tongue is the most anterior tip, which rests against the inside surfaces of the front teeth. The **body** (*corpus*) is the bulk of the tongue that extends posteriorly from the apex to the root. The body is that part of the tongue that is visible by simple inspection: i.e., without the aid of a mirror. The posterior border of the body is arbitrarily located somewhere anterior to the tonsillar material of the tongue. Extending down the median line of the body is a groove, the **central** (*median*) **sulcus.** The **root** of the tongue is the most posterior portion. Its surface is primarily covered by the **lingual tonsil.**

Extending upward from the posterior margin of the root of the tongue is the **epiglottis.** On each side of the tongue are seen the oval **palatine tonsils.**

The dorsum of the tongue is covered with several kinds of projections called *papillae.* The cutout section is an enlarged portion of its surface to reveal

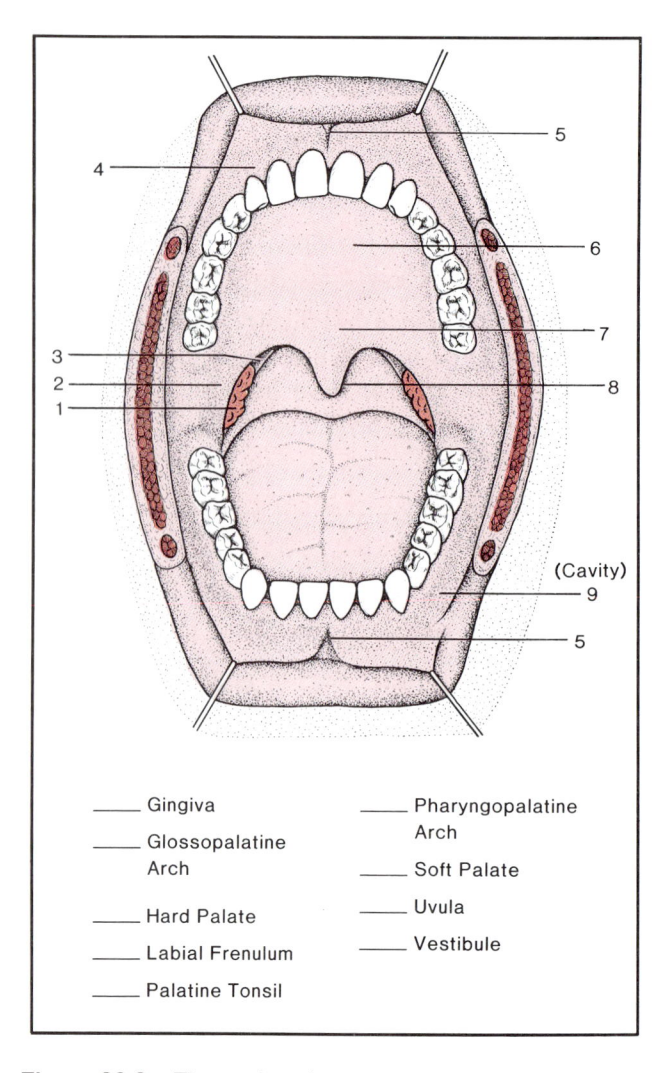

____ Gingiva	____ Pharyngopalatine Arch
____ Glossopalatine Arch	____ Soft Palate
____ Hard Palate	____ Uvula
____ Labial Frenulum	____ Vestibule
____ Palatine Tonsil	

Figure 36.2 The oral cavity.

the anatomical differences between these papillae. The majority of the projections have tapered points and are called **filiform papillae.** These projections are sensitive to touch and give the dorsum a rough texture. This roughness provides friction for the handling of food. Scattered among the filiform papillae are the larger rounded **fungiform papillae.** Two fungiform papillae are shown in the sectioned portion. A third type of papilla is the donut-shaped **vallate** (*circumvallate*) **papilla,** which is the largest of the three kinds. They are arranged in a "V" near the posterior margin of the dorsum. Although the exact number may vary in individuals, eight vallate papillae are shown.

The fungiform and vallate papillae contain **taste buds,** the receptors for taste. The circular furrow of the vallate papilla in the cutout section reveals the presence of these receptors. Comparatively speaking, the vallate papillae contain many more taste buds than the fungiform papillae.

A fourth type of papilla is the **foliate papilla.** These projections exist as vertical rows of folds of mucosa on each side of the tongue, posteriorly. A few taste buds are also scattered among these papillae.

Assignment:

Label figure 36.3.

The Salivary Glands

The salivary glands are grouped according to size. The largest glands, of which there are three pairs, are referred to as the *major salivary glands*. They are the parotids, submandibulars, and sublinguals. The smaller glands, which average only 2–5 mm in diameter, are the *minor salivary glands*.

Major Salivary Glands

Figure 36.4 illustrates the relative positions of the three major salivary glands as seen on the left side of the face. Since all of these glands are paired, it should be kept in mind that the other side of the face has another set of these glands.

The largest gland, which lies under the skin of the cheek in front of the ear, is the **parotid gland.** Note that it lies between the skin layer and the *masseter muscle.* Leading from this gland is the **parotid** (*Stensen's*) **duct,** which passes over the masseter and through the **buccinator muscle** into the oral cavity. The drainage opening of this duct usually exits near the upper second molar. The secretion of the parotid glands is a clear watery fluid that has a cleansing action in the mouth. It contains the digestive enzyme *salivary amylase,* which splits starch molecules into disaccharides (double sugar). The presence of sour (acid) substances in the mouth causes the gland to increase its secretion.

Inside the arch of the mandible lies the **submandibular** (*submaxillary*) **gland.** In figure 36.4 the mandible has been cut away to reveal two cut surfaces. Note that the lower margin of the submandibular gland extends down somewhat below the inferior border of the mandible. Also, note that a

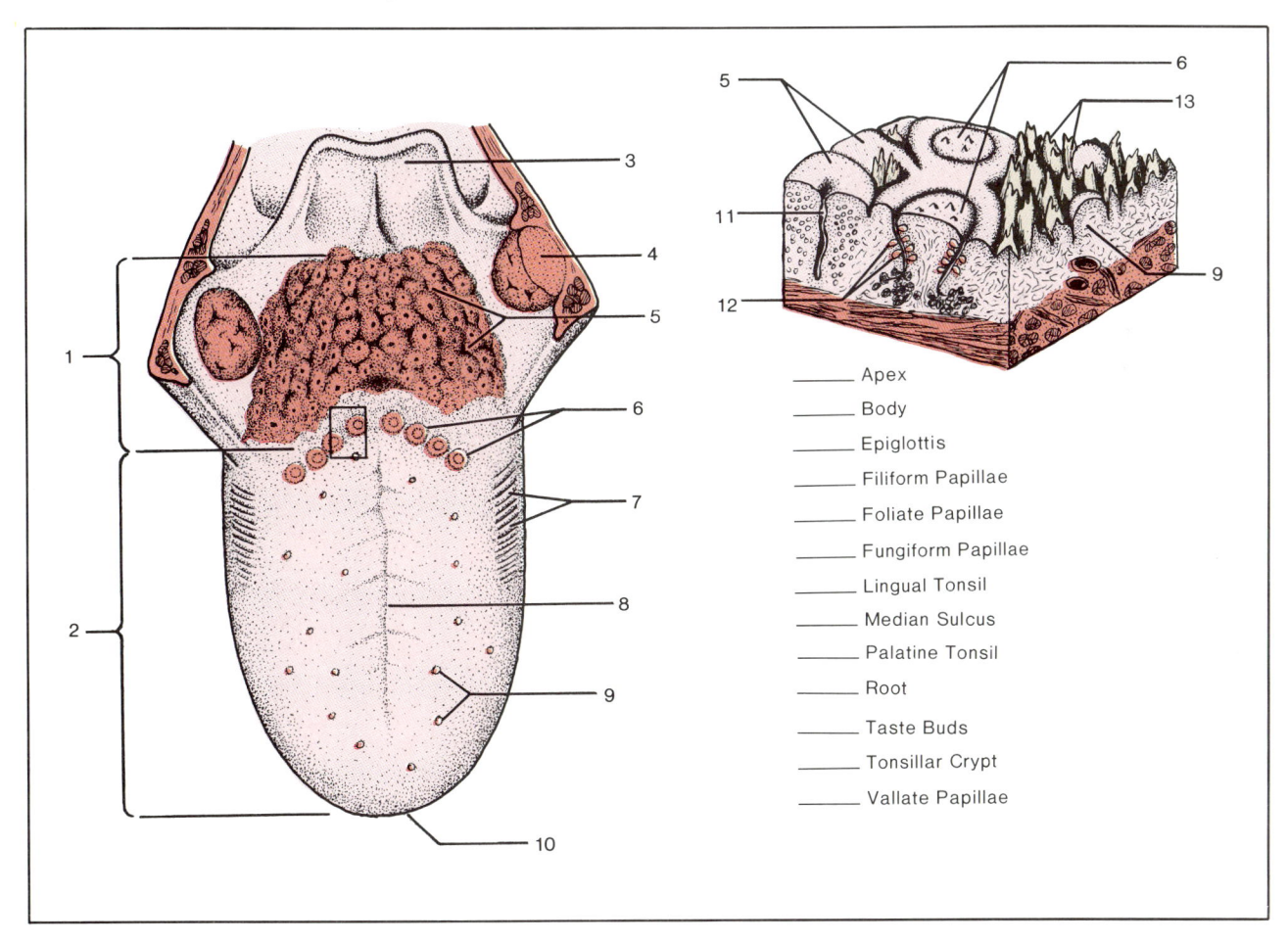

_____	Apex
_____	Body
_____	Epiglottis
_____	Filiform Papillae
_____	Foliate Papillae
_____	Fungiform Papillae
_____	Lingual Tonsil
_____	Median Sulcus
_____	Palatine Tonsil
_____	Root
_____	Taste Buds
_____	Tonsillar Crypt
_____	Vallate Papillae

Figure 36.3   Tongue anatomy.

flat muscle, the *mylohyoid,* extends somewhat into the gland. The secretions of this gland empty into the oral cavity through the **submandibular** (*Wharton's*) **duct.** The **opening of the submandibular duct** is located under the tongue near the lingual frenulum. The **lingual frenulum** is a mucosal fold on the median line between the tongue and the floor of the mouth. It is shown in figure 36.4 as a triangular membrane. The secretion of the submandibulars is quite similar in consistency to that of the parotid glands, except that it is slightly more viscous due to the presence of some mucin. This ingredient of saliva aids in holding the food together in a bolus. Bland substances such as bread and milk stimulate this gland.

The **sublingual gland** is the smallest of the three major salivary glands. As its name would imply, it

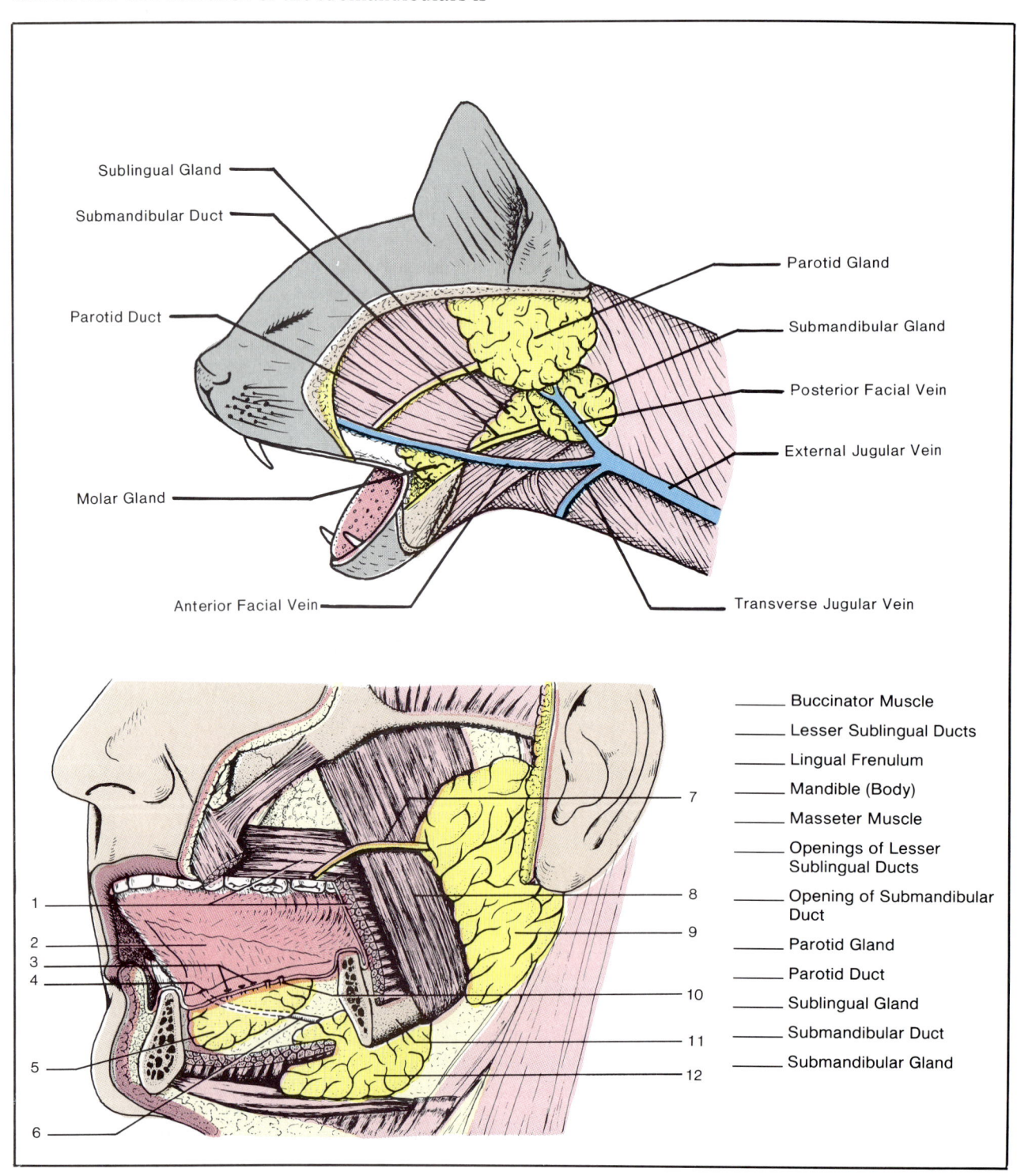

Figure 36.4 Major salivary glands, cat and human.

is located under the tongue in the floor of the mouth. It is encased in a fold of mucosa, the **sublingual fold,** under the tongue. This fold is shown in figure 36.5 (label 5). Drainage of this gland is through several **lesser sublingual ducts** (*ducts of Rivinus*). The number of openings is variable in different individuals. The gland differs from the other two in that it is primarily a mucous gland. The high mucin content of its secretion lends a certain degree of ropiness to it.

Minor Salivary Glands

There are four principal groups of these smaller salivary glands in the mouth: the palatine, lingual, buccal, and labial glands. In illustration A, figure 36.5, the palatine mucosa has been removed to reveal the closely packed nature of the **palatine glands.** These glands, which are about 2–4 mm in diameter, almost completely cover the roof of the oral cavity. Where the mucosa has been removed near the lower third molar we see that the glands occur even next to the teeth. The glands in this particular area are called **retromolar glands.**

Illustration B in figure 36.5 shows the oral cavity with the tongue pointed upward and the in-ferior surface partially removed. The gland exposed in this area of the tongue is the **anterior lingual gland.**

The **buccal glands** cover the majority of the inner surface of the cheeks, and the **labial glands** are found under the inner surface of the lips. All of the minor glands except for the palatine glands, produce salivary amylase. The palatine glands are primarily mucous glands.

Assignment:

Label figures 36.4 and 36.5.

The Teeth

Every individual develops two sets of teeth during the first twenty-one years of life. The first set, which begins to appear at approximately six months of age, are the *deciduous* teeth. Various other terms such as *primary, baby,* or *milk* teeth are also used in reference to these teeth. The second set of teeth, known as *permanent* or *secondary,* teeth, begin to appear when the child is about six years of age. As a result of normal growth from the sixth year on, the jaws enlarge, the secondary teeth begin to exert

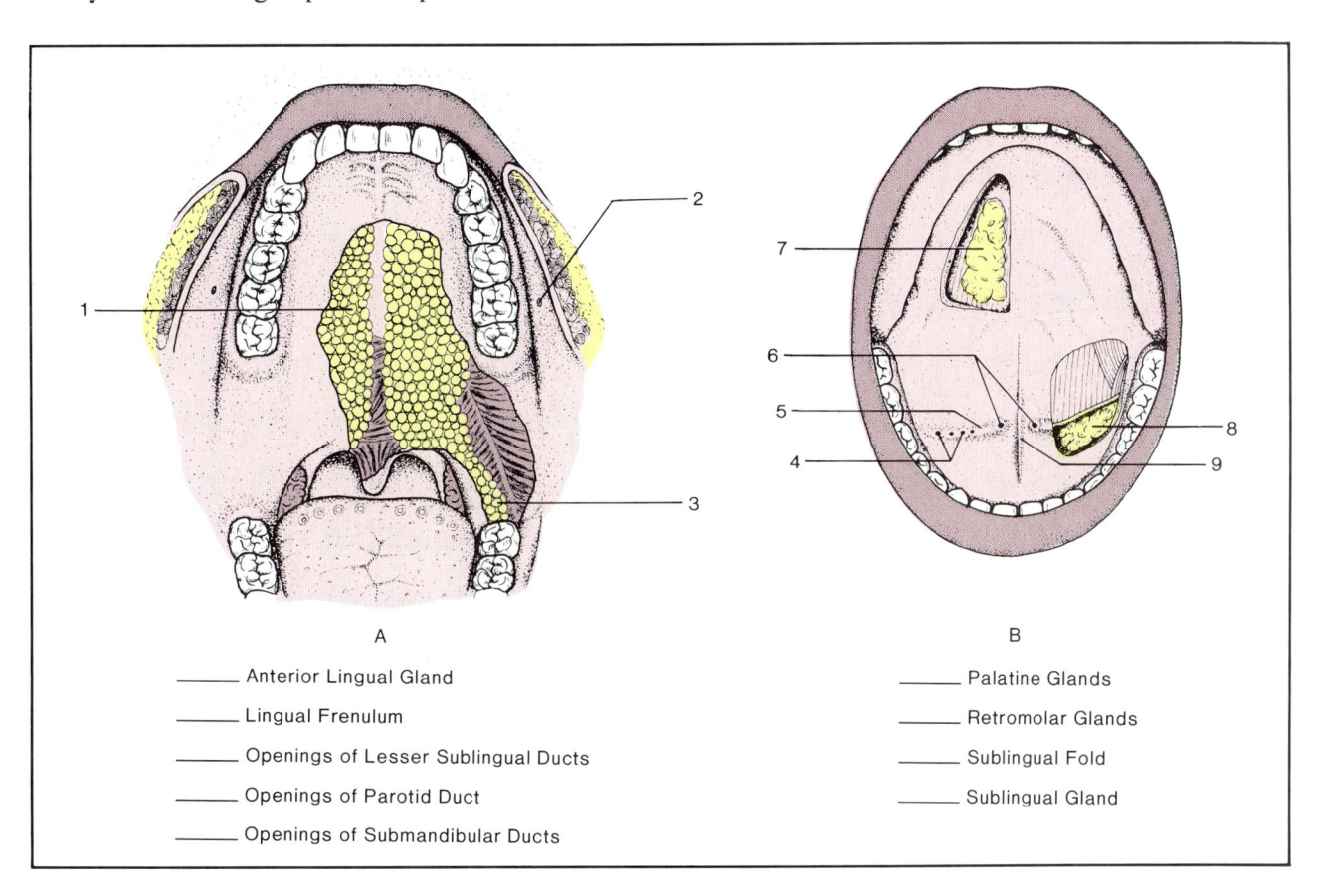

A

_____ Anterior Lingual Gland

_____ Lingual Frenulum

_____ Openings of Lesser Sublingual Ducts

_____ Openings of Parotid Duct

_____ Openings of Submandibular Ducts

B

_____ Palatine Glands

_____ Retromolar Glands

_____ Sublingual Fold

_____ Sublingual Gland

Figure 36.5   Minor salivary glands.

pressure on the primary teeth, and *exfoliation,* or shedding, of the deciduous dentition occurs.

The Deciduous Teeth

The deciduous teeth number twenty in all—five in each quadrant of the jaws. Normally, all twenty have erupted by the time the child is two years old. Starting with the first tooth at the median line, they are named as follows: **central incisor, lateral incisor, cuspid** (*canine*), **first molar,** and **second molar.** The naming of the lower teeth follows the same sequence.

Once the two-year-old child has all of the deciduous teeth, no visible change in the teeth occurs until around the sixth year. At this time the first permanent molars begin to erupt.

The Permanent Teeth

For approximately five years (seventh to twelfth year) the child will have a *mixed dentition,* consisting of both deciduous and permanent teeth. As the submerged permanent teeth enlarge in the tissues, the roots of the deciduous teeth undergo *re-*

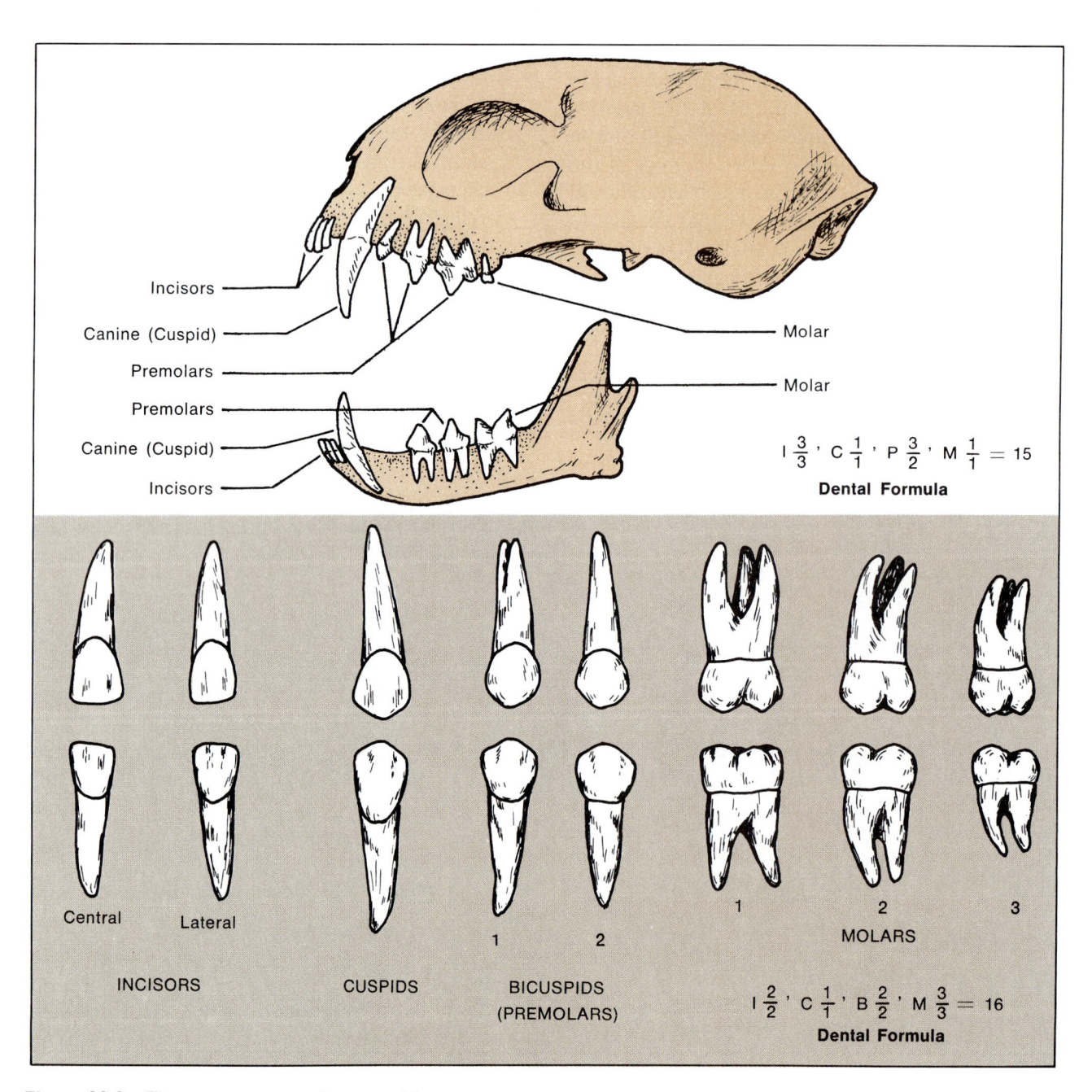

$$I \frac{3}{3}, \; C \frac{1}{1}, \; P \frac{3}{2}, \; M \frac{1}{1} = 15$$
Dental Formula

$$I \frac{2}{2}, \; C \frac{1}{1}, \; B \frac{2}{2}, \; M \frac{3}{3} = 16$$
Dental Formula

Figure 36.6 The permanent teeth, cat and human.

sorption. This removal of the underpinnings of the deciduous teeth results eventually in exfoliation.

Figure 36.6 illustrates the permanent dentition. Note that there are sixteen teeth in one half of the mouth—thus, a total of thirty-two teeth. Naming them in sequence from the median line of the mouth they are **central incisor, lateral incisor, cuspid** (*canine*), **first bicuspid, second bicuspid, first molar, second molar,** and **third molar.** The third molar is also called the *wisdom tooth.*

Comparisons of the teeth in figure 36.6 reveal that the anterior teeth have single roots and the posterior teeth may have several roots. Of the bicuspids, the only ones that have two roots (*bifurcated*) are the maxillary first bicuspids. Although all of the maxillary molars are shown with three roots (*trifurcated*) there may be considerable variability, particularly with respect to the third molar. The roots of the mandibular molars are generally bifurcated. The longest roots are seen on the maxillary cuspids.

Assignment:

Identify the teeth of skulls that are available in the laboratory.

Tooth Anatomy

The anatomy of an individual tooth is shown in figure 36.7. Longitudinally, it is divided into two portions, the crown and root. The line where these two parts meet is the **cervical line** or *cemento-enamel juncture.*

The dentist sees the crown from two aspects: the anatomical and clinical crowns. The **anatomical crown** is the portion of the tooth that is covered with enamel. The **clinical crown,** on the other hand, is the portion of the crown that is exposed in the mouth. The structure and physical condition of the soft tissues around the neck of the tooth will determine the size of the clinical crown.

The tooth is composed of four tissues: the enamel, dentin, pulp, and cementum. **Enamel** is the most densely mineralized and hardest material in the body. Ninety-six percent of enamel is mineral. The remaining 4 % is a carbohydrate-protein complex. Calcium and phosphorus make up over 50% of the chemical structure of enamel. Microscopically, this tissue is made up of very fine rods or prisms that lie approximately perpendicular to the outer surface of the crown. It has been estimated that the upper molars may have as many as twelve

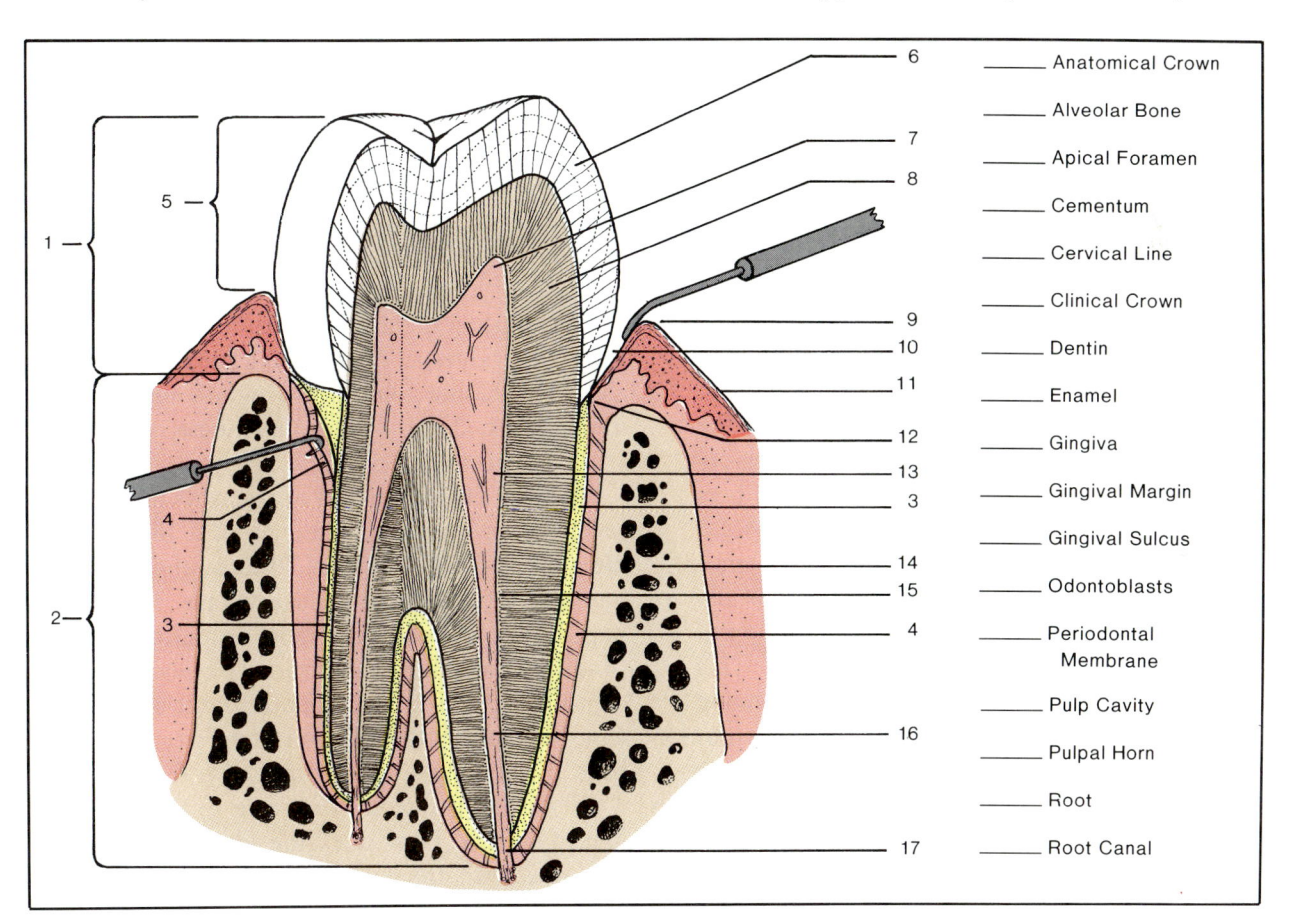

6	Anatomical Crown
	Alveolar Bone
7	Apical Foramen
8	Cementum
	Cervical Line
	Clinical Crown
9	Dentin
10	Enamel
11	Gingiva
12	Gingival Margin
13	Gingival Sulcus
3	Odontoblasts
14	Periodontal Membrane
15	Pulp Cavity
4	Pulpal Horn
16	Root
17	Root Canal

Figure 36.7 Tooth anatomy.

million of these small prisms per tooth. The hardness of enamel enables the tooth to withstand the abrasive action of one tooth against another.

Dentin is the material which makes up the bulk of the tooth and lies beneath the enamel. It is not as hard or brittle as the enamel and resembles bone in composition and hardness. This tissue is produced by a layer of **odontoblasts** (label 15) that lies in the outer margin of the pulp cavity.

Cementum is the hard dental tissue that covers the anatomical root of the tooth. It is a modified bone tissue, somewhat resembling osseous tissue. It is produced by cells called *cementocytes,* which are very similar to osteocytes. The primary function of the cementum is to provide attachment of the tooth to surrounding tissues in the alveolus.

The cavity that occupies the central portion of the tooth is called the **pulp cavity.** Extending down into the roots, this cavity becomes the **root canals.** Where this chamber extends up into the cusps of the crown, it forms the **pulpal horns.** The tissue of the pulp is essentially loose connective tissue. It consists of fibroblasts, intercellular ground substance, and white fibers. Permeating this tissue are blood vessels, lymphatic vessels, and nerve fibers. The functions of the pulp are to (1) provide nourishment for the living cells of the tooth, (2) provide some sensation to the tooth, and (3) produce dentin. The blood vessels and nerve fibers that enter the pulp cavity do so through openings, the **apical foramina,** in the tips of the roots. Inflammation of the pulp, or *pulpitis,* may result in the destruction of the blood vessels and nerves producing a dead or *devitalized* tooth.

Between the cementum and the alveolar bone lies a vascular layer of connective tissue, the **periodontal membrane.** On the left side of figure 36.7, it is shown pulled away from the root. One of the principal functions of this membrane is tooth retention. The membrane consists of bundles of fibers that extend from the cementum to the alveolar bone, firmly holding the tooth in place. Its presence also acts as a cushion to reduce the trauma of occlusal action. Another very important function of this membrane is tooth sensitivity to touch. This sensitivity is due to the presence of free nerve ending receptors in the membrane. The slightest touch at the surface of the tooth is transmitted to these nerve endings through the medium of the periodontal membrane. Even if the apical parts of the membrane are removed, as in root tip resection, the sense of touch is not impaired.

To demonstrate the depth of the **gingival sulcus,** a probe is seen on the right side of figure 36.7. This crevice is frequently a site for bacterial putrefaction and the origin of *gingivitis.* The upper edge of the gingiva is called the **gingival margin.** The portion of the gingiva that lies over the alveolar bone is called the *alveolar mucosa.*

Assignment:

Label figure 36.7.

Cat Dissection

Since the anatomical study of the circulatory, respiratory, and digestive systems of the cat cannot be studied independently of each other, it is very likely that this dissection may be performed simultaneously with the study of the other two systems. It is because of these interrelationships that there will be some repetition of discussion of anatomical structures.

Oral Cavity

If Exercise 35 has already been completed, you will have identified the *oral cavity, nasal cavity, nasopharynx, oropharynx, soft palate, hard palate, palatine tonsils, auditory tube aperture, esophagus, larynx,* and *trachea.* If you have not studied these organs previously, refer to page 215 to identify these structures. It will be necessary for some specimens to be cut along the medial line with a bone saw, as described on page 217, to reveal some of these structures.

In addition to the above structures, identify the transverse ridges, or **rugae,** of the hard palate, which assist in holding food in the mouth during swallowing. Also identify the **oral vestibule,** which is the space between the teeth and lips.

Lift up the tongue and examine its inferior surface. Do you see any evidence of a **lingual frenulum?** The cat has distinct **filiform** and **fungiform papillae** on the tongue's dorsal surface. The filiform papillae are spinelike and more numerous than the fungiform papillae. In addition to being tactile receptors, the filiform papillae also act as scrapers. Can you locate the **circumvallate papillae** at the back of the tongue? How many are there?

Examine the teeth, referring to figure 36.6 to identify them. How does the number of **incisors** compare with the human? Note how extremely small they are. The important anterior teeth on the cat are the **canines.** They function to kill small prey and tear away portions of food. Note that there are three upper and two lower **premolars** in the cat. Observe how insignificant the upper **molar** is compared to the lower molar. Since cats are carnivores and swallow chunks of meat without chewing it, the posterior teeth act as shears rather than grinders. No flat occlusal surfaces are seen on the cat's posterior teeth.

Salivary Glands

Remove the skin and platysma muscle from the left side of the head if this has not already been done. Any lymph nodes that obscure the anterior facial vein should be removed. Referring to figure 36.4 identify the **parotid, submandibular** and **sublingual glands.** What gland is seen on the cat that is lacking in humans? Can you locate the **parotid** and **submandibular ducts?** A fifth gland, the **infraorbital gland,** exists in the floor of each eye orbit but cannot be seen unless the eye is removed.

Esophagus

Force a probe into the upper end of the esophagus and stretch its walls laterally. Note how much it can be distended. Trace it down to where it penetrates the diaphragm and liver to enter the stomach.

Abdominal Organs

If the circulatory system has already been studied, the abdominal cavity will be open for the re-mainder of this study. If the abdomen has not been opened yet, make an incision with scissors along the median line from the thoracic region to the symphysis pubis. Also, make additional cuts laterally from the median line in the pubic region so that the muscle of the abdominal wall can be pulled aside to expose all the organs.

The two most prominent structures revealed by removing the abdominal wall are the liver and the greater omentum. Examine the **greater omentum.** It is a double sheet of peritoneum that is attached to the greater curvature of the stomach and to the dorsal body wall. Only a small segment of it is revealed in figure 36.9, because most of it has been cut away to expose the intestines which lie under it. Lift up the greater omentum and examine both surfaces. Note that the potential space (*omental bursa*) between its two layers of peritoneum is filled with fat. Cut a slit into its surface to confirm its structure. That portion of the greater omentum between the stomach and spleen is called the **gastrosplenic ligament.** Identify this latter ligament as well as the **spleen** and **stomach.** Cut away and discard most of the greater omentum so that it will not be in the way.

Identify the right medial, right lateral, left medial, and left lateral **lobes of the liver.** Also, locate the soft greenish **gallbladder.** By referring to figure 36.8, identify the falciform and round ligaments. The **falciform ligament** is a sickle-shaped (Latin: *falx, falcis,* sickle) double-layered peritoneal fold that lies in the notch between the right and left

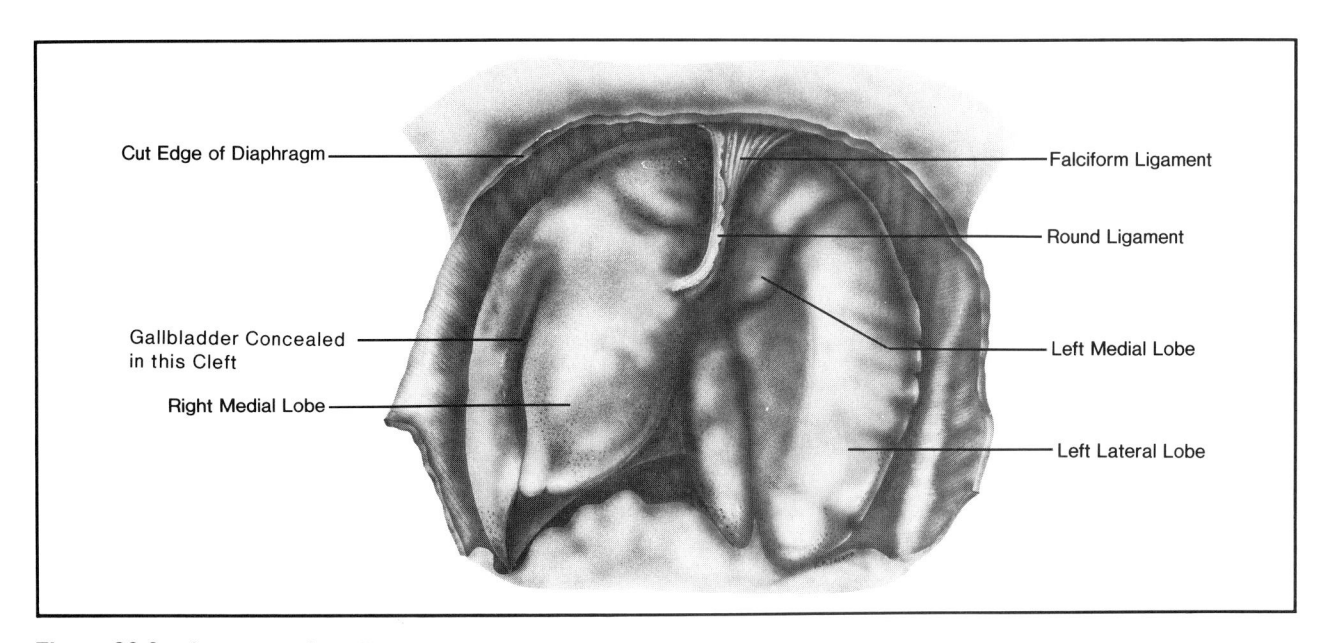

Figure 36.8 Anatomy of cat liver, anterior view.

medial lobes of the liver. Spread apart these lobes and lift this membrane out with a pair of forceps. Note that its left margin is attached to the diaphragm. Its free margin contains a thickened structure, the **round ligament.** This ligament is a vestige of the umbilical vein that functioned during prenatal existence.

Identify the **lesser omentum,** which extends from the liver to the lesser curvature of the stomach and a portion of the duodenum. The common bile duct, hepatic artery, and portal vein lie within the lateral border of the lesser omentum. Dissect into this region to see if these latter structures can be seen.

Probe into the space under the right medial lobe of the liver and locate the **cystic duct,** which leads from the gallbladder into the **common bile duct.**

Raise the liver sufficiently to see where the esophagus enters the stomach. Identify the **fundus, body,** and **pylorus** of the stomach. That portion of the stomach where the esophagus joins it is called the **cardiac portion.** Open up the stomach by making the incision along its long axis. Observe that its lining has long folds called **rugae.**

Identify the **duodenum.** Note that it passes posteriorly about 3 inches and then doubles back on itself for another 3 or 4 inches. Within this duodenal loop lies the duodenal portion of the **pancreas.** The pancreas is quite long in that it extends from the duodenum over to the spleen. The mesentery which supports the duodenum and pancreas in this region is called the *mesoduodenum.*

Expose the **pancreatic duct** by dissecting away some of the pancreatic tissue. This duct lies

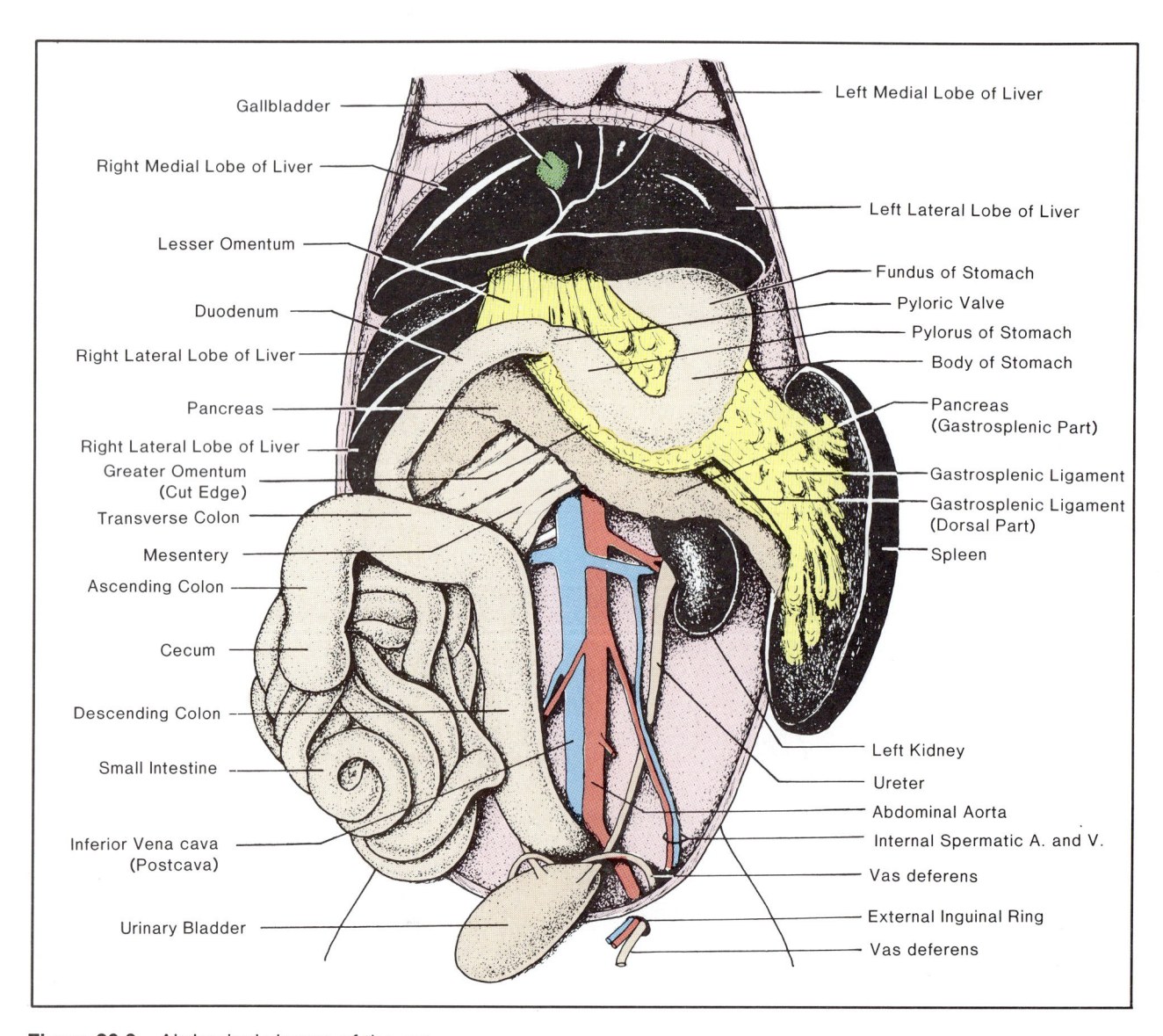

Figure 36.9 Abdominal viscera of the cat.

embedded in the gland. It joins the common bile duct to form a short duct, the **ampulla of Vater,** that empties into the duodenum. A small **accessory pancreatic duct** is often seen entering the duodenum about two centimeters caudad to the ampulla of Vater. It is often confused with small arteries in this region.

The remainder of the small intestine is divided, arbitrarily, into a proximal half, the **jejunum,** and a distal half, the **ileum.** Trace the ileum to where it enters the cecum.

Remove a two-inch section of the ileum or jejunum, slit it open longitudinally, and wash out its interior. Examine its inner lining with a dissecting microscope or hand lens, looking for the minute tubular projections called *villi.*

The large intestine consists of the **cecum, ascending colon, transverse colon,** and **descending colon.** The descending colon empties into the **rectum** which exits through the **anus.** Identify all these structures. Make an incision through the wall of the cecum on the side opposite where the ilium enters it to reveal the **ileocecal valve.**

Histological Studies

Make a systematic histological study of the organs of the digestive system, using the Histology Atlas for reference.

Materials:

Prepared slides of:

taste buds (H5.120, H5.121),
salivary glands (H5.131, H5.133, H5.134),
esophagus (5.311), stomach (H5.415),
duodenum, jejunum, and ileum (H5.58),
colon (H5.613), appendix (H5.65),
anal canal (H5.67)
tooth embryology (H5.1176, H5.1184)

Salivary Glands Examine slides of the three salivary glands, using figure HA-18 to note the histological differences between them.

Taste Buds Examine slides of vallate or foliate papillae. Identify the structures shown on figure HA-19.

Tooth Embryology Read the legend on figure HA-20 and examine slides to identify the structures shown in figure HA-20. Note in particular what cells give rise to dentin and enamel.

Esophagus Identify the four coats that make up the wall of the esophagus. Note in particular the type of epithelial tissue that lines the esophagus. Use figure HA-21 for reference.

Stomach Wall Examine a slide of the fundus of the stomach and compare it to illustrations C and D of figure HA-21. Study the deep cells within the pits and differentiate the **parietal** and **chief cells.** How do these cells differ in function? How does the mucosa of the stomach differ from the mucosa of the esophagus?

Small Intestine Study a slide that has all three sections of the small intestine. Use figures HA-22 and HA-23 for reference. Note the differences that exist between the duodenal and intestinal glands. How do these glands differ in function? What is the function of the lacteal in a villus? Look for lymphoidal tissue (**Peyer's patches**) in the ileum (see illustration D, figure HA-27). This tissue makes up the gut-associated lymphoid tissue (GALT) of the digestive tract, an important part of the immune system.

Large Intestine Examine a slide of the colon and refer to illustrations A and B, figure HA-24. What is lacking on the mucosa of the colon that is seen in the small intestine? Identify all structures.

Appendix Refer to illustration C, figure HA-24 while studying a slide of the appendix. Compare its structure with the colon. What function would lymph nodules perform here?

Liver and Pancreas When examining slides of the liver and pancreas, read the legend on figure HA-25 which explains the significance of the structures labeled in the four illustrations.

Gallbladder Refer to illustrations A and B, figure HA-26, while studying a slide of the gallbladder. How does the mucosa of the gallbladder resemble the small intestine? How does it differ?

Anal Canal Determine what kind of tissue makes up the mucosa in this region. Consult illustration D, figure HA-24.

Laboratory Report

Complete the Laboratory Report for this exercise.

37 The Urinary System

This study consists of three parts: (1) cat dissection, (2) sheep kidney dissection, and (3) microscopic studies. Although the anatomy of the cat's kidneys will be studied, the sheep kidney is also included here for dissection because of its more generous size. A general description of the human urinary system will precede these laboratory activities.

Organs of the Urinary System

Figure 37.1 illustrates the components of the urinary system with its principal blood supply. It consists of two kidneys, two ureters, the urinary bladder, and a urethra. The **kidneys** are somewhat bean-shaped, of dark brown color, and located behind the peritoneum. The right kidney is usually positioned somewhat lower than the left one, probably because of its displacement by the liver. Each kidney is supplied blood through a **renal artery** that is a branch off the **abdominal aorta.** Blood leaves each kidney through a **renal vein** that empties into the **inferior vena cava.**

Urine passes from each kidney to the **urinary bladder** through a **ureter.** The upper end of each ureter is enlarged to form a funnellike *pelvis.* The lower end of each ureter enters the posterior surface of the bladder.

Leading from the urinary bladder to the exterior is a short tube, the **urethra.** In the male the urethra is about 20 centimeters long; in females it is approximately 4 centimeters in length.

The exit of urine from the bladder is called *micturition.* The passage of urine from the bladder is controlled by two sphincter muscles, the sphincter vesicae and the sphincter urethrae. The **sphincter vesicae** is a smooth muscle sphincter that is near the exit of the bladder. When approximately 300 ml of urine has accumulated in the bladder, the muscular walls of the bladder are stretched sufficiently to initiate a parasympathetic reflex that causes the bladder wall to contract. These contractions force urine past the sphincter vesicae into the urethra above the **sphincter urethrae.** This second sphincter, which is located approximately 1–3 centimeters below the sphincter vesicae, consists of skeletal muscle fibers and is voluntarily controlled. The presence of urine in the urethra above this sphincter creates the desire to micturate;

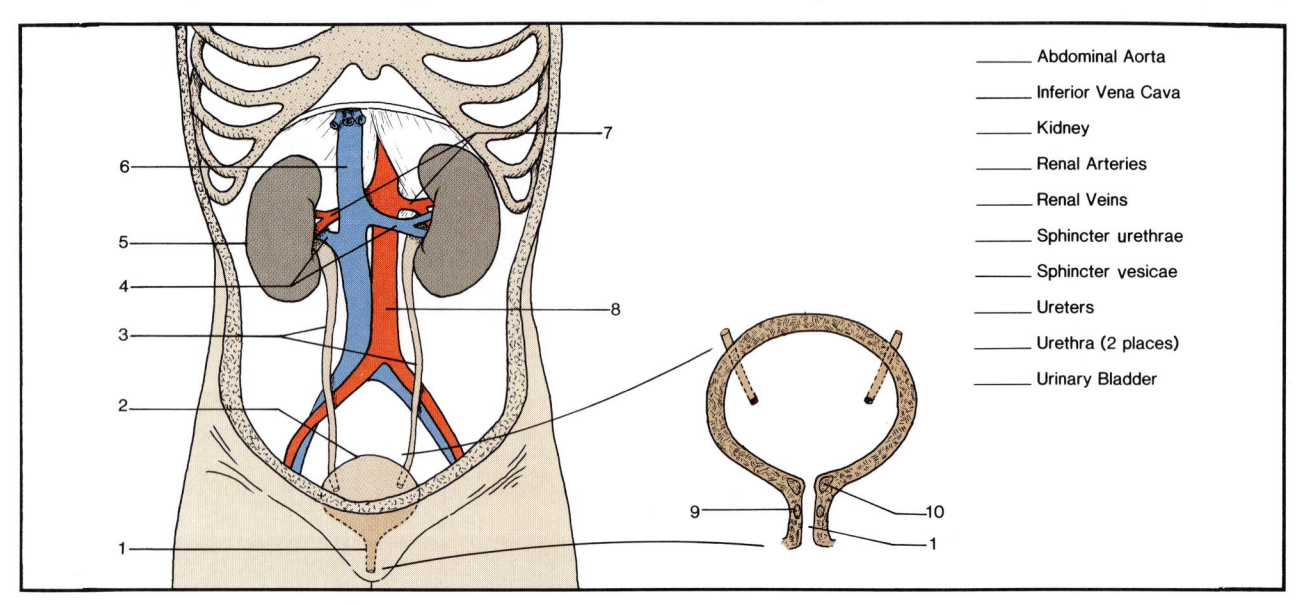

_____ Abdominal Aorta
_____ Inferior Vena Cava
_____ Kidney
_____ Renal Arteries
_____ Renal Veins
_____ Sphincter urethrae
_____ Sphincter vesicae
_____ Ureters
_____ Urethra (2 places)
_____ Urinary Bladder

Figure 37.1   The urinary system.

however, since the valve is under voluntary control, micturition can be inhibited. When both sphincters are relaxed, urine passes from the body.

Assignment:

Label figure 37.1.

Kidney Anatomy

Figure 37.2 reveals a frontal section of a human kidney. Its outer surface is covered with a thin fibrous **renal capsule** (label 8). In addition to this thin covering, the kidney is provided support and protection by a fatty capsule which completely encases it. The latter is not shown in figures 37.1 or 37.2.

Immediately under the capsule is the **cortex** of the kidney. The cortex is reddish-brown due to its great blood supply. The lighter inner portion is called the **medulla.** The medulla is divided into cone-shaped **renal pyramids.** Nine of these pyramids are seen in figure 37.2. Cortical tissue, in the form of **renal columns,** extends down between the pyramids. Each renal pyramid terminates as a **renal papilla,** which projects into a calyx. The **calyces** are short tubes that receive urine from the renal papillae; they empty into the large funnellike **renal pelvis.**

Nephrons

The basic functioning unit of the kidney is the *nephron.* The enlarged section in figure 37.2 reveals two nephrons. Figure 37.3 illustrates a single nephron in greater detail. It has been estimated that

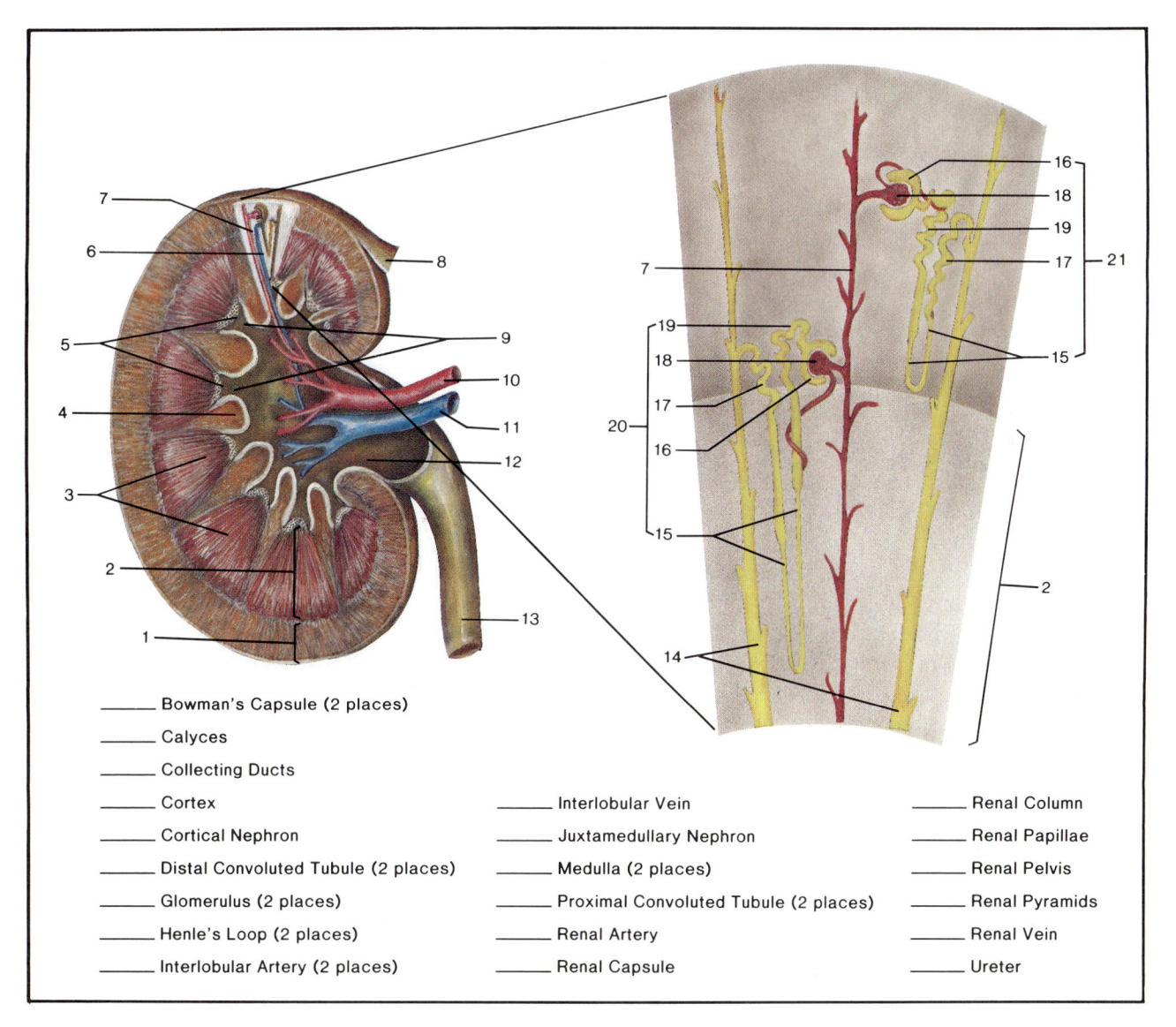

_____ Bowman's Capsule (2 places)		
_____ Calyces		
_____ Collecting Ducts		
_____ Cortex	_____ Interlobular Vein	_____ Renal Column
_____ Cortical Nephron	_____ Juxtamedullary Nephron	_____ Renal Papillae
_____ Distal Convoluted Tubule (2 places)	_____ Medulla (2 places)	_____ Renal Pelvis
_____ Glomerulus (2 places)	_____ Proximal Convoluted Tubule (2 places)	_____ Renal Pyramids
_____ Henle's Loop (2 places)	_____ Renal Artery	_____ Renal Vein
_____ Interlobular Artery (2 places)	_____ Renal Capsule	_____ Ureter

Figure 37.2 Anatomy of the kidney.

there are around one million nephrons in each kidney. Approximately 80% of the nephrons are located in the cortex; these are designated as **cortical nephrons.** The remainder, or **juxtamedullary nephrons** (label 20, figure 37.2), are located partially in the cortex and partially in the medulla.

The formation of urine by the nephron results from three physiological activities that occur in different regions of the nephron: (1) filtration, (2) reabsorption, and (3) secretion. Because of the differing functions of various regions of the nephron, the fluid that first forms at the beginning of the nephron is quite unlike the urine that enters the calyces of the kidney.

Note that each nephron consists of an enlarged end, the **renal corpuscle,** and a long tubule that empties eventually into the calyx of the kidney. Each renal corpuscle has two parts: an inner tuft of capillaries, the **glomerulus,** and an outer double-walled caplike structure, the **glomerular** (*Bowman's*) **capsule.** Blood that enters the kidney through the **renal artery** reaches each nephron through an **interlobular artery** (label 2, figure 37.3). A short **afferent arteriole** conveys blood into the glomerulus from the interlobular artery. Blood exits from the glomerulus through the **efferent arteriole,** which has a much smaller diameter than the afferent vessel.

The high intraglomerular blood pressure forces a highly dilute fluid, the *glomerular filtrate,* to pass into the glomerular capsule. This fluid consists of glucose, amino acids, urea, salts, and a great deal of water.

This filtrate passes next through the **proximal convoluted tubule** (label 8), the **descending limb of Henle's loop** (label 12), the **ascending limb of Henle's loop,** and the **distal convoluted tubule** (label 10) before emptying into the large **collecting duct** on the right side of the diagram. A single collecting duct may have several nephrons emptying into it.

As the filtrate moves through these various regions, water, glucose, amino acids, and other substances are reabsorbed back into the blood of the **peritubular capillaries** that enmesh the entire route. Eighty percent of the water is reabsorbed through the walls of the proximal convoluted tubules. Water reabsorption is facilitated by the *antidiuretic hormone* of the posterior pituitary and *aldosterone* of the adrenal cortex. Cells lining the collecting ducts alter urine composition by secreting ammonia, uric acid, and other substances into the lumen of the duct.

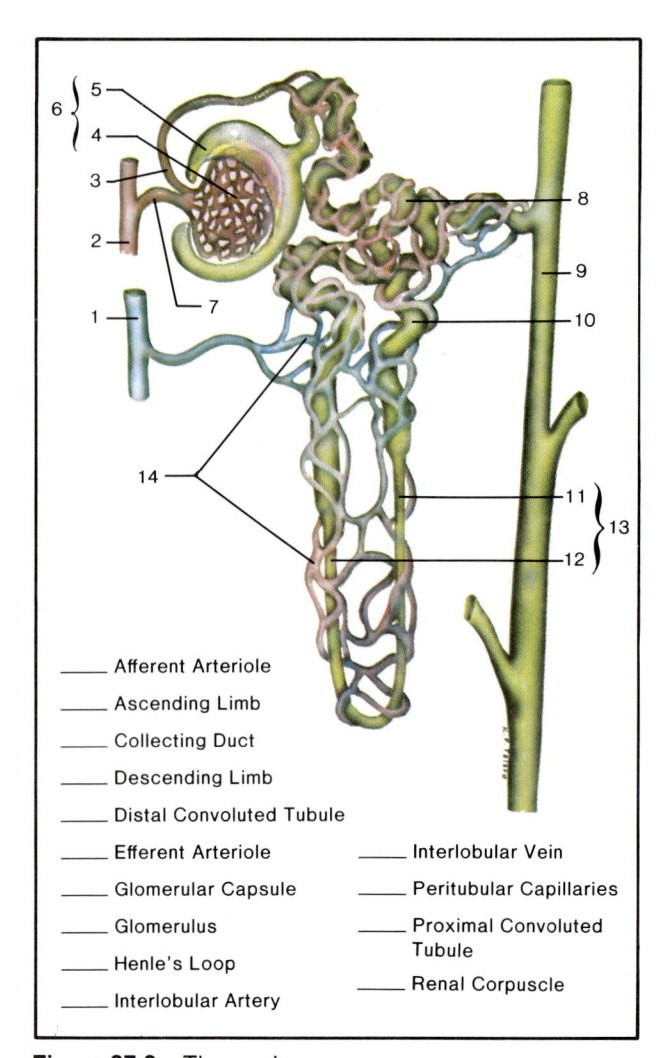

_____ Afferent Arteriole

_____ Ascending Limb

_____ Collecting Duct

_____ Descending Limb

_____ Distal Convoluted Tubule

_____ Efferent Arteriole   _____ Interlobular Vein

_____ Glomerular Capsule   _____ Peritubular Capillaries

_____ Glomerulus   _____ Proximal Convoluted Tubule

_____ Henle's Loop

_____ Interlobular Artery   _____ Renal Corpuscle

Figure 37.3 The nephron.

Assignment:

Label figures 37.2 and 37.3.

Histological Study

Materials:

Prepared slides of:
kidney tissue (H9.11, H9.115, or H9.14)
ureter (H9.16), urinary bladder (H9.21)

Examine slides of the **kidney cortex, kidney medulla, ureter,** and **urinary bladder,** and compare them to figures HA-29, HA-30, HA-26 (illus. C and D), and HA-33 (illus. A and B). Note the differences in kinds of tissue seen in the tubules, calyx, urinary bladder, and ureters.

Sheep Kidney Dissection

Dissection of the sheep kidney may be combined with the cat dissection to provide greater anatomical clarity. Although the injected cat kidney may illustrate better the blood supply, the fresh sheep kidney will reveal more vividly some of the lifelike characteristics of the kidney.

Materials:

dissecting kit, tray, long knife
fresh sheep kidneys

1. If the kidneys are still encased in fat, peel it off carefully. As you lift the fat away from the kidney, look carefully for the **adrenal gland,** which should be embedded in the fat near one end of the kidney. Remove the adrenal gland from the fat and cut it in half. Note that the gland has a distinct outer **cortex** and inner **medulla.**
2. Probe into the surface of the kidney with a sharp dissecting needle to see if you can differentiate the **capsule** from the underlying tissue.
3. With a long knife, slice the kidney longitudinally to produce a frontal section similar to figure 37.2. Wash out the cut halves with running water.

4. Identify all the structures seen in the kidney section of figure 37.2.

Cat Dissection

The close association of the urinary and reproductive organs necessitates the study of the organs of these two systems together. Most emphasis, however, will be placed here on the urinary system. As you proceed through the following dissection, refer to figures 37.4 and 37.5 to identify the various organs. A more detailed study of the reproductive organs will be made in Exercise 39.

1. To expose the urogenital system, remove the liver, spleen, and stomach. With forceps and scalpel clear away excess fat, the peritoneum, and other connective tissue in the area. *Take care not to injure the internal spermatic (or ovarian) blood vessels and the ureters, which are embedded in fat.*
2. Note that the **kidneys** lie between the peritoneum and the body wall (*retroperitoneal*) and

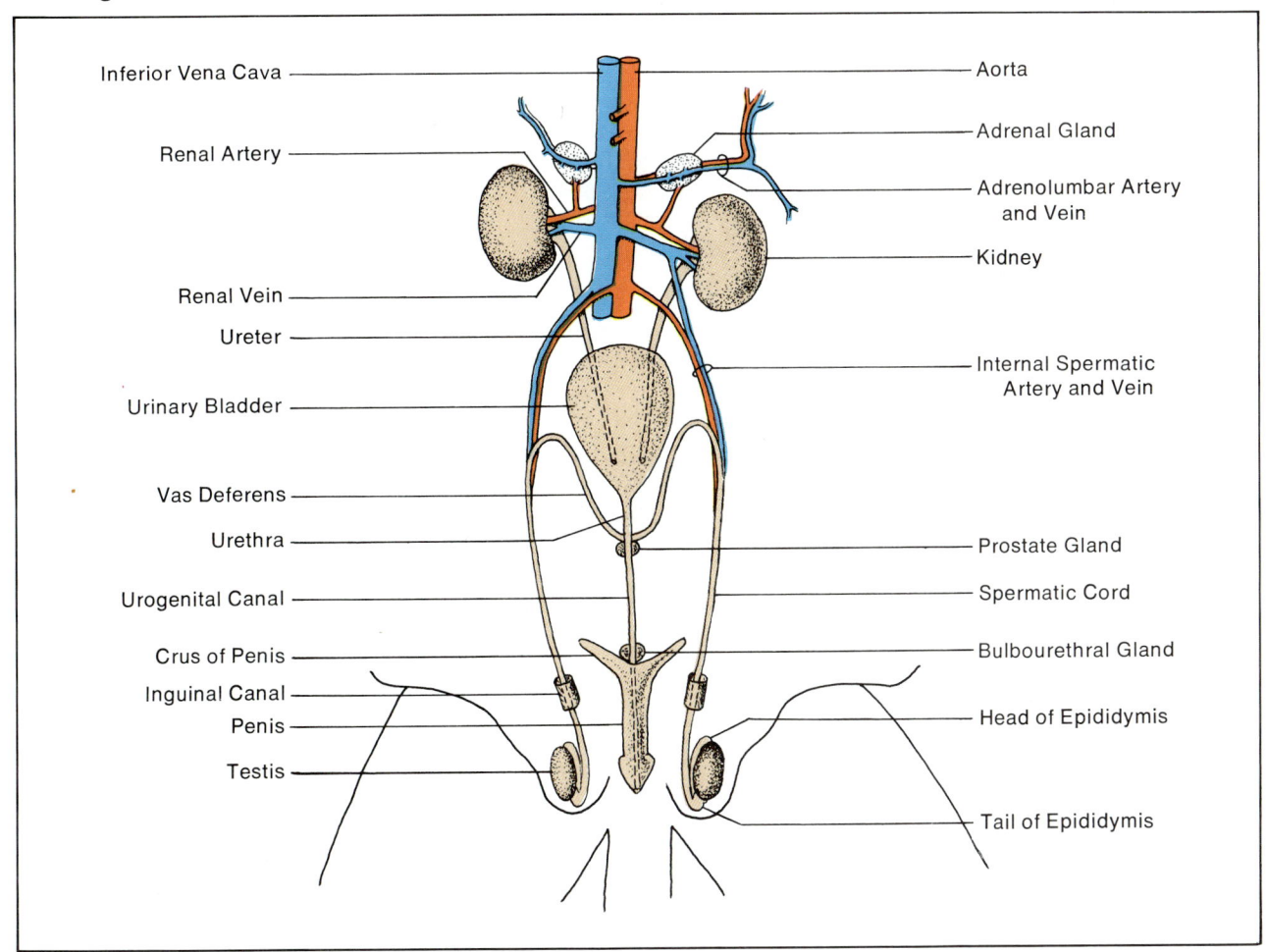

Figure 37.4 Urogenital system of the male cat.

that the left kidney is somewhat caudal to the right one.

3. Identify the two **adrenal glands,** which are embedded in connective tissue between the anterior ends of the kidneys and the large abdominal blood vessels (aorta and inferior vena cava).

4. Remove both kidneys. With a razor blade or sharp scalpel slice one longitudinally to produce a series of thin frontal sections revealing its internal structure. Slice the other kidney to produce a series of thin transverse sections. Identify the cortex, medulla, and papilla. Observe that there is only one renal papilla in the cat kidney emptying into the pelvis of the ureter. In the human there are approximately twelve papillae.

5. Trace the **ureter** of each kidney to the bladder where they enter the dorsal surface of the bladder.

6. Note that the bladder is also retroperitoneal. It is a musculomembranous sac attached to the abdomino-pelvic walls by ligaments formed from folds of peritoneum. The ventral side of the bladder is attached to the linea alba by the **medial ligament.** Two **lateral ligaments,** which contain sizable fat deposits, connect the sides of the bladder to the dorsal body wall. Make a linear ventral incision in the bladder with a scalpel and examine the inside wall. Locate the openings of the two ureters and urethra. Also, cut into the urethra where it joins the bladder. Do you see any evidence of **sphincter muscles** in this region?

7. Observe that the urethra of the female cat empties into a **urogenital sinus.** In the male it passes through the penis. Trade specimens with students that have the opposite sex of your specimen so that you can become familiar with the anatomy of both sexes.

Laboratory Report

Complete the Laboratory Report for this exercise.

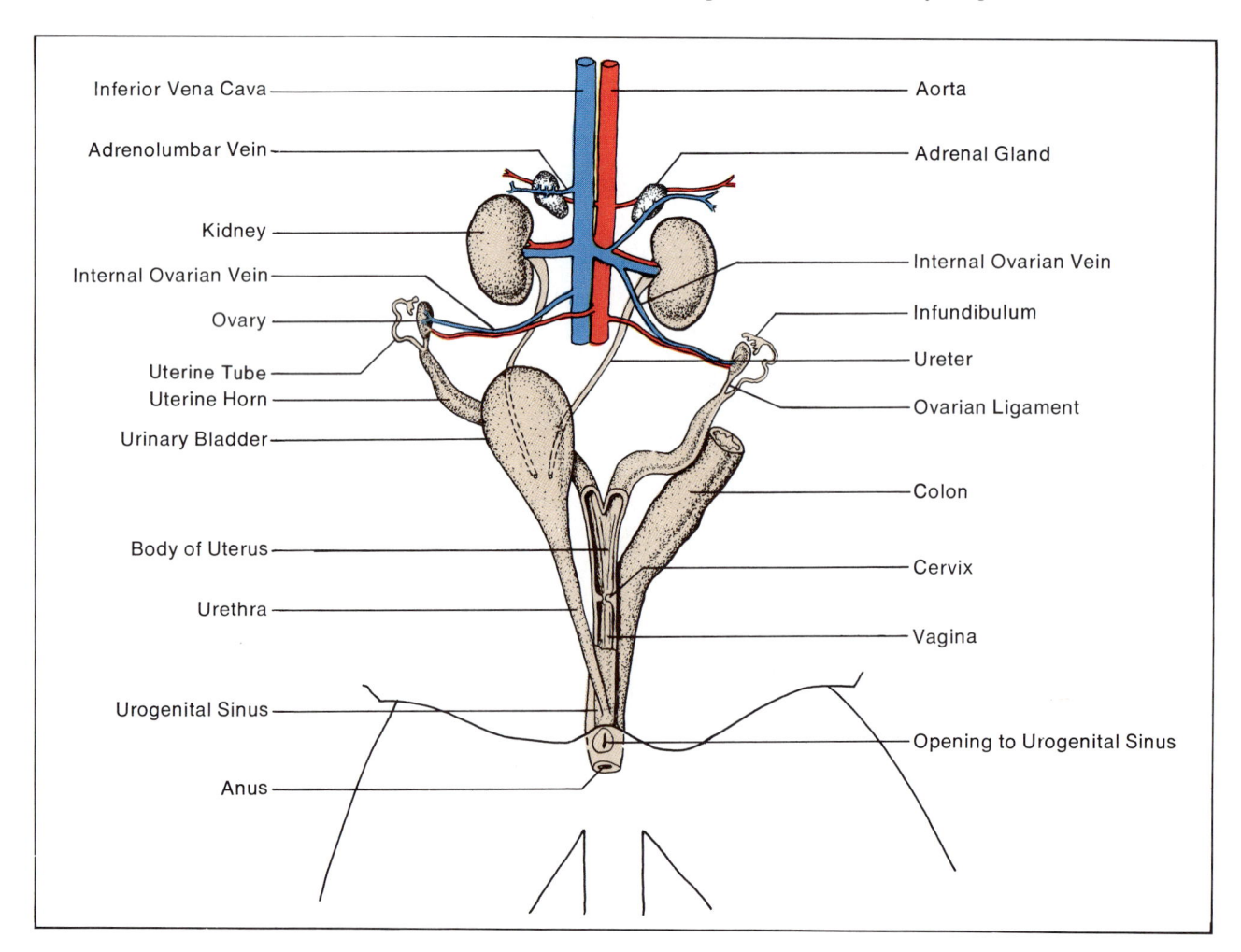

Figure 37.5 Urogenital system of the female cat.

Part 7 Endocrines and Reproduction

The regulatory action of the endocrine glands in the reproductive process logically places these two systems together. Exercise 38, which pertains to the endocrine glands, focuses in on the histological nature of the glands, and the specific hormones produced by each gland. Microscope slides of the various glands will be studied to locate the specific cells that produce the hormones. Since most of the glands have already been observed in previous dissections, no cat dissection will be performed here.

Exercise 39 pertains to the anatomy of the male and female reproductive organs. Spermatogenesis and oogenesis are also studied. The cat will be used for dissection.

The Endocrine Glands 38

In various dissections of previous exercises, endocrine glands have been encountered and discussed briefly. In this exercise all the glands will be studied in a unified manner to review what has been stated previously, and to explore more in depth the histology of each gland. By studying stained microscope slides of the various glands and comparing them with photomicrographs, you should have no difficulty identifying the specific cells in most glands that produce the various hormones. This laboratory experience should help to dispel some of the abstractness one usually encounters when attempting to assimilate a mass of endocrinological facts.

The Thyroid Gland

The thyroid gland consists of two lobes joined by a connecting isthmus. A posterior view of this gland is seen in figure 38.1. Note in figure 38.2 that, microscopically, it consists of large numbers of spherical sacs called **follicles.** These follicles are filled with a colloidal suspension of a glycoprotein, **thyroglobulin.** The principal hormones of this gland are the *thyroid hormone* and *calcitonin.*

The Thyroid Hormone

This hormone consists of thyroxine, triiodothyronine, and a small quantity of closely related iodinated hormones. They are formed within the thyroglobulin molecule, emerge from the molecule, and are absorbed by blood vessels in the gland. Once in the blood, the hormones combine with blood proteins and are carried to all tissues of the body for utilization. Excess hormones are stored in thyroglobulin.

Action The combined activity of thyroxine and triiodothyronine increases the metabolic activity of most tissues of the body. Bone growth in children is accelerated; carbohydrate metabolism is enhanced; cardiac output and heart rate are increased; respiratory rate is increased; and mental activity is increased.

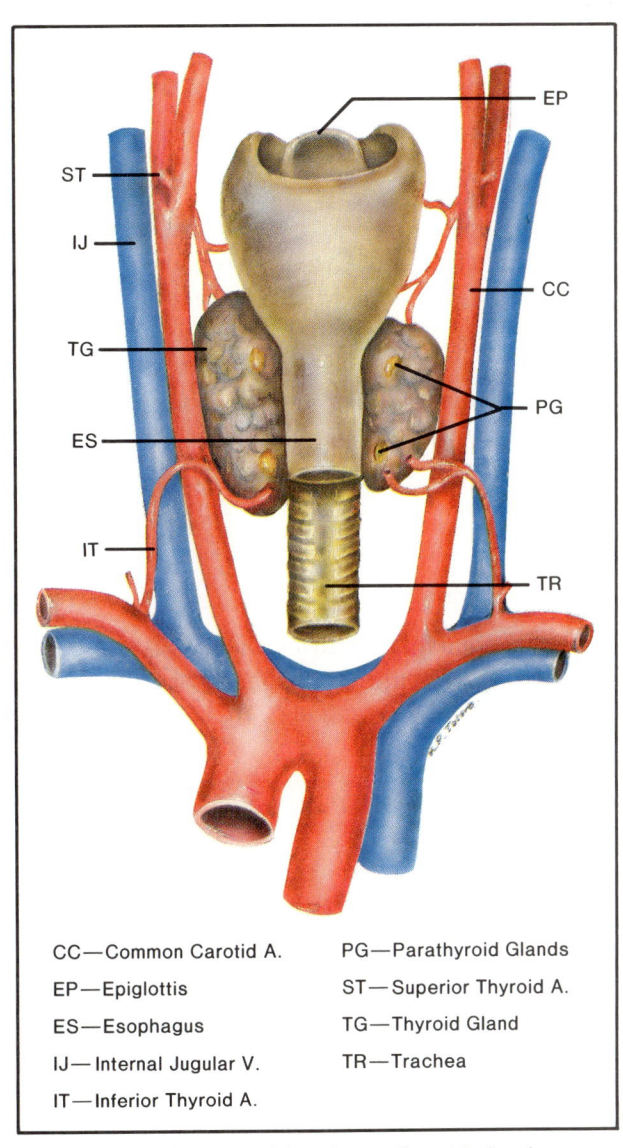

CC—Common Carotid A.   PG—Parathyroid Glands
EP—Epiglottis   ST—Superior Thyroid A.
ES—Esophagus   TG—Thyroid Gland
IJ—Internal Jugular V.   TR—Trachea
IT—Inferior Thyroid A.

Figure 38.1   The thyroid and parathyroid glands.

Deficiency Symptoms In children hypothyroidism may result in *cretinism,* a condition characterized by physical and mental retardation. In adults, severe long-term deficiency causes *myxedema,* which is characterized by obesity, slow pulse, lack of energy, and mental depression.

Oversecretion Symptoms Hyperthyroidism is characterized by weight loss, rapid pulse, intolerance to heat, nervousness, and inability to sleep. *Exophthalmos,* or eyeball protrusion, is often present.

Goiters Enlarged thyroid glands ("goiters") may be present in both hypo- and hyperthyroidism. Hypothyroid goiters may be due to iodine deficiency (*endemic goiter*) or some other unknown cause (*idiopathic nontoxic goiter*). Hyperthyroid goiters may, or may not, be due to malignancy of the gland.

Regulation Thyrotropin, which is produced by the anterior pituitary gland, stimulates the thyroid to produce the thyroid hormone.

Calcitonin

This hormone is produced by the parafollicular cells in the interstitium of the thyroid gland. When injected experimentally, calcitonin causes a decrease in blood calcium levels. This is due to increased osteoblastic and decreased osteoclastic activity.

It probably plays an important role in bone remodeling during growth in children, but in adults it appears to have very little, if any, effect on blood calcium levels over the long term.

The Parathyroid Glands

There are four small parathyroid glands embedded in the posterior surface of the thyroid gland. See figure 38.1. Occasionally, parathyroid tissue is seen outside of the thyroid gland in the neck region.

Two kinds of cells are seen in this gland: **chief** and **oxyphil cells.** Both cells are shown in figure 38.2. Note that the chief cells are more numerous, smaller, and arranged in cords. They produce the only hormone of this gland, which has been designated as the *parathyroid hormone.* The function of the larger oxyphil cells is unknown.

Action The parathyroid hormone raises blood calcium levels and lowers the phosphorous levels in the blood. This is accomplished by activating osteoclasts in the bone and impeding the reabsorption of phosphorus in the renal tubules. To prevent calcium loss in the kidneys, the hormone also promotes the reabsorption of calcium in the renal tubules. Removal of all parathyroid tissue results in *tetany* and death.

Regulation Production of this hormone is regulated by the level of calcium in the blood. Excess blood calcium levels inhibit hormone production; lowered blood calcium levels cause the gland to produce more of the hormone.

The Pancreas

Figure 38.3 illustrates the histology of this gland. The endocrine-secreting portion of the pancreas is performed by clusters of cells called **pancreatic**

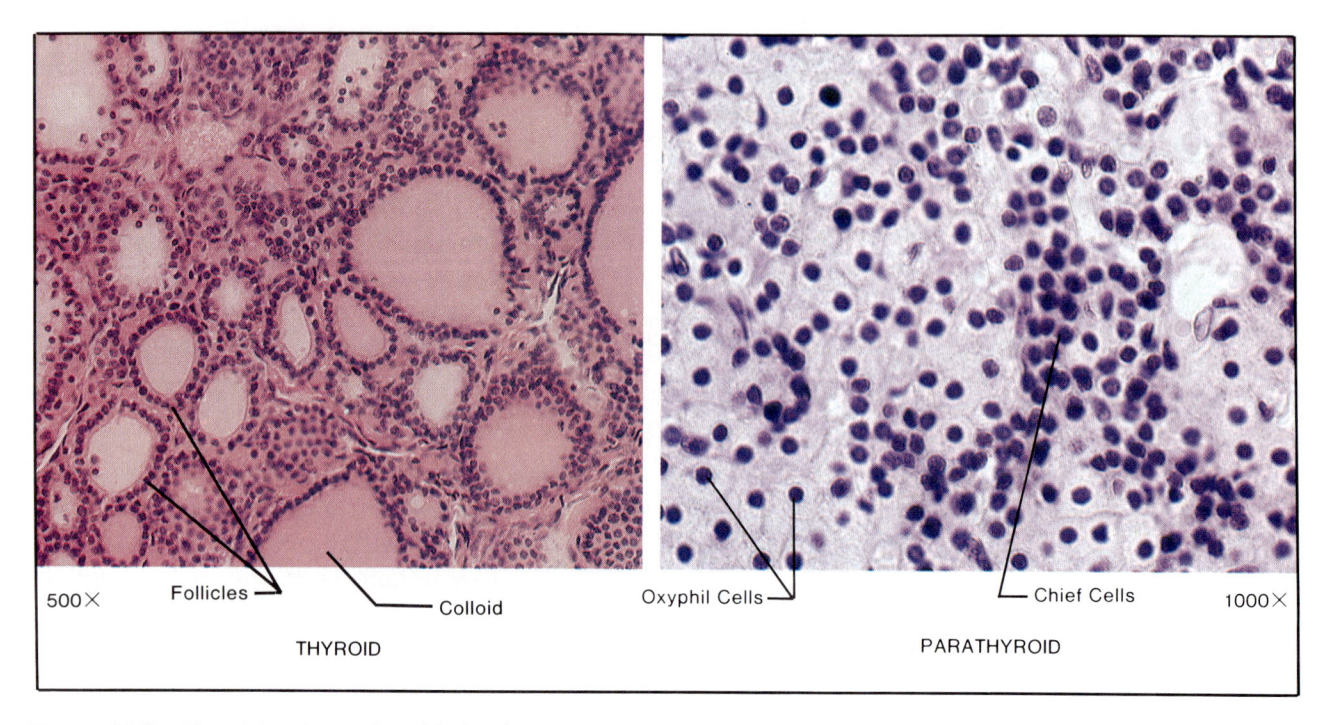

500× Follicles — Colloid
THYROID

Oxyphil Cells — Chief Cells 1000×
PARATHYROID

Figure 38.2 Thyroid and parathyroid glands.

islets (islets of Langerhans). These cells are located between the saclike glands (*acini*) that produce the pancreatic digestive enzymes. Insulin, glucagon, and somatostatin are produced by different types of cells in the islets.

Insulin

Insulin is an anabolic hormone that is produced by the **beta cells** of the pancreatic islets. These cells can be differentiated from other islet cells by the presence of many granules in the cytoplasm.

Insulin promotes the storage of glucose by converting it to glycogen. It also promotes the storage of fatty acids and amino acids. Insulin deficiency results in *diabetes mellitus* in which *hyperglycemia* (high blood sugar) is present.

Regulation Although a variety of stimulatory and inhibitory factors affect insulin production, feedback control by blood glucose levels on the beta cells is the major controlling factor. As glucose levels become elevated, insulin production is stepped up; when the glucose level is normal or low, the rate of insulin production is low.

Glucagon

Glucagon is a catabolic hormone produced by the **alpha cells** of the pancreatic islets. Its action is just the opposite of insulin in that it mobilizes glucose, fatty acids, and amino acids in tissues. Deficiency of this hormone will result in *hypoglycemia*. Glucagon also stimulates the production of the growth hormone, insulin, and pancreatic somatostatin.

Somatostatin

A third type of islet cells, called the **delta cells,** produce somatostatin, a growth-inhibiting hormone. With Mallory's stain the cytoplasm of these cells stains blue.

This hormone is growth inhibiting in that it inhibits the release of the growth hormone by the anterior pituitary gland. In addition, it inhibits the production of insulin and glucagon. Tumors involving the delta cells result in hyperglycemia and other diabetes-like symptoms. Removal of the tumors causes the symptoms to disappear.

The Adrenal Glands

Each adrenal gland has an outer **cortex** and inner **medulla.** Surrounding the entire gland is a **capsule** of fibrous connective tissue.

The embryological origins of the cortex and medulla explain their differences in function. The cells of the medulla originate from the neural crest of the embryo. This embryonic tissue also gives rise to ganglionic cells of the sympathetic nervous system; thus, we can expect a close kinship in function of the adrenal medulla and the sympathetic nervous system.

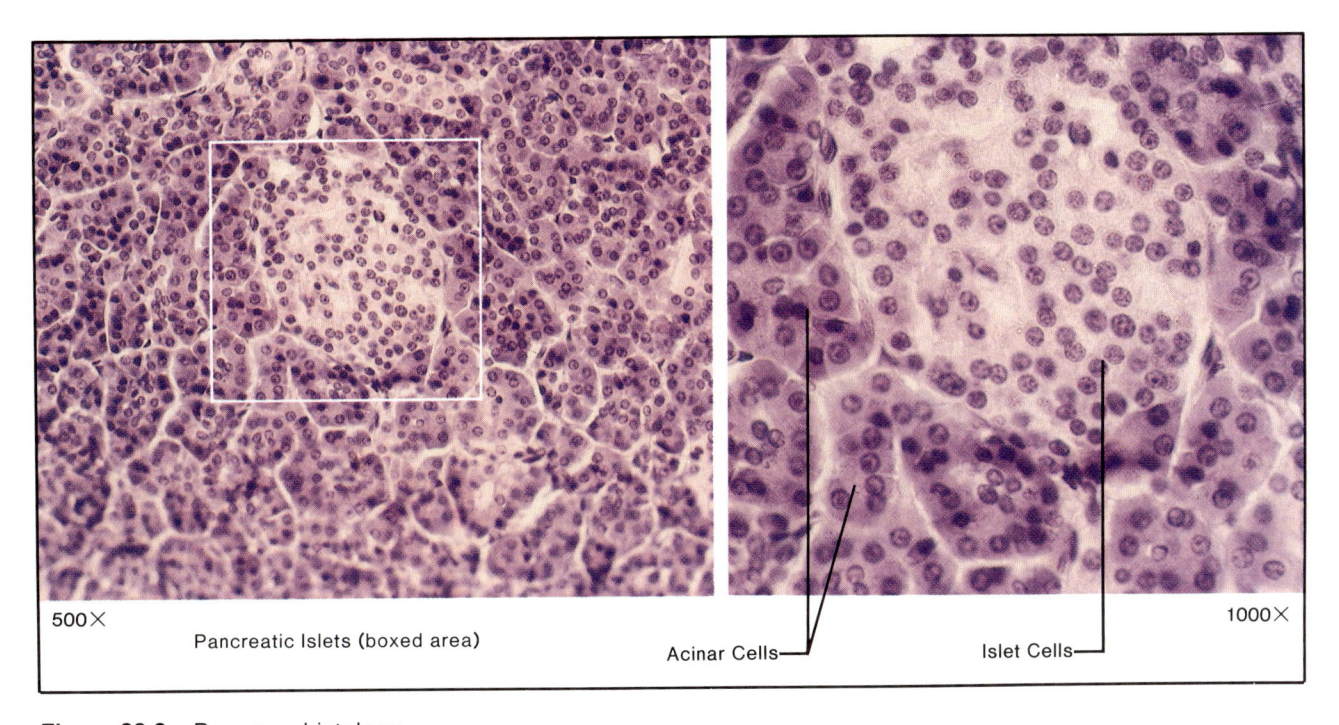

500×

Pancreatic Islets (boxed area)

1000×

Acinar Cells— Islet Cells—

Figure 38.3 Pancreas histology.

Cells of the cortex, on the other hand, arise from embryonic tissue associated with the gonads. Hormones having some relationship to the reproductive organs might, thus, be expected from the cortex.

The Adrenal Cortex

Figures 38.4 and 38.5 reveal the three layers of the cortex. Note that immediately under the capsule lies a layer called the **zona glomerulosa.** The innermost layer of cells, which interfaces with the medulla, is the **zona reticularis.** The middle layer, which is the thickest, is the **zona fasciculata.** In all the layers are seen vascular channels, called **sinusoids,** that are larger in diameter than capillaries, but resemble capillaries in that their walls are one cell thick. It is in these channels that the hormones collect prior to passing directly into the general circulation.

The adrenal cortex secretes many different hormones, all of which belong to a group of substances called *steroids.* Collectively, they are referred to as **corticosteroids.** All of them are synthesized from cholesterol and have similar molecular structures. While destruction of the adrenal medulla is more or less inconsequential to survival, obliteration of the adrenal cortex results in death.

The corticosteroids fall into three groups: the mineralocorticoids, the glucocorticoids, and the androgenic hormones. The *mineralocorticoids* are hormones that control the excretion of Na^+ and K^+, which affects the electrolyte balance. The *glucocorticoids* affect primarily the metabolism of glucose and protein. The *androgenic hormones* produce some of the same effects on the body as the male sex hormone testosterone. Of the 30 or more corticoids that are produced by the adrenal cortex, the most important two are aldosterone and cortisol. Descriptions of these two hormones follow.

Aldosterone This mineralocorticoid is produced by cells of the zona glomerulosa. The most important function of this hormone is to increase the rate of renal tubular absorption of sodium. Any condition that impairs the production of aldosterone will result in death within two weeks if salt replacement or mineralocorticoid therapy is not provided. In the absence of aldosterone the K^+ concentration in extracellular fluids rises, Na^+ and Cl^- concentrations decrease, and the total volume of body fluids be-

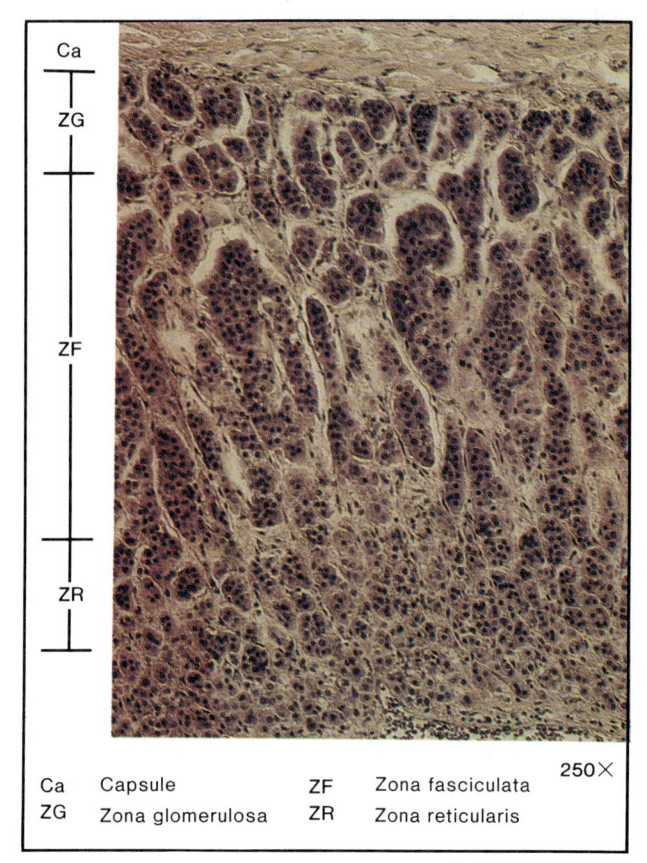

| Ca | Capsule | ZF | Zona fasciculata |
| ZG | Zona glomerulosa | ZR | Zona reticularis |

250×

Figure 38.4 The adrenal cortex.

comes greatly reduced. These conditions cause reduced cardiac output, shock, and death.

Factors that affect aldosterone production are ACTH, K^+ ion concentration, Na^+ ion concentration, and the renin-angiotensin system.

Cortisol (*Hydrocortisone, Compound F*)
Approximately 95% of the glucocorticoid activity results from the action of cortisol. This hormone is produced primarily by cells in the zona fasciculata; some of it is also produced by the zona reticularis.

When an excess of cortisol exists, the following physiological activities take place in the body: (1) the rate of glucogenesis is stepped up; (2) glucose utilization by cells is decreased; (3) protein catabolism in all cells except the liver is increased; (4) amino acid transport to muscle cells is decreased; and (5) fatty acids are mobilized from adipose tissue.

Cushing's syndrome is a condition in which many of the above reactions occur. It is caused by an *excess of glucocorticoids* induced by a pituitary tumor. Protein depletion in these patients causes them to have poorly developed muscles, weak bones due to bone dissolution, slow healing of wounds,

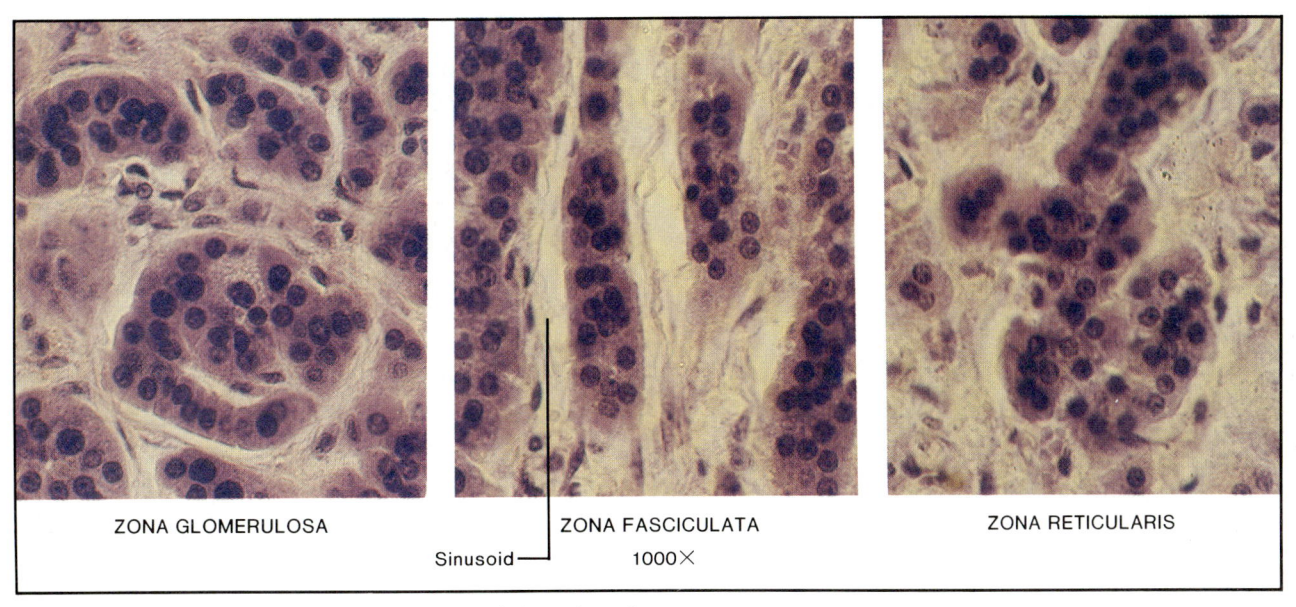

ZONA GLOMERULOSA

ZONA FASCICULATA

ZONA RETICULARIS

Sinusoid — | 1000×

Figure 38.5 Histology of the three layers of the adrenal cortex.

hyperglycemia, and hair that is thin and scraggly.

Addison's disease is a condition in which total *glucocorticoid insufficiency* exists. It can be caused by the destruction of the adrenal cortex by cancer, tuberculosis, or some other infectious agent.

Although several substances such as vasopressin, serotonin, and angiotensin II stimulate the adrenal cortex, it is primarily the action of ACTH that induces the cells of the zona fasciculata and zona reticularis to produce cortisol. ACTH production by the anterior pituitary is initiated by stress through the hypothalamus. Stress induces the hypothalamus to produce CRF, which passes to the anterior pituitary, causing the latter to produce ACTH.

The Adrenal Medulla

This portion of the adrenal gland produces the two catecholamines, *norepinephrine* and *epinephrine*. Although different cells in the medulla produce each of these hormones, cell differences are difficult to detect microscopically.

Approximately 80% of the medullary secretion is epinephrine; 20% is norepinephrine. Norepinephrine is also produced by the autonomic nervous system.

Action The effects of norepinephrine and epinephrine on different tissues depend on the types of receptors that exist in the tissues. There are two classes of adrenergic receptors: alpha and beta. Two types of alpha receptors are designated as α_1 and α_2; the beta receptors are β_1 and β_2.

Both norepinephrine and epinephrine increase the force and rate of contraction of the isolated heart. These reactions are mediated by β_1 receptors. Norepinephrine causes vasoconstriction in all organs through α_1 receptors. Epinephrine causes vasoconstriction everywhere except in the muscles and liver, where beta receptors bring about vasodilation. Increased mental alertness is also induced by both catecholamines, which may be induced by the increased blood pressure.

Blood glucose levels are increased by both hormones. This is accomplished by glycogenolysis (glycogen → glucose) in the liver. β_2 receptors account for this reaction.

Norepinephrine and epinephrine are equally potent in mobilizing free fatty acids through beta receptors. The metabolic rate is also increased by these hormones; how this takes place is not precisely understood at this time.

Control Production of both hormones is initiated when the adrenal medulla is stimulated by sympathetic nerve fibers.

The Thymus Gland

This gland consists of two long lobes and lies in the upper chest region above the heart. It is most highly developed before birth and during the growing years. After puberty it begins an involutionary process, which continues throughout life.

Histologically, this gland consists of a cortex and medulla. Figure 38.6 reveals its microscopic structure. The **cortex** consists of lymphoidlike tissue filled with a large number of lymphocytes. The **medulla** contains a smaller number of lymphocytes and structures called **thymic corpuscles** (Hassall's bodies) that are of unknown function.

Function It appears that the principal role of the thymus is to process lymphocytes into T-lymphocytes, as described on page 228. It is speculated that this gland produces one or more hormones that function in T-lymphocyte formation. Thymosin and several other extracts from this gland have been under study.

The Pineal Gland

The pineal gland is situated on the roof of the third ventricle under the posterior end of the corpus callosum. It is supported by a stalk that contains postganglionic sympathetic nerve fibers that do not seem to extend into the gland. The gland consists of neuroglial and parenchymal cells that suggest a secretory function. See figure 38.6.

In young animals and infants the gland is large and more glandlike; cells tend to be arranged in alveoli. Just before puberty the gland begins to regress and small concretions of calcium carbonate form that are called **pineal sand.** There is some evidence, though not conclusive, that the gland contains some gonadotropin peptides. Most attention, however, is on the production of melatonin by the gland.

Melatonin is an indole that is synthesized from serotonin. Its production appears to be regulated by daylight (circadian rhythm). During daylight its production is suppressed. At night the gland becomes active and produces considerable quantities of melatonin. Regulation occurs through the eyes. Light striking the retina sends messages to the pineal gland through a retina-hypothalamic pathway. Norepinephrine reaches the cells from the postganglionic sympathetic nerve endings in the pineal stalk. Beta adrenergic receptors in the cells are mediators in the inhibition of melatonin production. Although considerable speculation exists that melatonin inhibits the estrus cycle in humans, as it probably does in lower animals, there is no definitive proof at this time that this is the case.

The Testes

A section through the testis (figure 38.7) reveals that it consists of coils of **seminiferous tubules** where spermatozoa are produced, and **interstitial cells** where the male sex hormone, **testosterone,** is secreted. Note that the interstitial cells lie in the spaces between the seminiferous tubules.

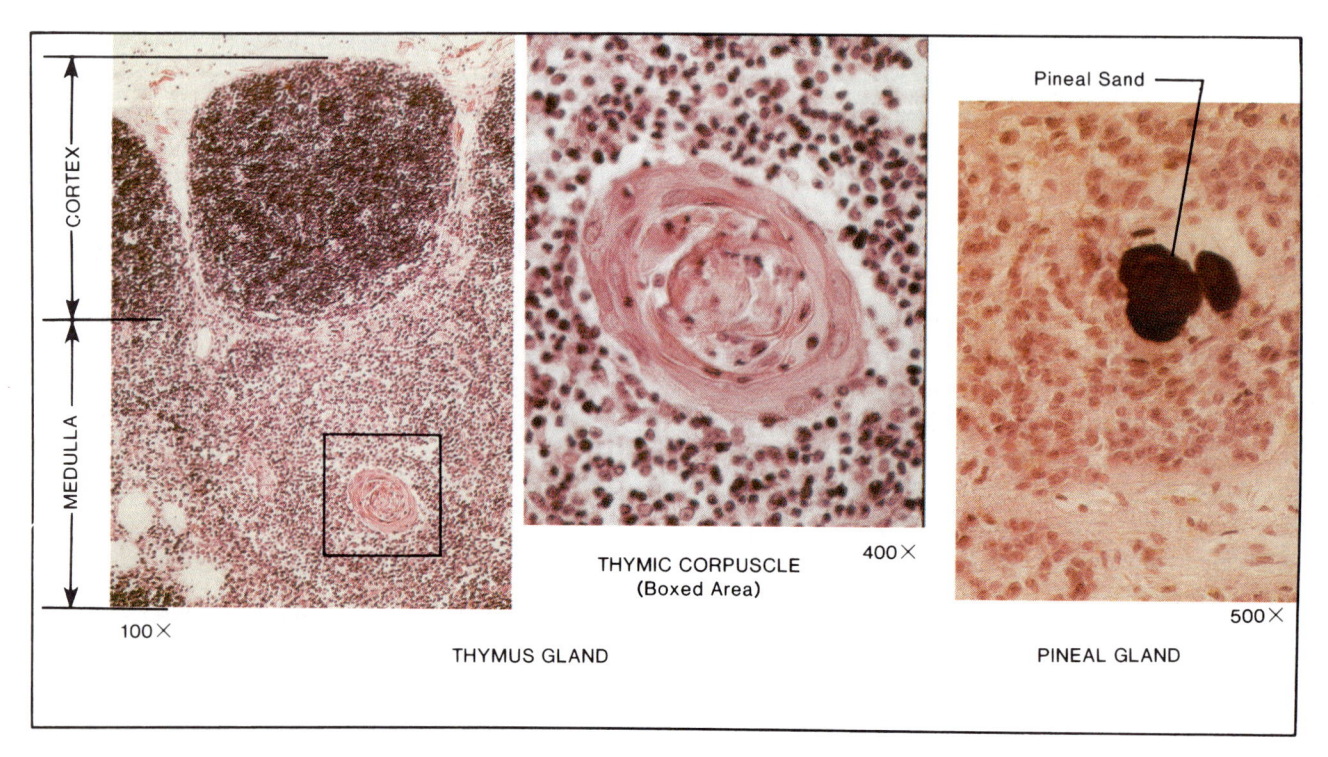

Figure 38.6 The thymus and pineal glands.

Testosterone is produced in considerable quantities during embryological development, but from early childhood to puberty very little of the hormone is produced. With the onset of puberty at the age of 10 or 11 years the testes begin to produce large quantities of testosterone as sexual maturity takes place.

During embryological development, testosterone is responsible for the development of the male sex organs. If the testes are removed from a fetus at an early stage, the fetus will develop a clitoris and vagina instead of a penis and scrotum, even though the fetus is a male. The hormone also controls the development of the prostate gland, seminal vesicles, and male ducts while suppressing the formation of female genitals.

Embryological development of the testes occurs within the body cavity. During the last two months of development the testes descend into the scrotum through the inguinal canals. The descent of the testes is controlled by testosterone.

During puberty the testes become larger and produce a great deal of testosterone, which causes considerable enlargement of the penis and scrotum. At the same time, the male secondary sexual characteristics develop. These characteristics are (1) the appearance of hair on the face, axillae, chest, and pubic region; (2) the enlargement of the larynx accompanied by a voice change; (3) increased skin thickness; (4) increased muscular development; (5) increased bone thickness and roughness; and (6) baldness.

During embryological development the production of testosterone is regulated by **chorionic gonadotropin,** a hormone produced by the placenta. At the onset of puberty the testes are stimulated to produce testosterone by the **luteinizing hormone (LH),** which is produced by the anterior lobe of the pituitary gland. This hormone stimulates the interstitial cells to produce testosterone. Maturation of spermatozoa in the testes is controlled by the **follicle-stimulating hormone (FSH),** which is also produced by the anterior pituitary gland. Testosterone assists FSH in this process.

The Ovaries

During fetal development small groups of cells move inward from the germinal epithelium of the ovary and develop into primordial follicles. As seen in figure 38.8, the **germinal epithelium** is the layer of cells near the surface of the ovary, and the **primordial follicles** are the small round bodies that contain *ova*. The ovaries of a young female at the onset of puberty are believed to contain between 100,000 and 400,000 of these immature follicles. During all the reproductive years of a woman only about 400 of these follicles will reach maturity and expel their ova.

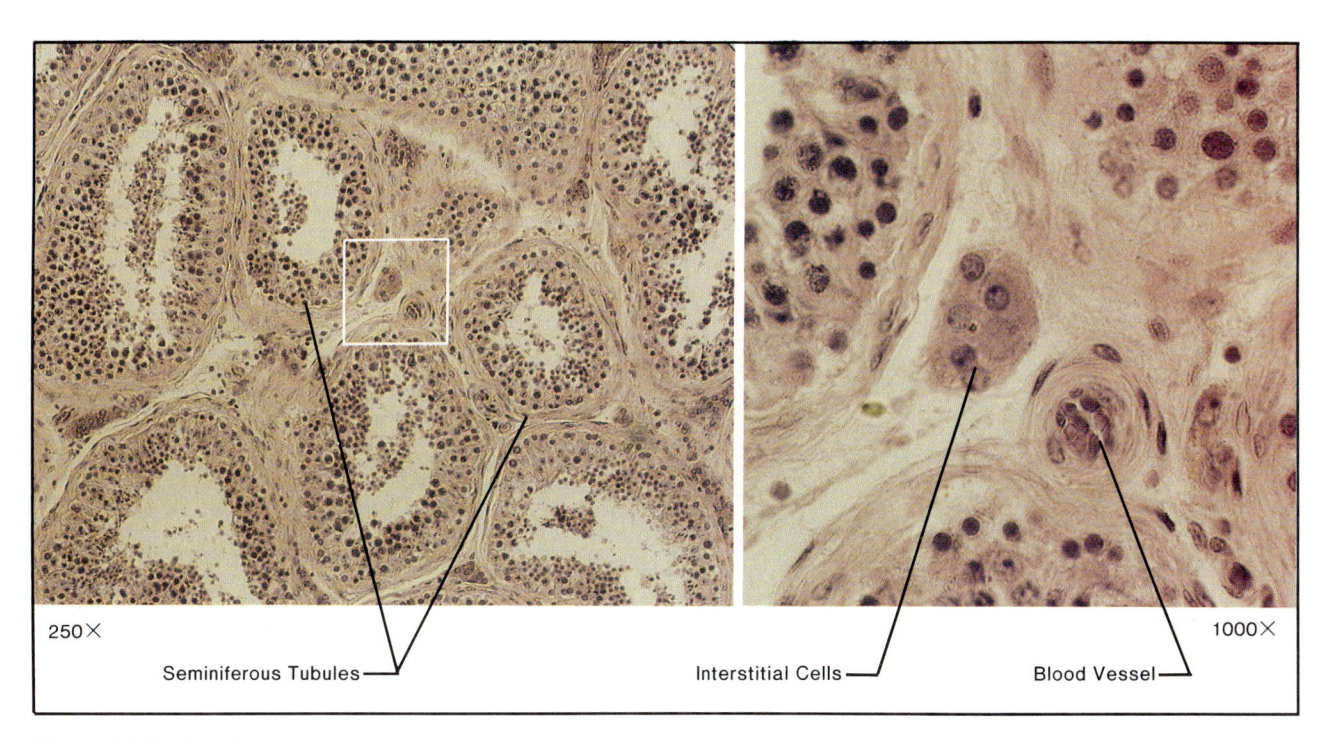

250✕   1000✕

Seminiferous Tubules — Interstitial Cells — Blood Vessel —

Figure 38.7   Testicular tissue.

During puberty selected primordial follicles enlarge to form **Graafian follicles,** and every 28 days a maturing Graafian follicle expels an ovum in the ovulation process. The development of these follicles and the subsequent corpus luteum results in the production of **estrogens** and **progesterone,** the principal female sex hormones.

Estrogens

The principal function of estrogens is to promote the growth of specific cells in the body and to control the development of female secondary sex characteristics. In addition to being produced in Graafian follicles, estrogens are also produced by the corpus luteum, placenta, adrenal cortex, and testes. The production of estrogens at puberty is initiated by the secretion of FSH by the anterior pituitary gland.

Of the six or seven estrogens that have been isolated from the plasma of women, β-**estradiol, estrone,** and **estriol** are the most abundant ones produced. The most potent of all the estrogens is β-**estradiol.**

During puberty when the estrogens are produced in large quantities the following changes occur: (1) the female sex organs become fully developed; (2) the vaginal epithelium changes from cuboidal to stratified epithelium; (3) the uterine lining (endometrium) becomes more glandular in preparation for implantation; (4) the breasts form;

(5) osteoblastic activity increases with more rapid bone growth; (6) calcification of the epiphyses in long bones is hastened; (7) pelvic bones enlarge and change shape, increasing the size of the pelvic outlet; (8) fat deposition under the skin, in the hips, buttocks, and thighs is increased; and (9) skin vascularization is increased.

Progesterone

Once ovulation takes place in the ovary the Graafian follicle is replaced by a **corpus luteum.** Progesterone is the principal hormone produced by this body. The ovary in figure 38.13 shows the development of Graafian follicles and the corpus luteum.

The most important function of this hormone is to promote secretory changes in the endometrium in preparation for implantation of the fertilized ovum. In addition, the hormone causes mucosal changes in the uterine tubes and promotes the proliferation of alveolar cells in the breasts in preparation for milk production.

When the plasma level of progesterone falls due to regression of the corpus luteum, deterioration of the endometrium takes place and menstruation occurs. If pregnancy occurs the corpus luteum enlarges and produces additional quantities of progesterone. The conversion of a Graafian follicle into a corpus luteum is completely dependent on LH production.

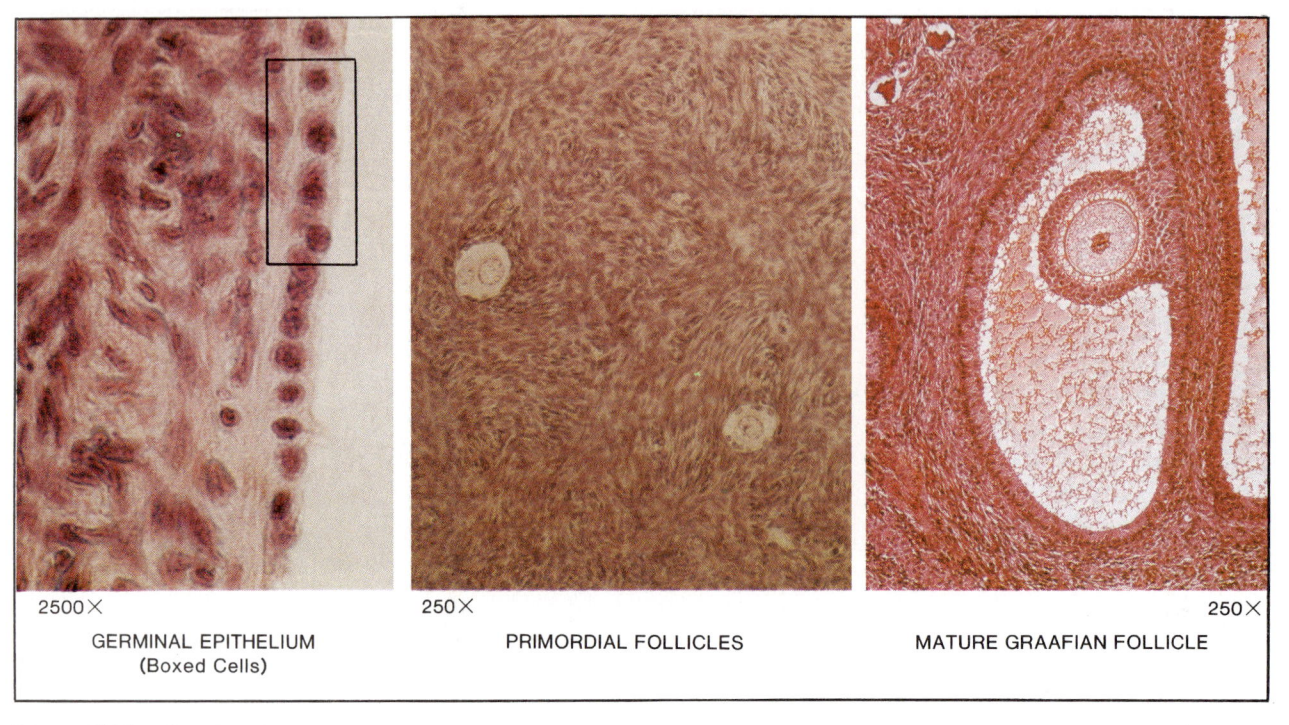

2500×	250×	250×
GERMINAL EPITHELIUM (Boxed Cells)	PRIMORDIAL FOLLICLES	MATURE GRAAFIAN FOLLICLE

Figure 38.8 Ovarian tissue.

The Pituitary Gland

The pituitary gland, or hypophysis, consists of two lobes: anterior and posterior. The anterior lobe, or **adenohypophysis,** develops from the roof of the oral cavity in the embryo. This part of the hypophysis is made up of glandular cells. The posterior lobe, or **neurohypophysis,** develops as an outgrowth of the floor of the brain during embryological development. Unlike the adenohypophysis, the cells of this lobe are nonsecretory and resemble neuroglial tissue. The entire gland is invested by an extension of the dura mater.

Figure 38.9 reveals portions of the two lobes. Note that the posterior lobe in this region consists of two parts: the **pars intermedia** and the **pars nervosa.**

The Adenohypophysis

Two basic types of glandular cells are seen in this portion of the hypophysis: chromophobes and chromophils. Both types of cells can be seen in figure 38.10. **Chromophobes** are cells that lack an affinity for routine dyes used in staining tissues. **Chromophils** stain readily and are of two types: acidophils and basophils. **Acidophils** take on the pink stain of eosin; **basophils,** on the other hand, stain readily with the basic stains, such as methylene blue and crystal violet.

Six hormones are produced by these various cells in the anterior lobe. Except for somatotropin, all these hormones are targeted specifically for glands. Production of the hormones is regulated by the hypothalamus. Between the hypothalamus and adenohypophysis is a vascular connection, the *hypophyseal portal system,* that transports *releasing factors* from the hypothalamus to the secretory cells. The releasing factors are secreted by cells in the hypothalamus.

Somatotropin (*SH*) This hormone, also called the **growth hormone** (*GH*), is produced by **somatotrophs,** a type of acidophil. In males and nonpregnant females most of the acidophils are of this type.

Somatotropin increases the growth rate of all cells in the body by enhancing amino acid uptake and protein synthesis. Excess production of the hormone during the growing years causes **gigantism** due to the stimulation of growth in the epiphyses of the long bones. An adult with excess SH production develops **acromegaly,** which is characterized by enlargement of the small bones of the hands and feet and the mandible and forehead. A deficiency of the hormone can cause **dwarfism.**

Prolactin (*Luteotropic Hormone, LTH*) This hormone is produced by another type of acidophil, called a **mammotroph.** With suitable staining methods it is possible to differentiate these cells from the somatotrophs.

Prolactin promotes the production of milk in the breasts after childbirth. The release of this hor-

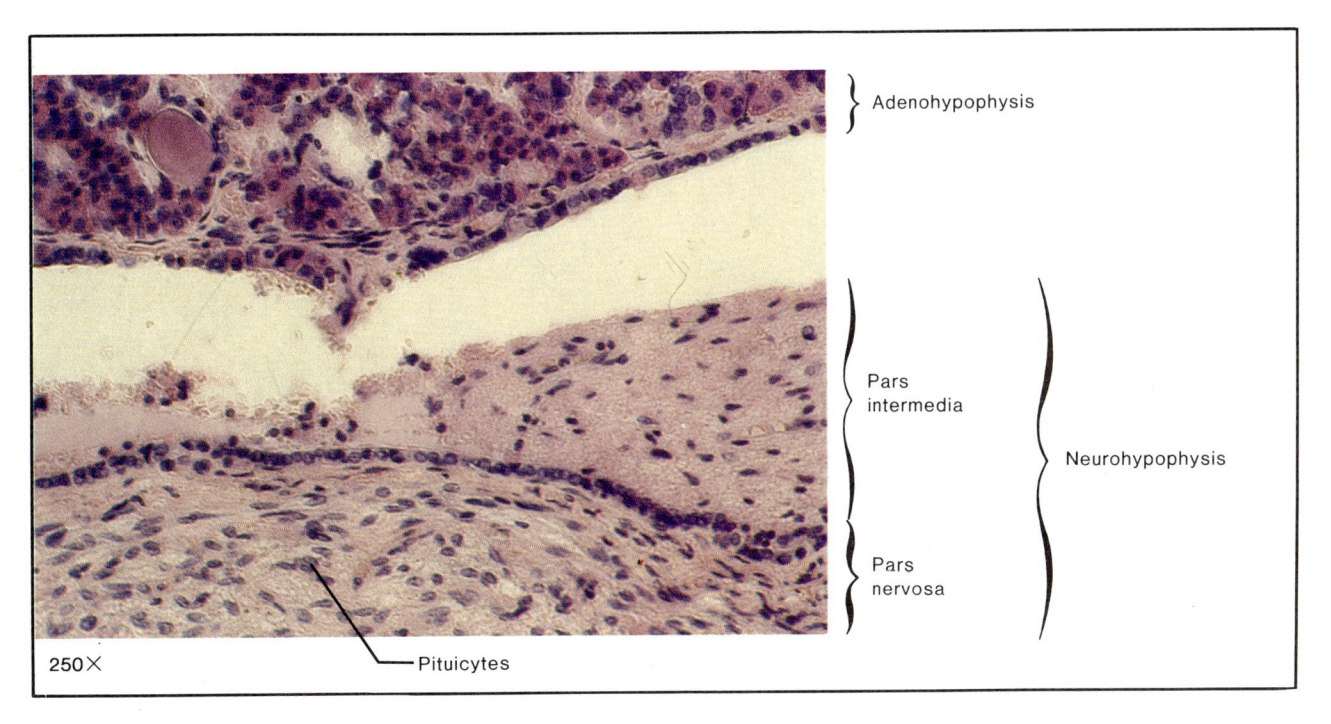

250×   Pituicytes

Adenohypophysis

Pars intermedia

Pars nervosa

Neurohypophysis

Figure 38.9 The pituitary gland.

mone prior to childbirth is inhibited by *PIF* (*prolactin inhibiting factor*), which is produced in the hypothalamus. The presence of large amounts of estrogens and progesterone prior to childbirth causes the hypothalamus to produce this inhibiting factor.

Thyrotropin (*TSH*) This hormone is produced by large irregular basophilic cells, called **thyrotrophs.** TSH regulates the rate of iodine uptake and the synthesis of the thyroid hormone by the thyroid gland. Excess amounts of TSH will cause hyperthyroidism. Hypothyroidism results from a deficiency of the hormone. TSH production is regulated by the hypothalamic *thyrotropin releasing factor* (*TRF*). TRF is secreted by nerve endings in the hypothalamus and passes through the hypophyseal portal system. Thyrotropin production is also regulated by a thyroid hormone feedback system.

Adrenocorticotropin (*ACTH*) This hormone is probably produced by a type of chromophobe. The suspected cell is a large chromophobe with large cytoplasmic granules, peripherally located. ACTH controls glucocorticoid production of the adrenal cortex. Its production is partially regulated by a glucocorticoid feedback mechanism.

Follicle-Stimulating Hormone (*FSH*) This hormone is produced by basophilic *gonadotrophs*. FSH promotes the development of Graafian follicles in the ovaries and the maturation of spermatozoa in the testes. FSH production by the adenohypophysis is regulated by estrogen and testosterone feedback mechanisms.

Luteinizing Hormone (*LH*) This hormone is produced by basophilic gonadotrophs that are somewhat larger than the FSH gonadotrophs. While the FSH cells tend to be located near the periphery of the gland, LH-producing cells are more generally distributed throughout the gland. Maturation of the Graafian follicles and ovulation during the menstrual cycle are dependent on this hormone. Although FSH contributes much to early follicle development, ovulation is entirely dependent on LH. The production of estrogens and progesterone is dependent on LH also.

In addition, this hormone stimulates the interstitial cells to produce testosterone; thus, it has been referred to as the **interstitial cell-stimulating hormone** (*ICSH*). LH production by the adenohypophysis is regulated by estrogen and progesterone feedback mechanisms.

The Neurohypophysis

The neuroglial-like cells in this portion of the hypophysis are called **pituicytes.** These cells are small and have numerous processes. Unlike neuroglia, pi-

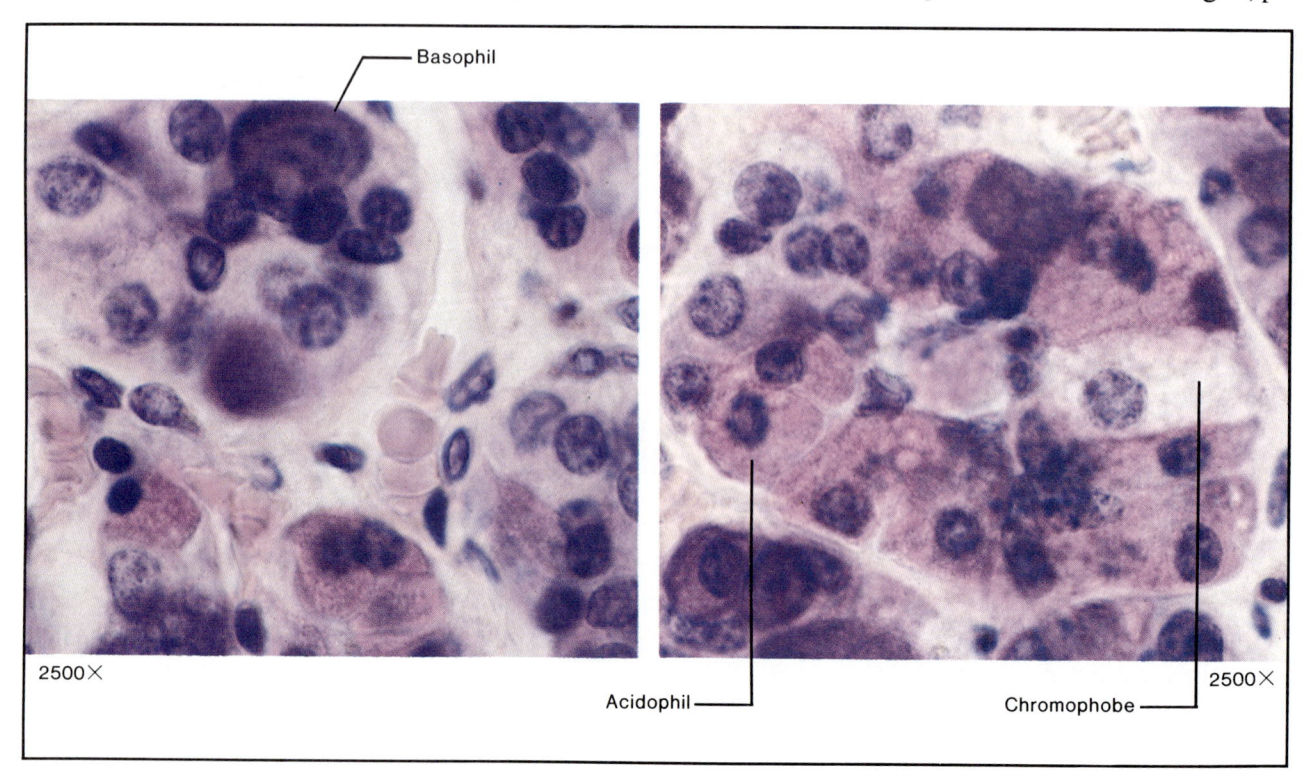

Figure 38.10 Cells of the adenohypophysis.

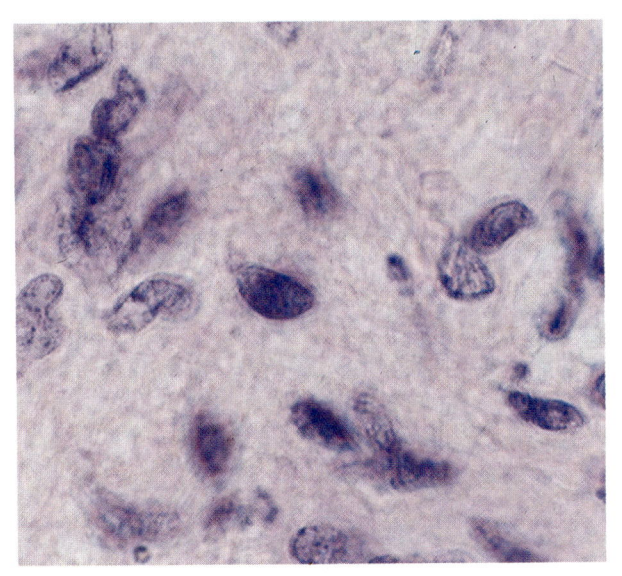

Figure 38.11 Pituicytes of the neurohypophysis (2500×).

tuicytes contain fat and pigment granules in their cytoplasm. Figure 38.11 is representative of these cells.

Pituicytes are nonsecretory. Their function is to provide support for nerve fibers from tracts that originate in the hypothalamus. Two hormones, the **antidiuretic hormone** and **oxytocin,** are liberated by the ends of these nerve tracts. The hormones are actually synthesized in the cell bodies of **neurosecretory neurons** of the hypothalamus and pass down the fibers into the neurohypophysis where they are released.

Antidiuretic Hormone (*ADH*) This hormone controls the permeability of collecting tubules in the nephrons to water reabsorption. When ADH is present in even minute amounts, water is easily reabsorbed back into the blood through the walls of the collecting tubules. When ADH is lacking, rapid water loss through the kidneys takes place. *Diabetes insipidus* is a disease in which the neurohypophysis fails to provide enough ADH. Without this hormone the osmotic balance of body fluids cannot remain stable very long.

Another function of ADH is to increase arterial blood pressure when a severe blood loss has reduced blood volume. A 25% loss of blood will increase ADH production by 25 to 50 times normal. ADH increases blood pressure by constricting arterioles. Because ADH has this potent pressor capability it is also called **vasopressin.** The mechanism for increased ADH production during blood loss lies in baroreceptors that are located in the carotid, aortic, and pulmonary regions.

Oxytocin Any substance that will cause uterine contractions during pregnancy is designated as being "oxytocic." During childbirth, pressure of the unborn child on the uterine cervix causes a neurogenic reflex to the neurohypophysis, stimulating it to produce the hormone oxytocin. This hormone, being oxytocic, increases the strength of uterine contractions to facilitate childbirth. Oxytocin also activates the myoepithelial cells of the mammary gland, resulting in the flow of milk.

Laboratory Assignment

Microscopic Studies

Do a systematic study of the various glands using the slides that are available. Make drawings, if required.

Materials:

prepared slides of the following glands:

thyroid (H14.11, H14.12, or H14.13)
parathyroid (H14.16)
thymus (H14.21 or H14.22)
adrenal (H14.26)
ovary (H9.310 or H9.3181)
testis (H9.415)
pituitary (H14.31)
pineal (H14.36)

While examining these slides, refer to the various photomicrographs in this exercise to identify the various kinds of cells that are mentioned in the text. Use low power for scanning and oil immersion wherever necessary.

Labeling

Figures 38.12 and 38.13 summarize many of the endocrinological facts learned in this exercise. Figure 38.12 pertains primarily to the various tissues that produce the hormones. Figure 38.13 depicts most of the hormones produced by the pituitary gland that regulate growth and glands of the body. It also includes many of the hormones produced by the glands that are regulated.

It will probably be necessary for you to refer back to various portions of the text in this exercise to seek out the various hormones. Once both of these diagrams are completed you should have a comprehensive picture of the endocrine system.

Laboratory Report

Complete the Laboratory Report for this exercise.

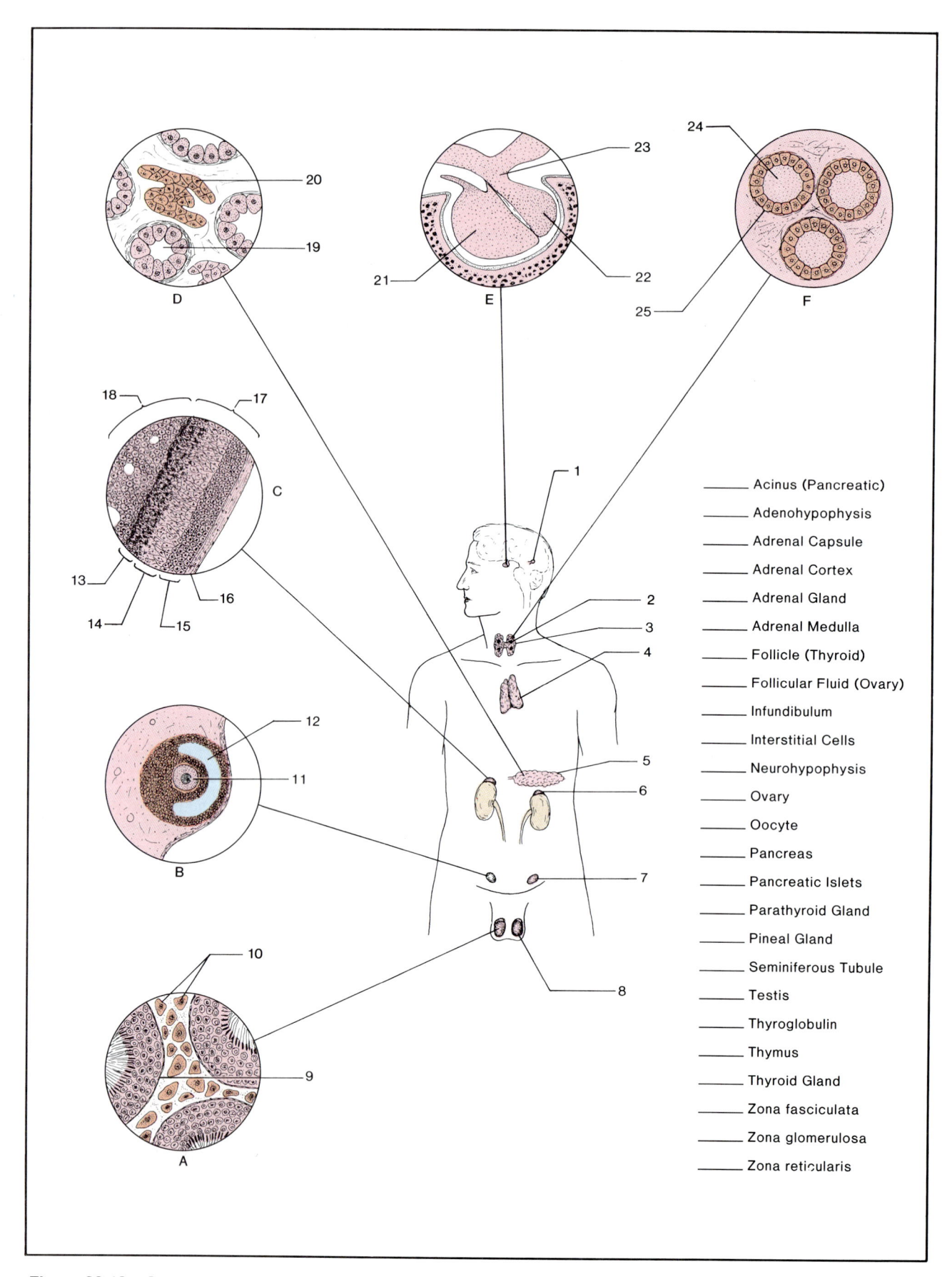

Acinus (Pancreatic)

Adenohypophysis

Adrenal Capsule

Adrenal Cortex

Adrenal Gland

Adrenal Medulla

Follicle (Thyroid)

Follicular Fluid (Ovary)

Infundibulum

Interstitial Cells

Neurohypophysis

Ovary

Oocyte

Pancreas

Pancreatic Islets

Parathyroid Gland

Pineal Gland

Seminiferous Tubule

Testis

Thyroglobulin

Thymus

Thyroid Gland

Zona fasciculata

Zona glomerulosa

Zona reticularis

Figure 38.12 Secretory components of the endocrine system.

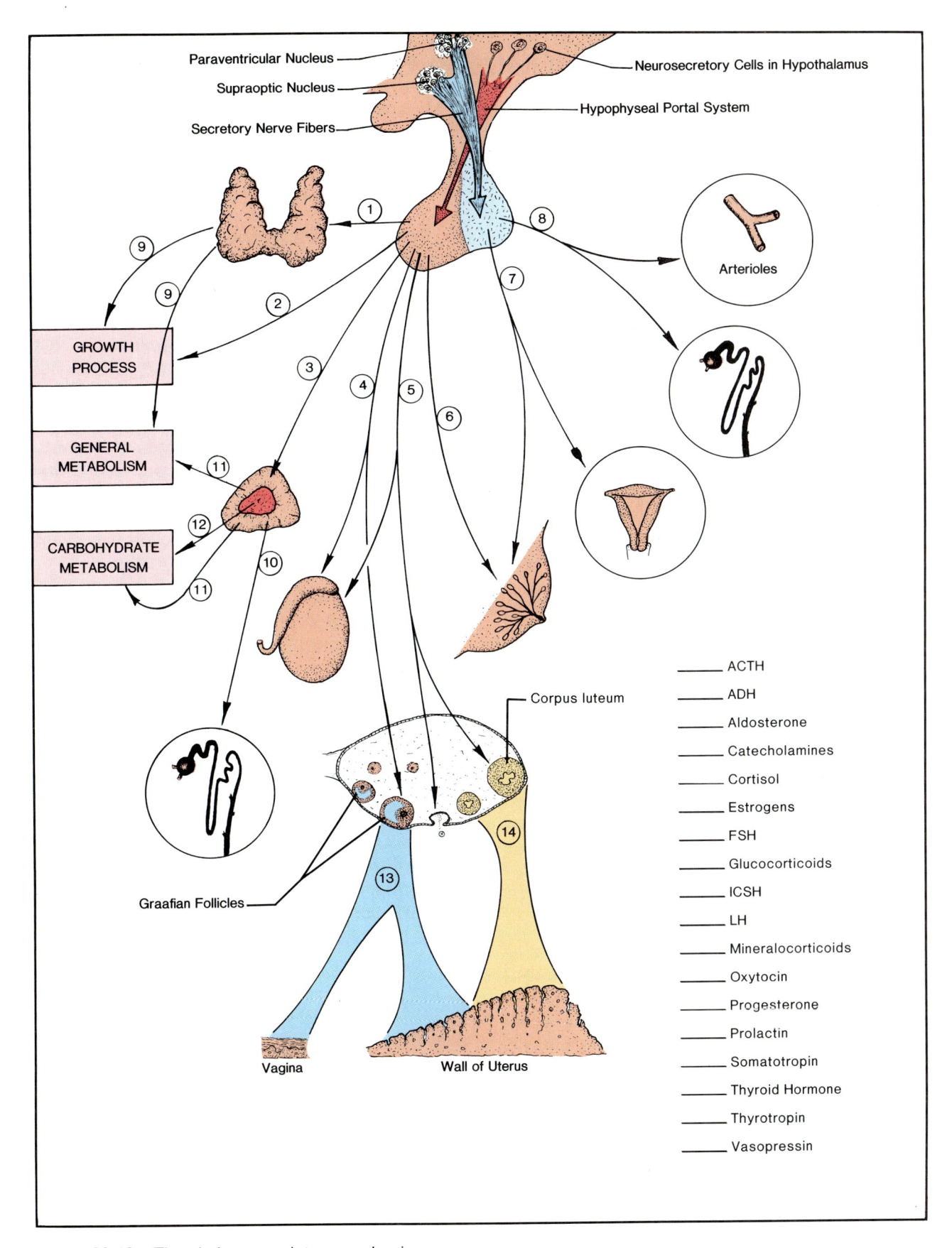

Figure 38.13 The pituitary regulatory mechanism.

39 The Reproductive System

This exercise on the reproductive system will include gross and histological studies of the reproductive organs, as well as dissection of the cat. The cytological nature and significance of spermatogenesis and oogenesis will also be studied.

Materials:

> models of human reproductive organs
> prepared slides of human testis
> ocular micrometer
> cat and dissection instruments

The Male Organs

Figure 39.1 is a sagittal section of the male reproductive system. The primary sex organs are the paired oval **testes** (*testicles*), which lie enclosed in a sac, the **scrotum.** The external nature of the testes provides a slightly lower temperature (94°–95° F), which favors the development of mature spermatozoa.

Lying over the superior and posterior surfaces of each testis is an elongated, flattened body, the **epididymis,** where immature sperm are stored after they leave the testis. The cutaway section of the testis in figure 39.1 reveals the relationship of the epididymis to the testis. Each testis is divided up into several chambers by partitions, or **septa,** that contain coiled-up **seminiferous tubules.** A single seminiferous tubule is shown held out of one of the compartments. All the seminiferous tubules anastomose to form a network of tubules called the **rete testis.** Cilia within the rete testis move the immature spermatozoa through this maze of tubules into 10 or 15 **vasa efferentia** that lead directly into the epididymis. The outer wall, or **tunica albuginea,** that surrounds each testis consists of fibrous connective tissue.

In the act of ejaculation the spermatozoa leave the epididymis by way of the **vas deferens.** Tracing this duct upward, we see that it passes over the pubic bone and bladder into the pelvic cavity. The terminus of the vas deferens is enlarged to form the **ampulla of the vas deferens.** A pair of glands, the **seminal vesicles,** and the ampulla empty into the **common ejaculatory duct.** This latter duct passes through the prostate gland and empties into the **prostatic urethra.** From here the sperm pass through the **penile urethra** out of the body.

The prostate gland, seminal vesicles, and bulbourethral glands contribute alkaline secretions to the seminal fluid, which stimulates sperm motility. The **prostate gland** is the largest of these secondary sex glands. The **bulbourethral** (Cowper's) **glands** are the smallest of the three. These pea-sized glands have ducts about one inch long that empty into the urethra at the base of the penis. The secretion of these glands is a clear mucoid fluid that lubricates the end of the penis and prepares the urethra for seminal fluid.

The **penis** consists of three cylinders of erectile tissue: two corpora cavernosa and one corpus spongiosum. The **corpus spongiosum** is a cylinder of tissue that surrounds the penile urethra. The two **corpora cavernosa** are located in the dorsal part of the organ and are separated on the midline by a **septum.** The distal end of the corpus spongiosum is enlarged to form a cone-shaped **glans penis.** The enlarged portion of the urethra within the glans is the **navicular fossa.** Erection of the penis occurs when the spongelike tissue of the three corpora fills with blood.

Over the end of the glans penis lies a circular fold of skin, the **prepuce.** Around the neck of the glans, and on the inner surface of the prepuce, are scattered small *preputial glands.* These sebaceous glands produce a secretion of peculiar odor that readily undergoes decomposition to form a whitish substance called *smegma. Circumcision* is a surgical procedure that involves the removal of the prepuce to facilitate sanitation.

Assignment:

Label figure 39.1.

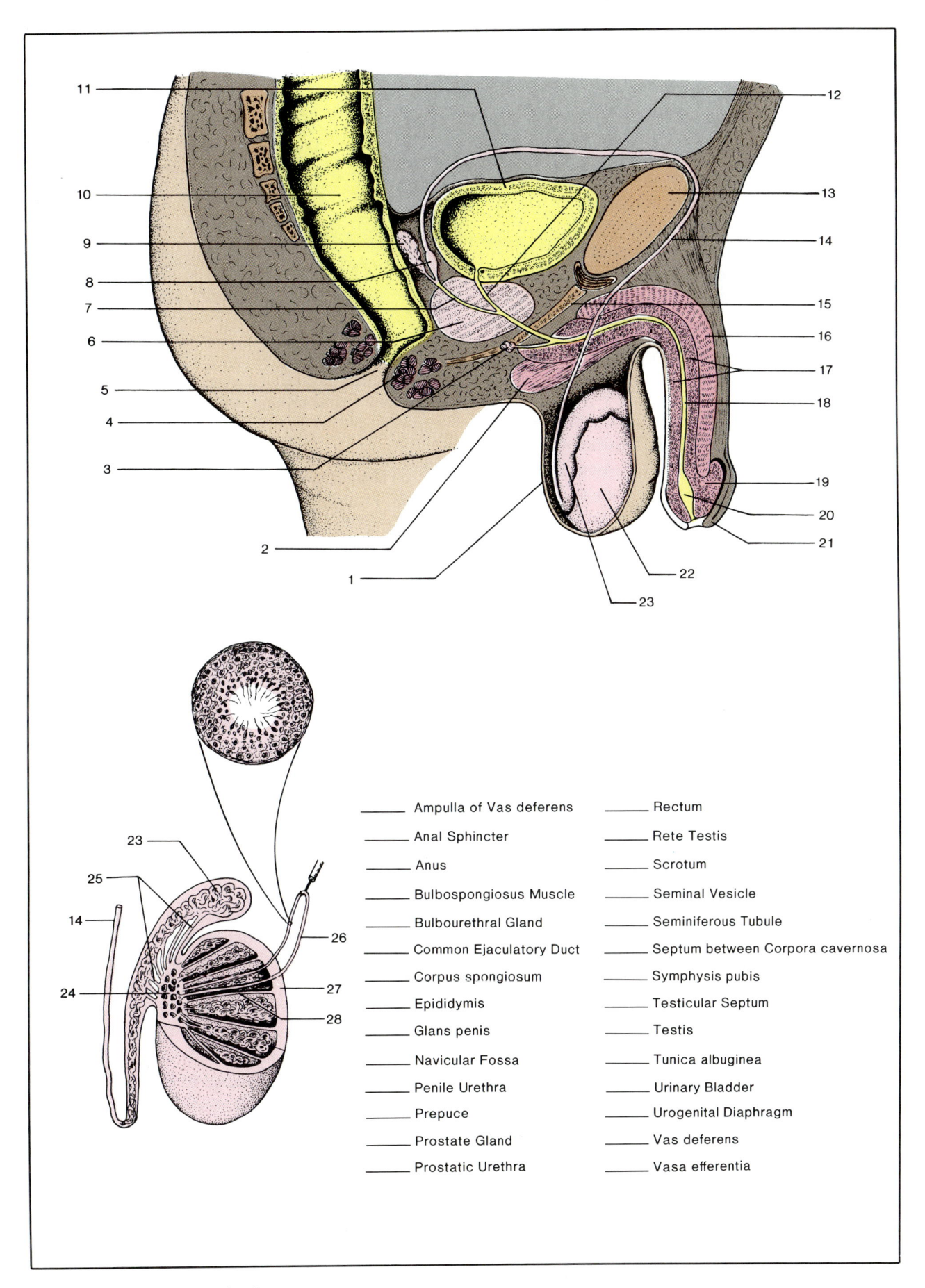

Ampulla of Vas deferens

Anal Sphincter

Anus

Bulbospongiosus Muscle

Bulbourethral Gland

Common Ejaculatory Duct

Corpus spongiosum

Epididymis

Glans penis

Navicular Fossa

Penile Urethra

Prepuce

Prostate Gland

Prostatic Urethra

Rectum

Rete Testis

Scrotum

Seminal Vesicle

Seminiferous Tubule

Septum between Corpora cavernosa

Symphysis pubis

Testicular Septum

Testis

Tunica albuginea

Urinary Bladder

Urogenital Diaphragm

Vas deferens

Vasa efferentia

Figure 39.1 Male reproductive organs.

Spermatogenesis

The process whereby spermatozoa are produced in the testes is known as *spermatogenesis*. This function of the testes begins at puberty and continues without interruption throughout life. Figure 39.2 illustrates a section of a seminiferous tubule and a diagram of the various stages in the development of mature spermatozoa. The formation of these germ cells takes place as the result of both mitosis and meiosis. In this study of spermatogenesis, slides of human testes will be studied under the microscope. Before examining the slides, however, familiarize yourself with the characteristic differences between meiosis and mitosis.

Mitosis

All spermatozoa originate from **spermatogonia** of the **primary germinal epithelium.** This layer of cells is located at the periphery of the seminiferous tubule. These cells contain the same number of chromosomes as other body cells (i.e., 23 pairs) and are said to be *diploid.* Mitotic division of these cells occurs constantly, producing other spermatogonia. As the spermatogonia move toward the center of the tubule they enlarge to form **primary spermatocytes.** In this stage the homologous chromosomes unite to form chromosomal units called *tetrads.* This union of homologous chromosomes is called *synapsis.*

Meiosis

Each primary spermatocyte divides further to produce two secondary spermatocytes. This division, however, occurs by meiosis instead of mitosis. *Meiosis,* or reduction division, results in the distribution of a *haploid* number of chromosomes to each **secondary spermatocyte.** The result is that each secondary spermatocyte has only twenty-three chromosomes instead of forty-six. The individual chromosomes of the secondary spermatocytes are formed by the splitting of the tetrads along the line of previous conjugation to form chromosomes called *dyads.* The second meiotic division occurs when each secondary spermatocyte divides to produce two haploid **spermatids.** In this division the dyads split to form single chromosomes, or *monads.* Each spermatid metamorphoses directly into a mature sperm cell. Note that four spermatozoa form from each spermatogonium.

Assignment:

Examine a slide of the human testis under low- and high-power magnifications. Refer to figure HA-36

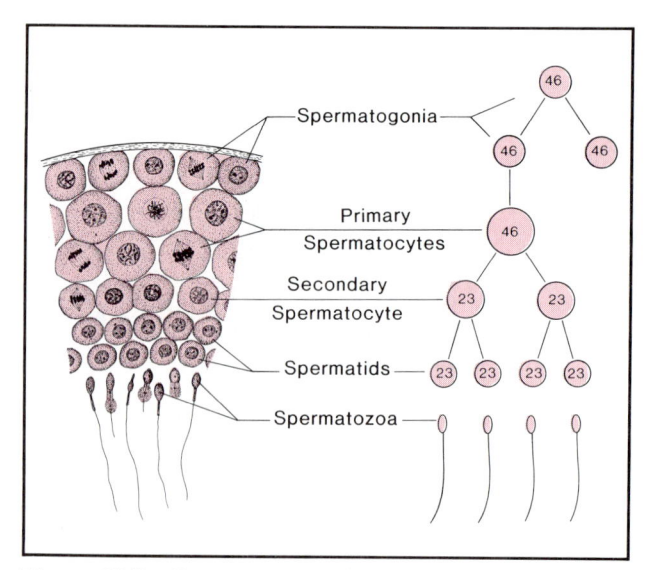

Figure 39.2 Spermatogenesis.

of the Histology Atlas to identify the various types of cells. Draw a representative section of a tubule, labeling all cell types.

The Female Organs

Figures 39.3, 39.4, and 39.5 illustrate the female reproductive organs. Models and wall charts will be helpful in identifying all the structures.

External Genitalia

The **vulva** of the external female reproductive organs includes the mons pubis, labia majora, labia minora, and hymen. All of these structures are shown in figure 39.3. The **mons pubis** (*mons veneris*) is the most anterior portion and consists of a firm cushionlike elevation over the symphysis pubis. It is covered with hair.

Two folds of skin on each side of the **vaginal orifice** (label 11) lie over the opening. The larger exterior folds are the **labia majora.** Their exterior surfaces are covered with hair; their inner surfaces are smooth and moist. The labia majora are homologous (of similar embryological origin) to the scrotum of the male. Medial to the labia majora are the smaller **labia minora.** These folds meet anteriorly on the median line to form a fold of skin, the **prepuce of the clitoris.** The **clitoris** is a small protuberance of erectile tissue under the prepuce that is homologous to the penis on the male. It is highly sensitive to sexual excitation. The fold of skin that extends from the clitoris to each labium minus is called the **frenulum of the clitoris.** Posteriorly, the labia minora join to form a transverse fold of skin, the **posterior commissure,** or *fourchette.* Between the anus and the posterior commissure is the **cen-**

condition or absence is not a determinant of virginity.

Assignment:

Label figure 39.3.

Internal Organs

Figure 39.4 is a posterior view of the female reproductive organs that shows the relationship of the vagina, uterus, ovaries, and uterine tubes. It also reveals many of the principal supporting ligaments.

The Uterus The uterus is a pear-shaped, thick-walled, hollow organ which consists of a fundus, corpus, and cervix. The **fundus** is the dome-shaped portion at the large end. The body, or **corpus,** extends from the fundus to the cervix. The **cervix,** or neck, of the uterus is the narrowest portion; it is about one inch long. Within the cervix is an **endocervical canal** that has an outer opening, the **external os,** that opens into the **vagina;** an inner opening, the **internal os,** opens into the cavity of the corpus.

The thick muscular portion of the uterine wall is called the **myometrium.** The inner lining, or **endometrium,** consists of mucosal tissue. The anterior and posterior surfaces of the corpus, as well as the fundus, are covered with peritoneum.

The Uterine (*Fallopian***) Tubes** Extending laterally from each side of the uterus is a uterine tube. The distal end of each tube is enlarged to form a funnel-shaped fimbriated **infundibulum** that surrounds an **ovary.** Although the infundibulum doesn't usually contact the ovary, one or more of the fingerlike **fimbriae** on the edge of the infundibulum usually do contact it. The infundibula and fimbriae receive oocytes produced by the ovaries.

The uterine tubes are lined with ciliated columnar cells that assist in transporting egg cells from the ovary into the uterus. The tubes also have a muscular wall that produces peristaltic movements that help to propel the egg cells. Fertilization usually occurs somewhere along the uterine tube. Note that each uterine tube narrows down to form an **isthmus** near the uterus.

The Urinary Bladder Figure 39.5 reveals the relationship of the urinary bladder to the reproductive organs. Note that it lies between the uterus and the **symphysis pubis.** The base of the bladder is in direct contact with the anterior vaginal wall. The **urethra** is positioned between the vagina and the

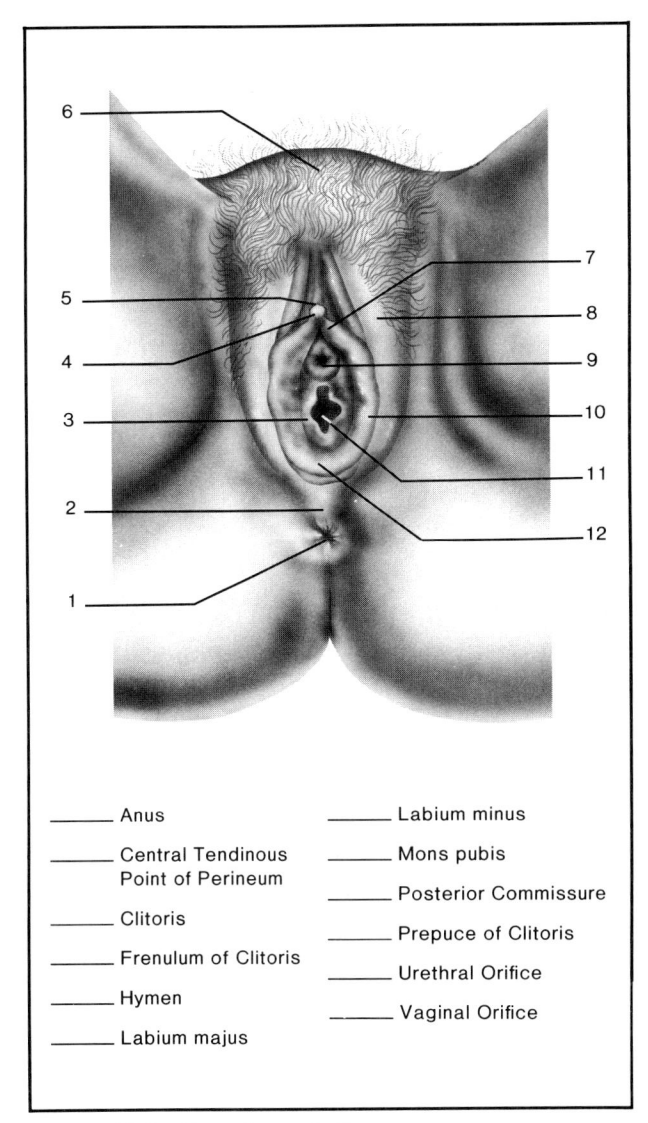

Figure 39.3 Female genitalia.

_____ Anus

_____ Central Tendinous Point of Perineum

_____ Clitoris

_____ Frenulum of Clitoris

_____ Hymen

_____ Labium majus

_____ Labium minus

_____ Mons pubis

_____ Posterior Commissure

_____ Prepuce of Clitoris

_____ Urethral Orifice

_____ Vaginal Orifice

tral tendinous point of the perineum. The **perineum** corresponds to the outlet of the pelvis.

The *vestibule* is the area between the labia minora, extending from the clitoris to the fourchette. Situated within the vestibule are the vaginal orifice, hymen, urethral orifice, and openings of the vestibular glands. The **urethral orifice** lies about 2–3 centimeters posterior to the clitoris. Many small **paraurethral glands** surround this opening. They are homologous to the prostate gland of the male. On either side of the vaginal orifice are openings from the two **greater vestibular (***Bartholin's***) glands.** These glands are homologous to the bulbourethral glands. They provide mucous secretion for vaginal lubrication. The **hymen** is a thin fold of mucous membrane that separates the vagina from the vestibule. It may be completely absent or cover the vaginal orifice partially or completely. Its

symphysis pubis. The neck of the bladder lies on the superior surface of the **urogenital diaphragm** (label 25, figure 39.5).

The superior surface of the bladder is covered with peritoneum that is continuous with the peritoneum on the anterior face of the uterus. The small cavity lined with peritoneum between the bladder and uterus is known as the **anterior cul-de-sac.** The space between the uterus and rectum is the **recto-uterine pouch** (*pouch of Douglas*).

Ligaments The uterus, ovaries, and uterine tubes are held in place and supported by various ligaments formed from the peritoneum and connective and muscular tissue. Figure 39.4 reveals the majority of them. A few are shown in figure 39.5.

The largest supporting structure is the **broad ligament** (label 3, figure 39.4). It is an extension of the peritoneal layers that cover the fundus and corpus of the uterus. It extends up over the fundus and corpus of the uterus. It extends up over the uterine tubes to form a mesentery, the **mesosalpinx,** on each side of the uterus. This portion of the

broad ligament, which is shown in figure 39.4 between the ovary and uterine tube, contains blood vessels that supply nutrients to the uterine tube.

Attached to the cervical region of the uterus are two **sacrouterine ligaments** that anchor the uterus to the sacral wall of the pelvic cavity. A **round ligament** (label 16, figure 39.5) extends from each side of the uterus to the body wall. This ligament is not shown in figure 39.4 because it is anterior in position.

Each ovary is held in place by ovarian and suspensory ligaments. The **ovarian ligament** extends from the medial surface of the ovary to the uterus. The **suspensory ligament** is a peritoneal fold on the other side of the ovary that attaches the ovary to the uterine tube.

Each uterine tube is held in place by an **infundibulopelvic ligament** that is attached to the posterior surface of the infundibulum.

Assignment:

Label figures 39.4 and 39.5.

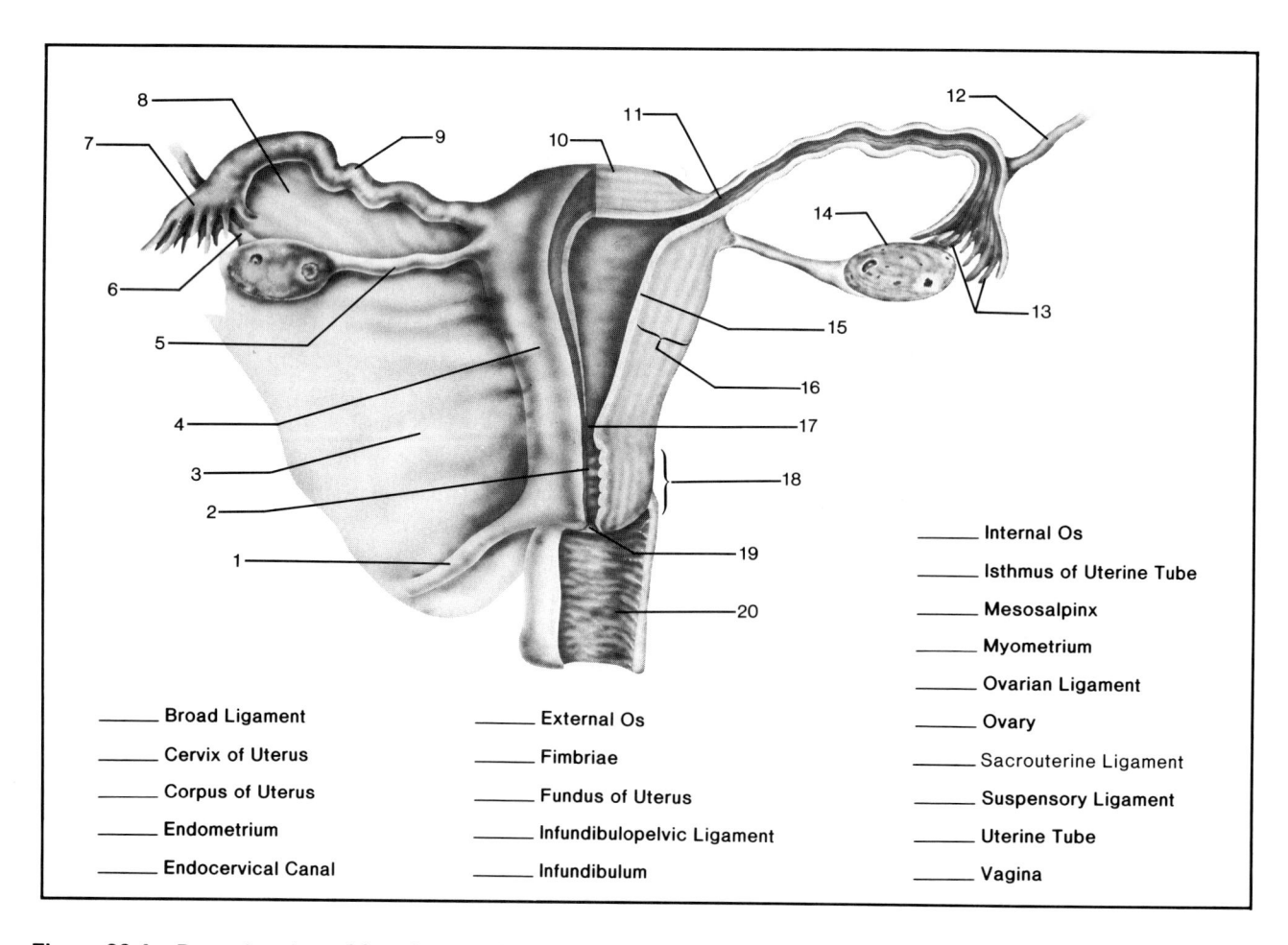

_____ Internal Os
_____ Isthmus of Uterine Tube
_____ Mesosalpinx
_____ Myometrium
_____ Ovarian Ligament
_____ Ovary
_____ Sacrouterine Ligament
_____ Suspensory Ligament
_____ Uterine Tube
_____ Vagina

_____ Broad Ligament
_____ Cervix of Uterus
_____ Corpus of Uterus
_____ Endometrium
_____ Endocervical Canal

_____ External Os
_____ Fimbriae
_____ Fundus of Uterus
_____ Infundibulopelvic Ligament
_____ Infundibulum

Figure 39.4 Posterior view of female reproductive organs.

Oogenesis

The development of egg cells in the ovary is called *oogenesis.* It was pointed out on page 261 that as many as 400,000 immature follicles develop in the ovaries from the germinal epithelium. At the onset of puberty all the potential ova in these follicles contain 46 chromosomes and are designated as **primary oocytes.** Only about 400 of these oocytes will mature during the reproductive lifetime of a woman.

Note in figure 39.6 that the primary oocyte, which forms from an oogonium of the germinal epithelium during embryological development, has 46 chromosomes. In the prophase stage of a dividing oocyte double-stranded chromosomes (dyads) unite to form 23 homologous pairs of chromosomes during synapsis. Each pair is made up of four chromatids; thus, it is called a tetrad. When the primary oocyte divides in the first meiotic division, each dyad member of each homologous pair enters a different cell. The first meiotic division produces a **secondary oocyte** with all the yolk of the primary oocyte and a **polar body** with no yolk. The secondary oocyte and polar body each contain 23 dyads.

The second meiotic division produces a **mature ovum** with 23 chromosomes that are *monads;* that is, each chromosome consists of a single chromatid. Another polar body is also formed in this division. The first polar body divides also to produce two new polar bodies with monads. The result is that one primary oocyte produces one mature ovum and three polar bodies. The polar bodies never serve any direct function in the fertilization process.

When ovulation takes place the "ovum" is a secondary oocyte. Usually, it is necessary for the sperm to penetrate the cell to trigger the second meiotic division. When the 23 chromosomes in the sperm unite with the chromosomes of the mature ovum, a **zygote** of 46 chromosomes is formed.

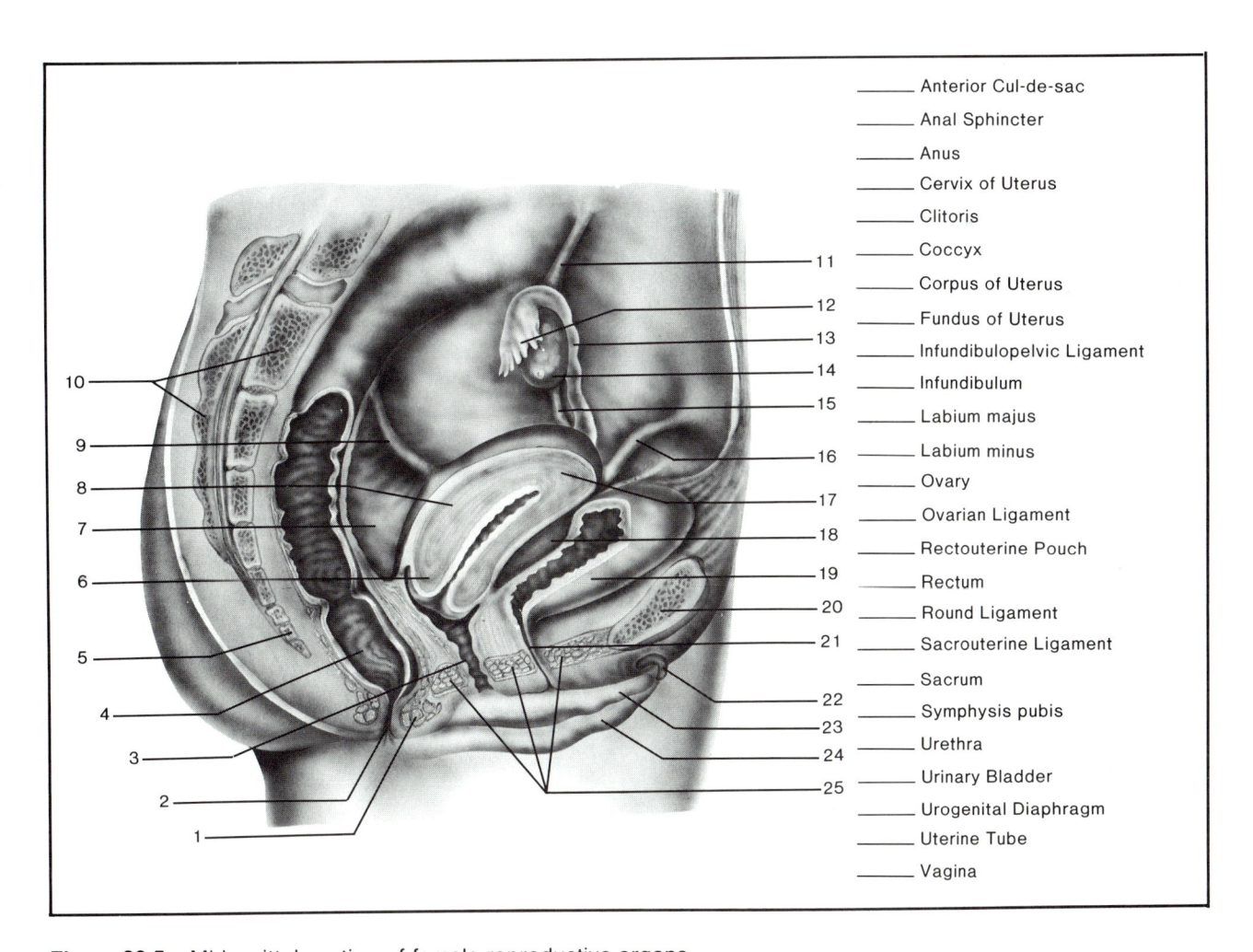

Labels at right:
_____ Anterior Cul-de-sac
_____ Anal Sphincter
_____ Anus
_____ Cervix of Uterus
_____ Clitoris
_____ Coccyx
_____ Corpus of Uterus
_____ Fundus of Uterus
_____ Infundibulopelvic Ligament
_____ Infundibulum
_____ Labium majus
_____ Labium minus
_____ Ovary
_____ Ovarian Ligament
_____ Rectouterine Pouch
_____ Rectum
_____ Round Ligament
_____ Sacrouterine Ligament
_____ Sacrum
_____ Symphysis pubis
_____ Urethra
_____ Urinary Bladder
_____ Urogenital Diaphragm
_____ Uterine Tube
_____ Vagina

Figure 39.5 Midsagittal section of female reproductive organs.

Assignment:

Study figures 39.6 and 38.8 thoroughly to familiarize yourself with the terminology and kinds of divisions. Several questions on the Laboratory Report pertain to this phenomenon.

Cat Dissection

In Exercise 37 the study of the urinary system necessitated a cursory examination of the reproductive organs in the cat. It will now be necessary to study these organs in greater detail. It may be desirable to refer back to figures 37.4 and 37.5 in some instances in this study, as well as to figures 39.7 and 39.8 on these pages when identifying the various organs in this dissection.

Male Reproductive System

This dissection will begin with an examination of the penis and necessitate the eventual removal of the right hind leg to reveal the inner structures. Proceed as follows:

1. Locate the **penis.** The skin that forms the sheath around the organ is called the **prepuce.** Pull back the prepuce to expose the enlarged distal end, which is the **glans.** The glans in the cat is covered with minute horny papillae.

2. Remove the **scrotum,** which is the skin that encloses the testes. Note that each testis is covered by a *fascial sac.* Do not open this sac at this time.

3. Trace the **spermatic cord** from one of the testes to the body wall. It is composed of the **vas deferens** (ductus deferens), blood vessels, nerves, and lymphatics that supply and drain the testis. Note that the covering of the spermatic cord is continuous with the fascial sac of the testis.

4. The vas deferens and vessels pass through the abdominal wall via the *inguinal canal.* From the inguinal canal the vas deferens passes up over the ureter and enters the penis near the prostate gland.

   To be able to study the structures shown in figure 39.7, remove the right leg near the hip joint. To do this it will be necessary to cut through the symphysis pubis. It will also be necessary to cut through the hipbone above the acetabulum. Clear away the pelvic muscles to expose the structures as shown in figure 39.7.

5. Locate the **prostate gland** where the vas deferens joins the urethra. The tube leading from the prostate through the penis is the **urogenital canal** (penile urethra). At the base of the penis will be seen a pair of **bulbourethral glands.**

6. Cut through the penis to produce a transverse section. Identify the two **corpora cavernosa** that cause erection. Near the symphysis pubis the two corpora diverge forming the **right** and **left crura** (*crus,* singular). Each crus is attached to a part of the ischium. Refer to figure 37.4 to see both crura.

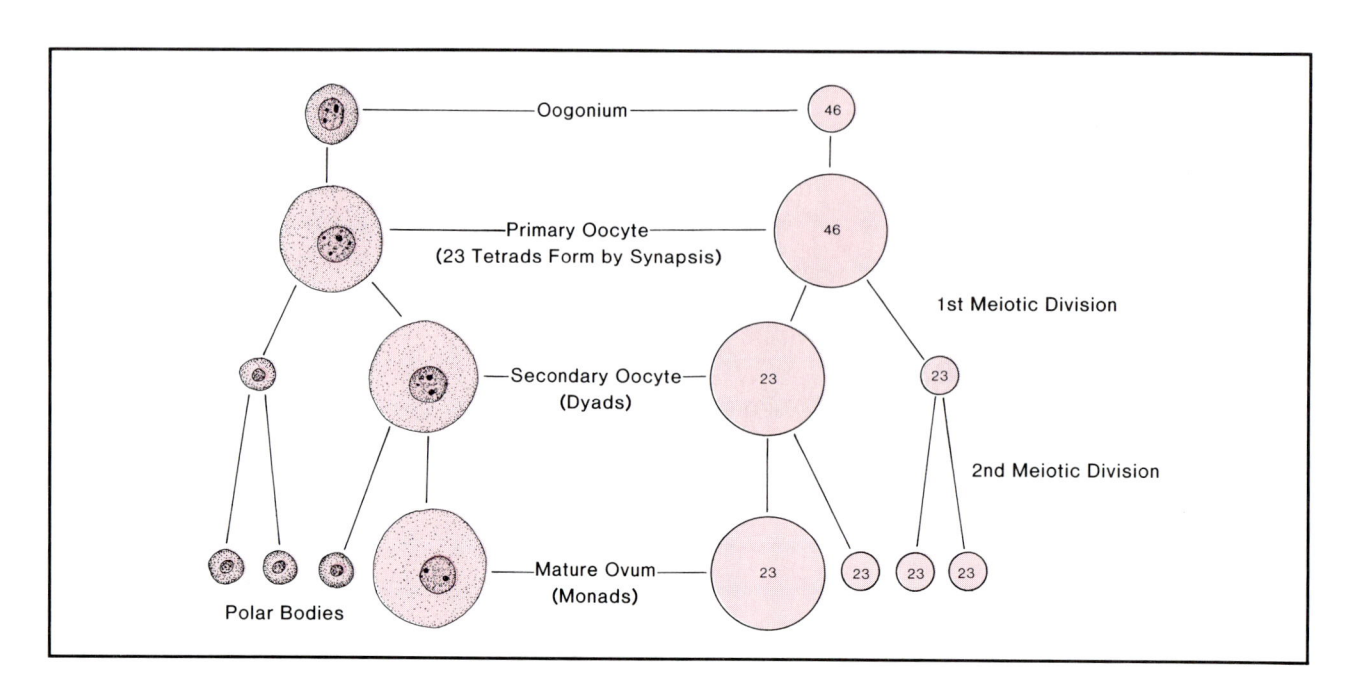

Figure 39.6 Oogenesis.

7. Cut through the fascial sac, exposing the testis. The space between this sac and the testis is called the *vaginal sac*. This cavity is a downward extension of the peritoneal cavity.

8. Trim away the fascial sac and trace the vas deferens toward the testis, noting its convoluted nature. Identify the **epididymis,** which lies on the dorsal side of the testis and is continuous with the vas deferens.

9. With a sharp scalpel or razor blade cut through the testis and epididymis to produce a section similar to the lower illustration in figure 39.1. Identify the structures revealed.

Female Reproductive System

Examination of the female reproductive organs will begin with the ovaries. Figure 37.5 will be useful for this portion of the study. Examination of the lower portion of the reproductive tract, however, will necessitate removal of the right leg, and figure 39.8 will then be used to identify structures in this region. Proceed as follows:

1. Identify the small, light colored oval **ovaries,** which lie posterior to the kidneys. Note that they are held by a fold of tissue to the dorsal body wall. This peritoneal fold is called the **mesovarium.** Note, also, that the ovary is attached to the uterine horn by the **ovarian ligament.**

2. Identify the **uterine tube** (oviduct) with its enlarged funnellike terminis, the **infundibulum** (*abdominal ostium*). Note that the perimeter of the infundibulum has many irregular projections called *fimbriae*. When ova leave the ovary they are drawn into the oviduct through the infundibulum by ciliated epithelium on the tissues of the area.

3. Observe that the uterus is Y-shaped, having two horns and a body. The **uterine horns** lie along each side of the abdominal cavity. The **uterine body** lies between the urinary bladder and the rectum (see figure 39.8).

4. To be able to observe the relationship of the vagina to other structures, as shown in figure

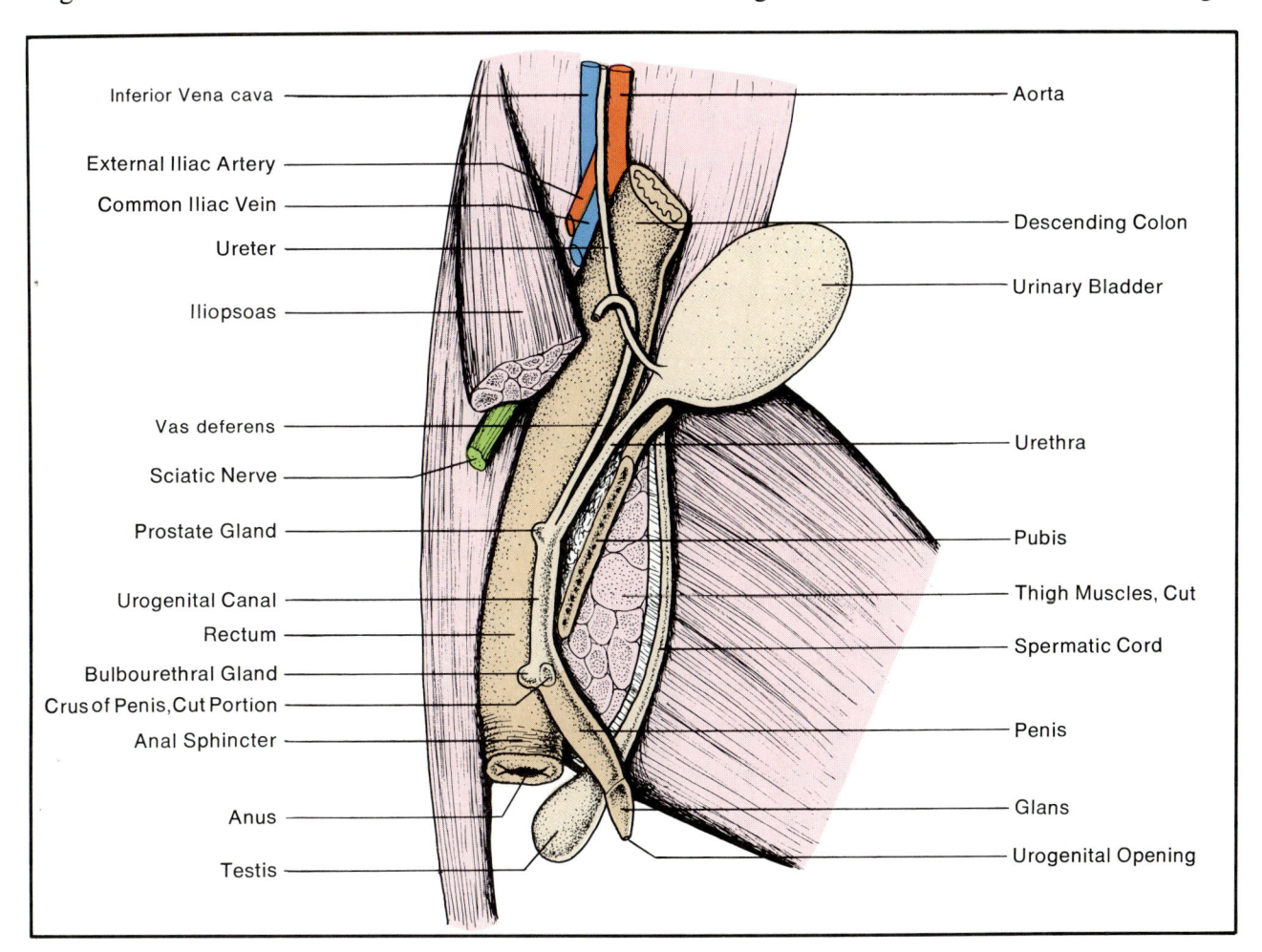

Figure 39.7   Lateral view of male cat urogenital system.

39.8, remove the right leg near the hip joint. To do this, it will be necessary to cut through the hipbone above the acetabulum. Remove the cut portion of the hipbone and clear away the pelvis muscles to expose the structures, as shown in figure 39.8. Preserve the blood vessels as much as possible.

5. Identify the general areas of the uterine body, vagina, and urogenital sinus. Remove the entire female reproductive tract and open it to reveal the inner structures shown in figure 37.5 (**cervix, vagina,** and **urogenital sinus**).

Histological Study

Assuming that spermatogenesis slides have been previously studied (page 270), we will focus here, primarily, on a histological study of the various reproductive organs of both sexes. Appropriate pages of the Histology Atlas and some of the illustrations in Exercise 38 will be used for reference.

Materials:

> prepared slides:
> > ovary (H9.310 or H9.3181)
> > uterus (H9.331), vagina (H9.341)
> > uterine tube (H9.321)
> > vas deferens (H9.432)
> > penis (H9.462), prostate gland (H9.443)
> > seminal vesicle (H9.442)

Ovary Study various slides of the ovary to identify **primordial follicles,** the **germinal epithelium,** and **Graafian follicles.** Since the ovaries are not included in the Histology Atlas, use figure 38.8, page 262 for reference.

Note that the developing ova in primordial follicles are surrounded by an incomplete layer of low cuboidal or flattened epithelium; the ova in developing follicles, on the other hand, are larger and are surrounded by two or more layers of cuboidal follicular cells.

Uterus When studying a slide of the uterus, take into consideration the phase of the menstrual cycle

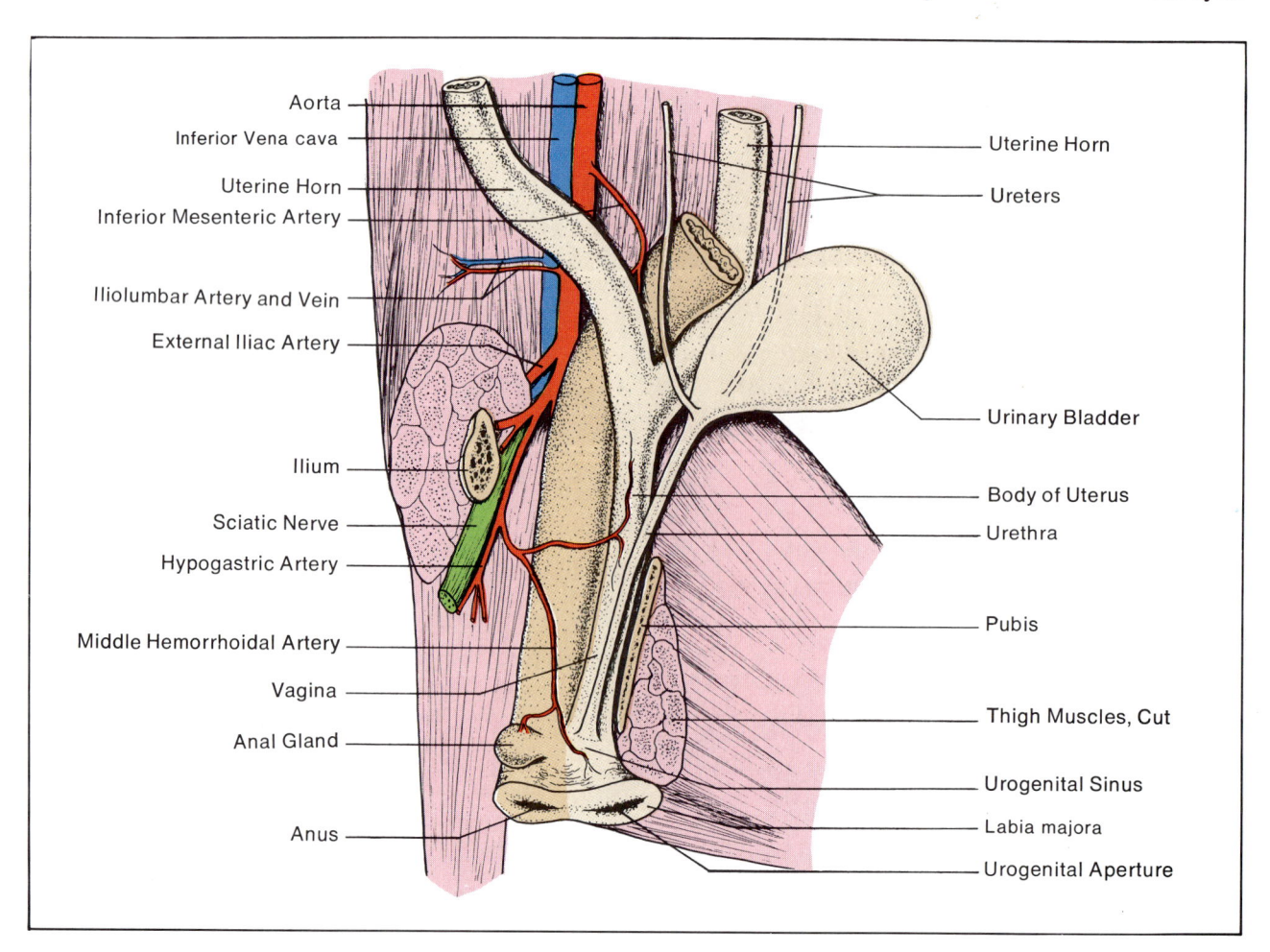

Figure 39.8 Lateral view of female cat urogenital system.

that is represented on the slide. The photomicrographs in figure HA-31 were made of Turtox slide H9.331, which represents about the third week in the cycle. Both the endometrium and myometrium will look much different in the earlier and later phases.

Differentiate the **endometrium** from the **myometrium.** Identify the **uterine glands** and endometrial **epithelium.**

Uterine Tube Scan a slide of the uterine tube with the low-power objective to find the lumen of the tube. Refer to illustrations C and D, figure HA-31. Note the extremely irregular outline of the mucosa, which consists of a mixture of ciliated and nonciliated columnar epithelium. How many layers of smooth muscle tissue do you find in the muscularis?

Vagina Examine a slide of the mucosa of the vagina and compare it to illustration C, figure HA-32. How does the vaginal mucosa differ from the skin? What function do the lymphocytes perform in the lamina propria?

Uterine Cervix Study a longitudinal section through the cervical area of the uterus which shows where the vaginal lining meets the cervical region. Consult illustration A, figure HA-32. Note the large number of spaces, or **cervical crypts,** that lie deep in the cervical tissue. Read the legend in figure HA-32 that pertains to the significance of these crypts.

Vas Deferens Examine a cross-sectional slide of the vas deferens, using minimum magnification to study the entire structure. Compare your slide with figure HA-34. Note that between its inner **epithelium** and the outer **adventitia** are three layers of smooth muscle tissue: an inner longitudinal layer, an outer longitudinal layer, and a middle layer of circular fibers. Note what the legend states about the **stereocilia** that are seen on the epithelium.

Penis Examine a cross-sectional preparation of the penis. The photomicrographs in illustrations C and D, HA-33, were made from an H9.462 Turtox slide. Examine the epithelium under high-dry magnification. Does the epithelium on your slide look like illustration D? If not, why not? Read the comments in the legend that pertain to epithelial differences.

Seminal Vesicle A cross section of a portion of a seminal vesicle is seen in illustrations A and B, figure HA-35. Examine a slide first with low-power magnification and note the striking way in which the mucosa is folded upon itself to produce a maze of pockets. Examine the epithelium under high-dry or oil immersion. What is the nature and function of the seminal fluid?

Prostate Gland Examine a slide of the gland under low power first to identify the structures seen in illustration C, figure HA-35. Note the large number of **tubulo-alveolar glands** that secrete the prostatic fluid. Why does the prostate gland tend to become hardened and restrict micturition in older men?

Laboratory Report

Complete the Laboratory Report for this exercise.

Student: _____

Desk No: _____ Section: _____

Anatomical Terminology, Body Cavities, and Membranes

A. Illustration Labels

Record the label numbers for all the illustrations in the appropriate places in the answer columns.

B. Terminology

From the list of positions, sections, and membranes, select those that are applicable to the following statements. In some cases more than one answer may apply.

Relative Positions		*Sections*	*Membranes*
anterior—1	lateral—7	frontal—13	mesentery—17
caudal—2	medial—8	midsagittal—14	pericardium, parietal—18
cranial—3	posterior—9	sagittal—15	pericardium, visceral—19
distal—4	proximal—10	transverse—16	peritoneum, parietal—20
dorsal—5	superior—11		peritoneum, visceral—21
inferior—6	ventral—12		pleura, parietal—22
			pleura, pulmonary—23

Sections:

1. Divides body into front and back portions.
2. Divides body into unequal right and left sides.
3. Three sections that are longitudinal.
4. Divides body into equal right and left sides.
5. Two sections that expose both lungs and heart in each section.

Positions:

6. The tongue is _____ to the palate.
7. The shoulder of a dog is _____ to its hip.
8. A hat is worn on the _____ surface of the head.
9. The cheeks are _____ to the tongue.
10. The fingertips are _____ to all structures of the hand.
11. The human shoulder is _____ to the hip.
12. The shoulder is the _____ (*proximal, distal*) portion of the arm.

Membranes:

13. Serous membrane attached to lung surface.
14. Serous membrane attached to thoracic wall.
15. Double-layered membrane that holds abdominal organs in place.
16. Double-layered membrane that surrounds the heart.

Select the surfaces on which the following are located:

17. Ear
18. Adam's apple
19. Kneecap
20. Palm of hand

Answers

Terms	Fig. 1.1
1. _____	_____
2. _____	_____
3. _____	_____
4. _____	_____
5. _____	_____
6. _____	_____
7. _____	_____
8. _____	_____
9. _____	_____
10. _____	_____
11. _____	_____
12. _____	_____
13. _____	_____
14. _____	_____
15. _____	_____
16. _____	_____
17. _____	_____
18. _____	_____
19. _____	_____
20. _____	_____

Fig. 2.1	Fig. 1.3
_____	_____
_____	_____
_____	_____
_____	_____
_____	_____
_____	_____
_____	_____
_____	_____
_____	_____
_____	_____
_____	_____
_____	_____

C. Localized Areas

Identify the specific areas of the body described by the following statements.

antebrachium—1	calf—6	gluteal—11	iliac—16
antecubital—2	costal—7	groin—12	lumbar—17
axilla—3	cubital—8	ham—13	plantar—18
brachium—4	epigastric—9	hypochondriac—14	pectoral—19
buttocks—5	flank—10	hypogastric—15	popliteal—20
			umbilical—21

1. The elbow area.
2. The "rump" area.
3. The underarm area.
4. The sole of the foot.
5. The upper arm.
6. The forearm.
7. Upper chest region.
8. Depression on back of leg behind knee.
9. Side of abdomen between lower edge of rib cage and upper edge of hipbone.
10. Back portion of abdominal body wall that extends from lower edge of rib cage to hipbone.
11. Area over the ribs on the dorsum.
12. Posterior portion of lower leg.
13. Anterior surface of the elbow.
14. Abdominal area that surrounds the navel.
15. Abdominal area which is lateral to pubic region.
16. Area of abdominal wall that covers the stomach.
17. Abdominal area which is lateral to epigastric area.
18. Abdominal area which is lateral to umbilical area.
19. Area of arm on opposite side of elbow.
20. Abdominal areas between the transpyloric and transtubercular planes.

D. Body Cavities

From the following list of cavities select those applicable to the following statements.

abdominal—1	dorsal—4	spinal—8
abdominopelvic—2	pelvic—5	thoracic—9
cranial—3	pericardial—6	ventral—10
	pleural—7	

1. Cavity that consists of cranial and spinal cavities.
2. Most inferior portion of the abdominopelvic cavity.
3. Cavity separated into two major divisions by the diaphragm.
4. Cavity inferior to the diaphragm that consists of two parts.

Select the cavity in which the following organs are located:

5. Kidneys	9. Rectum	13. Spleen
6. Duodenum	10. Pancreas	14. Spinal cord
7. Brain	11. Lungs and heart	15. Urinary bladder
8. Heart	12. Liver	16. Stomach

Answers

Areas	Fig. 1.2
1. _____	_____
2. _____	_____
3. _____	_____
4. _____	_____
5. _____	_____
6. _____	_____
7. _____	_____
8. _____	_____
9. _____	_____
10. _____	_____
11. _____	_____
12. _____	_____
13. _____	_____
14. _____	_____
15. _____	_____
16. _____	_____
17. _____	_____
18. _____	_____
19. _____	**Fig. 2.2**
20. _____	_____

Cavities	
1. _____	_____
2. _____	_____
3. _____	_____
4. _____	_____
5. _____	_____
6. _____	_____
7. _____	_____
8. _____	**Fig. 2.3**
9. _____	_____
10. _____	_____
11. _____	_____
12. _____	_____
13. _____	_____
14. _____	_____
15. _____	_____
16. _____	_____

Student: _____

Desk No: _____ Section: _____

Organ Systems: Rat Dissection

A. System Functions

Select the system (or systems) that perform the following functions in the body. Record the numbers in the answer column. More than one answer may apply.

circulatory—1	lymphatic—5	respiratory—9
digestive—2	muscular—6	reticuloendothelial—10
endocrine—3	nervous—7	skeletal—11
integumentary—4	reproductive—8	urinary—12

1. Removes carbon dioxide from the blood.
2. Provides a shield of protection for vital organs such as the brain and heart.
3. Movement of ribs in breathing.
4. Carries heat from the muscles to the surface of the body for dissipation.
5. Provides rigid support for the attachment of muscles.
6. Transportation of food from the intestines to all parts of the body.
7. Disposes of urea, uric acid, and other cellular wastes.
8. Movement of arms and legs.
9. Helps to maintain normal body temperature by dissipating excess heat.
10. Destroys microorganisms once they break through the skin.
11. Phagocytic cells of this system remove bacteria from lymph.
12. Carries messages from receptors to centers of interpretation.
13. Controls the rate of growth.
14. Returns tissue fluid to the blood.
15. Produces various kinds of blood cells.
16. Enables the body to adjust to changing internal and external environmental conditions.
17. Ensures continuity of the species.
18. Eliminates excess water from the body.
19. Carries hormones from glands to all tissues.
20. Acts as a shield against invasion by bacteria.
21. Carries fats from the intestines to the blood.
22. Coordination of all body movements.
23. Breaks food particles down into small molecules.
24. Controls the development of the ovaries and testes.
25. Production of spermatozoa and ova.

Answers

System Functions

1. _____
2. _____
3. _____
4. _____
5. _____
6. _____
7. _____
8. _____
9. _____
10. _____
11. _____
12. _____
13. _____
14. _____
15. _____
16. _____
17. _____
18. _____
19. _____
20. _____
21. _____
22. _____
23. _____
24. _____
25. _____

B. *Organ Placement*

Select the system at the right that includes the following organs.

1. Bones
2. Brain
3. Bronchi
4. Dermis
5. Esophagus
6. Hair
7. Heart
8. Kidneys
9. Lungs
10. Pancreas
11. Spleen
12. Stomach
13. Teeth
14. Trachea
15. Toenails
16. Tonsils
17. Thyroid
18. Ureters
19. Uterus
20. Veins

circulatory—1
digestive—2
endocrine—3
integumentary—4
lymphatic—5
muscular—6
nervous—7
reproductive—8
respiratory—9
skeletal—10
urinary—11

Answers
Organ Placement

1. _____
2. _____
3. _____
4. _____
5. _____
6. _____
7. _____
8. _____
9. _____
10. _____
11. _____
12. _____
13. _____
14. _____
15. _____
16. _____
17. _____
18. _____
19. _____
20. _____

4

Student: _____

Desk No: _____ Section: _____

Microscopy

A. Completion Questions

Record the answers to the following questions in the column at the right.

1. List three fluids that may be used for cleaning lenses.
2. How can one greatly increase the bulb life on a microscope lamp if the voltage is variable?
3. What characteristic of a microscope enables one to switch from one objective to another without altering the focus?
4. What effect (*increase* or *decrease*) does closing the diaphragm have on the following?
   a. Image brightness
   b. Image contrast
   c. Resolution
5. In general, at what position should the condenser be kept?
6. Express the maximum resolution of the compound microscope in terms of micrometers (μm).
7. If you are getting $225\times$ magnification with a $45\times$ high-dry objective, what would be the power of the eyepiece?
8. What is the magnification of objects observed through a $100\times$ oil immersion objective with a $7.5\times$ eyepiece?
9. Immersion oil must have the same refractive index as _____ to be of any value.
10. Substage filters should be of a _____ color to get the maximum resolution of the optical system.

B. True–False

Record these statements as True or False in the answer column.

1. Eyepieces are of such simple construction that almost anyone can safely disassemble them for cleaning.
2. Lenses can be safely cleaned with almost any kind of tissue or cloth.
3. When swinging the oil immersion objective into position after using high-dry, one should always increase the distance between the lens and slide to prevent damaging the oil immersion lens.
4. Instead of starting first with the oil immersion lens, it is best to use one of the lower magnifications first, and then swing the oil immersion into position.
5. The $45\times$ and $100\times$ objectives have shorter working distances than the $10\times$ objective.

Answers

Completion

1a. _____

b. _____

c. _____

2. _____

3. _____

4a. _____

b. _____

c. _____

5. _____

6. _____

7. _____

8. _____

9. _____

10. _____

True–False

1. _____

2. _____

3. _____

4. _____

5. _____

C. Multiple Choice
Select the best answer for the following statements.

1. The resolution of a microscope is increased by
   1. using blue light.
   2. stopping down the diaphragm.
   3. lowering the condenser.
   4. raising the condenser to its highest point.
   5. Both 1 and 4 are correct.

2. The magnification of an object seen through the $10\times$ objective with a $10\times$ ocular is
   1. ten times.
   2. twenty times.
   3. 1000 times.
   4. None of these are correct.

3. The most commonly used ocular is
   1. $5\times$.
   2. $10\times$.
   3. $15\times$.
   4. $20\times$.

4. Microscope lenses may be cleaned with
   1. lens tissue.
   2. a soft linen handkerchief.
   3. an air syringe.
   4. Both 1 and 3 are correct.
   5. 1, 2, and 3 are correct.

5. When changing from low power to high power, it is generally necessary to
   1. lower the condenser.
   2. open the diaphragm.
   3. close the diaphragm.
   4. Both 1 and 2 are correct.
   5. Both 1 and 3 are correct.

Answers
Multiple Choice
1. _____
2. _____
3. _____
4. _____
5. _____

Cytology: Basic Cell Structure and Mitosis

A. Figure 5.1

Record the labels for figure 5.1 in the answer column.

B. Cell Drawings

Sketch in the space below one or two epithelial cells as seen under high-dry magnification. Label the **nucleus, cytoplasm,** and **cell membrane.** If mitosis drawings are to be made, put them on a separate sheet of paper.

C. Cell Structure

From the list of structures below, select those that are described by the following statements. More than one structure may apply to some of the statements.

centrosome—1	Golgi apparatus—7	microtubules—12	polyribosomes—17
chromatin granules—2	lysosome—8	nuclear envelope—13	RER—18
cilia—3	microvilli—9	nucleolus—14	ribosomes—19
condensing vacuoles—4	mitochondria—10	nucleus—15	secretory granules—20
cytoplasm—5	microfilaments—11	plasma membrane—16	SER—21
flagellum—6			

1. Prominent body in nucleus that produces ribosomes.
2. Trilaminar unit membrane structure.
3. Outer membrane of the cell.
4. A nonmembranous organelle consisting of two bundles of microtubules.
5. Bodies within the nucleus that represent chromosomal material.
6. ER that lacks ribosomes.
7. Double-layered unit membrane structure.
8. Small bodies of RNA and protein attached to surfaces of the RER.
9. Extensive system of tubules, vesicles, and sacs within the cytoplasm.
10. All protoplasmic material between the plasma membrane and nucleus.
11. Sacs in the cytoplasm that contain digestive enzymes.
12. A unit membrane organelle in the cytoplasm that contains cristae.
13. Short, hairlike appendages on the surface of some cells.
14. ER that is covered by ribosomes.
15. Chains and rosettes of small bodies scattered throughout the cytoplasm.
16. Unit membrane structure that is continuous with the plasma and nuclear membranes.
17. Extranuclear bodies that possess DNA and are able to replicate themselves.
18. A layered concave structure in the cytoplasm that is similar to the basic structure of SER.
19. Surface protuberances that form a delicate brush border.
20. Bodies produced by Golgi and exocytosed by the cell.

Answers

Cell Structure	Fig. 5.1
1. _____	_____
2. _____	_____
3. _____	_____
4. _____	_____
5. _____	_____
6. _____	_____
7. _____	_____
8. _____	
9. _____	
10. _____	
11. _____	
12. _____	
13. _____	
14. _____	_____
15. _____	_____
16. _____	
17. _____	
18. _____	
19. _____	
20. _____	

D. Organelle Functions

Select the organelles that perform the following functions. More than one structure may apply to some statements.

centrosome—1	microvilli—5	plasma membrane—9
flagellum—2	mitochondrion—6	polyribosomes—10
Golgi apparatus—3	nucleolus—7	RER—11
lysosome—4	nucleus—8	SER—12

1. Forms asters during mitosis.
2. Produces ribonucleoprotein for ribosomes.
3. The microcirculatory system of the cell.
4. Contains genetic code of the cell.
5. Place where oxidative respiration occurs.
6. Synthesize protein for endogenous use.
7. Brings about rapid hydrolysis (digestion) of cell after death.
8. Place where ATP is synthesized and stored.
9. Regulates the flow of materials into and out of cell.
10. Synthesizes protein for extracellular distribution.
11. Disposal organelles in cytoplasm that digest protein.
12. Increases absorptive area of the cell.
13. Synthesis, packaging, and transportation of substances.
14. Plays a role in flagellar development.
15. Accomplishes some motile function for some cells.

E. True–False

Evaluate the validity of the following statements concerning cell structure and function.

1. Secretory cells have well-developed Golgi.
2. Mitochondria are able to replicate themselves.
3. Practically all molecules that pass through the plasma membrane are actively assisted by the membrane.
4. Ribosomes are found in the cytoplasm, mitochondria, RER, and SER.
5. The inner and outer layers of the plasma membrane are essentially lipoidal in nature with scattered molecules of protein and glycoprotein.
6. A "brush border" consists of microvilli.
7. Spermatozoa move with cilia.
8. Ribosomes are primarily involved in oxidative respiration.
9. Cilia form from basal bodies derived from centrioles.
10. Asters develop from mitochondria.

F. Mitosis (Ex. 6)

Select the phase in which the following events occur.

1. Nuclear membrane disappears.
2. Cleavage furrow forms.
3. Spindle fibers begin to form.
4. New nuclear membrane forms.
5. Asters form from centrioles.
6. Centriole replication occurs.
7. Replication of DNA occurs.
8. Sister chromosomes separate and pass to opposite poles.
9. Formed after telophase is completed.
10. Chromosomes become oriented on equatorial plane.

interphase—1
prophase—2
metaphase—3
anaphase—4
telophase—5
daughter cells—6

Answers

Functions

1. _____
2. _____
3. _____
4. _____
5. _____
6. _____
7. _____
8. _____
9. _____
10. _____
11. _____
12. _____
13. _____
14. _____
15. _____

True–False

1. _____
2. _____
3. _____
4. _____
5. _____
6. _____
7. _____
8. _____
9. _____
10. _____

Mitosis

1. _____
2. _____
3. _____
4. _____
5. _____
6. _____
7. _____
8. _____
9. _____
10. _____

9

Student: _____

Desk No: _____ Section: _____

The Integument

A. Figure 9.1

Record the labels for this illustration in the answer column.

B. Microscopic Study

If the space provided below is adequate for your histology drawings, use it. Use a separate sheet of paper if the space is inadequate.

C. Questions

Select the answer that completes the following statements. Only one answer applies for each question.

1. Granules of the stratum granulosum consist of
   (1) melanin.   (2) keratin.   (3) eleidin.

2. Pacinian corpuscles are sensitive to
   (1) temperature.   (2) pressure.   (3) touch.

3. Meissner's corpuscles are sensitive to
   (1) temperature.   (2) pressure.   (3) touch.

4. The epidermis consists of the following number of distinct layers:
   (1) three.   (2) four.   (3) five.   (4) six.

5. The papillary layer is a part of the
   (1) dermis.   (2) epidermis.   (3) stratum spinosum.

6. Melanin granules are produced by the
   (1) stratum granulosum.   (2) melanocytes.
   (3) corium.   (4) stratum corneum.

7. New cells of the epidermis originate in the
   (1) dermis.   (2) stratum germinativum.
   (3) stratum corneum.   (4) corium.

8. The outermost layer of the epidermis is the
   (1) stratum corneum.   (2) stratum germinativum.
   (3) stratum lucidum.   (4) stratum spinosum.

Answers

Fig. 9.1

_____
_____
_____
_____
_____
_____
_____
_____
_____
_____
_____
_____
_____
_____
_____
_____
_____

Questions

1. _____
2. _____
3. _____
4. _____
5. _____
6. _____
7. _____
8. _____

9. The secretions of the apocrine glands usually empty
   (1) into a hair follicle.   (2) directly out through skin surface.
   (3) Both 1 and 2   (4) None of these are correct.
10. Sebum is secreted by
   (1) sweat glands.   (2) eccrine glands.
   (3) apocrine glands.   (4) None of these are correct.
11. Keratin's function is primarily to
   (1) destroy bacteria.   (2) provide waterproofing.   (3) cool the body.
12. Meissner's corpuscles are located in the
   (1) papillary layer.   (2) reticular layer.   (3) hypodermis.
13. Arrector pili assist in
   (1) maintaining skin tonus.   (2) limiting excessive sweating.
   (3) forcing out sebum.   (4) None of these are correct.
14. The hair follicle is
   (1) a shaft of hair.   (2) the root of a hair.
   (3) a tube in the skin.   (4) None of these are correct.
15. Pacinian corpuscles are located in the
   (1) papillary layer.   (2) reticular layer.   (3) hypodermis.
16. Sweat is produced by
   (1) sebaceous glands.   (2) eccrine glands.
   (3) ceruminous glands.   (4) None of these are correct.
17. The coiled-up portion of an apocrine gland is located in the
   (1) hair follicle.   (2) dermis.   (3) epidermis.   (4) hypodermis.
18. Apocrine glands are located
   (1) in the axillae.   (2) on the scrotum.
   (3) in the ear canal.   (4) All of these are correct.

Answers
Questions
9. _____
10. _____
11. _____
12. _____
13. _____
14. _____
15. _____
16. _____
17. _____
18. _____

The Appendicular Skeleton

A. Illustrations
Record the labels for the illustrations of this exercise in the answer columns.

B. Shoulder
Identify the parts of the scapula and humerus that are described by the following statements. Refer to figures 13.1 and 13.2 for assistance.

axillary margin—1	glenoid cavity—5	lesser tubercle—9
acromion process—2	greater tubercle—6	scapular spine—10
coracoid process—3	head of humerus—7	vertebral margin—11
deltoid tuberosity—4	inferior angle—8	

1. Part of humerus that articulates with scapula.
2. Depression on scapula that articulates with humerus.
3. Process on humerus to which the deltoid muscle is attached.
4. Process on scapula that is anterior to glenoid cavity.
5. Most inferior tip of scapula.
6. Large lateral process near head of humerus.
7. Edge of scapula that is nearest to vertebral column.
8. Process on scapula that articulates with clavicle.
9. Lateral margin of scapula that extends from glenoid cavity to inferior angle.
10. Small process just above surgical neck of humerus.
11. Long oblique ridge on posterior surface of scapula that extends from the lateral border to the acromion.

C. Arm
By referring to figures 13.2 and 13.3 identify the following parts of the arm.

capitulum—1	medial epicondyle—5	radial notch—9
coronoid process—2	olecranon fossa—6	radial tuberosity—10
head of radius—3	olecranon process—7	styloid process—11
lateral epicondyle—4	semilunar notch—8	trochlea—12

1. Distal medial condyle of humerus.
2. Distal lateral condyle of humerus.
3. Part of radius that articulates with humerus.
4. Small distal medial process of ulna.
5. Process on radius for biceps brachii attachment.
6. Depression on proximal end of ulna that articulates with trochlea of humerus.
7. Depression on ulna that is in contact with head of radius.
8. Condyle of humerus that articulates with ulna.
9. Fossa on distal posterior surface of humerus.
10. Distal lateral prominence of radius.
11. Condyle of humerus that articulates with radius.
12. Process on anterior surface of ulna just below the semilunar notch.
13. Epicondyle adjacent to capitulum.
14. Proximal posterior process of ulna, sometimes called the "funny bone."
15. Epicondyle of humerus adjacent to trochlea.

Answers

Shoulder	Fig. 13.1
1. _____	_____
2. _____	_____
3. _____	_____
4. _____	_____
5. _____	_____
6. _____	_____
7. _____	_____
8. _____	_____
9. _____	_____
10. _____	_____
11. _____	_____
	_____

Arm	Fig. 13.2
1. _____	_____
2. _____	_____
3. _____	_____
4. _____	_____
5. _____	_____
6. _____	_____
7. _____	_____
8. _____	_____
9. _____	_____
10. _____	_____
11. _____	_____
12. _____	_____
13. _____	_____
14. _____	_____
15. _____	_____

D. Hand

By referring to figure 13.3 identify the parts of the wrist and hand described by these statements.

1. Part of ulna that articulates with fibrocartilaginous disk of the wrist.
2. Two carpal bones that articulate with radius.
3. Bone which articulates with the 4th and 5th metacarpals.
4. Two carpal bones that articulate with thumb.
5. Bones of the fingers.
6. List the four distal carpal bones from lateral to medial.
7. Bones that make up the palm of the hand.
8. List the four proximal carpal bones from lateral to medial.

capitate—1
hamate—2
head—3
lunate—4
metacarpals—5
navicular—6
phalanges—7
pisiform—8
trapezium—9
trapezoid—10
triquetral—11

E. Pelvis

By studying figures 13.4 and 13.5 identify the following parts of the pelvis.

1. Three bones of os coxa.
2. Upper bone of os coxa.
3. Anterior bone of os coxa.
4. Part of os coxa that one sits on.
5. Uppermost process on posterior edge of ischium.
6. Superior ridge of hipbone.
7. Prominent fossa on lateral surface of os coxa.
8. Large foramen on os coxa.
9. Joint between os coxa and sacrum.
10. Large prominent process of ischium.
11. Joint between two ossa coxae on the median line.
12. Lower posterior bone of os coxa.

acetabulum—1
iliac crest—2
ilium—3
ischial spine—4
ischium—5
obturator foramen—6
posterior inferior spine—7
posterior superior spine—8
pubis—9
sacroiliac joint—10
symphysis pubis—11
tuberosity of ischium—12

F. Comparisons

Compare the male and female pelves side-by-side to determine the validity (true or false) of these statements.

1. The aperture of the female pelvis is heart-shaped.
2. The greater pelvis (concavity of the expanded iliac bones above the pelvic brim) of the male is narrower than in the female.
3. The male sacrum and coccyx are more curved.
4. The obturator foramina of the female pelvis tend toward being triangular and smaller than in the male.
5. The aperture of the female pelvis is larger and more oval than the male pelvis.
6. The muscular impressions on the female pelvis are less distinct (bone is smoother).
7. The iliac crests of the female pelvis protrude outward more than in the male.
8. The acetabula of the female face more anteriorly.
9. The sacrum of the female pelvis is shorter and wider.
10. The obturator foramina of the female pelvis are rounder and larger than in the male.

Answers

Hand	Fig. 13.3
1. _____	_____
2. _____	_____
3. _____	_____
4. _____	_____
5. _____	_____
6. _____	_____
7. _____	_____
8. _____	_____

Pelvis	
	_____
1. _____	_____
2. _____	_____
3. _____	_____
4. _____	_____
5. _____	_____
6. _____	_____
7. _____	_____
8. _____	_____
9. _____	_____
10. _____	Fig. 13.4
11. _____	_____
12. _____	_____

Comparisons	
	_____
1. _____	_____
2. _____	_____
3. _____	_____
4. _____	_____
5. _____	_____
6. _____	_____
7. _____	_____
8. _____	_____
9. _____	_____
10. _____	_____

G. Leg

By referring to figures 13.5 and 13.6 identify the following parts of the leg.

femur—1
fibula—2
gluteal tuberosity—3
greater trochanter—4
head of femur—5
head of fibula—6
intertrochanteric crest—7
intertrochanteric line—8

lateral condyle—9
lateral malleolus—10
lesser trochanter—11
linea aspera—12
medial condyle—13
medial malleolus—14
tibia—15
tibial tuberosity—16

1. Distal lateral process of femur.
2. Distal medial process of femur.
3. Distal lateral process of fibula that forms outer anklebone.
4. Distal medial process of tibia that forms the inner prominence of the ankle.
5. Proximal lateral process of tibia that articulates with femur.
6. Proximal anterior process of tibia that protrudes below the kneecap.
7. Proximal medial process of tibia that articulates with femur.
8. Ridge on posterior surface of femur (upper portion).
9. Ridge on posterior surface of femur (lower portion).
10. Thin lateral bone of lower leg.
11. Strongest bone of lower leg.
12. Process just inferior to neck of femur on medial surface.
13. Oblique ridge between trochanters on posterior surface of femur.
14. Part of femur that fits into acetabulum.
15. Longest, heaviest bone of leg.
16. End of fibula that articulates with upper end of tibia.
17. Large process lateral to neck of femur.
18. Oblique ridge between trochanters on anterior surface of femur.

H. Foot

By referring to figure 13.6 identify the following parts of the foot.

calcaneous—1
cuboid—2
cuneiform—3
metatarsals—4

navicular—5
phalanges—6
talus—7

1. The heelbone.
2. Largest tarsal bone.
3. Tarsal bone that articulates with tibia.
4. Tarsal bone on side of foot in front of calcaneous.
5. Five elongated bones of foot that form instep.
6. Bones of toes.
7. Three similarly named tarsal bones anterior to navicular.
8. Tarsal bone anterior to talus and on medial side of foot.

Answers	
Leg	**Fig. 13.5**
1. _____	_____
2. _____	_____
3. _____	_____
4. _____	_____
5. _____	_____
6. _____	_____
7. _____	_____
8. _____	_____
9. _____	_____
10. _____	_____
11. _____	_____
12. _____	_____
13. _____	**Fig. 13.6**
14. _____	_____
15. _____	_____
16. _____	_____
17. _____	_____
18. _____	_____
Foot	
1. _____	_____
2. _____	_____
3. _____	_____
4. _____	_____
5. _____	_____
6. _____	_____
7. _____	_____
8. _____	_____

The Appendicular Skeleton

I. Numbers

Supply the correct numbers for the following statements.

1. Number of phalanges in large toe.
2. Total number of carpal bones in each wrist.
3. Total number of tarsal bones in each foot.
4. Total number of metatarsals in each foot.
5. Number of phalanges in thumb.
6. Number of phalanges on each of the other four fingers.
7. Number of phalanges in the 2nd, 3rd, 4th, and 5th toes.
8. Number designation for thumb metacarpal.
9. Number designation for the small toe metatarsal.
10. Number designation for little finger metacarpal.

Answers
Numbers
1. _____
2. _____
3. _____
4. _____
5. _____
6. _____
7. _____
8. _____
9. _____
10. _____

Student: _____

Desk No: _____ Section: _____

Articulations

A. Illustrations

Record the labels for the illustrations of this exercise in the answer columns.

B. Characteristics

Select the joints from the list on the right that have the following characteristics. More than one answer may apply in some cases.

1. Movement in all directions.
2. Slightly movable.
3. Immovable.
4. Freely movable in one plane only.
5. Freely movable in two planes.
6. Rotational movement only.
7. Condyle end in elliptical cavity.
8. Each bone end is concave in one direction and convex in another direction.
9. Held together with interosseous ligament.
10. Bone ends joined by fibrous connective tissue.
11. Bone ends are flat or slightly convex.
12. Fused joint of hyaline cartilage.
13. Contains fibrocartilaginous pad.

ball and socket—1
condyloid—2
gliding—3
hinge—4
pivot—5
saddle—6
sutures—7
symphysis—8
synchondrosis—9
syndesmosis—10

C. Joint Classification

By examining and manipulating the bones of a skeleton, classify the following joints. Two terms apply to each joint.

1. Elbow joint.
2. Knee joint.
3. Phalanges to metacarpals.
4. Phalanges to metatarsals.
5. Hip joint.
6. Shoulder joint.
7. Intervertebral joint (between vertebral bodies).
8. Metaphysis of long bone of child.
9. Interlocking joint between cranial bones.
10. Symphysis pubis.
11. Articulation between tibia and fibula at distal ends.
12. Atlas to skull.
13. Toe joints (between phalanges).
14. Finger joint (between phalanges).
15. Wrist (carpals to carpals).
16. Ankle (talus to tibia).
17. Ankle (tarsals to tarsals).
18. Axis-atlas rotation.

Basic Types
slightly movable—1
freely movable—2
immovable—3

Subtypes
ball and socket—4
condyloid—5
gliding—6
hinge—7
pivot—8
saddle—9
suture—10
symphysis—11
synchondrosis—12
syndesmosis—13

Answers

Characteristics	Fig. 14.1
1. _____	_____
2. _____	_____
3. _____	_____
4. _____	_____
5. _____	_____
6. _____	_____
7. _____	_____
8. _____	_____
9. _____	_____
10. _____	_____
11. _____	**Fig. 14.2**
12. _____	_____
13. _____	_____

Classification	
1. _____	_____
2. _____	_____
3. _____	_____
4. _____	_____
5. _____	_____
6. _____	_____
7. _____	_____
8. _____	_____
9. _____	
10. _____	
11. _____	
12. _____	
13. _____	
14. _____	
15. _____	
16. _____	
17. _____	
18. _____	

D. True–False

Evaluate the validity of the following statements concerning joints.

1. Bursae are sacs of synovial membrane.
2. When the cartilage is removed from a knee joint by surgical means, it is usually the hyaline type that is removed.
3. The ligamentum teres femoris is primarily nutritional in function.
4. The depth of the acetabulum is increased by the acetabular labrum.
5. Freely movable joints are lubricated with serum.
6. The capsule around a joint consists of a ligament lined with synovial membrane.
7. The ends of amphiarthrotic and diarthrotic joints are covered with hyaline cartilage.
8. "Water on the knee" would involve the suprapatellar bursa.
9. The knee joint is substantially reinforced to withstand lateral forces.
10. The most highly stressed joint in the body is the hip joint.
11. Articular capsules consist of ligaments and tendons.
12. The strongest ligament holding the hip together is the ligamentum teres femoris.

E. Medical

Consult your lecture text, medical dictionary, or other source for the following.

ankylosis—1
bursitis—2
chronic fibrositis—3
dislocation—4
gouty arthritis—5
osteoarthritis—6
rheumatism—7
rheumatoid arthritis—8
sprain—9
strain—10
subluxation—11
tenosynovitis—12

1. Partial or incomplete dislocation.
2. Displacement of bones from normal orientation in a joint.
3. Inflammation of synovial bursa.
4. Inflammation of fibrous connective tissue causing tenderness and stiffness.
5. Injury to joint by displacement, resulting in swelling and discoloration.
6. Inflammation of tendon and its sheath.
7. Injury to joint in which ligaments are stretched without swelling or discoloration.
8. Arthritis of confusing etiology, characterized by deformity and immobility of joints; often treated with cortisone.
9. Arthritis due to excess levels of uric acid in blood.
10. Arthritis resulting from degenerative changes in joint (wear and tear).
11. Fixation or fusion of a joint; usually preceded by infection.
12. General term applied to soreness and stiffness in muscles and joints.

Answers

True–False	Fig. 14.3
1.	
2.	
3.	
4.	
5.	
6.	
7.	
8.	
9.	
10.	
11.	
12.	

Medical	Fig. 14.4
1.	
2.	
3.	
4.	
5.	
6.	
7.	
8.	
9.	
10.	
11.	
12.	

Student: _____

Desk No: _____ Section: _____

Head and Neck Muscles

A. Illustrations

Record the labels for the illustrations of this exercise in the answer column.

B. Facial Expressions

Consult figure 19.1 and the text to identify the muscles described in the following statements.

1. Smiling
2. Horror
3. Irony
4. Sadness
5. Contempt or disdain
6. Pouting lips
7. Blinking or squinting
8. Horizontal wrinkling of forehead

frontalis—1
orbicularis oculi—2
orbicularis oris—3
platysma—4
quadratus labii
　inferioris—5
quadratus labii
　superioris—6
triangularis—7
zygomaticus—8

Origins

9. On frontal bone.
10. On zygomatic bone.

Insertions

11. On lips.
12. On eyebrows.
13. On eyelid.

C. Mastication

Consult figure 19.1 and the text to identify the muscles that perform the following movements in mastication of food.

1. Lowers the mandible.
2. Raises the mandible.
3. Retracts the mandible.
4. Protrudes the mandible.
5. Holds food in place.

buccinator—1
external pterygoid—2
internal pterygoid—3
masseter—4
temporalis—5

Origins

6. On zygomatic arch.
7. On sphenoid only.
8. On frontal, parietal, and temporal bones.
9. On maxilla, mandible, and pteromandibular raphé.
10. On maxilla, sphenoid, and palatine bones.

Insertions

11. On orbicularis oris.
12. On coronoid process of mandible.
13. On medial surface of body of mandible.
14. On lateral surface of ramus and angle of mandible.
15. On neck of mandibular condyle and articular disk.

Answers

Facial	Fig. 19.1
1. _____	_____
2. _____	_____
3. _____	_____
4. _____	_____
5. _____	_____
6. _____	_____
7. _____	_____
8. _____	_____
9. _____	_____
10. _____	_____
11. _____	_____
12. _____	_____
13. _____	_____

Mastication	
1. _____	
2. _____	Fig. 19.2
3. _____	
4. _____	
5. _____	
6. _____	
7. _____	
8. _____	
9. _____	Fig. 19.3
10. _____	
11. _____	
12. _____	
13. _____	
14. _____	
15. _____	

D. Neck Muscles

Consult figures 19.2 and 19.3 and the text to identify the muscles of the neck that are described below.

digastricus—1
longissimus capitis—2
mylohyoideus—3
omohyoideus—4
platysma—5
semispinalis capitis—6

splenius capitis—7
sternocleidomastoideus—8
sternohyoideus—9
sternothyroideus—10
trapezius—11

1. Broad sheetlike muscle on side of neck just under the skin.
2. A broad triangular muscle of the back that functions only partially as a neck muscle.
3. Provides support for the floor of the mouth.
4. A V-shaped muscle attached to hyoid and mandibular bones.
5. Posterior neck muscles that insert on the mastoid process.
6. Anterior neck muscle that is attached to the thyroid cartilage and part of the sternum.
7. Anterior neck muscle that extends from the hyoid bone to the clavicle and manubrium.
8. Long muscle of the neck that extends from the mastoid process to the clavicle and sternum.
9. Muscles that pull the head backward (hyperextension).
10. Muscles that pull the head forward.

Answers
Neck Muscles
1. _____
2. _____
3. _____
4. _____
5. _____
6. _____
7. _____
8. _____
9. _____
10. _____

Student: _____

Desk No: _____ Section: _____

Trunk and Shoulder Muscles

A. Illustrations

Record the labels for the illustrations of this exercise in the answer columns.

B. Anterior Trunk Muscles

By referring to figure 20.1 and the text, identify the muscles described by the following statements.

Origins

1. On upper eight or nine ribs.
2. On scapular spine and clavicle.
3. On third, fourth, and fifth ribs.
4. On clavicle, sternum, and costal cartilages.

deltoideus—1
intercostalis externi—2
intercostalis interni—3
pectoralis major—4
pectoralis minor—5
serratus anterior—6
subscapularis—7

Insertions

5. On coracoid process.
6. On deltoid tuberosity of humerus.
7. On anterior surface of scapula.
8. On upper anterior end of humerus.

Actions

9. Pulls scapula forward, downward, and inward.
10. Rotates arm medially.
11. Raises ribs (inhaling).
12. Lowers ribs (exhaling).
13. Adducts arm; also, rotates it medially.
14. Abducts arm.

C. Posterior Trunk Muscles

By referring to figure 20.2 and the text, identify the muscles described by the following statements.

infraspinatus—1
latissimus dorsi—2
levator scapulae—3
rhomboideus major—4
rhomboideus minor—5
sacrospinalis—6
supraspinatus—7
teres major—8
teres minor—9
trapezius—10

Origins

1. Near inferior angle of scapula.
2. On lateral (axillary) margin of scapula.
3. On fossa of scapula above spine.
4. On infraspinous fossa of scapula.
5. On thoracic and lumbar vertebrae, sacrum, lower ribs, and iliac crest.
6. On lower part of ligamentum nuchae and first thoracic vertebra.
7. On transverse processes of first four cervical vertebrae.

Answers	
Anterior	**Fig. 20.1**
1. _____	_____
2. _____	_____
3. _____	_____
4. _____	_____
5. _____	_____
6. _____	_____
7. _____	_____
8. _____	**Fig. 20.2**
9. _____	_____
10. _____	_____
11. _____	_____
12. _____	_____
13. _____	_____
14. _____	_____
Posterior	_____
1. _____	_____
2. _____	_____
3. _____	_____
4. _____	_____
5. _____	_____
6. _____	_____
7. _____	

Trunk and Shoulder Muscles

infraspinatus—1 rhomboideus minor—5 teres major—8
latissimus dorsi—2 sacrospinalis—6 teres minor—9
levator scapulae—3 supraspinatus—7 trapezius—10
rhomboideus major—4

Insertions
8. On lower third vertebral border of scapula.
9. On vertebral border of scapula near origin of scapular spine.
10. On crest of lesser tubercle of humerus.
11. On intertubercular groove of humerus.
12. On middle facet of greater tubercle of humerus.
13. On ribs and vertebrae.

Actions
14. Abducts arm.
15. Raises scapula and draws it medially.
16. Extends spine to maintain erectness.
17. Adducts and rotates arm medially.
18. Adducts and rotates arm laterally.

Answers
Posterior
8. _____
9. _____
10. _____
11. _____
12. _____
13. _____
14. _____
15. _____
16. _____
17. _____
18. _____

Student: _____

Desk No: _____ Section: _____

Upper Extremity Muscles

A. Illustrations

Record the labels for figures 21.1 and 21.2 in the answer column.

B. Arm Movements

Consult figure 21.1 to select the muscles that apply to the following statements. Verify your answers by referring to the text material.

1. Extends the forearm.
2. Adducts the arm.
3. Flexes the forearm.
4. Carries the arm forward in flexion.
5. Flexes forearm and rotates the radius outward to supinate the hand.

coracobrachialis—1
biceps brachii—2
brachialis—3
brachioradialis—4
triceps brachii—5

Origins

6. On lower half of humerus.
7. On coracoid process of scapula.
8. Above the lateral epicondyle of the humerus.
9. Three heads: One on scapula, another on posterior surface of humerus, and the third just below the radial groove of humerus.
10. Two heads: One on coracoid process; other on supraglenoid tubercle of humerus.

Insertions

11. On the olecranon process.
12. On the radial tuberosity.
13. Near the middle, medial surface of humerus.
14. On front surface of coronoid process of ulna.
15. On the lateral surface of the radius just above the styloid process.

C. Hand Movements

Consult figure 21.2 to select the muscles that apply to the following statements. Verify as above.

1. Supinates the hand.
2. Pronates the hand.
3. Flexes and abducts hand.
4. Extends wrist and hand.
5. Flexes the thumb.
6. Extends all fingers except thumb.
7. Abducts the thumb.
8. Flexes all distal phalanges except the thumb.
9. Flexes all fingers except thumb.
10. Extends thumb.

abductor pollicis—1
extensor carpi radialis brevis—2
extensor carpi radialis longus—3
extensor carpi ulnaris—4
extensor digitorum communis—5
extensor pollicis longus—6
flexor carpi radialis—7
flexor carpi ulnaris—8
flexor digitorum profundus—9
flexor digitorum superficialis—10
flexor pollicis longus—11
pronator quadratus—12
pronator teres—13
supinator—14

Answers

Arm Movements	Fig. 21.1
1. _____	_____
2. _____	_____
3. _____	_____
4. _____	_____
5. _____	_____
6. _____	**Fig. 21.2**
7. _____	_____
8. _____	_____
9. _____	_____
10. _____	_____
11. _____	_____
12. _____	_____
13. _____	_____
14. _____	**Fig. 21.3**
15. _____	_____
Hand Movements	_____
1. _____	_____
2. _____	_____
3. _____	_____
4. _____	_____
5. _____	_____
6. _____	
7. _____	
8. _____	
9. _____	
10. _____	

C. Hand Movements (continued)

abductor pollicis—1
extensor carpi radialis brevis—2
extensor carpi radialis longus—3
extensor carpi ulnaris—4
extensor digitorum communis—5
extensor pollicis longus—6
flexor carpi radialis—7

flexor carpi ulnaris—8
flexor digitorum profundus—9
flexor digitorum superficialis—10
flexor pollicis longus—11
pronator quadratus—12
pronator teres—13
supinator—14

Origins

11. On interosseous membrane between radius and ulna.
12. On radius, ulna, and interosseous membrane.
13. On lateral epicondyle of humerus and part of ulna.
14. On humerus, ulna, and radius.
15. On medial epicondyle of humerus.

Insertions

16. On distal phalanges of second, third, fourth, and fifth fingers.
17. On distal phalanx of thumb.
18. On middle phalanges of second, third, fourth, and fifth fingers.
19. On radial tuberosity and oblique line of radius.
20. On upper lateral surface of radius.
21. On first metacarpal and trapezium.
22. On second metacarpal.
23. On proximal portion of second and third metacarpals.
24. On middle metacarpal.
25. On fifth metacarpal.

Answers
Hand Movements
11. _____
12. _____
13. _____
14. _____
15. _____
16. _____
17. _____
18. _____
19. _____
20. _____
21. _____
22. _____
23. _____
24. _____
25. _____

Abdominal, Pelvic, and Intercostal Muscles
(Ex. 22)

A. Illustrations
Record the labels for figures 22.1 and 22.2 in the answer column.

B. Abdomen
Consult figure 22.1 to identify the muscles that apply to the following statements. Verify your selections from the text.

external oblique—1   rectus abdominis—3
internal oblique—2   transversus abdominis—4

1. Flexion of spine in lumbar region.
2. Maintain intraabdominal pressure.
3. Antagonists of diaphragm.

Origins
4. On pubic bone.
5. On external surface of lower eight ribs.
6. On lateral half of inguinal ligament and anterior two-thirds of iliac crest.
7. On inguinal ligament, iliac crest, and costal cartilages of lower six ribs.

Insertions
8. On linea alba and crest of pubis.
9. On cartilages of fifth, sixth, and seventh ribs.
10. On the linea alba where fibers of the aponeurosis interlace.
11. On costal cartilages of lower three ribs, linea alba, and crest of pubis.

C. Pelvic Region
Consult figure 22.3 to identify the muscles that apply to the following statements. Verify your selections from the text.

iliacus—1
psoas major—2
quadratus lumborum—3

1. Flexes femur on trunk.
2. Flexes lumbar region of vertebral column.
3. Extension of spine at lumbar vertebrae.

Origins
4. On lumbar vertebrae.
5. On iliac crest, iliolumbar ligament, and transverse processes of lower four lumbar vertebrae.
6. On iliac fossa.

Insertions
7. On inferior margin of last rib and transverse processes of upper four lumbar vertebrae.
8. On lesser trochanter of femur.

Answers	
Abdomen	**Fig. 22.1**
1. _____	_____
2. _____	_____
3. _____	_____
4. _____	_____
5. _____	_____
6. _____	_____
7. _____	_____
8. _____	**Fig. 22.3**
9. _____	_____
10. _____	_____
11. _____	_____
Pelvic	_____
1. _____	_____
2. _____	_____
3. _____	
4. _____	
5. _____	
6. _____	
7. _____	
8. _____	

Lower Extremity Muscles (Ex. 23)

A. Illustrations
Record the labels for this exercise in the answer column.

B. Thigh Movements
Consult figure 23.1 to select the muscles that apply to the following statements. More than one muscle may apply to a statement.

1. Gluteus muscle that extends femur.
2. Gluteus muscles that abduct femur.
3. Three muscles that pull femur toward median line.
4. Gluteus muscle that rotates femur outward.
5. Three muscles attached to linea aspera that flex femur.
6. Small muscle that abducts, extends, and rotates femur.

adductor brevis—1
adductor longus—2
adductor magnus—3
gluteus maximus—4
gluteus medius—5
gluteus minimus—6
piriformis—7

Origins
7. On anterior surface of sacrum.
8. On the pubis.
9. On external surface of ilium.
10. On ilium, sacrum, and coccyx.
11. On inferior surface of ischium and portion of pubis.

Insertions
12. On linea aspera of femur.
13. On anterior border of greater trochanter.
14. On upper border of greater trochanter of femur.
15. On lateral part of greater trochanter of femur.
16. On iliotibial tract and posterior part of femur.

C. Thigh Muscles
Identify the muscles of the thigh that are described by the following statements.

biceps femoris—1
gracilis—2
rectus femoris—3
sartorius—4
semimembranosus—5
semitendinosus—6
tensor fasciae latae—7
vastus intermedius—8
vastus lateralis—9
vastus medialis—10

1. The largest quadriceps muscle that is located on the side of the thigh.
2. That portion of the quadriceps that lies beneath the rectus femoris.
3. Portion of the quadriceps that is on the medial surface of the thigh.
4. Hamstring muscle that is on the lateral surface of the thigh.
5. The longest muscle of the thigh.
6. The most medial component of the hamstring muscles.
7. The smallest hamstring muscle.
8. A superficial muscle on the medial surface of the thigh that inserts with the sartorius on the tibia.
9. Four muscles of a group that extend the leg.
10. Flexes the thigh upon the pelvis.
11. Two muscles other than parts of quadriceps that rotate the thigh medially (inward).
12. Rotates the thigh laterally (outward).
13. Adducts the thigh.

Answers

Thigh Movements	Fig. 23.1	Fig. 23.10 Anterior

(Thigh Muscles, Fig. 23.2, Fig. 23.3, Fig. 23.4, Fig. 23.10 Posterior answer columns)

312

D. Lower Leg and Foot Muscles

Identify the muscles of the lower leg and foot that are described by the following statements. In some instances several answers are applicable.

extensor digitorum longus—1
extensor hallucis longus—2
flexor digitorum longus—3
flexor hallucis longus—4
gastrocnemius—5
peroneus brevis—6
peroneus longus—7
peroneus tertius—8
soleus—9
tibialis anterior—10
tibialis posterior—11

1. Located on the front of the lower leg; causes dorsiflexion and inversion of the foot.
2. Deep portion of triceps surae.
3. Superficial portion of triceps surae.
4. Three muscles that originate on the fibula that cause various movements of the foot.
5. Two muscles that join to form the Achilles tendon.
6. Part of the triceps surae that originates on the femur.
7. Inserts on the proximal superior portion of the fifth metatarsal bone of the foot.
8. Inserts on the proximal inferior portion of the fifth metatarsal bone of the foot.
9. Flexes the great toe.
10. On the posterior surfaces of the tibia and fibula; causes plantar flexion and inversion of foot.
11. Originates on the tibia and fascia of the tibialis posterior; causes flexion of 2nd, 3rd, 4th, and 5th toes.
12. Flexes the calf on the thigh.
13. Originates on the tibia, fibula, and interosseous membrane; extends toes (dorsiflexion) and inverts foot.
14. Two muscles that insert on the calcaneous.
15. Peroneus muscle that causes dorsiflexion and eversion of foot.
16. Two peroneus muscles that cause plantar flexion.
17. Muscle on tibia that provides support for foot arches.

E. General Questions

Record the answers to the following questions in the answer column.
1. List the four muscles that are collectively referred to as the quadriceps femoris.
2. List two muscles associated with the iliotibial tract.
3. List three muscles that constitute the hamstrings.
4. What two muscles are associated with the Achilles tendon?
5. What two muscles constitute the triceps surae?

F. Figure 17.1

Refer back to figure 17.1 and identify the muscles that cause each type of movement. Record answers in column.

Answers

Lower Leg and Foot

1. _____ 10. _____
2. _____ 11. _____
3. _____ 12. _____
4. _____ 13. _____
5. _____ 14. _____
6. _____ 15. _____
7. _____ 16. _____
8. _____ 17. _____
9. _____

General Questions

1a. _____
b. _____
c. _____
d. _____
2a. _____
b. _____
3a. _____
b. _____
c. _____
4a. _____
b. _____
5a. _____
b. _____

Figure 17.1

A. _____
B. _____
C. _____
D. _____
E. _____
F. _____
G. _____
H. _____
I. _____
J. _____
K. _____
L. _____
M. _____

Nerve Tissue

A. Cell Drawings
On a separate sheet of paper, sketch representative cells of the various types of neurons and muscle cells from slides that are available. Staple the drawings to this report when it is handed in for grading.

B. Figure 24.1
Record the label numbers for this illustration in the answer column.

C. Nerve Cell Types
From the list of cells below, select those that are described by the following statements. More than one cell may apply in some cases.

1. Afferent neurons.
2. Efferent neurons.
3. Specialized cells of retina.
4. Pseudounipolar neurons.
5. Multipolar neurons.
6. Ganglion cells.
7. Golgi Type II cells.
8. Neurons lacking in axons.
9. Predominant neurons in cerebellar cortex.
10. Linkage cells between Purkinje cells.
11. Linkage cells between pyramidal cells.
12. Linkage cells between sensory and motor neurons.
13. Predominant type of neuron in cerebral cortex.
14. Small cells covering the perikaryon of a sensory neuron.

amacrine cells—1
basket cells—2
interneurons—3
motor neuron—4
neurolemmocytes—5
Purkinje cells—6
pyramidal cells—7
satellite cells—8
sensory neuron—9
stellate cells—10

D. True–False
Indicate whether the following statements concerning nerve cells are true or false.

1. Neuroglial cells do not carry nerve impulses.
2. Perikarya of afferent neurons are located in the spinal ganglia.
3. Most neurons have many dendrites with only a single axon.
4. Perikarya of motor neurons are located in the white matter of the spinal cord.
5. Myelinated fibers carry nerve impulses at a slower speed than unmyelinated ones.
6. Unmyelinated fibers lack neurolemmocytes.
7. Part of the axon of a sensory neuron functions like a dendrite.
8. Some neurons lack axons.
9. Both the myelin sheath and neurolemma are formed by neurolemmocytes.
10. Motor neurons carry nerve impulses away from the CNS.

Answers

Nerve Cell Types	Fig. 24.1
1. _____	_____
2. _____	_____
3. _____	_____
4. _____	_____
5. _____	_____
6. _____	_____
7. _____	_____
8. _____	_____
9. _____	_____
10. _____	_____
11. _____	_____
12. _____	_____
13. _____	_____
14. _____	_____

True-False	
1. _____	_____
2. _____	_____
3. _____	_____
4. _____	_____
5. _____	
6. _____	
7. _____	
8. _____	
9. _____	
10. _____	

E. Neuron Structure

From the list of neuron structures select those that are described by the following statements. More than one structure may apply in some cases.

1. Nerve cell body.
2. Side branch of an axon.
3. Long process on motor neuron.
4. Short process on motor neuron.
5. Lacking on unmyelinated nerve fibers.
6. Process that receives nerve impulses.
7. Slender filaments in perikaryon.
8. Formed by neurolemmocytes.
9. Synonym for neurolemmal sheath.
10. Interruptions in neurolemma.
11. Outer membrane covering myelin sheath.
12. Bodies on the ER that synthesize protein.
13. Promotes regeneration of damaged nerve fiber.
14. Facilitate the speed of nerve impulse transmission.
15. Bodies in perikaryon that stain well with basic aniline dyes.
16. Process that carries nerve impulses away from perikaryon.

axis cylinder—1
axon—2
collateral—3
dendrite—4
myelin sheath—5
neurolemma—6
neurolemmocytes—7
neurofibrils—8
Nissl bodies—9
nodes of Ranvier—10
perikaryon—11

Answers

Structure

1. _____
2. _____
3. _____
4. _____
5. _____
6. _____
7. _____
8. _____
9. _____
10. _____
11. _____
12. _____
13. _____
14. _____
15. _____
16. _____

Student: _____

Desk No: _____ Section: _____

The Spinal Cord, Spinal Nerves, and Reflex Arcs

A. Illustrations

Record the labels for figures 25.1, 25.2, and 25.4 in the answer columns.

B. Completion Questions

Supply the information that is necessary to complete the following statements.

1. The dural sac of the spinal cord is continuous with the _____ mater that surrounds the brain.
2. The caudal end of the spinal cord is called the _____ .
3. The caudal end of the spinal cord terminates at the lower border of the _____ lumbar vertebra.
4. The cluster of nerves that extend downward from the end of the spinal cord is called the _____ .
5. The coccygeal nerve emerges from the _____ plexus.
6. The femoral nerve is formed by the union of the following three lumbar nerves: _____ , _____ , and

   _____ .
7. The largest nerve emerging from the sacral plexus is the _____ nerve.
8. The iliohypogastric and ilioinguinal nerves are branches of the first _____ nerve.
9. The innermost meninx surrounding the spinal cord is the _____ mater.
10. The meninx that lies just within the dura mater is the

    _____ .
11. The spinal ganglion is an enlargement of the _____ root.
12. The central canal of the spinal cord is lined with _____ ependymal cells.
13. The cavity within the spinal cord that is continuous with the ventricles of the brain is called the _____ canal.
14. The inner portion of the spinal cord, forming the pattern of a butterfly, consists of _____ matter.
15. The space between the dura mater and vertebral bone is called the _____ space.
16. _____ (*vertebral* or *collateral*) ganglia are usually located close to the organ that is innervated.
17. A somatic reflex arc with one or more interneurons is said to be

    _____ .
18. Cell bodies of afferent neurons of visceral reflexes are located in _____ ganglia.
19. If a somatic reflex lacks an interneuron it is said to be

    _____ .
20. List the two divisions of the autonomic nervous system.

Answers

Completion

1. _____
2. _____
3. _____
4. _____
5. _____
6. _____
7. _____
8. _____
9. _____
10. _____
11. _____
12. _____
13. _____
14. _____
15. _____
16. _____
17. _____
18. _____
19. _____
20. _____

Figure 25.1

_____	_____
_____	_____
_____	_____
_____	_____
_____	_____
_____	_____
_____	_____
_____	_____
_____	_____
_____	_____
_____	_____

C. True–False

Indicate the validity of the following statements with a T or F.

1. The spinal cord during fetal life fills the entire length of the spinal cavity.
2. The lumbar plexus is formed by the union of L_1, L_2, L_3, and most of L_4 nerves.
3. The brachial plexus is formed by the union of the lower four cervical nerves and the first thoracic nerve.
4. The cervical plexus is formed by the union of the first three pairs of cervical nerves.
5. The filum terminale externa is a downward extension of the filum terminale interna.
6. The innermost fiber of the cauda equina (on the median line) is the filum terminale interna.
7. Cerebrospinal fluid fills the subarachnoid space.
8. The white matter of the spinal cord consists of myelinated fibers of nerve cells.
9. The posterior cutaneous nerve emerges from the lumbar plexus.
10. The sacral plexus is formed by the union of the femoral and sciatic nerves.
11. The effector in a somatic reflex is always skeletal muscle.
12. Most organs of the body are innervated by fibers of the sympathetic and parasympathetic divisions of the autonomic nervous system.
13. Collateral ganglia of the autonomic nervous system are united to form a chain along the vertebral column.
14. All visceral reflex arcs have two afferent neurons.
15. The central canal of the spinal cord is continuous with the ventricles of the brain.
16. The dura mater of the spinal cord extends peripherally to form a covering for spinal nerves.
17. The central canal of the spinal cord is lined with ciliated epithelium.
18. All somatic reflex arcs have at least one interneuron.
19. All visceral reflex arcs have two efferent neurons.
20. Spinal ganglia are located in the anterior roots of spinal nerves.

D. Numbers

Indicate the number of pairs of the following that are normally present.

1. Cervical nerves
2. Thoracic nerves
3. Lumbar nerves
4. Sacral nerves
5. Coccygeal nerves

Answers

True–False, Fig. 25.2, 1–20; Fig. 25.4; Numbers 1–5.

318

Student: _____

Desk No: _____ Section: _____

Brain Anatomy: External

A. Illustrations

Record the labels for all the illustrations of this exercise in the answer columns.

B. Brain Dissections

Answer the following questions that pertain to your observations of the sheep brain dissections.

1. Does the arachnoid mater appear to be attached to the dura mater? _____ to the brain? _____

2. Describe the appearance of the dura mater.

   _____

   _____

   _____

3. Within what structure is the sagittal sinus enclosed?

   _____

4. Differentiate:

   Gyrus: _____

   Sulcus: _____

5. Of what value are the sulci and gyri of the cerebrum?

   _____

   _____

6. List five structures that you were able to identify on the dorsal surface of the midbrain: _____

   _____

   _____

7. Is the cerebellum of the sheep brain divided on the median line as is the case of the human brain? _____

   _____

8. What significance is there to the size differences of the olfactory bulbs on the sheep and human brains?

   _____

   _____

   _____

9. Which cranial nerve is the largest in diameter? _____

Answers

Fig. 26.1	Fig. 26.9
_____	_____
_____	_____
_____	_____
_____	_____
_____	_____
_____	_____
_____	_____
_____	_____
_____	_____
_____	_____
_____	_____
Fig. 26.7	_____
_____	_____
_____	_____
_____	_____
_____	_____
_____	**Fig. 26.10**
_____	_____
_____	_____
_____	_____
_____	_____
_____	_____
_____	_____
_____	

C. Meninges

Select the meninx or meningeal space described by the following statements.

1. Fibrous outer meninx.
2. The middle meninx.
3. Meninx that surrounds the sagittal sinus.
4. Meninx that forms the falx cerebri.
5. Meninx attached to the brain surface.
6. Space that contains cerebrospinal fluid.

arachnoid mater—1
dura mater—2
epidural space—3
pia mater—4
subarachnoid space—5
subdural space—6

D. Fissures and Sulci

Select the fissure or sulcus that is described by the following statements.

1. Between the frontal and parietal lobes.
2. On the median line between the two cerebral hemispheres.
3. Between the occipital and parietal lobes.
4. Between the temporal and parietal lobes.

anterior central sulcus—1
central sulcus—2
lateral cerebral fissure—3
longitudinal cerebral fissure—4
parieto-occipital fissure—5

E. Brain Functions

Select the part of the brain that is responsible for the following activities.

1. Maintenance of posture.
2. Cardiac control.
3. Respiratory control.
4. Vasomotor control.
5. Consciousness.
6. Voluntary muscular movements.
7. Brightness and sound discrimination (animals only).
8. Contains fibers that connect the two cerebral hemispheres.
9. Contains nuclei of fifth, sixth, seventh, and eighth cranial nerves.
10. Coordination of complex muscular movements.
11. Function in humans is unknown.

cerebellum—1
cerebrum—2
corpora quadrigemina—3
corpus callosum—4
medulla oblongata—5
midbrain—6
pineal body—7
pons Varolii—8

F. Cerebral Functional Localization

Select those areas of the cerebrum that are described by the following statements.

Location

1. On posterior central gyrus.
2. On parietal lobe.
3. On superior temporal gyrus.
4. On temporal lobe.
5. On frontal lobe.
6. On occipital lobe.
7. On anterior central gyrus.
8. On angular gyrus.
9. In area anterior to anterior central gyrus.

association area—1
auditory area—2
common integrative area—3
motor speech area—4
olfactory area—5
premotor area—6
somatomotor area—7
somatosensory area—8
visual area—9

Answers

Meninges: 1. _ 2. _ 3. _ 4. _ 5. _ 6. _

Fissures and Sulci: 1. _ 2. _ 3. _ 4. _

Fig. 26.11

Brain Functions: 1.–11. _

Localization: 1.–9. _

F. Cerebral Functional Localization (continued)

Function

10. Speech production.
11. Speech understanding.
12. Cutaneous sensibility.
13. Sight.
14. Sense of smell.
15. Visual interpretation.
16. Voluntary muscular movement.
17. Integration of sensory association areas.
18. Influences motor area function.

association area—1
auditory area—2
common integrative area—3
motor speech area—4
olfactory area—5
premotor area—6
somatomotor area—7
somatosensory area—8
visual area—9

G. Cranial Nerves

Record the number of the cranial nerve that applies to the following statements. More than one nerve may apply to some statements.

1. Sensory nerves.
2. Mixed nerves.
3. Emerges from midbrain.
4. Emerges from pons Varolii.
5. Emerges from medulla.

Structures Innervated

6. Cochlea of ear.
7. Heart.
8. Salivary glands.
9. Abdominal viscera.
10. Retina of eye.
11. Receptors in nasal membranes.
12. Taste buds at back of tongue.
13. Lateral rectus muscle of eye.
14. Taste buds of anterior two-thirds of tongue.
15. Semicircular canals of ear.
16. Thoracic viscera.
17. Three extrinsic eye muscles (superior rectus, medial rectus, inferior oblique) and levator palpebrae.
18. Superior oblique muscle of eye.
19. Pharynx, upper larynx, uvula, and palate.

1. Olfactory
2. Optic
3. Oculomotor
4. Trochlear
5. Trigeminal
6. Abducens
7. Facial
8. Vestibulocochlear
9. Glossopharyngeal
10. Vagus
11. Accessory
12. Hypoglossal

H. Trigeminal Nerve

Select the branch of the trigeminal nerve that innervates the following structures.

1. All lower teeth.
2. All upper teeth.
3. Tongue.
4. Lacrimal gland.
5. Outer surface of nose.
6. Buccal gum tissues of mandible.
7. Lower teeth, tongue, muscles of mastication, and gum surfaces.

incisive—1
infraorbital—2
inferior alveolar—3
lingual—4
long buccal—5
mandibular—6
maxillary—7
ophthalmic—8

Answers
Localization
10. _____
11. _____
12. _____
13. _____
14. _____
15. _____
16. _____
17. _____
18. _____

Cranial Nerves
1. _____
2. _____
3. _____
4. _____
5. _____
6. _____
7. _____
8. _____
9. _____
10. _____
11. _____
12. _____
13. _____
14. _____
15. _____
16. _____
17. _____
18. _____
19. _____

Trigeminal Nerve
1. _____
2. _____
3. _____
4. _____
5. _____
6. _____
7. _____

I. General Questions

Select the correct answers that complete the following statements.

1. Shallow furrows on the surface of the cerebrum are called
   (1) sulci.   (2) fissures.   (3) gyri.

2. Deep furrows on the surface of the cerebrum are called
   (1) sulci.   (2) fissures.   (3) gyri.

3. The infundibulum supports the
   (1) mammillary body.   (2) hypophysis.   (3) hypothalamus.

4. The mammillary bodies are a part of the
   (1) medulla.   (2) midbrain.   (3) hypothalamus.

5. The corpora quadrigemina are located on the
   (1) cerebrum.   (2) medulla.   (3) midbrain.

6. The major ganglion of the trigeminal nerve is the
   (1) gasserian.   (2) sphenopalatine.   (3) ciliary.

7. Convolutions on the surface of the cerebrum are called
   (1) sulci.   (2) fissures.   (3) gyri.

8. The hypophysis is located on the inferior surface of the
   (1) medulla.   (2) midbrain.   (3) hypothalamus.

9. The spinal bulb is the
   (1) medulla oblongata.   (2) pons Varolii.   (3) midbrain.

10. The pineal gland is located on the
    (1) medulla.   (2) pons Varolii.   (3) midbrain.

Answers
General Questions
1. _____
2. _____
3. _____
4. _____
5. _____
6. _____
7. _____
8. _____
9. _____
10. _____

Brain Anatomy: Internal

A. Illustrations

Record the labels for all the illustrations of this exercise in the answer columns.

B. Location

Identify that part of the brain in which the following structures are located.

cerebellum—1
cerebrum—2
diencephalon—3

medulla oblongata—4
midbrain—5
pons Varolii—6

1. Aqueduct of Sylvius
2. Caudate nuclei
3. Cerebral peduncles
4. Corpus callosum
5. Fornix
6. Globus pallidus
7. Hypothalamus

8. Lateral ventricles
9. Mammillary bodies
10. Putamen
11. Rhinencephalon
12. Thalamus
13. Third ventricle

C. Functions

Identify the structures that perform the following functions.

aqueduct of Sylvius—1
arachnoid granulations—2
caudate nuclei—3
cerebral peduncles—4
choroid plexus—5
corpus callosum—6
fornix—7
foramen of Monro—8

hypothalamus—9
infundibulum—10
intermediate mass—11
lateral aperture—12
lentiform nucleus—13
median aperture—14
rhinencephalon—15
thalamus—16

1. Relay station for all messages to cerebrum.
2. Temperature regulation.
3. Entire olfactory mechanism of cerebrum.
4. Assists in muscular coordination.
5. Fiber tracts of olfactory mechanism.
6. Connects the two halves of the thalamus.
7. Exerts steadying effect on voluntary movements.
8. Allows cerebrospinal fluid to pass from third to fourth ventricle.
9. Consists of ascending and descending tracts.
10. Supporting stalk of hypophysis.
11. Allows cerebrospinal fluid to return to blood.
12. A commissure which unites the cerebral hemispheres.
13. Secretes cerebrospinal fluid into ventricle.
14. Coordinates autonomic nervous system.

D. General Questions

Select the best answer that completes the following statements.

1. The brain stem consists of the
   (1) cerebrum, pons, midbrain, and medulla.
   (2) cerebellum, medulla, and pons.
   (3) pons, medulla, and midbrain.
2. The lateral ventricles are separated by the
   (1) thalamus.   (2) fornix.   (3) septum pellucidum.

Answers

Location	Fig. 27.2
1. _____	_____
2. _____	_____
3. _____	_____
4. _____	_____
5. _____	_____
6. _____	_____
7. _____	_____
8. _____	_____
9. _____	_____
10. _____	_____
11. _____	_____
12. _____	_____
13. _____	_____

Functions	
1. _____	_____
2. _____	_____
3. _____	_____
4. _____	_____
5. _____	_____
6. _____	Fig. 27.3
7. _____	_____
8. _____	_____
9. _____	_____
10. _____	_____
11. _____	_____
12. _____	_____
13. _____	_____
14. _____	_____

General	
1. _____	_____
2. _____	_____

3. Pain is perceived in the
   (1) somatomotor area.   (2) thalamus.   (3) pons.
4. The hypothalamus regulates
   (1) the hypophysis, appetite, and wakefulness.
   (2) body temperature, hypophysis, and vision.
   (3) reproductive functions, body temperature, and voluntary movements.
5. Feelings of pleasantness and unpleasantness appear to be associated with the
   (1) somatomotor area.   (2) hypothalamus.   (3) thalamus.
   (4) medulla oblongata.
6. The reticular formation consists of
   (1) gray matter.   (2) white matter.
   (3) an interlacement of white and gray matter.
7. Alert consciousness is partially regulated by
   (1) caudate nuclei.   (2) lentiform nuclei.
   (3) nuclei of the reticular formation.
8. The intermediate mass passes through the
   (1) midbrain.   (2) third ventricle.   (3) hypothalamus.
9. The reticular formation is seen in the
   (1) spinal cord.   (2) cerebrum.   (3) brain stem.
   (4) spinal cord, brain stem, and diencephalon.
10. Centers for vomiting, coughing, swallowing, and sneezing are located in the
    (1) pons.   (2) medulla.   (3) midbrain.   (4) thalamus.

E. Cerebrospinal Fluid

You should be able to trace the path of the cerebrospinal fluid from its point of origin to where it is reabsorbed into the blood. If you can complete the following paragraph without referring to the text, you know the sequence fairly well. If you can state the sequence from memory, better yet.

Ventricles	*Structures*
lateral—1	arachnoid granulations—10
third—2	cerebellum—11
fourth—3	cerebrum—12
Passageways	choroid plexus—13
acoustic meatus—4	cisterna cerebellomedullaris—14
aqueduct of Sylvius—5	cisterna superior—15
foramen magnum—6	dura mater—16
foramen of Monro—7	sagittal sinus—17
lateral aperture—8	septum pellucidum—18
median aperture—9	subarachnoid space—19

Cerebrospinal fluid is secreted into each ventricle by a ___1___ . From the ___2___ ventricles, which are located in the cerebral hemispheres, the fluid passes to the ___3___ ventricle through an opening called the ___4___ . A canal, called the ___5___ , allows the fluid to pass from the latter ventricle to the ___6___ ventricle. From this last ventricle the cerebrospinal fluid passes into a subarachnoid space called the ___7___ through three foramina: one ___8___ and two ___9___ . From this cavity the fluid passes over the cerebellum into another subarachnoid space called the ___10___ . It also passes ___11___ (*up, down*) the posterior side of the spinal cord and ___12___ (*up, down*) the anterior side of the spinal cord. From the cisterna superior the cerebrospinal fluid passes to the subarachnoid space around the ___13___ . This fluid is reabsorbed back into the blood through delicate structures called the ___14___ . The blood vessel that receives the cerebrospinal fluid is the ___15___ .

Answers

General	Fig. 27.4
3. _____	_____
4. _____	_____
5. _____	_____
6. _____	_____
7. _____	_____
8. _____	_____
9. _____	_____
10. _____	_____

Cerebrospinal Fluid

1. _____
2. _____
3. _____
4. _____
5. _____
6. _____
7. _____
8. _____
9. _____
10. _____
11. _____
12. _____
13. _____
14. _____
15. _____

Student: _____

Desk No: _____ Section: _____

The Eye

A. Illustrations
Record the labels from figures 28.1, 28.2, and 28.3 in the answer columns.

B. Structures
Identify the structures described by the following statements.

1. Small nonphotosensitive area on retina.
2. Small pit in retina of eye.
3. Outer layer of wall of eye.
4. Fluid between lens and retina.
5. Fluid between lens and cornea.
6. Inner light sensitive layer.
7. Round yellow spot on retina.
8. Delicate membrane that lines eyelids.
9. Middle vascular layer of wall of eyeball.
10. Drainage tubes for tears in eyelids.
11. Clear transparent portion of front of eyeball.
12. Tube that drains tears from lacrimal sac.
13. Chamber between iris and cornea.
14. Conical body in medial corner of the eye.

anterior chamber—1
aqueous humor—2
blind spot—3
caruncula—4
choroid coat—5
ciliary body—6
cornea—7
conjunctiva—8
fovea centralis—9
iris—10
lacrimal ducts—11
lacrimal sac—12
macula lutea—13
medial canthus—14
nasolacrimal duct—15
plica semilunaris—16
posterior chamber—17
pupil—18
retina—19
scleroid coat—20
suspensory ligament—21
trochlea—22
vitreous body—23

15. Chamber between the iris and lens.
16. Circular color band between lens and cornea.
17. Circular band of smooth muscle tissue surrounding lens.
18. Cartilaginous loop through which superior oblique muscle acts.
19. Connective tissue between lens perimeter and surrounding muscle.
20. A semicircular fold of conjunctiva in the medial canthus of the eye.

C. Extrinsic Muscles
Select the muscles of the eye that are described by the following statements.

1. Inserted on top of eyeball.
2. Inserted on side of eyeball.
3. Inserted on medial surface.
4. Inserted on bottom of eyeball.
5. Inserted on eyelid.
6. Raises the eyelid.
7. Rotates eyeball inward.
8. Rotates eyeball downward.
9. Rotates eyeball outward.
10. Rotates eyeball upward.

inferior oblique—1
inferior rectus—2
lateral rectus—3
medial rectus—4
superior levator palpebrae—5
superior oblique—6
superior rectus—7

Answers

Structures	Fig. 28.1
1. _____	_____
2. _____	_____
3. _____	_____
4. _____	_____
5. _____	_____
6. _____	_____
7. _____	_____
8. _____	_____
9. _____	_____
10. _____	_____
11. _____	_____
12. _____	
13. _____	Fig. 28.2
14. _____	_____
15. _____	_____
16. _____	_____
17. _____	_____
18. _____	_____
19. _____	_____
20. _____	_____

Muscles	
1. _____	_____
2. _____	_____
3. _____	_____
4. _____	_____
5. _____	_____
6. _____	_____
7. _____	_____
8. _____	_____
9. _____	_____
10. _____	_____
	_____

D. Functions

Select the part of the eye that performs the following functions. More than one answer may apply in some cases.

aqueous humor—1
blind spot—2
choroid coat—3
ciliary body—4
conjunctiva—5
iris—6
lacrimal ducts—7
lacrimal puncta—8
lacrimal sac—9
macula lutea—10

nasolacrimal duct—11
pupil—12
retina—13
scleral venous sinus—14
scleroid coat—15
suspensory ligament—16
trabeculae—17
trochlea—18
vitreous body—19

1. Place where nerve fibers of retina leave eyeball.
2. Furnishes blood supply to retina and sclera.
3. Large vessel in wall of the eye that collects aqueous humor from trabeculae.
4. Exerts force on the lens, changing its contour.
5. Controls the amount of light that enters the eye.
6. Maintains firmness and roundness of eyeball.
7. Part of retina where critical vision occurs.
8. Provides most of the strength to the wall of the eyeball.

Answers	
Functions	Fig. 28.3
1. _____	_____
	_____
2. _____	_____
	_____
3. _____	_____
	_____
4. _____	_____
	_____
5. _____	_____
	_____
6. _____	
7. _____	
8. _____	

E. Beef Eye Dissection

Answer the following questions that pertain to the dissection of the beef eye.

1. What is the shape of the pupil? _____

2. Why do you suppose it is so difficult to penetrate the sclera with a sharp scalpel?

   _____

3. What is the function of the black pigment in the eye?

   _____

   _____

4. Compare the consistency of the two fluids in the eye.

   aqueous humor: _____

   vitreous humor: _____

5. When you hold the lens up and look through it, what is unusual about the image?

   _____

6. Does the lens magnify printed matter when placed directly on it? _____

7. Compare the consistencies of the following portions of the lens.

   center: _____

   edge: _____

8. What is the reflective portion of the choroid coat called? _____

9. Is there a macula lutea on the retina of the beef eye? _____

F. Ophthalmoscopy

Record your ophthalmoscope measurements here, and answer the questions.

1. **Diopter Measurements**

   The diopter value of a lens is the reciprocal of its focal length (f) in meters, or $D=\frac{1}{f}$.

   A lens of one diopter (1D) has a focal length of 1 meter, $(D=\frac{1}{f}=\frac{1}{1}=1)$; a 2D lens has a focal length of .5 meter, or $\frac{1}{f}=\frac{1}{.5}=2$; etc.

   Record here your measurements for: 5D_____; 10D_____; 20D_____; and 40D_____.

   Calculated diopter distances: 5D_____; 10D_____; 20D_____; and 40D_____.

   Do your calculations match the measured distances? _____

2. If you were able to examine your laboratory partner's eye with "0" in the diopter window of the ophthalmoscope, what would this indicate about the curvature of the lens of your eye? _____ about your laboratory partner's eye? _____

Student: _____

Desk No: _____ Section: _____

The Ear

A. Illustrations

Record the labels for two illustrations in the answer columns.

B. Auditory Components

Identify the auditory structures of the ear that are described by the following statements.

basilar membrane—1
endolymph—2
hair cells—3
helicotrema—4
incus—5

malleus—6
perilymph—7
reticular lamina—8
rods of Corti—9
scala media—10
scala tympani—11

scala vestibuli—12
stapes—13
tectorial membrane—14
tympanic membrane—15
vestibular membrane—16

1. Membrane set in vibration by sound waves in the air.
2. Ossicle activated by tympanic membrane.
3. Ossicle that fits in oval window.
4. Chamber of cochlea into which oval window opens.
5. Chamber of cochlea into which round window opens.
6. Two fluids found in cochlea.
7. Fluid within cochlear duct.
8. Fluid within scala tympani.
9. Fluid within scala vestibuli.
10. Parts of organ of Corti.
11. Membrane that contains 20,000 fibers of varying lengths.
12. Membrane in which hair tips of hair cells are embedded.
13. Transfers vibrations from basilar membrane to reticular lamina.
14. Receptors that initiate action potentials in cochlear nerve.
15. Opening between scala vestibuli and scala tympani.

C. Mechanics of Hearing

Supply the correct terms to complete the following statements concerning the mechanics of hearing.

Sound waves in the air strike the tympanic membrane, causing it to vibrate and activate the three ___1___ of the middle ear. The vibrational movement of the ___2___, which fits in the oval window, responds to these forces by transferring the energy first to the scala ___3___ and then through a small opening, the ___4___, of the cochlea into the scala ___5___. The sound wave energy in the cochlea activates specific areas of the ___6___ membrane, which contains about 20,000 fibers of different lengths that are capable of vibrating in harmony with specific wavelenghs of sound. Vibration in specific spots of this latter membrane causes the ___7___ cells of the organ of ___8___ to vibrate, and nerve impulses to be sent along the ___9___ nerve fibers to the brain. The short fibers within this membrane are activated by sound waves of ___10___ frequency, and the longer fibers are activated by ___11___ frequency sounds. Equalization of air pressure in the middle ear is maintained through the ___12___ tube.

Answers

Figure 29.2

_____   _____
_____   _____
_____   _____
_____   _____
_____   _____
_____   _____
_____   _____
_____   _____
_____   _____
_____   _____
_____   _____
_____   _____

Auditory Components

1. _____   9. _____
2. _____   10. _____
3. _____   11. _____
4. _____   12. _____
5. _____   13. _____
6. _____   14. _____
7. _____   15. _____
8. _____

Mechanics

1. _____
2. _____
3. _____
4. _____
5. _____
6. _____
7. _____
8. _____
9. _____
10. _____
11. _____
12. _____

D. Vestibular Components

Identify the hearing components of the ear that are described by the following statements.

1. What are the sensory receptors for static equilibrium called?

2. Where are the static equilibrium sensory receptors located (two places)?

3. What are the small calcium carbonate crystals of the macula called?

4. Where are the sensory receptors of dynamic equilibrium located?

5. What nerve branch of the eighth cranial nerve supplies the vestibular apparatus?

6. What part of the vestibular apparatus connects directly to the cochlear duct?

7. What is the name of the fluid within the vestibular apparatus?

8. What structures in joints prevent a sense of malequilibrium when one tilts the head to one side?

9. What fluid lies between the semicircular ducts and the surrounding bone of the semicircular canals?

10. Within how many planes do the semicircular ducts lie?

Answers		
Vestibular Components		**Figure 29.4**
1. _____		____
2. _____		____
_____		____
3. _____		____
4. _____		____
5. _____		____
6. _____		____
7. _____		____
8. _____		____
9. _____		____
10. _____		____

Student: _____

Desk No: _____ Section: _____

The Blood

A. Cell Count Results

As you move the slide in the pattern indicated in figure 30.4, record all the different types of cells in the following table. Refer to figures 30.1 and 30.2 for cell identification. Use this method of tabulation: ~~THL~~ ~~THL~~ 11. Identify and tabulate 100 leukocytes. Divide the total of each kind of cell by 100 to determine percentages.

Neutrophils	Lymphocytes	Monocytes	Eosinophils	Basophils
Totals				
Percent				

B. Questions

Record the answers to the following questions in the answer column at the right.

1. Which type of leukocyte is most numerous in the blood?
2. Which type of leukocyte is most difficult to find on a slide?
3. Which leukocytes are classified as agranulocytes?
4. Name three leukocytes that are classified as granulocytes.
5. Which type of leukocyte increases in the blood when one has an infection such as appendicitis?
6. Which leukocytes increase in numbers when one has whooping cough or viral infections?
7. A deficiency in neutrophils is called _____ .

Answers

1. _____
2. _____
3. _____
   _____
4. _____
   _____
   _____
5. _____
6. _____
7. _____

LABORATORY REPORT 31

The Heart

A. Illustrations

Record the labels for figures 31.1 and 31.2 in the answer columns.

B. Structures

Identify the structures of the heart described by the following statements.

aorta—1	myocardium—13
aortic semilunar valve—2	papillary muscles—14
bicuspid valve—3	parietal pericardium—15
chordae tendineae—4	pulmonary artery—16
endocardium—5	pulmonic semilunar valve—17
epicardium—6	right atrium—18
inferior vena cava—7	right pulmonary artery—19
left atrium—8	right ventricle—20
left pulmonary artery—9	superior vena cava—21
left ventricle—10	tricuspid valve—22
ligamentum arteriosum—11	ventricular septum—23
mitral valve—12	visceral pericardium—24

1. Lining of the heart.
2. Partition between right and left ventricles.
3. Fibroserous saclike structure surrounding the heart.
4. Two chambers of the heart that contain deoxygenated blood.
5. Large artery that carries blood from the right ventricle.
6. Blood vessel that returns blood to heart from head and arms.
7. Remnant of a functional prenatal vessel between the pulmonary artery and the aorta.
8. Structure formed from ductus arteriosum.
9. Valve at the base of the pulmonary artery.
10. Two arteries that are branches of the pulmonary artery.
11. Synonym for bicuspid valve.
12. Structures on the cardiac wall to which the chordae tendineae are attached.
13. Muscular portion of cardiac wall.
14. Thin covering on surface of heart (2 names).
15. Large vein that empties blood into top of right atrium.
16. Two chambers of the heart that contain oxygenated blood.
17. Chamber of the heart that receives blood from the lungs.
18. Large artery that carries blood out from left ventricle.
19. Large vein that empties blood into the lower part of the right atrium.
20. Atrioventricular valves.
21. Valve at the base of the aorta.
22. Blood vessel in which openings to the coronary arteries are located.
23. Atrium into which the coronary sinus empties.
24. Valvular restraints that prevent the atrioventricular valve cusps from being forced back into the atria.

Answers

Structures	Fig. 31.1
1. _____	_____
2. _____	_____
3. _____	_____
4. _____	_____
5. _____	_____
6. _____	_____
7. _____	_____
8. _____	_____
9. _____	_____
10. _____	_____
11. _____	_____
12. _____	_____
13. _____	_____
14. _____	_____
15. _____	_____
16. _____	_____
17. _____	_____
18. _____	_____
19. _____	_____
20. _____	_____
21. _____	_____
22. _____	_____
23. _____	_____
24. _____	_____

C. Coronary Circulation

Identify the arteries and veins of the coronary circulatory system that are described by the following statements.

anterior interventricular artery—1
circumflex artery—2
coronary sinus—3
great cardiac vein—4
left coronary artery—5
middle cardiac vein—6
posterior descending right coronary artery—7
posterior interventricular vein—8
right coronary artery—9
small cardiac vein—10

1. Two principal branches of the left coronary artery.
2. Coronary vein that lies in the anterior interventricular sulcus.
3. Coronary artery that lies in the right atrioventricular sulcus.
4. Vein that receives blood from the great cardiac vein.
5. Vein that lies in the posterior interventricular sulcus.
6. Two major coronary arteries that take their origins in the wall of the aorta.
7. Large coronary vessel that empties into the right atrium.
8. Coronary vein that parallels the right coronary artery in the right atrioventricular sulcus.
9. Branch of the right coronary artery on the posterior surface of the heart.
10. Vein that lies alongside of the posterior descending right coronary artery.

D. Sheep Heart Dissection

After completing the sheep heart dissection answer the following questions. Some of these questions were encountered during the dissection; others pertain to structures not shown in figures 31.1 and 31.2.

1. Identify the following structures:

   Pectinate muscle: _____

   _____

   Moderator band: _____

   _____

   Ligamentum arteriosum: _____

   _____

2. How many papillary muscles did you find in the

   right ventricle? _____ left ventricle? _____

3. How many pouches are present in each of the following?

   pulmonary semilunar valve: _____

   aortic semilunar valve: _____

4. Where does blood enter the myocardium? _____

   _____

5. Where does blood leave the myocardium and return to the circulatory system? _____

Answers	
Coronary Circulation	**Fig. 31.2 Anterior**
1. _____	_____
2. _____	_____
3. _____	_____
4. _____	_____
5. _____	_____
6. _____	_____
7. _____	_____
8. _____	_____
9. _____	_____
10. _____	_____
Fig. 31.2 Posterior	_____
_____	_____
_____	_____
_____	_____
_____	_____
_____	_____
_____	_____
_____	
_____	
_____	
_____	
_____	
_____	
_____	

Student: _____

Desk No: _____ Section: _____

The Arteries and Veins

A. Illustrations

Record the labels for figures 32.2 and 32.3 in the answer columns. Note that the labels for figure 32.2 are on both sides of this sheet.

B. Arteries

Refer to the left-hand illustration in figure 31.2 to identify the arteries described by the following statements.

anterior tibial—1	internal iliac—13
aorta—2	left common carotid—14
aortic arch—3	left subclavian—15
axillary—4	popliteal—16
brachial—5	posterior tibial—17
celiac—6	radial—18
common iliac—7	renal—19
deep femoral—8	right common carotid—20
external iliac—9	subclavian—21
femoral—10	superior mesenteric—22
inferior mesenteric—11	ulnar—23
innominate—12	

1. Artery of the shoulder.
2. Artery of upper arm.
3. Artery of the armpit.
4. Gives rise to right common carotid and right subclavian.
5. Lateral artery of the forearm.
6. Medial artery of the forearm.
7. Three branches of the aortic arch.
8. Gives rise to femoral artery.
9. Major artery of the thigh.
10. Artery of knee region.
11. Artery of calf region.
12. Large branch of common iliac.
13. Small branch of common iliac.
14. Supplies the stomach, spleen, and liver.
15. Major artery of chest and abdomen.
16. Supplies the kidney.
17. Also known as the hypogastric artery.
18. Supplies blood to most of small intestines and part of colon.
19. Artery in interior portion of lower leg.
20. Branch of femoral that parallels medial surface of femur.
21. Curved vessel that receives blood from left ventricle.
22. Supplies the large intestine and rectum.

Answers

Arteries	Fig. 32.2 Arteries
1. _____	_____
2. _____	_____
3. _____	_____
4. _____	_____
5. _____	_____
6. _____	_____
7. _____	_____
8. _____	_____
9. _____	_____
10. _____	_____
11. _____	_____
12. _____	_____
13. _____	_____
14. _____	_____
15. _____	_____
16. _____	_____
17. _____	_____
18. _____	_____
19. _____	_____
20. _____	_____
21. _____	_____
22. _____	_____

C. Veins

Refer to the right-hand illustration in figure 32.2 and to figure 32.3 to identify the veins described by the following statements.

accessory cephalic—1
axillary—2
basilic—3
brachial—4
cephalic—5
common iliac—6
coronary—7
dorsal venous arch—8
external iliac—9
external jugular—10
femoral—11
great saphenous—12
hepatic—13
inferior vena cava—14
innominate—15
inferior mesenteric—16
internal iliac—17
internal jugular—18
median cubital—19
popliteal—20
portal—21
posterior tibial—22
pyloric—23
subclavian—24
superior mesenteric—25
superior vena cava—26

1. Largest vein in neck.

2. Small vein in neck.

3. Vein of armpit.

4. Empty into innominate veins.

5. Collects blood from veins of head and arms.

6. Short vein between basilic and cephalic veins.

7. Collects blood from veins of chest, abdomen, and legs.

8. On posterior surface of humerus.

9. Large veins that unite to form the inferior vena cava.

10. On medial surface of upper arm.

11. On lateral portion of forearm.

12. On lateral portion of upper arm.

13. Vein from liver to inferior vena cava.

14. Receives blood from descending colon and rectum.

15. Empties into popliteal.

16. Collects blood from two innominate veins.

17. Collects blood from top of foot.

18. Superficial vein on medial surface of leg.

19. Vein of knee region.

20. Collects blood from intestines, stomach, and colon.

21. Vein that receives blood from posterior tibial.

22. Receives blood from ascending colon and part of ileum.

23. Empties into great saphenous.

24. Small vein that empties into common iliac at juncture of external iliac.

25. Vein that great saphenous empties into.

26. Two veins that drain blood from stomach into portal vein.

Answers

	Veins	Fig. 32.2 Veins
1.	_____	_____
2.	_____	_____
3.	_____	_____
4.	_____	_____
5.	_____	_____
6.	_____	_____
7.	_____	_____
8.	_____	_____
9.	_____	_____
10.	_____	_____
11.	_____	_____
12.	_____	_____
13.	_____	_____
14.	_____	_____
15.	_____	_____
16.	_____	_____
17.	_____	_____
18.	_____	_____
19.	_____	_____
20.	_____	_____
21.	_____	_____
22.	_____	_____
23.	_____	_____
24.	_____	_____
25.	_____	**Fig. 32.3**
26.	_____	_____
		_____
		_____
		_____
		_____
		_____
		_____
		_____
		_____
		_____
		_____

Student: _____ _____

Desk No: _____ Section: _____

Fetal Circulation (Ex. 33)

A. Figure 33.1
Record the labels for this illustration in the answer column.

B. Questions
Record the answers for the following questions in the answer column.

1. What blood vessel in the umbilical cord supplies the fetus with nutrients?
2. What blood vessel in the umbilical cord returns blood to the placenta from the fetus?
3. What blood vessel shunts blood from the pulmonary artery to the aorta?
4. What vessel in the liver carries blood from the umbilical vein to the inferior vena cava?
5. What structure in the liver is formed from the ductus venosus?
6. What structure forms from the ductus arteriosus?
7. What structure forms from the umbilical vein?
8. What structure enables blood to flow from the right atrium to the left atrium before birth?
9. Give two occurrences at childbirth that prevent excessive blood loss by the infant through the cut umbilical cord.
10. What structures near the bladder form from the hypogastric arteries?

The Lymphatic System and the Immune Response (Ex. 34)

A. Figure 34.1
Record the labels for this illustration in the answer column.

B. Components
By referring to figures 34.1 and 34.2 identify the following structures in the lymphatic system.

1. Large vessel in thorax and abdomen that collects lymph from lower extremities.
2. Short vessel that collects lymph from right arm and right side of head.
3. Microscopic lymphatic vessels situated among cells of tissues.
4. Saclike structure that receives chyle from intestine.
5. Blood vessel that receives fluid from thoracic duct.
6. Filters of the lymphatic system.
7. Vessels of arms and legs that convey lymph to collecting ducts.
8. Depression in lymph node through which blood vessels enter node.
9. Outer covering of lymph node.
10. Structural units of lymph node that are packed with lymphocytes.
11. Cells involved in organ transplant rejections.
12. Cells that produce antibodies.

capsule—1
cisterna chyli—2
germinal centers—3
hilum—4
left subclavian vein—5
lymphatics—6
lymph capillaries—7
lymphoblasts—8
lymph nodes—9
plasma cells—10
right lymphatic duct—11
thoracic duct—12
none of these—13

Answers

Questions

1. _____
2. _____
3. _____
4. _____
5. _____
6. _____
7. _____
8. _____
9a. _____
b. _____
10. _____

Components	Fig. 33.1
1. _____	_____
2. _____	_____
3. _____	_____
4. _____	_____
5. _____	_____
6. _____	_____
7. _____	_____
8. _____	_____
9. _____	_____
10. _____	_____
11. _____	_____
12. _____	_____

C. Questions

1. List three forces that move lymph through the lymphatic vessels:

   a. _____

   b. _____ c. _____

2. How does lymph in the lymphatics of the legs differ in composition from the lymph in the thoracic duct?

   _____

   _____

3. Where do stem cells for all lymphocytes originate? _____

   _____

4. Give the cell type that accounts for each type of immunity:

   Humoral immunity: _____

   Cellular immunity: _____

5. What tissues program stem cells for

   Humoral immunity: _____

   Cellular immunity: _____

6. What type of tissue is common to the thymus gland and bursal tissues?

   _____

Answers

Fig. 34.1

Student: _____

Desk No: _____ Section: _____

The Respiratory System

A. Illustrations

Record the labels for the illustrations of this exercise in the answer column.

B. Cat Dissection

After completing the dissection of the cat, answer the following questions. Both of these questions are asked in the course of the dissection.

1. Are the cartilaginous rings of the trachea continuous all the

   way around the organ? _____

2. Which lung has four lobes? _____

   . . . three lobes? _____

C. Sheep Pluck Dissection

After completing the sheep pluck dissection, answer the following questions.

1. Are the cartilaginous rings of the trachea continuous all the

   way around the organ? _____

2. Describe the texture of the surface of the lung. _____

   _____

   _____

3. How many lobes exist on the right lung? _____

   . . . on the left lung? _____

4. Why does lung tissue collapse so readily when you quit blowing

   into it with a straw? _____

   _____

   _____

5. What does the "pulmonary membrane" consist of? _____

   _____

   _____

   _____

D. Histological Study

On a separate sheet of plain paper make drawings, as required by your instructor, of nasal, tracheal, and lung tissues.

Answers	
Fig. 35.1	**Fig. 35.3**
_____	_____
_____	_____
_____	_____
_____	_____
_____	_____
_____	_____
_____	_____
_____	_____
_____	_____
_____	_____
_____	_____
_____	_____
_____	_____
Fig. 35.2	_____
_____	_____
_____	_____
_____	_____
_____	_____
_____	_____
_____	_____
_____	_____
_____	_____
_____	_____

E. Organ Identification

Identify the respiratory structures according to the following statements.

alveoli—1
bronchioles—2
bronchi—3
cricoid cartilage—4
epiglottis—5
hard palate—6
larynx—7
lingual tonsils—8
nasal cavity—9
nasal conchae—10

nasopharynx—11
oral cavity proper—12
oral vestibule—13
oropharynx—14
palatine tonsils—15
pharyngeal tonsils—16
pleural cavity—17
soft palate—18
thyroid cartilage—19
trachea—20

1. Partition between nasal and oral cavities.
2. Cartilage of Adam's apple.
3. Small air sacs of lung tissue.
4. Cavity above soft palate.
5. Cavity above hard palate.
6. Cavity that contains the tongue.
7. Cavity near palatine tonsils.
8. Voice box.
9. Small tubes leading into alveoli.
10. Another name for adenoids.
11. Tube between larynx and bronchi.
12. Fleshy lobes in nasal cavity.
13. Cavity between lips and teeth.
14. Tonsils located on sides of pharynx.
15. Tonsils attached to base of tongue.
16. Flexible flaplike cartilage over larynx.
17. Most inferior cartilaginous ring of larynx.
18. Tubes formed by bifurcation of trachea.
19. Potential cavity between lung and thoracic wall.

F. Organ Function

Select the structures in the above list that perform the following functions.

1. Initiates swallowing.
2. Prevents food from entering the larynx when swallowing.
3. Provides supporting walls for vocal folds.
4. Assists in destruction of harmful bacteria in the oral region.
5. Warms the air as it passes through the nasal cavity.
6. Prevents food from entering nasal cavity during chewing and swallowing.
7. Provides surface for gas exchange in the lungs.
8. Essential for speech.

Answers

Organ Identification

1. _____
2. _____
3. _____
4. _____
5. _____
6. _____
7. _____
8. _____
9. _____
10. _____
11. _____
12. _____
13. _____
14. _____
15. _____
16. _____
17. _____
18. _____
19. _____

Organ Function

1. _____
2. _____
3. _____
4. _____
5. _____
6. _____
7. _____
8. _____

Student: _____

Desk No: _____ Section: _____

The Digestive System

A. Illustrations
Record the labels for the illustrations of this exercise in the answer columns.

B. Microscopic Studies
Record here the drawings of the microscopic examinations that are required for this exercise. If there is insufficient space for all required drawings, utilize a separate sheet of paper for all of them.

Answers

Fig. 36.1	Fig. 36.2
_____	_____
_____	_____
_____	_____
_____	_____
_____	_____
_____	_____
_____	_____
_____	_____
_____	**Fig. 36.3**
_____	_____
_____	_____
_____	_____
_____	_____
_____	_____
_____	_____
_____	_____
_____	_____
_____	_____
_____	_____
_____	
_____	

C. Alimentary Canal

Identify the parts of the digestive system described by the following statements.

anus—1	esophagus—10
cecum—2	ileum—11
colon—3	pharynx—12
colon, sigmoid—4	rectum—13
duct, common bile—5	stomach, fundus—14
duct, cystic—6	stomach, pyloric portion—15
duct, hepatic—7	valve, cardiac—16
duct, pancreatic—8	valve, ileocecal—17
duodenum—9	valve, pyloric—18

1. Place where swallowing (peristalsis) begins.
2. Entrance opening of stomach.
3. Exit opening of stomach.
4. Tube between mouth and stomach.
5. Distal coiled portion of small intestine.
6. First twelve inches of small intestine.
7. Proximal pouch or compartment of large intestine.
8. Section of large intestine between descending colon and rectum.
9. Most active portion of stomach.
10. Duct that drains the liver.
11. Valve between small and large intestines.
12. Duct that drains the gallbladder.
13. Part of small intestine where most digestion occurs.
14. Part of small intestine where most absorption occurs.
15. Duct that joins the common bile duct before entering the intestine.
16. Structure on which appendix is located.
17. Duct that conveys bile to intestine.
18. Exit of alimentary canal.
19. Part of tract where most water absorption (conservation) occurs.
20. Last six inches of alimentary canal.

Answers

Alimentary Canal	Fig. 36.4
1. _____	_____
2. _____	_____
3. _____	_____
4. _____	_____
5. _____	_____
6. _____	_____
7. _____	_____
8. _____	_____
9. _____	_____
10. _____	_____
11. _____	_____
12. _____	_____
13. _____	
14. _____	
15. _____	
16. _____	
17. _____	
18. _____	
19. _____	
20. _____	

D. Oral Cavity

Identify the structures of the mouth that are described by the following statements.

arch, glossopalatine—1
arch, pharyngopalatine—2
buccae—3
duct, parotid—4
duct, submandibular—5
ducts, lesser sublingual—6
frenulum, labial—7
frenulum, lingual—8
gingiva—9
glands, parotid—10
glands, sublingual—11
glands, submandibular—12
mucosa—13
papillae, filiform—14
papillae, foliate—15
papillae, fungiform—16
papillae, vallate—17
tonsil, lingual—18
tonsil, palatine—19
tonsil, pharyngeal—20
uvula—21

1. Lining of the mouth.
2. Name for the cheeks.
3. Duct that drains the parotid gland.
4. Fold of skin between the lip and gums.
5. Duct that drains the submandibular gland.
6. Fold of skin between the tongue and floor of mouth.
7. Portion of mucosa around the teeth.
8. Tonsils seen at back of mouth.
9. Tonsils located at root of tongue.
10. Fingerlike projection at end of soft palate.
11. Vertical ridges on side of tongue.
12. Rounded papillae on dorsum of tongue.
13. Small tactile papillae on surface of tongue.
14. Large papillae at back of tongue.
15. Ducts that drain sublingual gland.
16. Place where taste buds are located.
17. Salivary glands located inside and below the mandible.
18. Membrane located in front of palatine tonsil.
19. Membrane located in back of palatine tonsil.
20. Salivary glands located under the tongue.
21. Salivary glands located in cheeks.

E. The Teeth

Select the correct answer that completes each of the following statements.

1. All deciduous teeth usually erupt by the time a child is
   (1) one year. (2) two years. (3) four years old.
2. A complete set of primary teeth consists of
   (1) ten teeth. (2) twenty teeth. (3) thirty-two teeth.
3. The permanent teeth with the longest roots are the
   (1) incisors. (2) cuspids. (3) molars.
4. The smallest permanent molars are the
   (1) first molars. (2) second molars. (3) third molars.
5. A complete set of permanent teeth consists of
   (1) twenty-four teeth. (2) twenty-eight teeth.
   (3) thirty-two teeth.
6. The primary dentition lacks
   (1) molars. (2) incisors. (3) bicuspids.

Answers

Oral Cavity	Fig. 36.5
1. _____	_____
2. _____	_____
3. _____	_____
4. _____	_____
5. _____	_____
6. _____	_____
7. _____	_____
8. _____	_____
9. _____	_____
10. _____	_____
	Fig. 36.7
11. _____	_____
12. _____	_____
13. _____	_____
14. _____	_____
15. _____	_____
16. _____	_____
17. _____	_____
18. _____	_____
19. _____	_____
20. _____	_____
21. _____	_____
	_____
Teeth	_____
1. _____	_____
2. _____	_____
3. _____	_____
4. _____	_____
5. _____	_____
6. _____	

343

7. A child's first permanent tooth usually erupts during the
   (1) second year.   (2) third year.
   (3) fifth year.   (4) sixth year.
8. Trifurcated roots exist on
   (1) upper cuspids.   (2) upper molars.   (3) lower molars.
9. Bifurcated roots exist on
   (1) upper first bicuspids and lower molars.
   (2) cuspids and lower bicuspids.   (3) all molars.
10. A tooth is considered "dead" or devitalized if
    (1) the enamel is destroyed.   (2) the pulp is destroyed.
    (3) the periodontal membrane is infected.
11. Dentin is produced by cells called
    (1) odontoblasts.   (2) ameloblasts.   (3) cementocytes.
12. Cementum is secreted by cells called
    (1) odontoblasts.   (2) ameloblasts.   (3) cementocytes.
13. The wisdom tooth is
    (1) a supernumerary tooth.   (2) a succedaneous tooth.
    (3) the third molar.
14. Caries (cavities) are caused primarily by
    (1) using the wrong toothpaste.   (2) acid production by bacteria.   (3) fluorides in water.
15. Most teeth that have to be extracted have become useless because of
    (1) caries.   (2) gingivitis.   (3) periodontitis (pyorrhea).
16. Enamel covers the
    (1) entire tooth.   (2) clinical crown only.
    (3) anatomical crown only.
17. The tooth receives nourishment through
    (1) the apical foramen.   (2) the periodontal membrane.
    (3) both the apical foramen and the periodontal membrane.
18. The tooth is held in the alveolus by
    (1) bone.   (2) dentin.   (3) periodontal membrane.

Answers
Teeth
7. _____
8. _____
9. _____
10. _____
11. _____
12. _____
13. _____
14. _____
15. _____
16. _____
17. _____
18. _____

LABORATORY REPORT **37**

Student: _____

Desk No: _____   Section: _____

The Urinary System

A. Illustrations

Record the labels for the three illustrations of this exercise in the answer columns. Note that figure 37.2 is on the reverse side of this sheet.

B. Microscopy

If the space provided below is adequate for your histology drawings, use it. Use a separate sheet of paper if several sketches are to be made.

C. Anatomy

Identify the structures of the urinary system that are described by the following statements.

calyces—1	medulla—6	renal pelvis—11
collecting tubule—2	nephron—7	renal pyramids—12
cortex—3	renal capsule—8	ureters—13
glomerular capsule—4	renal column—9	urethra—14
glomerulus—5	renal papilla—10	

1. Tubes that drain the kidneys.
2. Tube that drains the urinary bladder.
3. Portion of kidney that contains renal corpuscles.
4. Cone-shaped areas of medulla.
5. Portion of kidney that consists primarily of collecting tubules.
6. Basic functioning unit of the kidney.
7. Two portions of renal corpuscle.
8. Distal tip of renal pyramid.
9. Short tubes that receive urine from renal papillae.
10. Funnellike structure that collects urine from calyces of each kidney.
11. Structure that receives urine from several nephrons.
12. Cup-shaped membranous structure that surrounds glomerulus.
13. Thin fibrous outer covering of kidney.
14. Cortical tissue between renal pyramids.
15. Tuft of capillaries that produces dilute urine.

Answers

Anatomy	Fig. 37.1
1. _____	_____
2. _____	_____
3. _____	_____
4. _____	_____
5. _____	_____
6. _____	_____
7. _____	_____
8. _____	_____
9. _____	_____
10. _____	_____
11. _____	Fig. 37.3
12. _____	_____
13. _____	_____
14. _____	_____
15. _____	_____

D. Physiology

Select the best answer that completes the following statements concerning the physiology of urine production. For definitions of medical terms consult a medical dictionary or your lecture text.

1. Blood enters the glomerulus through the
   (1) efferent arteriole.   (2) arcuate artery.
   (3) afferent arteriole.   (4) None of these are correct.

2. Surgical removal of a kidney is called
   (1) nephrectomy.   (2) nephrotomy.   (3) nephrolithotomy.

3. Water reabsorption from the glomerular filtrate into the peritubular blood is facilitated by
   (1) antidiuretic hormone.   (2) renin.
   (3) aldosterone.   (4) Both 1 and 3 are correct.

4. The following substances are reabsorbed through the walls of the nephron into the peritubular blood:
   (1) glucose and water.   (2) urea and water.
   (3) glucose, amino acids, salts, and water.
   (4) glucose, amino acids, urea, salts, and water.

5. The amount of urine produced is affected by
   (1) blood pressure.
   (2) environmental temperature.
   (3) amount of solute in glomerular filtrate.
   (4) 1, 2, 3 and additional factors are correct.

6. The amount of urine normally produced in 24 hours is about
   (1) 100 ml.   (2) 500 ml.   (3) 1.5 liters.   (4) 4.5 liters.

7. The reabsorption of sodium ions from the glomerular filtrate into the peritubular blood draws the following back into the blood:
   (1) potassium ions.   (2) chloride ions.
   (3) water.   (4) chloride ions and water.

8. Cells of the walls of collecting tubules secrete the following substances into urine:
   (1) amino acids.   (2) uric acid.
   (3) ammonia.   (4) Both 2 and 3 are correct.

9. Renal diabetes is due to
   (1) a lack of ADH.   (2) a lack of insulin.
   (3) faulty reabsorption of glucose in the nephron.
   (4) Both 1 and 2 are correct.

10. The presence of glucose in the urine and a low level of insulin in the blood would be diagnosed as
    (1) diabetes insipidus.   (2) diabetes mellitus.
    (3) renal diabetes.   (4) None of these are correct.

11. Approximately eighty percent of water in the glomerular filtrate is reabsorbed in the
    (1) proximal convoluted tubule.   (2) Henle's loop.
    (3) distal convoluted tubule.   (4) None of these are correct.

12. The desire to micturate normally occurs when the following amount of urine is present in the bladder:
    (1) 100 ml.   (2) 200 ml.   (3) 300 ml.   (4) 400 ml.

13. Removal of calculus (kidney stones) is called
    (1) nephrectomy.   (2) nephrotomy.
    (3) nephrolithotomy.   (4) Both 2 and 3 are correct.

Answers

Physiology

1. _____
2. _____
3. _____
4. _____
5. _____
6. _____
7. _____
8. _____
9. _____
10. _____
11. _____
12. _____
13. _____

Fig. 37.2

_____
_____
_____
_____
_____
_____
_____
_____
_____
_____
_____
_____
_____
_____
_____
_____
_____

Student: _____

Desk No: _____ Section: _____

The Endocrine Glands

A. Illustrations
Record the labels for figures 38.12 and 38.13 in the answer columns.

B. Microscopy
Make the drawings of the various microscopic studies on separate drawing paper. Include these drawings with the Laboratory Report.

C. Sources
Select the glandular tissues that produce the following hormones.

1. ACTH
2. ADH
3. Aldosterone
4. Calcitonin
5. Chorionic gonadotropin
6. Cortisol
7. Epinephrine
8. Estrogens
9. FSH
10. Glucagon
11. ICSH
12. Insulin
13. LH
14. Melatonin
15. Norepinephrine
16. Oxytocin
17. Parathyroid hormone
18. PIF
19. Prolactin
20. Progesterone
21. Somatostatin
22. Testosterone
23. Thymosin
24. Thyrotropin
25. Thyroxine
26. Triiodothyronine
27. Vasopressin

adrenal cortex
 zona fasciculata—1
 zona glomerulosa—2
 zona reticularis—3
adrenal medulla—4
hypothalamus—5
ovary
 corpus luteum—6
 Graafian follicle—7
pancreas
 alpha cells—8
 beta cells—9
 delta cells—10
 acini cells—11
parathyroid gland—12
pineal gland—13
pituitary gland
 adenohypophysis—14
 neurohypophysis—15
placenta—16
testis—17
thymus gland—18
thyroid gland
 follicular cells—19
 parafollicular cells—20

D. Physiology
Select the hormones that produce the following physiological effects. Note that a separate list of hormones is provided for each group.

GROUP I

1. Increases metabolism.
2. Increases blood pressure.
3. Increases strength of heartbeat.
4. Promotes sodium absorption in nephron.
5. Promotes gluconeogenesis.
6. Causes vasoconstriction in all organs.
7. Causes vasoconstriction in all organs except muscles and liver.
8. Causes vasodilation in skeletal muscles.
9. Inhibits the estrus cycle in lower animals.

aldosterone—1
epinephrine—2
glucocorticoids—3
melatonin—4
norepinephrine—5
none of these—6

Answers

Sources	Fig. 38.12
1. _____	_____
2. _____	_____
3. _____	_____
4. _____	_____
5. _____	_____
6. _____	_____
7. _____	_____
8. _____	_____
9. _____	_____
10. _____	_____
11. _____	_____
12. _____	_____
13. _____	_____
14. _____	_____
15. _____	_____
16. _____	_____
17. _____	_____
18. _____	_____
19. _____	_____
20. _____	_____
21. _____	_____
22. _____	_____
23. _____	_____
24. _____	_____
25. _____	_____
26. _____	
27. _____	

Physiology Group I
1. _____
2. _____
3. _____
4. _____
5. _____
6. _____
7. _____
8. _____
9. _____

D. Physiology (continued)

Select the hormones that produce the following physiological effects.

GROUP II

1. Inhibits insulin production.
2. Inhibits production of SH.
3. Stimulates osteoclasts.
4. Mobilizes fatty acids.
5. Inhibits glucagon production.
6. Raises blood calcium level.
7. Increases cardiac output and respiratory rate.
8. Impedes phosphorus reabsorption in renal tubules.
9. Promotes storage of glucose, fatty acids, and amino acids.
10. Mobilizes glucose, fatty acids, and amino acids.
11. Stimulates metabolism of all cells in body.
12. Lowers blood phosphorus levels.
13. Decreases blood calcium when injected intravenously.

calcitonin—1
glucagon—2
insulin—3
parathyroid hormone—4
somatostatin—5
thyroid hormone—6
none of these—7

GROUP III

1. Promotes breast enlargement.
2. Promotes rapid bone growth.
3. Stimulates testicular descent.
4. Causes milk ejection from breasts.
5. Promotes maturation of spermatozoa.
6. Causes constriction of arterioles.
7. Stimulates production of thyroxine.
8. Stimulates glucocorticoid production.
9. Inhibits prolactin production.
10. Causes thickening and vascularization of endometrium.
11. Causes interstitial cells to produce testosterone.
12. Causes myometrium contraction during childbirth.
13. Promotes milk production after childbirth.
14. Promotes stratification of vaginal epithelium.
15. Suppresses development of female genitalia in male.
16. Prepares the endometrium for egg cell implantation.
17. Promotes growth of all cells in the body.

ACTH—1
ADH—2
chorionic gonadotropin—3
estrogens—4
FSH—5
LH—6
oxytocin—7
PIF—8
progesterone—9
somatotropin—10
testosterone—11
thyrotropin—12
none of these—13

E. Hormonal Imbalance

Select the hormones that are responsible for the following disorders. After each hormone number indicate with a (+) or (−) whether the condition is due to *excess* (+) or *deficiency* (−). More than one hormone may apply in some cases.

1. Acromegaly
2. Addison's disease
3. Cretinism
4. Cushing's syndrome
5. Diabetes insipidus
6. Diabetes mellitus
7. Dwarfism
8. Exophthalmos
9. Gigantism
10. Hyperglycemia
11. Hypothyroidism
12. Myxedema
13. Tetany

ADH—1
glucagon—2
glucocorticoids—3
insulin—4
mineralocorticoids—5
parathyroid hormone—6
somatotropin—7
thyroid hormone—8
none of these—9

Answers

Physiology Group II	Fig. 38.13
1. _____	_____
2. _____	_____
3. _____	_____
4. _____	_____
5. _____	_____
6. _____	_____
7. _____	_____
8. _____	_____
9. _____	_____
10. _____	_____
11. _____	_____
12. _____	_____
13. _____	_____

Group III	
1. _____	
2. _____	
3. _____	
4. _____	
5. _____	**Imbalance**
6. _____	1. _____
7. _____	2. _____
8. _____	3. _____
9. _____	4. _____
10. _____	5. _____
11. _____	6. _____
12. _____	7. _____
13. _____	8. _____
14. _____	9. _____
15. _____	10. _____
16. _____	11. _____
17. _____	12. _____
	13. _____

Student: _____

Desk No: _____ Section: _____

The Reproductive System

A. Labels
Record the labels for the illustrations of this exercise in the answer columns.

B. Microscopy
Draw the various stages of spermatogenesis on a separate piece of paper to be included with this Laboratory Report.

C. Male Organs
Identify the structures described by the following statements.

common ejaculatory duct—1
corpora cavernosa—2
corpus spongiosum—3
Cowper's gland—4
epididymis—5
glans penis—6
penis—7

prepuce—8
prostate gland—9
prostatic urethra—10
seminal vesicle—11
seminiferous tubule—12
testes—13
vas deferens—14

1. Copulatory organ of male.
2. Source of spermatozoa.
3. Erectile tissue of penis (3).
4. Fold of skin over end of penis.
5. Structure that stores spermatozoa.
6. Contribute fluids to semen (3).
7. Duct that passes from urinary bladder through the prostate gland.
8. Coiled up structures in testes where spermatozoa originate.
9. Tube that carries sperm from epididymis to ejaculatory duct.
10. Distal end of penis.

D. Female Organs
Identify the structures described by the following statements.

cervix—1
clitoris—2
external os—3
fimbriae—4
greater vestibular glands—5
hymen—6
infundibulum—7
internal os—8

labia majora—9
labia minora—10
mons pubis—11
myometrium—12
paraurethral glands—13
ovaries—14
uterine tubes—15
vagina—16

1. Copulatory organ of female.
2. Source of ova in female.
3. Muscular wall of uterus.
4. Neck of uterus.
5. Provides vaginal lubrication during coitus.
6. Fingerlike projections around edge of infundibulum.
7. Protuberance of erectile tissue sensitive to sexual excitation.
8. Entrance to uterus at vaginal end.
9. Homologous to Cowper's glands of male.
10. Homologous to penis of male.
11. Homologous to scrotum of male.
12. Homologous to prostate gland of male.
13. Ducts that convey ovum to uterus.
14. Membranous fold of tissue surrounding entrance to vagina.
15. Open funnellike end of uterine tube.

Answers	
Male Organs	**Fig. 39.1**
1. _____	_____
2. _____	_____
3. _____	_____
4. _____	_____
5. _____	_____
6. _____	_____
7. _____	
8. _____	
9. _____	
10. _____	
Female Organs	
1. _____	_____
2. _____	_____
3. _____	_____
4. _____	_____
5. _____	_____
6. _____	_____
7. _____	_____
8. _____	_____
9. _____	_____
10. _____	_____
11. _____	_____
12. _____	_____
13. _____	_____
14. _____	_____
15. _____	_____
	_____

E. Ligaments

Identify the following supporting structures that hold the ovaries, uterus, and uterine tubes in place.

broad ligament—1
infundibulopelvic ligament—2
mesosalpinx—3
ovarian ligament—4

round ligament—5
sacrouterine ligament—6
suspensory ligament—7
none of these—8

1. A ligament that extends from the uterus to the ovary.
2. Ligament between the cervix and sacral part of the pelvic wall.
3. A ligament that extends from the infundibulum to the wall of the pelvic cavity.
4. A ligament that extends from the corpus of the uterus to the body wall.
5. A large flat ligament of peritoneal tissue that extends from the uterine tube to the cervical part of the uterus.
6. A mesentery between the ovary and uterine tubes that contains blood vessels leading to the uterine tube.
7. A fold of peritoneum that attaches the ovary to the uterine tube.

F. Germ Cells

Identify the types of cells of oogenesis and spermatogenesis described by the following statements. More than one answer may apply.

Spermatogenesis
primary spermatocyte—1
secondary spermatocyte—2
spermatids—3
spermatogonia—4
spermatozoa—5

Oogenesis
oogonia—6
polar bodies—7
primary oocyte—8
secondary oocyte—9

1. Cells that are haploid.
2. Cells that contain tetrads.
3. Cells that contain monads.
4. Cells that contain dyads.
5. Cells that are diploid.
6. Cells at periphery of ovary that produce all ova.
7. Cells that undergo mitosis.
8. Cells in which first meiotic division occurs.
9. Cells at periphery of seminiferous tubule that give rise to all spermatozoa.
10. Cells that develop directly into mature spermatozoa.
11. Cells in which second meiotic division occurs.

G. Physiology of Reproduction and Development

Select the best answer that completes the following statements.

1. The ovum gets from the ovary to the uterus by
   (1) amoeboid movement. (2) ciliary action.
   (3) peristalsis and ciliary action of uterine tube.
2. The vaginal lining is normally
   (1) alkaline. (2) acid. (3) neutral.
3. The seminal vesicle secretion is
   (1) alkaline. (2) acid. (3) neutral.
4. The birth canal consists of the
   (1) vagina. (2) uterus. (3) the vagina and uterus.
5. Spermatozoan viability is enhanced by a temperature that is
   (1) 98.6° F. (2) above 98.6° F. (3) below 98.6° F.
6. The prostatic secretion is
   (1) alkaline. (2) acid. (3) neutral.

Answers

Ligaments	Fig. 39.3
1. _____	_____
2. _____	_____
3. _____	_____
4. _____	_____
5. _____	_____
6. _____	_____
7. _____	_____

Germ Cells	
1. _____	_____
2. _____	_____
3. _____	_____
4. _____	Fig. 39.4
5. _____	_____
6. _____	_____
7. _____	_____
8. _____	_____
9. _____	_____
10. _____	_____
11. _____	_____

Physiology	
1. _____	_____
2. _____	_____
3. _____	_____
4. _____	_____
5. _____	_____
6. _____	_____

7. The fetal stage of the human is
   (1) the first 8 weeks.   (2) from the ninth week until birth.
   (3) the entire prenatal term.

8. Circumcision involves excisement of the
   (1) prepuce.   (2) perineum.   (3) glans penis.

9. Fertilization of the human ovum usually occurs in the
   (1) uterus.   (2) vagina.   (3) uterine tube.

10. Implantation of the fertilized ovum occurs usually
    (1) within 2 days after fertilization.
    (2) within 6 to 8 days after fertilization.
    (3) after 10 days.

11. The innermost fetal membrane surrounding the embryo is the
    (1) amnion.   (2) chorion.   (3) decidua.

12. The life span of an ovum without fertilization is
    (1) 6 hours.   (2) 24–28 hours.   (3) 7 days.

13. Uterine muscle consists of
    (1) smooth muscle.   (2) striated muscle.
    (3) both smooth and striated muscle.

14. The outermost fetal membrane surrounding the embryo is the
    (1) amnion.   (2) chorion.   (3) decidua.

15. The lining of the uterus is the
    (1) myometrium.   (2) endometrium.   (3) epimetrium.

16. Milk production by the breasts usually occurs
    (1) immediately after birth.   (2) on the second day.
    (3) on the third or fourth day.

17. The afterbirth refers to the
    (1) placenta.   (2) damaged uterus.
    (3) the placenta, umbilical vessels, and fetal membranes.

18. Parturition is the
    (1) process of giving birth.   (2) period of pregnancy.
    (3) first few days of postnatal life.

19. The following substances pass from the mother to the fetus through the placenta:
    (1) nutrients, gases, and blood cells.
    (2) nutrients and all blood cells except red blood cells.
    (3) nutrients, gases, hormones, and antibodies.

20. Abortion is correctly known as
    (1) criminal emptying of the uterus.
    (2) interruption of pregnancy during fetal life.
    (3) interruption of pregnancy during embryonic life.

H. Menstrual Cycle

Select the correct answer to the following statements.

1. The cessation of menstrual flow in a woman in her late forties is known as
   (1) menarche.   (2) menopause.   (3) amenorrhea.

2. The first menstrual flow is known as
   (1) menarche.   (2) climacteric.   (3) menopause.

3. A distinct rise in the basal body temperature usually occurs
   (1) at ovulation.   (2) during the proliferative phase.
   (3) during the quiescent period.

Answers

Physiology	Fig. 39.5
7. _____	_____
8. _____	_____
9. _____	_____
10. _____	_____
11. _____	_____
12. _____	_____
13. _____	_____
14. _____	_____
15. _____	_____
16. _____	_____
17. _____	_____
18. _____	_____
19. _____	_____
20. _____	_____

Menstrual Cycle	
1. _____	_____
2. _____	_____
3. _____	_____

4. Menstrual flow is the result of
   (1) a deficiency of progesterone and estrogen.
   (2) a deficiency of estrogen.
   (3) an excess of progesterone and estrogen.
5. Ovulation usually (not always) occurs the following number of days before the next menstrual period:
   (1) three.   (2) seven.   (3) fourteen.   (4) eighteen.
6. Pain during ovulation, as experienced by some women, is known as
   (1) dysmenorrhea.   (2) oligomenorrhea.
   (3) mittleschmerz.
7. The proliferative phase in the menstrual cycle begins at about the
   (1) second day.   (2) fifth day.   (3) seventh day of menstrual cycle.
8. Repair of the endometrium after menstruation is due to
   (1) estrogen.   (2) progesterone.   (3) luteinizing hormone.
9. Progesterone secretion ceases entirely within the following number of days after the onset of menses:
   (1) ten.   (2) fourteen.   (3) twenty-six.   (4) twenty-eight.
10. Excessive blood flow during menstruation is known as
   (1) oligomenorrhea.   (2) dysmenorrhea.   (3) menorrhagia.
11. Excessive discomfort and pain during menstruation is known as
   (1) dysmenorrhea.   (2) oligomenorrhea.   (3) menorrhagia.
12. Occasional or irregular menses is known as
   (1) amenorrhea.   (2) oligomenorrhea.   (3) dysmenorrhea.
13. Absence of menstruation is called
   (1) dysmenorrhea.   (2) oligomenorrhea.   (3) amenorrhea.

I. Medical

Select the type of surgery or condition that is described by the following statements.

anteflexion—1
cryptorchidism—2
endometritis—3
episiotomy—4
gonorrhea—5
hysterectomy—6
mastectomy—7
oophorectomy—8
oophorhysterectomy—9
oophoroma—10
retroflexion—11
salpingitis—12
salpingectomy—13
syphilis—14
vasectomy—15

1. Surgical removal of breast.
2. Failure of testes to descend into scrotum.
3. Surgical removal of uterus.
4. Spirochaetal sexually transmitted disease.
5. Sterilization procedure in males.
6. Type of incision made in perineum at childbirth to prevent excessive damage to anal sphincter.
7. Surgical removal of one or both ovaries.
8. Ovarian malignancy.
9. Sexually transmitted disease that affects the mucous membranes rather than the blood.
10. Surgical removal or sectioning of uterine tubes.
11. Most common sexually transmitted disease.
12. Inflammation of uterine wall.
13. Malpositioned uterus (2 types).
14. Sexually transmitted disease caused by a coccoidal (spherical) organism.
15. Surgical removal of ovaries and uterus.

Answers

Menstrual Cycle

4. _____
5. _____
6. _____
7. _____
8. _____
9. _____
10. _____
11. _____
12. _____
13. _____

Medical

1. _____
2. _____
3. _____
4. _____
5. _____
6. _____
7. _____
8. _____
9. _____
10. _____
11. _____
12. _____
13. _____
14. _____
15. _____